D1273710

Principles of Nutrition

4th Edition

Principles of Nutrition

Eva D. Wilson

Professor Emerita
Ohio State University

Katherine H. Fisher

Writer and Consultant on Nutrition

Pilar A. Garcia

Professor Iowa State University

John Wiley & Sons
New York / Chichester
Brisbane / Toronto

Library of Congress Cataloging in Publication Data:

Wilson, Eva D.
  Principles of nutrition.

  Includes indexes.
  1. Nutrition. I. Fisher, Katherine H., joint
author. II. Garcia, Pilar A., joint author.
III. Title.

QP141.W52 1979   641.1   78-11710
ISBN 0-471-02695-6

Printed in the United States of America

Dedicated to

Wylle B. McNeal,

early leader in home economics, a
friend who inspired the writing
of the first edition of this book

Preface to Fourth Edition

Many things are happening in nutrition and these have been included within the scope of the book and limits of space. One of the goals of the book is to stimulate and foster interest in nutrition by including accurate information documented by published research studies. Basic information—the long accepted as well as the recent breakthroughs—are presented as well as some controversial points and unsolved questions.

The following new sections have been added to this edition:

Concepts in biology and chemistry—to make the more technical discussions clearly understandable.

The ADA Exchange List for Meal Planning—to provide a scheme for introducing variety in meals without changing the energy value or content of the energy nutrients.

Nutrition during the life cycle has been expanded to include young adulthood and middle age—to make the picture more complete.

The following changes have been made:

Digestion, absorption, and metabolism are discussed with basic understandings in nutrition; specific aspects of these topics are presented in Part Two.

The relationship between over- and under-nutrition to energy are discussed in Chapter 8.

Nutrients and their importance to diet and dental health are discussed in Chapters 13 and 14.

Each chapter outlines the content at the beginning and summarizes the important points at the end.

The chapters provide an explanation of abbreviations and contain a glossary of terms that are most likely unfamiliar.

Pilar A. Garcia, Professor of Food and Nutrition, Iowa State University, replaces Mary E. Fuqua as coauthor in this edition of the book.

We are particularly grateful to Hazel M. Hatcher and M. Colleen McCann whose suggestions helped to improve the usefulness of the book. We express appreciation to personnel of the Division of Consumer Studies and Bureau of Foods of the Food and Drug Administration, the National Center for Health Statistics of the Public Health Service, the Consumer and Food Economics Institute of the Agricultural Research Service, and the National Institutes of Health for their cooperative attention to our requests for information and materials.

We are grateful to the staff of John Wiley and Sons, Inc. for their contributions to the development and completion of this fourth edition.

Eva D. Wilson
Katherine H. Fisher
Pilar A. Garcia

A Note
to Students

The objective of this book is to provide accurate up-to-date information on nutrition. It is an introduction to nutrition, requiring no university science prerequisite. However, if you believe that your background in science needs some bolstering, turn to Chapter Two where some basic concepts in Biology and Chemistry appear.

To facilitate your study of the book, each chapter opens with an outline of its content and closes with a summary of the important points; any abbreviations used are explained; all terms thought to be new to you appear in a glossary at the end of the chapter. To assist in review of the material, study questions have been prepared and to aid you in making practical use of the information, activities suggested; both are found near the end of each chapter. Statements made in the book are based on published research; the specific citations appear in the reference list at the end of each chapter.

In the Appendix is a new food composition table (1977) with the foods arranged in alphabetical order for your convenience. Also included are tables of height, weight, and skinfolds for easy comparison of your own measurements.

To know what constitutes an adequate diet and to put that know-how into practice is much of what nutrition is about. Actually, there is considerable flexibility in choosing an adequate diet. Guides are given to help you select foods that will meet your energy and nutrient needs.

This book was written with you in mind; we hope that it serves you well.

Eva D. Wilson
Katherine H. Fisher
Pilar A. Garcia

Contents

Appendix
Tables

1

Introduction to the Study of Nutrition

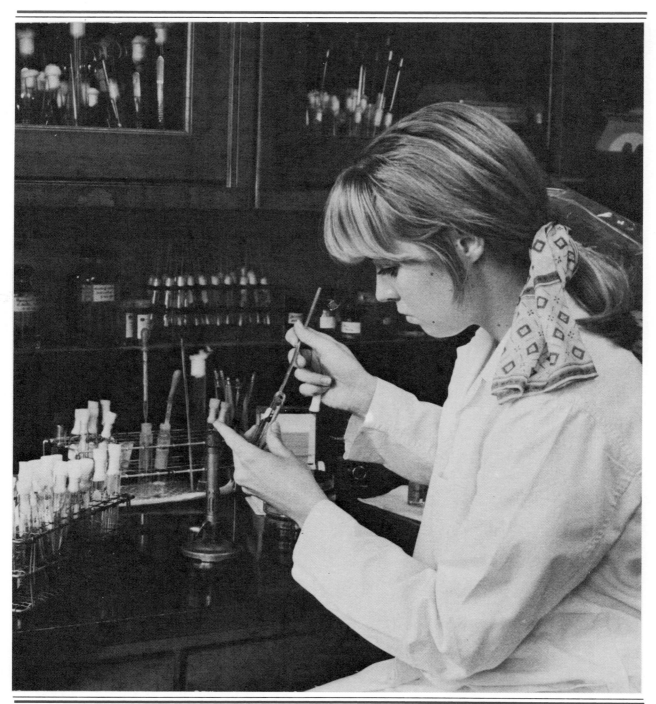

Nutritional Findings come from laboratory studies.

Chapter 1

Introduction to Nutrition

The Science of Nutrition

The science of nutrition is the science of *nourishing* the body. To function, the body needs certain chemical substances, for which the general term is *nutrients*. Some of the nutrients cannot be *synthesized* by the body—at least not in amounts sufficient to satisfy the need for them; others the body can produce. Food is the source of the nutrients the body cannot synthesize (except for vitamin D; see chapter 9) and the source of the chemical elements to produce the others. Nutrition deals with the nutrients: their characteristics, functions, the body's quantitative need for them, and food sources; the effects of an inadequate intake and, for some nutrients, of an excessive intake; with the digestion of food, absorption of the end products, and their utilization in the body; the interrelationships that occur among some nutrients; and the systems that salvage nutrients for reuse or eliminate them as waste. An introduction to each of these phases of nutrition is presented in the chapters that follow.

Food: The Source of Nutrients

Foods provide six major classes of nutrients: carbohydrates, *lipids*, proteins, minerals, vitamins, and water, each serving specific functions in the body. Some nutrients supply energy. All of them build and maintain cells and tissues and regulate body processes.

The primary function of food is to supply energy for the body. The energy nutrients—those that yield energy upon *oxidation*—are carbohydrates, fats, and proteins. Because of the large amount of carbohydrates normally eaten, they are usually the chief source of energy. Fat is typically the second source, followed by protein. In 1977, in the United States, 46 percent of the energy available for consumption was provided by carbohydrates, 42 percent by fat, and 12 percent by protein (3). Although this general pattern of distribution of the energy nutrients is found in most cultural groups around the world, there are occasional exceptions.

Proteins, minerals, and water are the principal structural materials of the body. In addition, lipid-containing compounds, such as the *phospholipids* and *cholesterol*, are found in the membranes of the body cells. *Glycolipids* (carbohydrate-containing lipids) are a part of brain tissue. Vitamin A is a structural substance in the *retina* of the eye. With the exception of certain vitamins, all nutrients function as structural materials.

Proteins, carbohydrates, lipids, minerals, vitamins, and water all help to regulate body processes. Each performs certain functions essential to normal body *metabolism*, such as the movements of fluids, the control of balance between acid and base, the coagulation of blood, the *activation of enzymes*, the maintenance of normal body temperatures, the release of useful energy, and the synthesis of body proteins.

The Roots of Nutrition

A Few Historical Points The first recorded efforts to probe the mysteries of nourishing the body occurred in ancient times (prior to A.D. 476) (2, 4). Ever since, the search has continued (6). The Greek philosopher Hippocrates (460–359 B.C.), without advantage of experiment, propounded some beliefs that are sustained today, such as this aphorism translated as "Persons who are naturally very fat are apt to die earlier than those who are slender" (2).

After the Middle Ages (476–1453), a period in history regarded as "intellectually barren," there arose in the Italian Renaissance a genius of many talents—Leonardo da Vinci (1452–1519). He was an artist, anatomist, biologist, and aeronautical engineer. He made statements about nutrition that have a present-day connotation: ". . . if you do not supply nourishment equal to the nourishment departed, life will fail in vigor; and if you take away this nourishment, life is utterly destroyed" (2).

4

Born shortly after the death of Leonardo, Sanctorius (1561–1636), a professor at Padua, Italy, spent much of his life weighing himself. He found that he lost weight during periods "when no additional food or drink was taken and no sensible evacuations from the body occurred." He termed this loss in his era, as it is today, "insensible perspiration."

About a century after Sanctorious' death, Joseph Priestley (1733–1804), a Unitarian clergyman in England, and Karl Wilhelm Scheele (1742–1786), a Swedish apothecary and chemist, discovered oxygen independently at about the same time. It was Antoine Laurent Lavoisier (1743–1794) who brought together the findings of his predecessors to explain the phenomenon of respiration. He become known as the "father of nutrition."

The achievements that led to the modern era of nutrition often did not bring honor to the men with the brilliant minds. Priestley, unhappy with the reception of his work on the continent, came to America in 1794 and made his home in Northumberland, Pennsylvania, where he spent the remainder of his life. Lavoisier was executed at the age of 51 for alleged criminal acts during the French Revolution.

The nineteenth century yielded notable discoveries in nutrition based on laboratory findings and witnessed attempts to make applications for serving the needs of the people. Claude Bernard (1857) isolated *glycogen*; chemical methods for analysis of foodstuffs were developed (1864); a number of amino acids were isolated; Emil Fischer began classic studies of protein composition (1899), and energy studies in small animals (1883) and farm animals (1887) were initiated. Efforts to use nutrition findings in solving the needs of people were made. In 1851, there was an attempt to provide cheap, nutritious diets in almhouses, prisons, and hospitals in New York (6). At the time of the siege of France by Germany (1870–1871), milk was scarce, so the French scientist Dumas (1800–1884) prepared an artificial milk, using all the then-identified nutrients—proteins, fats, carbohydrates, and minerals—but the children who drank the milk did not grow. Dumas concluded that some as yet unidentified essential component was missing from artificial milk (4). It was, of course, the vitamins; the first one was discovered early in the twentieth century.

Spectacular advances in nutrition have been made in the twentieth century and continue to be made as the century moves into its last 25 years. The vitamins were discovered, the essential amino acids identified, certain minerals were found to be essential, proposals were made for the quantitative needs for nutrients, and further food composition analyses were made. The development in this century of new instruments and new methods has made possible important new discoveries. The *electron microscope* (1933), which reveals the details of cell structure, made possible the study of nutrition at the cellular level, the place where metabolic action takes place. *Radioactive isotopes*, which are tags or markers, made it possible to follow the progress of elements and compounds in the body and discern their functions. The *radioimmunoassay* method used for measuring insulin developed by Dr. Rosalyn Yalow, and for which she was awarded the 1977 Nobel Prize for medicine, makes possible the determination of insulin in the blood.

The one-world concept emerged in the twentieth century. Hunger anywhere in the world is of concern to us. The importance of nutrition education was recognized in this era with the founding of the Nutrition Education Society in 1971.

Sciences Related to the Origin and Development of Nutrition

The roots of the science of nutrition can be traced to biochemistry and human physiology. As research in these and other related sciences progressed, research in nutrition also made strides. The findings revealed interrelationships between

5

nutrition and a number of sciences including molecular biology, genetics, microbiology, and histology. Food habits and eating behavior are rooted in social sciences, that is, anthropology, sociology, and psychology.

Biochemistry The first biochemistry course to be inaugurated in the United States (then known as physiological chemistry) was at Yale University in 1874. Among the faculty of the program in biochemistry that developed at Yale were Professor Russell H. Chittenden (1856–1943) and Professor Lafayette B. Mendel (1872–1935), both of whom became pioneers in nutrition as well as in biochemistry; the areas of their research and teaching — human protein requirements and the nutritive quality of protein, respectively — were distinctly nutrition oriented.

Biochemistry is defined as "an attempt to describe life in chemical terms" (1). It deals with components of living matter — how they are formed and how they are broken down — and how *chemical reactions* in living bodies proceed and are controlled to allow for growth in the young, maintenance in the mature, and degeneration in the old.

Human Physiology Physiology deals with the functioning of the body and its mechanisms for maintaining the constancy of the composition of the fluids that surround the cells (*extracellular fluids*). There are highly sensitive and perfectly coordinated processes that maintain a constant state (*homeostasis*) within the body regardless of most extremes of the environment. Adjustments can be made for lack of food, severe climatic conditions, and other abuses to the body unless the insult extends far beyond the body's regulatory capacities.

Professor George R. Cowgill of Yale University was a noted physiologist who became a pioneer in nutrition. His early research was on the vitamin B complex.

Cell Biology To nourish the body is to nourish the individual cells that make up the organism as a whole. Within the cell the body uses food nutrients, transforms them into new substances, stores them, or expels them. The cell exists as a separate unit by virtue of its membrane that sets it apart from its environment (5). The membrane is the virtual gateway to and from the cell and functions as a barrier to the passage of certain molecules. The cell's nutrients all come from outside the body. Eventually they enter the cell and are used to construct, to repair, to provide energy, and to help regulate various functions. (See p. 16 for discussion of structural parts of the cell).

Other Biological Sciences Genetics is important to nutrition because nutrient needs are determined genetically and this information is transmitted to succeeding generations. Microbiology is important because certain vitamins are synthesized by bacteria in the intestine. In the area of histology, understanding the structure of the tissues in relation to their function is important for nutrition; for example, the histological structure of the long bones shows a pattern for calcium deposit to yield maximum strength.

Social Sciences From the biological standpoint, the kinds of nutrients needed by human beings are not very different from those needed by other mammals. However, eating habits of the human are affected by cultural background, by social group, and by the psychological significance of food for the person. The sciences of anthropology, sociology, and psychology help us to understand why people eat as they do, and hence the sciences are basic to effective nutrition education.

Food in the Lives of People

The urge to eat is basic in the human. When deprivation has been severe, the urge to obtain food overrides all else. However, under less acute physiological conditions other needs for food, more subtle but none-the-less real, seek satisfaction; these needs arise from the individual's cultural background and are manifested in social customs and psychological behavior. Only a few citations are noted here; excellent sources for information may be found in Ritchie (3), Lowenberg et al. (2), and Gifft, Washbon, and Harrison (1).

Food and Social Customs

Warmth and friendship are expressed through sharing food, giving gifts of food, and inviting persons to dine. These foods are usually not just ordinary foods but special ones—those that the recipient particularly likes or that may be traditional for the occasion. And when company is invited for dinner, "company food" is served. Family members who return home after having been away for a time are served their favorite foods.

Invariably, food is part of the celebration of happy occasions, such as birthdays, weddings, and anniversaries. And when a friend stops by for even a short visit, something is served. At times of sadness, food is served as a solace to the grieving ones by friends and neighbors. At a business meeting, the break is usually enlivened with a bit of food or beverage. At a university, food is served at many social events—banquets, athletic award dinners, parties, and meetings of all kinds. At these affairs, food acts indirectly as an instrument to develop social rapport.

Food may help one to achieve status. The food itself or the way it is served may connote distinction. When eating out, some places are more prestigious than others, conferring a certain status on those who dine there.

In some countries, because of the adult male's higher status he is given more and better food than the women and children are given. This preferential treatment may explain why in a Nigerian hospital more girls than boys die of infectious diseases, and why in Jordan (and perhaps elsewhere as well) the prevalence of malnutrition is higher among female than male children (3).

Food and Psychological Associations

For every person there are emotional associations with eating. There are happy occasions to be remembered—winter evenings with popcorn and apples—or the unhappy time when you ate so much of your favorite tapioca pudding that it became a heartily disliked food from then on.

Many people like to try new foods, but most enjoy familiar foods best. In the era when diets for diabetics were low carbohydrate and high fat, special calculations were made for the diets of the diabetic children at the University of Iowa hospital so that on Christmas Day they could have a special treat of mashed potato. Not one child wanted the unfamiliar potatoes; they all preferred spinach, which was their usual fare.

Food is a tool often used for influencing behavior in children. "Good" behavior is rewarded by giving the child his favorite food, and "bad" behavior is punished by depriving him of the food. Almost without exception, favorite foods are sweets.

Children try to influence their parents by reacting negatively to food. Refusal to eat is a forceful weapon in the hands of a child; he thereby gets the attention he is seeking. Refusal to eat is a weapon for adults as well; for them, it is invariably an expression of protest.

An important means to a psychological end is eating to relieve anxiety and frustration. Many people who feel unloved, or who are lonely, bored, or unhappy, use food to assuage these feelings. On the other hand, some people refuse to eat normally under frustrating or lonely conditions.

Age and Changing Interests in Food

There are several fairly well-defined periods in the human life cycle with respect to nutrition. For the infant, food with an admixture of sleep and

7

attention comprise his concerns in life. After the period of infancy, the child delights in his newly won independence through locomotion. He extends this independence to his eating habits as well — he wants to eat very little and only what he likes. In the early school years, playing with friends is more important than eating. The pre-adolescent likes to eat, but he is much too busy to do so; he would prefer to eat on the run. For the adolescent, eating is important because he is very hungry. However, both young men and young women care about their physical appearance, and so they may modify their eating habits accordingly. And they like to eat whatever their friends are having.

Adults have many different interests in food. The pregnant woman is concerned about her unborn child. The businessman may want to control his weight and his blood cholesterol level. Poor people may want only to satisfy their hunger. Those doing heavy work may be largely concerned with the energy value of food. For the obese, food may be a torment — a pleasure tainted with remorse. Some elderly persons may want foods they cannot have because of economic reasons, medical restrictions, or constraints imposed by their living arrangement.

Who Needs Nutrition Information?

The community nutritionist, the dietitian (or food service director), the nutrition researcher, and the university professor of nutrition need a thorough knowledge of the subject; basic understanding is needed by professionals in related areas — the elementary-school teacher, home economics teacher, nurse, food scientist, pharmacist, health education teacher, and physician. Parents and lay persons also need nutrition information.

The community nutritionist helps families plan for the best use of their resources to provide a good diet; the nutritionist may be employed by an agricultural extension service, a public health nursing association, or a social agency.

The dietitian (or food service director) plans adequate diets for dormitory residents (if he or she is a university food service director), for hospital patients (if a hospital dietitian), for school children (if a school lunch supervisor), or for restaurant, cafeteria, or other public eating place patrons (if a manager of a public eating place). The hospital dietitian teaches nutrition — sometimes to medical students, regularly to nurses — and guides patients in an understanding of nutrition relative to their particular dietary needs.

The nutrition researcher attempts to discover new facts of nutrition, seeks to identify problems and to find solutions for them, or may look for basic truths without being concerned about the immediate utility of the findings.

The elementary-school teacher is interested in the development of the whole child, including the status of his nutrition.

The home economics teacher educates high-school or elementary-school children in nutrition.

The nurse conveys to her patients in the hospital and to her clients in public health the essentials of a good diet and its importance in obtaining and maintaining health.

The food scientist does research in new-product development and plans the operations that are required to put new processed food products on the market.

The pharmacist knows the nutrient concentrates that are available for use when foods cannot supply the individual's requirements.

The health education teacher informs his or her students about the essentials of an adequate diet to help them keep physically fit and capable of superior performance.

The physician prescribes diets that help to prevent or treat certain diseases.

Parents, although not professionals, play a most responsible role in determining the food habits of their children. Persons free to choose their food need to know how to make good selections. All lay persons need enough information to assess the validity of claims made for products on the market and the soundness of nutrition advice available to them.

Food for the People of the World

In some parts of the world, the shortage of food makes chronic and seasonal hunger a part of life. In preparation for the World Food Conference in 1974, the United Nations reassessed the world food situation and estimated that approximately 460 million persons were undernourished (1, 6).

The existence of hunger is not unique to our times; mankind throughout history has struggled for enough food. Starting in the decade of the 1940s, however, a new factor was introduced — overpopulation. A falling death rate in the developing regions with no decline in birthrate caused an unprecedented population increase (3). The heavy tolls on life from malaria, cholera, smallpox, typhoid, and other diseases had been brought under better control. The increase in population was disproportionate, occurring chiefly in the developing regions (Table 1.1).

Table 1.1 Population Growth Rates

Region or country	Population (millions) 1960	Population (millions) 1975	Growth rate (percentage) 1960–1970	Growth rate (percentage) 1970–1975
More developed regions	976	1,133	1.05	0.88
Developing regions	2,019	2,855	2.28	2.36
World	2,995	3,988	1.90	1.93
Europe	425	473	0.77	0.64
U.S.S.R.	214	255	1.25	0.99
North America	199	237	1.31	0.90
South Asia	865	1,268	2.50	2.64
China	654	838	1.70	1.64
Japan	94	111	1.03	1.26
Africa	272	402	2.58	2.66
Latin America	216	326	2.74	2.73

From M. Moulik, *Billions More to Feed*. Rome: FAO, 1977, p. 5.

The problems of inadequate available food supply and population increase are inseparable (4). Actually, for more than a decade, total food production has been increasing in both developed and developing countries and at similar rates. However, the increase per capita has been largely nullified in the less developed countries because of the rapid population growth (2).

Projections made by the Food and Agricultural Organization (FAO) indicate that even if the supply of food were made sufficient to meet the demand by increases in domestic production, food aid, and commercial imports, the number of persons suffering from malnutrition would not fall. Inadequate purchasing power to obtain the food available would be the reason. Poverty is an underlying cause of undernutrition. Almost everyone agrees that there must be some changes in social and political systems to reduce poverty (5).

The demand for food in the developing countries is expected to rise at a rate of 3.6 percent per year until 1985, whereas the rise in food production in these countries increased by only 2.6 percent per year between 1961 and 1973. The concern for today and until the end of this century is to maintain a reasonable balance between supply and demand (7). For the long run, experts appear to be in agreement that developing countries have the capability of producing several times more food than they are producing at present. New lands can be opened for cultivation and the lands currently under cultivation can be made more productive by employing more modern methods. Hopefully, as FAO projects, "it is clear that the task of banishing hunger from the world is not an insuperable one."

Summary

The science of nutrition is the science of nourishing the body. To function, the body needs certain chemical substances known as nutrients; some of them the body is unable to synthesize, others it can. Food is the source of the nutrients the body cannot synthesize and the source of the elements for the synthesis of the others.

Nutrition is concerned with the nutrients: their characteristics, functions, the body's quantitative need for them, and food sources; the effects of an inadequate intake and, for some nutrients, of an excessive intake; with the digestion of food, absorption of the endproducts, and their utilization in the body; the metabolic interrelationships that occur among some nutrients; and the systems that salvage nutrients for reuse or eliminate them as waste.

Six major classes of nutrients are found in foods: carbohydrates, lipids, proteins, vitamins, and minerals, and water, each serving specific functions in the body. Some nutrients supply energy. All of them build and maintain cells and tissues and regulate body processes.

The beginnings of the science of nutrition extend back to ancient times. It was the philosophers who initially propounded beliefs about the mystery of nourishing the body. Chemists in the eighteenth century, joined by physiologists in the nineteenth, made discoveries basic to the development of modern nutrition. In the twentieth century, the use of the electron microscope made possible the study of nutrition at the cellular level where the processes actually take place. The one-world concept emerged in the twentieth century, making hunger anywhere a matter of universal concern. During this last quarter of the twentieth century, nutrition education has moved to the fore as an important part of human nutrition.

In addition to biochemistry and human physiology, nutrition is related to other biological sciences, including molecular biology, genetics, microbiology, and histology. Food habits and eating behavior are rooted in social sciences, that is, anthropology, sociology, and psychology.

Food plays an important role in the lives of people. The urge to eat is basic in the human. When deprivation has been severe, the urge to obtain food overrides all else. However, under less acute physiological conditions other needs for food, more subtle but none-the-less real, seek satisfaction; these needs come from the individual's cultural background and are manifested in social customs and psychological behavior.

Eating is universal, so the need for sound nutrition information is also universal. Professionals in the area of nutrition need a thorough knowledge of the subject; these include the community nutritionist, the dietitian (or food service director), the nutrition researcher, and the university professor. Basic understanding is needed by professionals in related areas—the elementary-school teacher, home economics teacher, nurse, food scientist, pharmacist, health education teacher, and physician. Parents and lay persons need sound practical information that can direct their choice of food to provide an adequate diet.

In some parts of the world, the shortage of food makes chronic and seasonal hunger a part of life. Poverty is the universal underlying cause of almost all undernutrition. The developing countries, experts believe, have the capacity to increase their production several times over what it is today. FAO projects that "it is clear that the task of banishing hunger from the world is not an insuperable one" (1).

Glossary

activation of enzymes: some enzymes function independently; others require either loosely or tightly attached to them a metal, such as magnesium, or a nonmetal group or both for the enzyme to function.

chemical reaction: a process in which one substance is changed into another.

cholesterol: an alcohol with fatlike properties that occurs in animal tissue.

electron microscope: developed in 1933; available for use in general research about 1940; magnifies from 150,000 to 300,000 times, permitting visualization of cell structure.

extracellular fluid: fluid outside the cell; comprises about one-third of the total body fluid; includes tissue fluid, blood plasma, cerebrospinal fluid, fluid in the eye, and fluid of the gastrointestinal tract.

glycogen: the chief carbohydrate storage material in man and animal.

glycolipid: any lipid containing a carbohydrate.

homeostasis: maintenance of static, or constant, conditions within the body; for example, the lungs provide oxygen as it is required by the cells; the kidneys, through the process of elimination, help to maintain the normal blood composition.

lipids: a heterogeneous collection of compounds with the common feature of being sparingly soluble in water and soluble in such solvents as alcohol and ether; they are widely distributed in nature both in plant and animal tissue.

metabolism: the sum total of all the chemical and physical changes that occur in a living system, which may be a cell, a tissue, or an organ.

nourish: to provide food or other substances necessary for life and growth.

nutrient: a substance that promotes the growth, maintenance, function, and reproduction of a cell or an organism.

oxidation: the change in an atom, a group of atoms, or a molecule that involves one or more of the following: (a) gain of oxygen, (b) loss of hydrogen, (c) loss of electrons.

phospholipid: a lipid that contains one or more phosphate groups
$$\left[-O-\overset{\overset{\displaystyle H}{\overset{\displaystyle |}{\overset{\displaystyle O}{|}}}}{\underset{\underset{\displaystyle H}{\underset{\displaystyle |}{\underset{\displaystyle O}{|}}}}{P}}=O \right];$$
of great importance for the structure and functioning of biological membranes.

radioactive isotope, also radioisotope: a chemical element that has been changed into another with the emission of radiations.

radioimmunoassay: a method for determining hormones, such as insulin, by means of a radioactive-labeled substance that reacts with the substance under test.

retina: the light-sensitive portion of the eye.

synthesize: the production of a more complex substance from simpler substances.

Study Questions and Activities

1. Does man know instinctively how to nourish himself well? Is there a difference between men and other animals in this respect? Support your answer with evidence.

2. Explain what is meant by an essential dietary nutrient. Give an example.

3. When the food supply is not sufficient to satisfy all physiological needs, which need is given priority?

4. The use of food to satisfy social and psychological needs is a highly individual matter. Are you aware that you use food for such ends? Make a list of some of these social and psychological uses.

References

The Science of Nutrition

1. Banks, P., W. Bartley, and L. M. Birt (1976). *The Biochemistry of the Tissues.* 2nd ed. New York: John Wiley and Sons, Inc., p. 1.
2. Lusk, G. (1933). *Nutrition.* New York: Häfner Publ. Co.
3. Marston, R., and B. Friend (1978). Nutrient content of the national food supply. *National Food Review,* NFR-1 (January) 13.
4. McCollum, E. V. (1957). *A History of Nutrition.* Boston: Houghton Mifflin Co.
5. Swanson, C. P. (1969). *The Cell.* 3rd ed. Englewood Cliffs, N.J.: Prentice-Hall.
6. Todhunter, E. N. (1976). Chronology of some events in the development and application of the science of nutrition. *Nutrition Rev.,* **34:** 353.

Food in the Lives of People

1. Gifft, H. H., M. B. Washbon, and G. G. Harrison (1972). *Nutrition, Behavior, and Change.* Englewood Cliffs, N.J.: Prentice-Hall.
2. Lowenberg, M. E., E. N. Todhunter, E. D. Wilson, J. R. Savage, and J. L. Lubaueski (1979). *Food and People.* 3rd ed. New York: John Wiley and Sons, Inc.

11

3. Ritchie, J. A. S. (1967). *Learning Better Nutrition.* FAO Nutritional Studies No. 20. Rome: Food and Agr. Organ., pp. 31, 32.

Food for the People of the World

1. *Assessment of the World Food Situation, Present and Future* (1974). New York: The United Nations.
2. *Billions More to Feed* (1977). Rome: Food and Agr. Organ.
3. Duncan, E. R., ed. (1977). *Dimensions of World Food Problems.* Ames, Ia.: Iowa State University Press, p. XI.
4. Duncan, E. R. (1977). A review of population and trends. In *Dimensions of World Food Problems,* edited by E. R. Duncan. Ames, Ia.: Iowa State University Press, p. 3.
5. Fischer, L. K. (1977). Constraints to change — social, political, and economic. In *Dimensions of World Food Problems,* edited by E. R. Duncan. Ames, Ia.: Iowa State University Press, p. 202.
6. *Things To Come* (1974). The United Nations World Food Conference. New York: The United Nations.
7. Wortman, S. (1976). Food and agriculture. *Scientific American,* **235:**31.

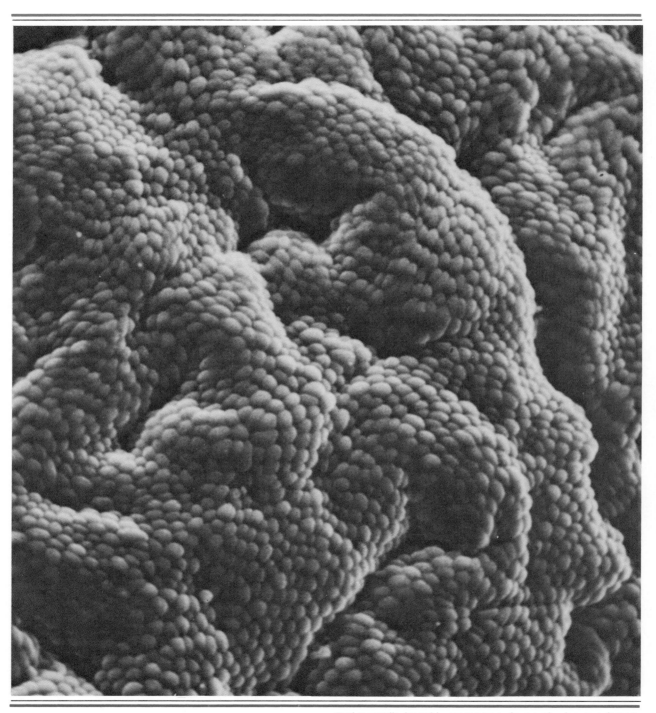

Food is partially digested by gastric juice in the stomach, whose inner lining is shown here in a scanning electron micrograph.

Chapter 2   Basic Understandings in Nutrition

Abbreviations

ATP: adenosine triphosphate
CoA: coenzyme A
DNA: deoxyribonucleic acid

RNA: ribonucleic acid
TAC: tricarboxylic acid cycle

Concepts in Biology and Chemistry

Biology

The study of nutrition begins with the cell. It is in the cell that the processes of nutrition (metabolism) take place, the building of compounds for use in the body (anabolism), and the breakdown of compounds into simpler units (catabolism) for new uses or for excretion if not useful. The release of energy by some substances and the acceptance of it by others occurs in the cell, providing energy for use whenever and wherever it may be needed.

Each of the many cells is specialized in some way to carry out the functions of the organism (body) of which it is a part. Cells serving the same general function, grouped together, form a tissue. There are muscle, nerve, epithelial, and connective tissues. Within each tissue category, there is further differentiation (specialization); for example, bone, adipose tissue, and blood are all of connective tissue origin. Structural units, made up of two or more tissues, serving a specific function or functions are organs; examples of organs are the heart, kidneys, and lungs.

Cells have several important parts; each part has a specific function and an appropriate structure. The two major parts of the cell are the nucleus and the protoplasm surrounding the nucleus, called cytoplasm (Fig. 2.1). The nucleus serves as the center of the cell, controlling its functions; the cytoplasm performs the cell's metabolic activities.

In the nucleus, the pattern for each of the different proteins is present as *deoxyribonucleic acid* (DNA). The information stored in DNA is put into action by *transcribing* it into *ribonucleic acid* (RNA), which directs the actual protein synthesis in the *ribosomes*. This process of transcription is the key to nutrition. (For a discussion of protein synthesis, see p. 88.)

All components for the formation of nutrients come from food. Genes determine which ones the body can synthesize and which it cannot; this truth was established by Beadle and Tatum (1), who were awarded the Nobel prize in Physiology and Medicine (1958) for the discovery. They observed that the diet which adequately nourished the mold *Neurospora crassa* (commonly used in genetic experiments) would no longer do so after exposure of the mold to irradiation. The new strains produced had different dietary needs (4); each nutrient deficiency that resulted was associated with a structural change (mutation) in a single gene. By supplementing the diet with nutrients, one by one, those needed to make the diet adequate were determined.

The cytoplasm of nearly all cells has a more or less continuous network of channels, which are bounded by a membrane. These small channels, called *endoplasmic reticulum*, transport nutrients and their breakdown products (metabolites) throughout the cytoplasm. The membranes surrounding the channels contain enzymes that function in the metabolism of the nutrients. Adhering to the membrane are many small particles of the compound *ribonucleoprotein*; some of the particles are free in the cytoplasm also. These particles, which are ribosomes, are associated together in clusters called polysomes

16

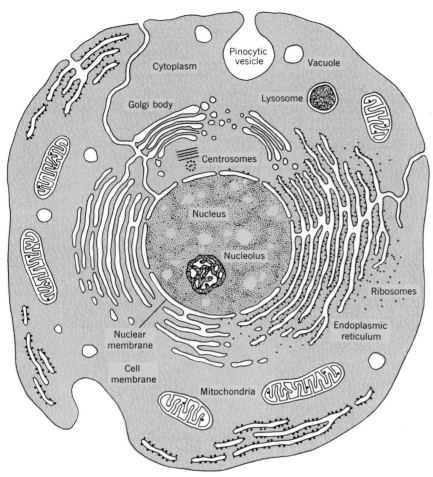

Fig. 2.1 Diagram of a typical cell based on electron micrographs. (Adapted from "The Living Cell" by J. Bracket. Copyright © 1961 by Scientific American, Inc. All rights reserved.)

(polyribosomes). Protein synthesis takes place on the polysomes. (Protein synthesis is discussed on p. 88.)

Also present in the cytoplasm are the mitochondria and the lysosomes. The mitochondria are the "power plants" of the cell; they release the energy stored in the carbohydrates, fats, and proteins and transfer it to an energy acceptor (primarily the chemical compound *adenosine triphosphate* [ATP]). The important character-

istic of ATP is that it can give up its energy to another compound of the cell at whatever place work is being done. Enzymes present in the mitochondria play an essential role in these reactions.

The lysosomes, limited by a membrane, contain enzymes that function in the breakdown of proteins and other compounds. Injured cells with a break in the membrane are digested by the released enzymes. Lysosomes play an important part also in the digestion of foreign matter that

17

may have entered the cell. Lysosomes appear to function as an intracellular digestive system for the cell.

Chemistry

The body and the food to nourish it are made of chemical elements. Some information about the elements and their behavior is basic to the study of nutrition.

Elements, Atoms, Molecules, Ions, Isotopes, and Compounds Chemical elements are fundamental units of matter, each with characteristic properties. The Periodic Table contains all of the elements — 106 are presently known, 92 of which occur in nature; the remainder are of synthetic origin. Oxygen, iron, and carbon are examples of elements.

Atoms are the constituent parts of elements. Atoms of one element may combine with atoms of another to form a compound. For example, the compound, sodium chloride (table salt) ($NaCl$) contains one atom of sodium and one of chloride; water (H_2O) contains two atoms of hydrogen and one of oxygen.

Smaller particles — protons, neutrons, and electrons — are parts of atoms. The proton, a positively charged particle, and the neutron, an uncharged particle, are located in the nucleus of the atom. The electron, a negatively charged particle, occurs in shells (orbits) around the nucleus.

A molecule is a basic unit composed of one or more elements which are present in the form of atoms. Examples of molecules that contain only one element are hydrogen (H_2) with two atoms, and oxygen (O_2) with two atoms; examples of those made up of at least two elements are potassium chloride (KCl) with one atom of potassium and one of chloride, and magnesium sulfate (epsom salts) ($MgSO_4$) made up one atom of magnesium, one of sulfur, and four atoms of oxygen.

An ion is an electrically charged atom, group, or molecule. If positively charged, it is a cation; if negatively charged, it is an anion. An example

of a positive atom is K^+; of a negative atom, Cl^-; a positive group, NH_4^+; a negative group, NO_3^-; a positive molecule, H_2^+; a negative molecule, N_2^-.

Ionization is a chemical change by which ions are formed from a neutral molecule. Sodium chloride ($NaCl$) is a neutral compound which, when dissolved in water, ionizes to form the cation Na^+ and the anion Cl^-.

An isotope is an element that has the same number of protons in the nucleus as another form of the same element but with a different atomic weight. The atomic weight of carbon, for example, is 12; an isotope of carbon has an atomic weight of 14 (^{14}C).

A radioisotope (radioactive isotope) is an unstable form of an element with emissions of energy or particles. The ^{14}C isotope of carbon is naturally radioactive. The nuclei of many stable elements are made radioactive artificially. Radioisotopes, such as carbon, hydrogen, iron, and calcium, have been used in nutrition studies. Normally, radioactive elements do not occur in the body, consequently the radioisotope can be distinguished and its behavior in the body followed.

Inorganic Compounds and Organic Compounds An inorganic compound is one that does not contain the element carbon (C) in its structure. There are some exceptions, such as carbon dioxide (CO_2), sodium bicarbonate ($NaHCO_3$) as in baking soda, and calcium carbonate ($CaCO_3$) as in toothpaste; these inorganic compounds contain carbon. The nutrients, water and minerals, are inorganic substances.

An organic compound contains the element carbon in its structure. There are some exceptions as just noted. Carbohydrates, fats, proteins, hormones, enzymes, and vitamins are all organic compounds.

Acids, Bases, Hydrogen Ion Concentration An acid is a chemical compound which yields hydrogen ions (H^+) when dissolved in water. There are two general types of acids, inorganic acids and organic acids. Hydrochloric (HCl), sulfuric (H_2SO_4), and phosphoric (H_3PO_4) are examples of inorganic acids. Phosphoric acid (H_3PO_4), for example, yields the phosphate group ($\equiv PO_4$) which is necessary for the phosphorylation of organic compounds in the cells; an example is the phosphorylation of the vitamin thiamin (see p. 69). Later in this chapter the function of hydrochloric acid in digestion will be discussed. Organic or carboxylic acids contain one or more carboxyl groups (COOH) in their structure. Acetic acid (CH_3COOH), found in vinegar, and oxalic acid $\left(\begin{array}{c}COOH \\ | \\ COOH\end{array}\right)$, found in spinach leaves, are examples of organic acids. In nutrition, fatty acids and amino acids are important organic acids.

A base is a chemical compound which yields hydroxyl ions (OH^-) when dissolved in water. Sodium hydroxide (NaOH) is an example of a base.

Hydrogen-ion concentration is the amount of hydrogen ion (H^+) per unit volume of an aqueous (water) solution. The acidic or basic reaction of a solution depends upon its concentration of hydrogen ions. The symbol pH (potential of hydrogen) was devised for simplicity in expressing hydrogen-ion concentration (to avoid using large fractional numbers); it is the negative logarithm of the hydrogen-ion concentration. The pH scale ranges from 0 to 14.0, with the midpoint (7.0) neutral. The scale is acid from 0 to 7.0 and base from 7.0 to 14.0. The lower the pH number, the greater the hydrogen-ion concentration (and thus the greater the acidity); the higher the pH number, the lower the hydrogen-ion concentration (and thus the greater the basicity).

Some Chemical Reactions

1. Salt formation: a salt is one of the products formed from the reaction of an acid and a base.

$$\underset{\text{acid}}{HCl} + \underset{\text{base}}{KOH} \rightarrow \underset{\text{salt}}{KCl} + \underset{\text{water}}{H_2O}$$

In this equation hydrochloric acid reacts with potassium hydroxide, producing potassium chloride and water.

2. Ester formation: esters are commonly formed by the reaction of an organic acid with an alcohol. An example is the reaction of fatty acids with glycerol (an alcohol) to form a fat (an ester). This reaction is shown on page 69.

3. Oxidation–reduction: oxidation is always accompanied by reduction; electrons are transferred from one atom to another. The atom that receives the electron is reduced and the atom that gives up the electron is oxidized. An example of an oxidation–reduction reaction is the reduction of the form of iron found in the foods of the diet (ferric iron) to the form used by body cells (ferrous iron) by vitamin C.

$$\underset{\text{ferric iron}}{Fe^{+++}} + \underset{\text{of vitamin C}}{\text{reduced form}} \rightleftarrows \underset{\text{ferrous iron}}{Fe^{++}} + \underset{\text{of vitamin C}}{\text{oxidized form}}$$

4. Hydrolysis: the reaction of water with another compound involving the uptake of a molecule of water. The breakdown of carbohydrates, fats, and proteins to simpler compounds in digestion is by hydrolysis, catalyzed by enzymes. An example is the breakdown of white or brown sugar (sucrose) during digestion by the intestinal enzyme sucrase to yield two simple sugars (glucose and fructose) and water (H_2O).

5. Phosphorylation: a chemical reaction in which a phosphate group is introduced into an organic compound. In oxidative phosphorylation, adenosine triphosphate (ATP) with three phosphate groups, two of which are held by high energy bonds (designated in this manner $\sim [P—P \sim P]$), is formed from adenosine diphosphate (ADP) by the addition of phosphate. Energy released from the oxidation of glucose makes possible the conversion of ADP to ATP, the compound that furnishes the energy needed for many of the chemical reactions that take place in the body.

19

6. Synthesis: the process whereby a more complex substance is produced from simpler substances by a reaction or series of reactions. Examples of synthesis are the formation of proteins from amino acids (see pp. 88–89) and the formation of glycogen from molecules of glucose (see p. 51).

7. Degradation: the gradual breakdown in steps of complex substances to simpler ones. The breakdown of proteins to the constituent amino acids and of glycogen to glucose are examples of degradation.

Digestion, Absorption, and Metabolism

When a hamburger or milkshake is eaten, nutrients that will ultimately nourish the cells of the body are being ingested. Yet, before these nutrients finally reach the cells, the foods themselves must be digested and the nutrients absorbed. Digestion involves subdividing the complex molecules into simple, soluble materials (the nutrients) that can pass through the lining of the digestive tract into the blood and lymph streams. Some nutrients are ingested ready for absorption, such as glucose and salt. After absorption, the nutrients enter into the chemical processes of the body known as metabolism.

Digestion

Beginning of the Study of Digestion The study of digestion began in quest of an answer to the mystery of *respiration*. The first notable contribution was made by René de Réaumur (1683–1757), a French scientist who studied changes of food in the stomach. For his experiments he used his pet buzzard—a bird that swallowed its food and later regurgitated the indigestible portions. Réaumur took advantage of this unique opportunity and trained his pet to swallow sponges. When the sponges were brought up, they were soaked with *gastric* juice. He found that the juice squeezed from the sponge would liquefy meat.

The next important investigations were made by Lazzaro Spallanzani (1729–1799), who studied the action of saliva on foodstuffs and also verified Réaumer's observations on gastric digestion. He performed a number of daring experiments on himself. He was impelled to use himself as a subject because of his conviction that certain observations ought to be made with man. Spallanzani swallowed little linen bags containing food. In the first experiment he placed masticated bread in the bag; after 23 hours the bag was excreted empty. He repeated the experiment with other foods, such as masticated meat; he also used bags made of several layers of cloth—always with similar results. He found to his satisfaction that in human beings digestion also takes place in the stomach and intestines.

Most important were the contributions of William Beaumont (1785–1853), a physician stationed at a military post in a forest in northern Michigan. Here, he had a patient, Alexis St. Martin, who had an unhealed opening (fistula) in his stomach that had been caused by a gunshot wound. For two years after the accident Beaumont tried to close the wound. Failing to do so, he realized that he could use this opportunity to study gastric digestion. It took infinite patience and ingenuity for Beaumont to maintain the cooperation of Alexis St. Martin for a number of years. Beaumont's epoch-making observations were of the movements of the stomach during digestion and of changes in the appearance of *gastric mucosa* in response to food or emotional states.

The Gastrointestinal Tract The digestion and absorption of food nutrients takes place along the *gastrointestinal* tract, a tube about 5.1 m (16.5 ft) in length, extending from the mouth to the anus (Fig. 2.2). The parts of the tract are the mouth, *esophagus*, stomach, small intestine, and large intestine. The esophagus is the passageway between the mouth and stomach. The stomach empties into the *duodenum*, the first section of the small intestine. Here secretions from the liver and pancreas enter the tract. The other two sections of the small intestine are called the *jejunum* and *ileum*. The large intestine (colon) begins at the end of the small intestine and forms the last part of the gastrointestinal tract.

The Processes of Digestion Certain nutrients in foods, such as simple carbohydrates, minerals,

and water, are not changed by the digestive processes because of their elementary chemical structure. The digestion of more complex food molecules, however, takes place in the gastrointestinal tract between the mouth and the end of the small intestine (Fig. 2.2). Digestion consists of both mechanical and chemical actions.

Cooking food actually begins the breakdown of some of its chemical compounds before it is ingested. *Cellulose* is softened and starch and *collagen* are partially broken down into simpler substances (hydrolyzed). Cooking also enhances

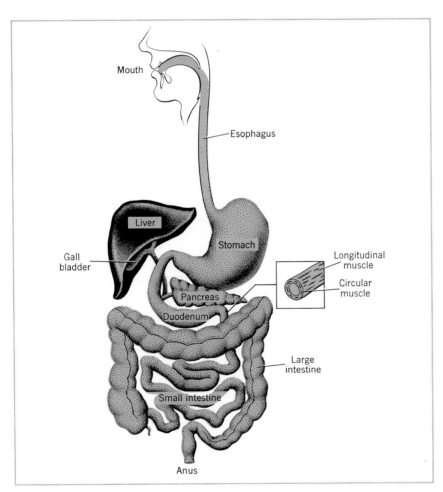

Mouth

Esophagus

Liver

Gall
bladder

Stomach

Longitudinal
muscle

Circular
muscle

Pancreas

Duodenum

Large
intestine

Small intestine

Anus

Fig. 2.2 The digestive tract.

the digestibility of some foods (egg white) and improves the texture of others (sweet potatoes). The aroma and taste of flavorful, well-prepared foods may initiate the chemical phase of digestion by stimulating certain digestive secretions.

The Mechanical Phase of Digestion The mechanical phase, which consists of the mixing, subdividing, and moving of food along the digestive tract, is accomplished by chewing in the mouth and by the muscular activity of the walls of the tract itself. These walls contain two types of muscular tissue: the fibers that run in a circular direction and the fibers that run in a longitudinal direction (Fig. 2.2). When the circular fibers contract, squeezing causes the food to be mixed and subdivided into smaller pieces. When the longitudinal fibers contract, the food mass is pushed through the tract. The coordinated movement of these two kinds of muscle fibers produces a wavelike motion (called *peristalsis*) all along the digestive tract. After food reaches the esophagus, it is moved along by peristalic waves, which continue through the stomach, small intestine, and large intestine. The increased peristalsis, produced after eating a meal, moves the fecal material along to the rectum, resulting in evacuation.

The peristaltic movements of the stomach can be affected by the emotional state of the individual. Sadness, depression, fear, or pain in any part of the body may decrease gastric peristalsis; anger and aggression may increase it. The effects of these reactions vary from person to person and are not always predictable. The entire gastrointestinal tract is affected by emotions. However, the stomach reactions have been studied more extensively than those of other parts of the gastrointestinal tract.

The Chemical Phase of Digestion In the chemical phase, the components of the food are broken down by *enzymes*. Enzymes are complex chemical substances that either "speed up" or "slow down" a chemical reaction without undergoing any change themselves. Fig. 2.3 illustrates how the enzyme maltase helps to break down the two-sugar maltose (*disaccharide*) into two molecules of glucose (*monosaccharide*).

Digestive Enzymes These are produced (synthesized) by the glands and organs of the digestive tract. They help to hydrolyze (break down) complex carbohydrates into *simple sugars*; fats or *lipids* into *glycerol*, *fatty acids*, and *glycerides*; and proteins into amino acids. A distinctive feature of an enzyme is that it is specific for a particular reaction: those that act on carbohydrates cannot act on fats and proteins, and vice versa. Even though an enzyme-naming system (*nomenclature*)

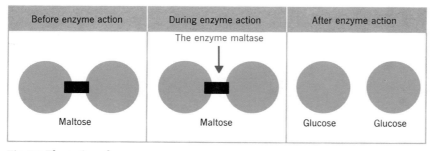

Fig. 2.3 The action of an enzyme.

Table 2.1 Representative examples of digestive enzymes

Source of the enzyme secretion	Site of enzyme reaction	Names of enzymes and the substances they act upon			
		Starches	Sugars	Fats	Proteins
Salivary glands	Mouth	Salivary amylase (ptyalin)			
Stomach	Stomach				Gastric protease (pepsin)
Pancreas	Small intestine	Pancreatic amylase		Pancreatic lipase	Pancreatic proteases
Wall of small intestine	Small intestine		Sucrase Maltase Lactase	Intestinal lipase	Intestinal proteases

has been adopted, certain traditional names are still used, such as *ptylan* and *pepsin*. In the new enzyme nomenclature the root of the enzyme name is derived from the substance that it acts upon (the substrate) and the suffix is "ase," the characteristic designation of an enzyme. Enzymes that break down a carbohydrate, a fat or lipid, or a protein are called carbohydrases, lipases, or proteases, respectively. For a specific carbohydrate, such as starch, the root of the enzyme name is derived from the word "amylum," meaning starch; thus amylase is the root of this enzyme name. However, the root names of the disaccharide-splitting enzymes are derived from the sugars themselves, that is, sucrase, maltase, and lactase. Because one nutrient may be digested in different parts of the digestive tract, an adjective indicating the source of the enzymatic secretion is used before the root word to complete the enzyme name (Table 2.1). For example, the fat-splitting enzyme that is secreted by the pancreas and acts in the small intestine is called pancreatic lipase.

Besides the digestive enzymes, there are thousands of other enzymes needed in the body to carry on its various functions. In subsequent chapters, some of these will be discussed.

The Passage of Food Through the Digestive Tract— The Mouth Food enters the gastrointestinal tract through the mouth where it is chewed into small pieces and mixed with saliva. Over a liter (qt) of saliva is produced daily. It is an alkaline solution (3). The salivary glands, located under the tongue, secrete the first digestive enzyme and mucin (a *glycoprotein*), the slippery substance that gives saliva its characteristic consistency. Mixed with water, mucin forms mucous, which has a lubricating action that helps food to be swallowed and pass through the esophagus to the stomach.

The Passage of Food Through the Digestive Tract— The Stomach When food enters the stomach, it remains temporarily in the upper portion where the action of the salivary enzyme continues until the mixture becomes sufficiently acid to stop the action of the enzyme.

Gastric juice, acid in reaction (pH 1.0–3.5), is a combination of secretions from the glands in the stomach (3). Along with digestive enzymes, gastric juice contains *hydrochloric acid*, an important factor in gastric digestion. Hydrochloric acid converts the inactive form of the protein-

23

splitting enzyme pepsinogen to the active enzyme pepsin; it creates an optimum acidity in the stomach for the action of pepsin; it destroys bacteria that may have entered with the food; it may break down (hydrolyze) some of the sugars (disaccharides) in food; and it increases the solubility of the minerals calcium and iron, leading to optimum absorption of these essential nutrients in the small intestine.

Gastric secretion is stimulated by eating. After a meal the rate of secretion may increase up to six times what it is when the stomach is empty. The concentration of acid and enzymes in the gastric secretion rises during the first hour after eating and declines during the following hours. Distending the stomach with food also increases the secretion, as does the type of food eaten: fat and carbohydrate provide little stimulation, whereas ethyl alcohol, *caffeine*, and protein provide a great deal. The secretion is reduced when the duodenum is distended and when there is acid or fat in the duodenum. About 2 liters (qt) of gastric juice is secreted each day (3).

The length of time that food remains in the stomach depends upon the composition of the diet, but it also varies widely even among people who have eaten the same thing. An ordinary meal leaves the stomach in 3 to 4½ hours. Carbohydrate foods leave the stomach most rapidly, followed by protein, and then by fat foods. The sensation of hunger occurs more quickly after a meal that is relatively high in carbohydrate than after a meal containing substantial protein and fat.

Because the membranes of the gastrointestinal tract are made up of proteins, why are they not digested by pepsin? The thick, viscous fluid of the mucous-secreting cells coat the walls of the stomach, helping to protect them. Also, the protein content of the mucous and its alkalinity tend to neutralize the acid in the immediate areas of the epithelial cell layer, thus forming a barrier between the highly acid content of the tract and the cell surface. In addition, the epithelial mucous cells lining the walls of the stomach are continuously being replaced. Despite these protective mechanisms, some persons still develop *gastric* or *duodenal ulcers* (2).

The Passage of Food Through the Digestive Tract—The Small Intestine After leaving the stomach, the semiliquid food mass (referred to as chyme) passes into the duodenum where bicarbonate ions and water secreted by the pancreatic juice neutralize the acid in the chyme (3). Into this area flow intestinal juices, pancreatic juices, and bile.

Bile, which contains no digestive enzymes, is secreted continually by the liver and stored in the gall bladder until needed to help emulsify fats so that they can be digested by the pancreatic lipase. It also aids in the absorption of the end products of fat digestion by increasing their solubility for passage through the gastrointestinal tract.

The secretions of the small intestine and the pancreas contain enzymes that will complete the digestion of carbohydrates, fats, and proteins.

The Passage of Food Through the Digestive Tract—The Large Intestine The material entering the large intestine (colon) contains undigested residues, some of the end products of digestion that escaped absorption, bile pigments, other waste materials, and water. The only important secretion in the large intestine is mucous, and the only absorption of consequence through the walls of the colon is of water and the mineral sodium. The mucous protects the intestinal wall against tear or wear and provides an adherent medium for holding the fecal matter together. Small amounts of certain vitamins are synthesized by bacteria in the large intestine and are absorbed there.

Absorption

Before the body can use the soluble products of digestion, the nutrients must be absorbed. Even though water, ethyl alcohol, and simple sugars

24

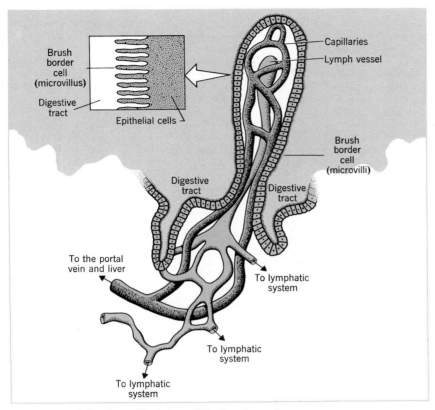

Fig. 2.4 Brush border cells (microvilli), the absorption organs of the small intestine.

may pass through the mucosa of the stomach directly into the bloodstream, most absorption takes place in the small intestine. The absorptive surface of this area is increased about 600 times by fingerlike projections in the lining of the small intestine called villi (2). Each villus contains a *lymph* vessel surrounded by a network of very small blood vessels (capillaries), and each cell in the surface area of the villus is composed of smaller units called brush border cells or microvilli (Fig. 2.4).

Substances or nutrients pass through the intestinal membrane in two ways—by *diffusion* and by *active transport*. Both of these processes are related to osmosis. Those substances that are found in the intestinal tract in higher concentration than across the membrane in the blood and lymph pass through by simple diffusion. The diffusion process is illustrated in Fig. 2.5; the sugar fructose, one of the substances absorbed by diffusion, is used as an example. On the other hand, substances that are absorbed from an area of lower concentration across a membrane to a higher one do so by active transport. This second process requires energy for the absorption and a "carrier" to transport the substance. The "carrier" substance appears to be protein or protein-related compound *(lipoprotein)*. Amino acids, the end product of protein digestion, are among the substances absorbed by active transport (Fig. 2.5).

25

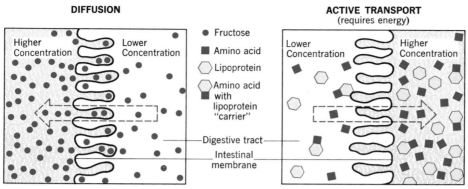

DIFFUSION

Higher Concentration   Lower Concentration

ACTIVE TRANSPORT
(requires energy)

Lower Concentration   Higher Concentration

● Fructose
■ Amino acid
⬡ Lipoprotein
⬡ Amino acid with lipoprotein "carrier"

Digestive tract
Intestinal membrane

Fig. 2.5 A sketch showing intestinal absorption by diffusion and active transport.

Daily, several hundred grams of carbohydrate, 100 g of fat, 50 to 100 g of amino acids, 50 to 100 g of mineral ions, 8 to 9 liters (qt) of water, and vitamins are absorbed from the small intestine (3). The nutrients that are absorbed into the lymph vessels (fatty acids and small amounts of *cholesterol* and other lipids) pass into the *lymphatic system*. All other nutrients are absorbed by the capillaries, empty into the *portal vein*, and are carried directly to the liver (Fig. 2.4). The lymph vessels begin in the spaces between the body tissues, and the lymph finally empties into the bloodstream in the area of the chest cavity.

Metabolism

Metabolism is a term used to describe all the chemical changes that take place after the end products of carbohydrate, fat, and protein digestion, the vitamins, the minerals, and water are absorbed into the body.

There are two phases of metabolism: anabolism and catabolism. Anabolism includes the chemical reactions by which the absorbed nutrients are used to replace worn-out body substances (this is called maintenance) and to form new cellular material (this is called growth). Catabolism includes the chemical reactions whereby cellular

material is broken down to smaller units. For example, an athlete uses food nutrients to build up stores of liver and muscle glycogen (anabolism), and these glycogen stores then will be broken down to supply energy for part of the physical activity involved in a sport (catabolism). In the body cells, anabolism and catabolism occur simultaneously.

In the beginning nutrition course, it is not possible to study all the details of metabolism. Yet there are several parts of metabolism that must be highlighted to make the subsequent study of the nutrients meaningful. Figure 2.6 is a simple sketch depicting several important steps in metabolism.

One substance formed in the metabolism of the absorbed end products of carbohydrate and/or protein digestion is pyruvic acid. For pyruvic acid to proceed to the next step in the metabolic chain, acetyl coenzyme A (acetyl CoA), the vitamin thiamin is needed. (If thiamin is missing from the diet, pyruvic acid accumulates in the body cells and causes symptoms of a thiamin deficiency.)

Because acetyl CoA is a very important compound in metabolism, it will be mentioned often in the nutrient chapters. Acetyl CoA has been called "the gateway to the tricarboxylic cycle." The tricarboxylic acid cycle (TAC) is a term used

26

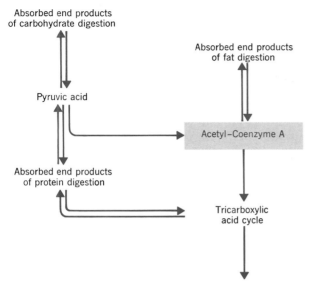

Fig. 2.6 A simple sketch depicting some important steps in metabolism.

to describe the final series of reactions where energy from food carbohydrate, fat, and protein is released for the body's use.

The energy released by the reactions of the TAC is contained (or stored) in a compound called ATP (adenosine triphosphate), which also will be discussed often in the study of the nutrients. The energy stored in ATP is used for "work," such as muscle contraction and the formation of body compounds, and for "heat" to maintain the body's ideal temperature.

In the following chapters the digestion, absorption, and metabolism of all the nutrients are presented to describe their roles in supplying energy, building and maintaining body tissue, and regulating body processes.

Summary

The study of nutrition begins with the cell; it is there that compounds for use in the body are synthesized and those no longer needed are broken down. The release of energy by some substances and the acceptance of it by others takes place in the cell, providing energy for use whenever and wherever it may be needed. Each cell has several characteristic parts, each with a structure appropriate for carrying out its specific function.

The body and the food to nourish it are constituted of chemical elements. Information about the elements and the forms they take and about some of the chemical reactions that take place in the body is basic to the study of nutrition.

The food one eats must undergo a series of mechanical and chemical processes (digestion) and pass through the lining of the gastrointestinal tract (absorption) before the nutrients become available to the body cells. The mechanical phase of digestion begins with food preparation and continues after the food is ingested and moved along the gastrointestinal tract. The chemical phase begins in the mouth and continues in the stomach and small intestine until the food nutrients are digested into simple units to pass through the gastrointestinal wall. After the nutrients are absorbed, they pass into the body cells by way of the lymphatic system or the portal vein.

In the metabolism of nutrients some reactions require energy and others yield energy. This energy comes from ATP and is used by the cells to perform such work as muscle contraction, the active transport of nutrients across cell membranes, and the formation of body compounds.

Glossary

active transport: the movement of substances across cell membranes, usually against a concentration gradient; it requires the expenditure of energy.

adenosine triphosphate: a compound that furnishes the energy needed for many of the reactions that take place in the body.

caffeine: a slightly bitter-tasting substance found in

coffee and tea that acts as a stimulant of the central nervous system.

cellulose: the structural carbohydrate in plants that passes undigested through the human digestive tract.

cholesterol: see page 79.

collagen: a comparatively insoluble protein that is found in the skin, tendons, bones, and cartilage.

deoxyribonucleic acid (DNA): the substance which constitutes the genetic material in most organisms.

diffusion: the process by which a molecule passes through a membrane from an area of high concentration to one of lower concentration.

disaccharide: a carbohydrate composed of two sugars.

duodenum: the first portion of the small intestine.

endoplasmic reticulum: continuous system of cavities (channels) bound by a membrane that passes throughout the cytoplasm of the cell.

enzyme: a protein formed in plant and animal cells that acts as an organic catalyst in initiating or speeding up specific chemical reactions.

esophagus: the hollow muscular tube extending from the mouth to the stomach.

fatty acids: organic acids, composed of carbon, hydrogen, and oxygen, which combine with glycerol to form fat.

gastric: pertaining to the stomach.

gastric mucosa: the membrane lining the stomach.

gastric or duodenal ulcers: a defect (ulceration) of the mucous membrane of the stomach or duodenum.

gastrointestinal: pertaining to the stomach and intestinal tract.

glyceride: a compound (ester) formed by the combination of glycerol and fatty acids and the loss of water from the ester linkage.

glycerol: the three-carbon atom alcohol derived from the hydrolysis of fat.

glycoprotein: a compound of a carbohydrate and protein.

hydrochloric acid: a normal constituent of the human gastric juice.

ileum: the distal section of the small intestine between the duodenum and the large intestine.

jejunum: the middle section of the small intestine between the duodenum and ileum.

lipids: see page 11.

lipoprotein: a compound composed of a lipid and a protein.

lymph: a fluid that circulates within the lymphatic vessels and is eventually added to the venous blood circulation.

lymphatic system: all the vessels and structures that carry lymph from the tissues to the blood.

monosaccharide: a carbohydrate composed of one sugar.

nomenclature: a system of technical terms; terminology.

pepsin: the protein-splitting enzyme of the gastric secretion.

peristalsis: the wavelike movement in the lining of the digestive tract that propels the food mass along by contraction and relaxation of the muscle fibers.

portal vein: the vein that carries blood from the wall of the intestine to the liver.

ptyalin: the starch-splitting enzyme of the saliva.

respiration: the exchange of oxygen and carbon dioxide in the lungs, between the cell and its environment, and in the metabolism of the cell.

ribonucleic acid (RNA): a compound that occurs in three major forms—ribosomal, transfer, and messenger ribonucleic acid—all of which function in the cell in the synthesis of proteins.

ribonucleoprotein: a substance composed of both protein and ribonucleic acid.

ribosomes: particles composed of approximately equal amounts of RNA and protein; they are the sites of protein synthesis in the cell.

simple sugars: the monosaccharides; glucose, fructose, and galactose.

transcribing: copying the genetic information of DNA (deoxyribonucleic acid) in the form of RNA.

Study Questions and Activities

1. Certain information about the cell is basic to an understanding of nutrition. Provide evidence to support or justify the foregoing statement.

2. Explain the following: atom, ion, compound, radioisotope, organic acid, hydrolysis, and synthesis.

3. Identify the following: enzyme, pepsin, anabolism, catabolism, microvilli, carbohydrase, lipase, protease, Alexis St. Martin, and peristalsis.

4. What happens in the mechanical phase of digestion?

5. How does hydrochloric acid function in the stomach?

6. What effects may fatigue, worry, or hurried meals have on the digestive processes?

7. Why are pyruvic acid, acetyl coenzyme A, and ATP (adenosine triphosphate) important factors in the body?

References

1. Beadle, G. W., and E. L. Tatum (1941). Genetic control of biochemical reactions in Neurospora. *Proc. Natl. Acad. Sci. (U.S), 27*:449.

2. Brobeck, J. R., ed. (1973). *Best and Taylor's Physiological Basis of Medical Practice. 9th ed.* Baltimore: Williams and Wilkins, Chapter 2.

3. Guyton, A. C. (1976). *Textbook of Medical Physiology.* 5th ed. Philadelphia: W. B. Saunders Co., Chapters 64 and 65.

4. Tatum, E. L. (1959). A case history in biological research. *Science,* **129:** 1711.

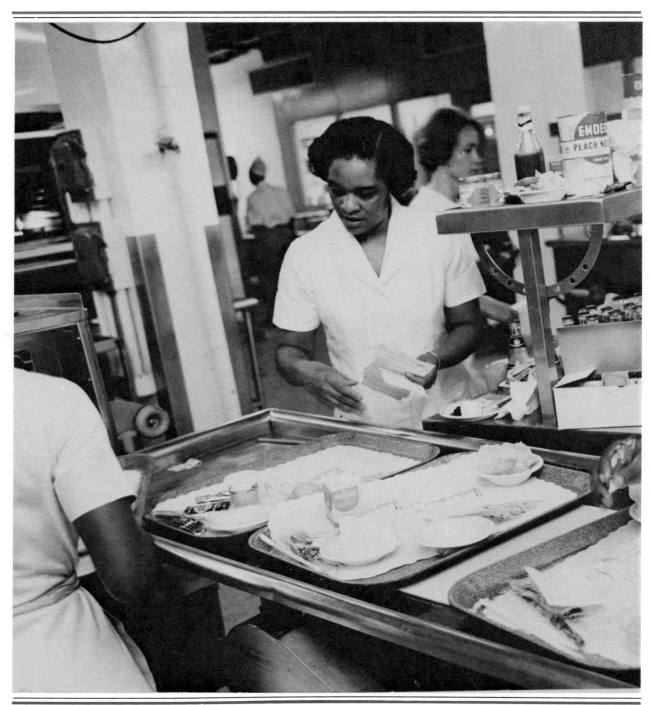

Dietitians need to know the nutrient needs of men and women of all ages (as well as any specific individual requirements) in order to plan appropriate diets for hospital patients.

Chapter 3

Dietary Allowances and Standards

Abbreviations

FAO/WHO: Food and Agriculture Organization/
World Health Organization
FDA: Food and Drug Administration
IU: International Unit
kcal: kilocalorie
kJ: kilojoule
MDR: Minimum Daily Requirement

NAS–NRC: National Academy Sciences–
National Research Council
RDA: Recommended Dietary Allowances
RE: retinol equivalent
μg: microgram
U.S. RDA: United States Recommended
Daily Allowance

The general term for describing man's nutritional needs is "dietary standard." It is a compilation (or summary) of nutrient requirements, stated quantitatively.

One of the early attempts to establish dietary standards was made by the Health Committee of the League of Nations in 1936. Since the member governments of the League wanted to be able to provide enough proper food for the whole world, the dietary standards of 1936 were formulated as a yardstick for making quantitative estimates.

United States Allowances

During the Depression of the 1930s both American consumers and producers requested information about dietary needs. Because of their limited spending capacity, consumers wanted to know about their minimum nutrient needs; and because producers wished to project production goals for food crops, they also wanted such information. In response to these demands, Stiebeling and Ward of the U. S. Department of Agriculture (13) planned diets at four levels of cost and nutritive content. Because there were no meaningful, published dietary standards at that time, Stiebeling and Ward evaluated the nutritive adequacy of their planned diets by utilizing certain data that had been reported in various research journals.

Recommended Dietary Allowances

In 1940 the *Food and Nutrition Board* of the *National Research Council*-National Academy of Sciences was established to advise the government on nutrition problems related to national defense. One of its first tasks was to establish dietary standards for people of different ages; the first set of standards was published in 1943. The term "Recommended Dietary Allowances" (RDA) (rather than "dietary standards") was adopted to show that the proposed values were not to be considered requirements but only value judgments based on existing knowledge. The Board wanted to convey the idea that these values were not final, but would be revised as new knowledge became available. These recommendations have been revised in 1945, 1948, 1953, 1958, 1963, 1968, and 1974 (10).

The RDAs are not requirements but "are levels of intake of essential nutrients, considered in the judgment of the Food and Nutrition Board on the basis of available scientific knowledge to be adequate to meet the known nutritional needs of practically all healthy persons" (10).

Recommendations have been made for the following nutrients: energy (*kcal, kJ*), protein (g), vitamin A activity (*IU* or *RE*),[1] vitamin D (IU), vita-

---

[1] Retinol equivalents.

Table 3.1. Recommended Daily Dietary Allowances[a] (designed for the maintenance of good nutrition of practically all healthy people in the U.S.A.)

	Years From up to	Weight (kg)	(lb)	Height (cm)	(in.)	Energy (kcal)[b]	Protein (g)	Vitamin A activity (RE)[c]	Vitamin A activity (IU)	Vita-min D activity[d] (IU)	Vita-min E activity[e] (IU)	Vita-min C (mg)	Fola-cin[f] (μg)	Nia-cin[g] (mg)	Ribo-flavin (mg)	Thia-min (mg)	Vita-min B-6 (mg)	Vita-min B-12 (μg)	Cal-cium (mg)	Phos-phorus (mg)	Iodine (μg)	Iron (mg)	Mag-nesium (mg)	Zinc (mg)
Infants	0.0–0.5	6	14	60	24	kg × 117	kg × 2.2	420[d]	1400	400	4	35	50	5	0.4	0.3	0.3	0.3	360	240	35	10	60	3
	0.5–1.0	9	20	71	28	kg × 108	kg × 2.0	400	2000	400	5	35	50	8	0.6	0.5	0.4	0.3	540	400	45	15	70	5
Children	1–3	13	28	86	34	1300	23	400	2000	400	7	40	100	9	0.8	0.7	0.6	1.0	800	800	60	15	150	10
	4–6	20	44	110	44	1800	30	500	2500	400	9	40	200	12	1.1	0.9	0.9	1.5	800	800	80	10	200	10
	7–10	30	66	135	54	2400	36	700	3300	400	10	40	300	16	1.2	1.2	1.2	2.0	800	800	110	10	250	10
Males	11–14	44	97	158	63	2800	44	1000	5000	400	12	45	400	18	1.5	1.4	1.6	3.0	1200	1200	130	18	350	15
	15–18	61	134	172	69	3000	54	1000	5000	400	15	45	400	20	1.8	1.5	2.0	3.0	1200	1200	150	18	400	15
	19–22	67	147	172	69	3000	54	1000	5000	400	15	45	400	20	1.8	1.5	2.0	3.0	800	800	140	10	350	15
	23–50	70	154	172	69	2700	56	1000	5000		15	45	400	18	1.6	1.4	2.0	3.0	800	800	130	10	350	15
	51+	70	154	172	69	2400	56	1000	5000		15	45	400	16	1.5	1.2	2.0	3.0	800	800	110	10	350	15
Females	11–14	44	97	155	62	2400	44	800	4000	400	12	45	400	16	1.3	1.2	1.6	3.0	1200	1200	115	18	300	15
	15–18	54	119	162	65	2100	48	800	4000	400	12	45	400	14	1.4	1.1	2.0	3.0	1200	1200	115	18	300	15
	19–22	58	128	162	65	2100	46	800	4000	400	12	45	400	14	1.4	1.1	2.0	3.0	800	800	100	18	300	15
	23–50	58	128	162	65	2000	46	800	4000		12	45	400	13	1.2	1.0	2.0	3.0	800	800	100	18	300	15
	51+	58	128	162	65	1800	46	800	4000		12	45	400	12	1.1	1.0	2.0	3.0	800	800	80	10	300	15
Pregnant						+300	+30	1000	5000	400	15	60	800	+2	+0.3	+0.3	2.5	4.0	1200	1200	125	18+[h]	450	20
Lactating						+500	+20	1200	6000	400	15	80	600	+4	+0.5	+0.3	2.5	4.0	1200	1200	150	18	450	25

[a] The allowances are intended to provide for individual variations among most normal persons as they live in the United States under usual environmental stresses. Diets should be based on a variety of common foods in order to provide other nutrients for which human requirements have been less well defined.

[b] Kilojoules (kJ) = 4.2 × kcal.

[c] Retinol equivalents.

[d] Assumed to be all as retinol in milk during the first six months of life. All subsequent intakes are assumed to be one-half as retinol and one-half as β-carotene when calculated from International Units. As retinol equivalents, three-fourths are as retinol and one-fourth as β-carotene.

[e] Total vitamin E activity, estimated to be 80 percent as α-tocopherol and 20 percent other tocopherols.

[f] The folacin allowances refer to dietary sources as determined by *Lactobacillus casei* assay. Pure forms of folacin may be effective in doses less than one-fourth of the RDA.

[g] Although allowances are expressed as niacin, it is recognized that on the average 1 mg of niacin is derived from each 60 mg of dietary tryptophan.

[h] This increased requirement cannot be met by ordinary diets; therefore, the use of supplemental iron is recommended.

From *Recommended Daily Dietary Allowances. Eighth Edition.* Washington, D.C.: Natl. Research Council. 1974.

33

min E activity (IU), vitamin C (mg), folacin (μg), niacin (mg), riboflavin (mg), thiamin (mg), vitamin B-6 (mg), vitamin B-12 (μg), calcium (mg), phosphorus (mg), iodine (μg), iron (mg), magnesium (mg), and zinc (mg). Allowances are given for each sex and for different age groups (Table 3.1).

United States
Recommended Daily Allowances

In 1973 the Food and Drug Administration established a new standard called the U.S. RDA for use in nutrition labeling (4, 8). The nutrients included in this allowance are eight that must be listed on the food label, protein, vitamin A, vitamin C, thiamin, riboflavin, niacin, calcium, and iron and 12 that may be listed vitamin D, vitamin E, vitamin B-6, folacin, vitamin B-12, phosphorus, iodine, magnesium, zinc, copper, biotin, and pantothenic acid (Table 3.2). Except for the calcium, phosphorus, zinc, copper, biotin, and pantothenic acid allowances, these values are the highest for each nutrient in the 1968 Recommended Dietary Allowances for males and for females (nonpregnant, nonlactating) four years of age and older (11). The U.S. RDA replaces the Minimum Daily Requirements (MDR), which had been used since 1941 in the labeling of food and vitamin products. The MDR represented the minimum amount of various nutrients that were believed to be necessary for maintaining health; the U.S. RDA represents the daily amounts felt to be needed by healthy people plus an additional 30 to 50 percent to allow for individual variations.

The information required when nutrition labeling is used includes serving size, servings per container, caloric (energy) content per serving, protein content per serving, carbohydrate content per serving, and percentage of U.S. RDA of protein, vitamins, and minerals per serving.

It is possible to use the U.S. RDA table to calculate the nutrient value of a food product. For example, an envelope containing a powdered food mix that is intended to be added to milk

Table 3.2 The U.S. Recommended Daily Allowance

	Nutrients	U.S. RDA
	Protein	65 g[a]
that	Vitamin A	5000 IU
must	Vitamin C (ascorbic acid)	60.0 mg
be	Thiamin (vitamin B$_1$)	1.5 mg
listed	Riboflavin (vitamin B$_2$)	1.7 mg
on	Niacin	20.0 mg
label	Calcium	1.0 g
	Iron	18.0 mg
that	Vitamin D	400 IU
may	Vitamin E	30 IU
be	Vitamin B-6	2.0 mg
listed	Folacin (folic acid)	0.4 mg
on	Vitamin B-12	6.0 μg
label	Phosphorus	1.0 g
	Iodine	150 μg
	Magnesium	400 mg
	Zinc	15 mg
	Copper	2.0 mg
	Biotin	0.3 mg
	Pantothenic acid	10.0 mg

From *Federal Register* **38**: No. 13 (January 19, 1973).
[a] 45 g for foods providing high-quality protein such as meat, fish, poultry, eggs, and milk.
[b] Peterkin, *Nutrition Labeling Tools for its Use.* Agr. Inf. Bult. No. 382, Washington, D.C.: U.S. Dept. Agr. 1975, p. 8.

states that its contents provide 27 percent of the U.S. RDA for thiamin, 31.5 percent for riboflavin, and 24 percent for iron. Using the values presented in Table 3.2 one can calculate that this portion of the food mix contains 0.41 mg of thiamin, 0.54 mg of riboflavin, and 4.3 mg of iron.

International Allowances

The accumulation of pertinent data on nutritive functions and requirements, as well as the experience gained from formulating and using statements on dietary needs for several decades, has led to the formulation of other standards. The best known ones are the Dietary Standard of Canada, the Recommended Intakes of Nutrients for the United Kingdom, and the FAO/WHO Recommended Intakes of Nutrients.

Dietary Standard for Canada

The Dietary Standard for Canada (revised in 1964) was prepared by a committee of the Canadian Council on Nutrition to be used in planning diets and food supplies for healthy persons or groups (1, 2). These standards are considered to be adequate for maintaining good health among most Canadians. The tables of nutrient intake recommendations give values for energy, protein, calcium, iron, vitamin A, vitamin D, vitamin C, thiamin, riboflavin, and niacin for infancy, childhood, adolescence, adulthood, pregnancy, and lactation. The daily energy needs for men and women (beyond the age of 19 years) are given in different degrees of physical activity and different body sizes. The end of adolescence is 19 years in these standards.

Recommended Intakes of Nutrients for the United Kingdom

The United Kingdom was one of the first nations to formulate and recommend a dietary standard for its population (1934). The standards recommended by the Committee on Nutrition of the British Medical Association in 1950 were reviewed and revised in 1968 by the Panel on Recommended Allowances of Nutrients, which was appointed by the Department of Health and Social Security. These recommended intakes are defined as "the amounts sufficient or more than sufficient for the nutritional needs of practically all healthy persons in a population" (12).

The same ten nutrients listed in the Canadian standards are recommended in the tables of Recommended Nutrient for the United Kingdom. Here again, nutrient levels are based on the physical activity level (sedentary, moderately active, and very active) of men and women from early

adulthood throughout life. The 18-year-old person in the United Kingdom is considered to be a young adult.

FAO/WHO Recommended Intakes of Nutrients

The *Handbook of Human Nutrition Requirements* is a compilation of data prepared by groups of international scientists in nutrition (9). It recommends intakes of energy, protein, vitamin A, vitamin D, thiamin, riboflavin, niacin, folic acid, vitamin B-12, vitamin C (ascorbic acid), calcium, and iron for people throughout the world. Requirements are given for children (up to 1 year, 1–3 years, 4–6 years, and 7–9 years), for male and female adolescents (10–12 years, 13–15 years, and 16–19 years), for adult men and women, and for women during pregnancy and lactation (Table 3.3).

The FAO/WHO Expert Committee on Energy and Protein Requirements (3) has taken a major step in assessing differences in physical activities throughout adult life. Energy needs are given for men and women of different body sizes according to different occupations (Table 3.4). These occupational categories are listed in Table 3.5. (Students and teachers, for example, have been listed under moderately active and light activity, respectively). After the age of 39 years, a decrease in the energy intake from the recommendation for the 20–39-year-old group is suggested: 40 to 49 years (5 percent less), 50–59 years (10 percent less), 60–69 years (20 percent less), and 70–79 years (30 percent less).

A Comparison of Standards

Both the RDA for the United States and the Recommended Intakes for the United Kingdom were intended to be more than adequate for good nutrition in "practically all healthy persons" (10, 12). The Canadian Dietary Standard is believed to be sufficient for maintaining good health "in the majority of Canadians" (1). The FAO/

Table 3.3 Recommended Intakes of Nutrients (FAO/WHO)

Age range	Body weight kg	Energy (a) kcal	Energy (a) MJ	Protein (a, b) g	Vitamin A (c, d) µg	Vitamin D (e, f) µg	Thiamine (c) mg	Riboflavine (c) mg	Niacin (c) mg	Folic acid (e) µg	Vitamin B12 (e) µg	Ascorbic acid (e) mg	Calcium (g) g	Iron (e, h) mg
Children														
< 1	7.3	820	3.4	14	300	10.0	0.3	0.5	5.4	60	0.3	20	0.5–0.6	5–10
1–3	13.4	1360	5.7	16	250	10.0	0.5	0.8	9.0	100	0.9	20	0.4–0.5	5–10
4–6	20.2	1830	7.6	20	300	10.0	0.7	1.1	12.1	100	1.5	20	0.4–0.5	5–10
7–9	28.1	2190	9.2	25	400	2.5	0.9	1.3	14.5	100	1.5	20	0.4–0.5	5–10
Male adolescents														
10–12	36.9	2600	10.9	30	575	2.5	1.0	1.6	17.2	100	2.0	20	0.6–0.7	5–10
13–15	51.3	2900	12.1	37	725	2.5	1.2	1.7	19.1	200	2.0	30	0.6–0.7	9–18
16–19	62.9	3070	12.8	38	750	2.5	1.2	1.8	20.3	200	2.0	30	0.5–0.6	5–9
Female adolescents														
10–12	38.0	2350	9.8	29	575	2.5	0.9	1.4	15.5	100	2.0	20	0.6–0.7	5–10
13–15	49.9	2490	10.4	31	725	2.5	1.0	1.5	16.4	200	2.0	30	0.6–0.7	12–24
16–19	54.4	2310	9.7	30	750	2.5	0.9	1.4	15.2	200	2.0	30	0.5–0.6	14–28
Adult man (moderately active)	65.0	3000	12.6	37	750	2.5	1.2	1.8	19.8	200	2.0	30	0.4–0.5	5–9
Adult woman (moderately active)	55.0	2200	9.2	29	750	2.5	0.9	1.3	14.5	200	2.0	30	0.4–0.5	14–28
Pregnancy (later half)		+350	+1.5	38	750	10.0	+0.1	+0.2	+2.3	400	3.0	30	1.0–1.2	(i)
Lactation (first 6 months)		+550	+2.3	46	1200	10.0	+0.2	+0.4	+3.7	300	2.5	30	1.0–1.2	(i)

[a] Energy and protein requirements. Report of a Joint FAO/WHO Expert Group, FAO, Rome, 1972.

[b] As egg or milk protein.

[c] Requirements of vitamin A, thiamine, riboflavin and niacin. Report of a Joint FAO/WHO Export Group, FAO, Rome, 1965.

[d] As retinol.

[e] Requirements of ascorbic acid, vitamin D, vitamin B12, folate and iron. Report of a Joint FAO/WHO Expert Group, FAO, Rome, 1970.

[f] As cholecalciferol.

[g] Calcium requirements. Report of a FAO/WHO Expert Group, FAO, Rome 1961.

[h] On each line the lower value applies when over 25 percent of calories in the diet come from animal foods, and the higher value when animal foods represent less than 10 percent of calories.

[i] For women whose iron intake throughout life has been at the level recommended in this table, the daily intake of iron during pregnancy and lactation should be the same as that recommended for nonpregnant, nonlactating women of childbearing age. For women whose iron status is not satisfactory at the beginning of pregnancy, the requirement is increased, and in the extreme situation of women with no iron stores, the requirement can probably not be met without supplementation.

From R. Passmore et al. *Handbook on Human Nutritional Requirements.* WHO Monogram Ser. No. 61. Geneva: World Health Organ., 1974.

Table 3.4 FAO/WHO Energy Requirements for Adults (30 years of age and over)

	Body weight, kg	Light activity		Moderately active		Very active		Exception- ally active	
		kcal	MJ	kcal	MJ	kcal	MJ	kcal	MJ
Men	50	2100	8.8	2300	9.6	2700	11.3	3100	13.0
	55	2310	9.7	2530	10.6	2970	12.4	3410	14.3
	60	2520	10.5	2760	11.5	3240	13.6	3720	15.6
	65	2700	11.3	3000	12.5	3500	14.6	4000	16.7
	70	2940	12.3	3220	13.5	3780	15.8	4340	18.2
	75	3150	13.2	3450	14.4	4050	16.9	4650	19.5
	80	3360	14.1	3680	15.4	4320	18.1	4960	20.8
Women	40	1440	6.0	1600	6.7	1880	7.9	2200	9.2
	45	1620	6.8	1800	7.5	2120	8.9	2480	10.4
	50	1800	7.5	2000	8.4	2350	9.8	2750	11.5
	55	2000	8.4	2200	9.2	2600	10.9	3000	12.6
	60	2160	9.0	2400	10.0	2820	11.8	3300	13.8
	65	2340	9.8	2600	10.9	3055	12.8	3575	15.0
	70	2520	10.5	2800	11.7	3290	13.8	3850	16.1

Pregnancy +150 kcal (628 kJ) per day in first trimester

+350 kcal (1464 kJ) per day in second and third trimesters

Lactation +550 kcal (2301 kJ) per day

Adapted from *Energy and Protein Requirements*, FAO Nutrition Meetings Rept. Series 52, and WHO Tech. Rept. Series 522 (Rome: Food and Agr. Organ., 1973), pp. 31, 36.

WHO Recommended Intakes are intended to apply to people in all countries and "when translated into terms of local foods, the figures can certainly be used as a practical guide for agricultural planning in all countries . . . especially those in which a large population growth is anticipated" (9).

The four standards also differ in their expression of energy values for men and women. Canada (1), the United Kingdom (12), and the FAO/WHO (9) give caloric allowances in terms of activities or occupational categories; the RDA of the United States (10) does not. The FAO/WHO standard, for example, includes the energy needs for those who are slightly active, moderately active, very active, and exceptionally active (see Table 3.4).

Other differences found in the four dietary standards are the number of nutrients recommended (18 for the United States, 12 for the FAO/WHO, and 10 each for Canada and United Kingdom); the amounts of the nutrients recommended (see Table 3.6); the cut-off year for the end of adolescence (19 years for Canada and the FAO/WHO, 18 years for the United States and United Kingdom); and the groupings by sex and age (the United States, for example, the values begin with the male and female groupings at age 11).

37

Table 3.5 Classification of the FAO/WHO Occupation Categories

	Men	Women
Light activity	Office workers, most professionals (doctors, teachers, etc.), shop workers	Office workers, teachers, most professionals, housewives using mechanical household appliances
Moderately active	Students, most workers in light industry, building workers, many farm workers, fishermen, military personnel not on active duty	Students, housewives without mechanical household appliances, workers in light industry, department store clerks
Very active	Some agricultural workers, unskilled laborers, forestry workers, military recruits and those on active duty, mine and steel workers, athletes	Some farm workers, dancers, athletes
Exceptionally active	Lumberjacks, blacksmiths, rickshaw-pullers	Construction workers

Adapted from *Energy and Protein Requirements*, FAO Nutrition Meetings Rept. Series 52, and WHO Tech. Rept. Series 522 (Rome: Food and Agr. Organ., 1973), p. 25.

An interesting comparison exists among the nutrient allowances recommended for college-age men and women in various countries. The example used here is the 19-year-old male and female student whose energy allowances vary from standard to standard (Table 3.6). Both the Canadian and international standards categorize 19-year-old as an older boy or girl rather than as a young adult as do the RDA for the United States and the Recommended Intakes of Nutrients for the United Kingdom. Thus Canada and the FAO/WHO have somewhat higher energy allowances than the United States or United Kingdom.

Table 3.6 presents differences in the recommendations for protein, iron, calcium, and vitamin C, indicated as units per 1000 kcal (4184 kJ). American college-age women have the largest allowance for iron (8.6 mg), calcium (380 mg), and vitamin C (21 mg) per 1000 kcal (4184 kJ); young men and women of the United Kingdom have the largest protein allowance (25 g per 1000 kcal [4184 kJ]).

Use of Dietary Allowances or Standards

Dietary allowances and standards may be used for several purposes (14). They enable one to calculate the approximate nutritional requirements of a group, as in establishing a ration; to evaluate the diet of a group by analyzing the total and average quantities of food eaten; to serve as a guide or goal for teaching the nutrient needs of different age–sex groups; to formulate regulations pertaining to the composition of foods, dietary supplements, or drugs, and the claims that can

Table 3.6 Protein, Iron, Calcium, and Vitamin C Allowances per 1000 kcal (4184 kJ) for 19-Year-Old Men and Women: the United States (10), United Kingdom (12), Canada (1, 2), and International (FAO/WHO) (9)

	Sex	Protein, g	Iron, mg	Calcium, mg	Vitamin C, mg
United States	M	18.0	3.3	267	15
	F	21.9	8.6	380	21
United Kingdom	M	25.0	3.3	167	10
	F	25.0	5.5	227	14
Canada	M	15.8	1.6	237	8
	F	20.4	4.1	367	12
International (FAO/WHO)	M	20.5[a]	1.6[b]	180	10
	F	21.6[a]	6.1[b]	238	13

[a] Based on the upper level of protein requirement (protein quality of 60 percent).
[b] Based on an intake of animal foods comprising more than 25 percent of the kilocalories.

be made about them; and to evaluate the diet of individuals by means of the food purchased or eaten.

It should be noted that the RDA and the nutritional standards of other countries are only approximate; they have been established to try to allow for individual variation in need and differences in the composition of foods eaten. In the case of some nutrients, the recommended intake is determined according to the consuming habits of a given population. For example, the average consumption of calcium is relatively high in the United States and so is the RDA for calcium. Failure to meet the RDA cannot, by itself, be interpreted as evidence of an inadequate intake of a specific nutrient.

Summary

Dietary allowances or standards for the United States, Canada, and the United Kingdom, and the FAO/WHO allowances for worldwide use are presented. The allowances differ in purpose, in number and amounts of nutrients recommended, in cut-off year for end of adolescence, and in groupings by sex and age.

There are differences between the RDA of the NAS–NRC and the U.S. RDA of the FDA. The 1974 RDA gives allowances for the intake of the essential nutrients to meet known nutritional needs of healthy persons in the United States, whereas the U.S. RDA is a standard used by the government for nutritional labeling of food products. The U.S. RDA, which is based on the 1968 edition of the RDA, has a somewhat higher vitamin C (ascorbic acid) value and includes nutrients not listed in the present RDA (copper, biotin, and pantothenic acid).

There are five ways that dietary allowances or standards may be used: to establish a ration for a group; to evaluate the diet of a group; to serve as a guide for teaching nutrient needs; to set up regulations for the composition of foods, dietary supplements, or drugs; and to evaluate the diet of individuals.

Do the RDAs fulfil the purposes for which they are intended? Some general criticisms are that the allowances are meaningless because the values for the nutrients are excessive, the allowances are inadequate because they do not provide for an "ideal diet," and/or the RDA bulletins are sociopolitical documents (5).

Hegsted has studied in depth the use and interpretation of the RDAs and has concluded that their two major purposes — the evaluation of food consumption records and the planning of diets and food supplies — cannot be accomplished with a single set of allowances. He recommends that "... these two purposes should be clearly recognized and the standards and instruction for their use for each purpose should be developed" (6).

The RDAs are not for amateurs is the theme employed by Leverton (7) to describe the pitfalls that may occur in their use. They are:

1. Placing too much emphasis on small differences between the food intake value and the allowance of a nutrient. (If a student's daily food intake of calcium, for example, is only 742 mg as compared to the RDA of 800 mg, this is not significant.)

2. Assessing a person's nutritional status by a comparison of the actual food intake value with the RDA. (When a college student, for example, ingests only 65 percent of the RDA for calcium, it cannot be concluded that the individual is malnourished.)

3. Attempting to make a value judgment at what intake level below the RDA nutritional risk may occur when the margin of safety for the various nutrients in the RDA are not known. (Some scientists believe that the RDAs exceed actual needs and so accept two-thirds or even one-half of the RDA values as adequate. When a diet in a national food consumption survey supplies less than two-thirds of the allowances for one or more nutrients, for example, the U.S. Department of Agriculture has labeled it "poor.")

4. Trying to develop a food pattern using the RDA, with its margin of safety for all nutrients except energy. This may result in unrealistic and unnecessary modifications of the diet, extra food expenditure, and concern about nutrient shortages. (The best example of this is planning a daily diet of 2100 kcal (8786 kJ) for college women, 19 to 22 years, and including 18 mg of food iron. Without a serving of liver, it becomes

necessary to include four or more servings of dark green vegetables and other foods rich in the nutrient.)

Glossary

Food and Agriculture Organization of the United Nations (FAO): established in 1945, the FAO's main purpose is to raise the levels of nutrition and the standards of living of the people of the UN member nations. Periodic estimates are made of the food available to each country in an attempt to improve production and distribution. Its headquarters is in Rome.

Food and Nutrition Board (National Academy of Sciences–National Research Council): established in 1940, this board serves as an advisory body to the government on food and nutrition. One of its functions has been the establishment and periodic revision of the Recommended Dietary Allowances.

gram (g): a metric unit of weight that is equivalent to about 1/28 of an ounce (1 oz = 28.4 g), 1/1000 of a kilogram, or 1000 milligrams.

International Unit (IU): a unit of measure used to express the value of vitamin A activity, vitamin D, and vitamin E activity.

kilocalorie (kcal): the quantity of heat required to raise the temperature of 1 kg of water 1°C (or more precisely, from 15°C to 16°C); 4.184 kJ.

kilogram (kg): a metric unit of weight that is equivalent to 2.2 pounds, or 1000 grams.

kilojoule (kJ): a metric unit of energy that is equivalent to 0.239 kcal.

megajoule (MJ): a metric unit of energy that is equal to 240 kcal, or 1000 kJ.

microgram (μg): a metric unit of weight that is equivalent to one-millionth of a gram, or 1/1000 of a milligram.

milligram (mg): a metric unit of weight that is equivalent to 1/1000 of a gram, or 1000 micrograms.

National Academy of Sciences (NAS): a scientific group founded over a century ago to serve science and the United States Government.

National Research Council (NRC): a scientific group

founded in 1916 by the National Academy of Sciences to work with the major American scientific and technical societies to coordinate their efforts in the service of science and the government.

retinol equivalents (RE): a unit now used to express vitamin A activity; 3.33 International Units equal one retinol equivalent.

World Health Organization of the United Nations (WHO): the specialized agency, located in Geneva, that is concerned with health on an international level.

Study Questions and Activities

1. Why have dietary allowances or standards been established?

2. Why do dietary standards vary from one country to another?

3. How are dietary standards used?

4. What is the difference between the NAS–NRC's Recommended Daily Dietary Allowances and the Food and Drug Administration's U.S. Recommended Daily Allowance? What purpose do they each serve?

5. Why have international dietary standards been established—first by the League of Nations and then by the FAO and FAO/WHO?

6. Select two foods or food products (for example, a breakfast cereal) that list the Food and Drug Administration's values for the U.S. Recommended Daily Allowance on the package. Calculate the actual quantity of given nutrients in the two products.

References

1. Dietary Standard for Canada (1964). *Can. Bull Nutrition,* **6:** No. 1.

2. Dietary Standard for Canada, protein revision 1968 (1969). *Can. Nutrition Notes,* **25:** 70.

3. *Energy and Protein Requirements* (1973). FAO Nutrition Meetings Rept. Series 52, and WHO Tech. Rept. Series 522. Rome: Food and Agr. Organ.

4. *Federal Register,* **38:** No. 13 (January 19, 1973).

5. Harper, A. E. (1974). Recommended Dietary Allowances: are they what we think they are? *J. Am. Dietet. Assoc.,* **64:** 151.

6. Hegsted, D. M. (1975). Dietary standards. *J. Am. Dietet. Assoc.* **66:** 13.

7. Leverton, R. M. (1975). The RDAs are not for amateurs. *J. Am. Dietet. Assoc.,* **66:** 9.

8. Nutrition labeling (1973). *Nutrition Rev.,* **31:** 36.

9. Passmore, R., B. M. Nicol, M. N. Rao, G. H. Beaton, and E. M. Demayer (1974). *Handbook on Human Nutritional Requirements.* WHO Monogram Ser. No. 61. Geneva: World Health Organ.

10. *Recommended Dietary Allowances, Eighth Edition* (1974). Washington, D.C.: Natl. Research Council.

11. *Recommended Dietary Allowances, Seventh Edition* (1968). Natl. Acad. Sci-Natl. Research Council Publ. No. 1694. Washington, D. C.: Natl. Research Council.

12. *Recommended Intakes of Nutrients for the United Kingdom* (1969). Department of Health and Social Security, Reports on Public Health and Medical Subjects No. 120. London: H. M. Stationery Office.

13. Stiebeling, H. K., and M. M. Ward (1933). *Diets at Four Levels of Nutritive Content and Cost.* U.S. Dept. Agr. Circular No. 296. Washington, D.C.: U.S. Dept. Agr.

14. Young, E. G. (1964). Dietary standards. In *Nutrition: A Comprehensive Treatise,* Vol. 2, edited by G. H. Beaton and E. W. McHenry. New York: Academic Press, p. 299.

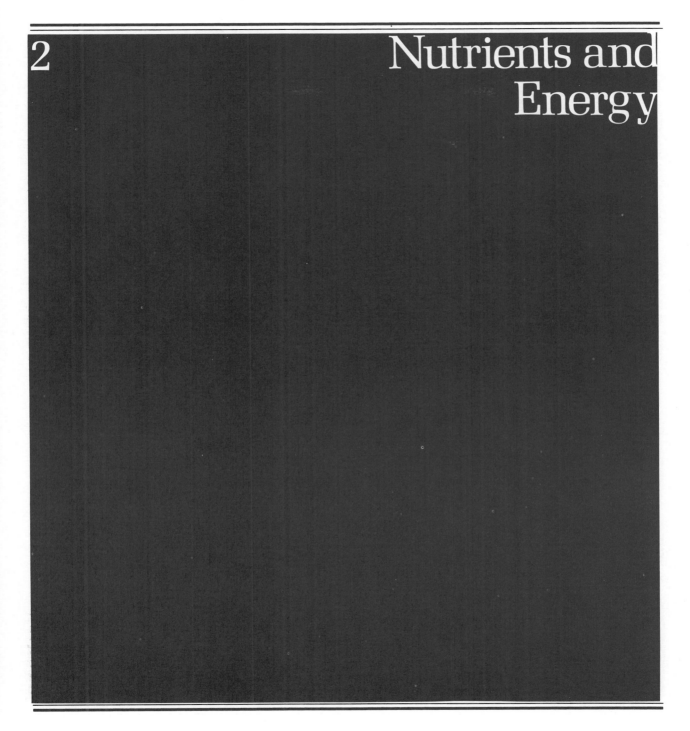

2

Nutrients and Energy

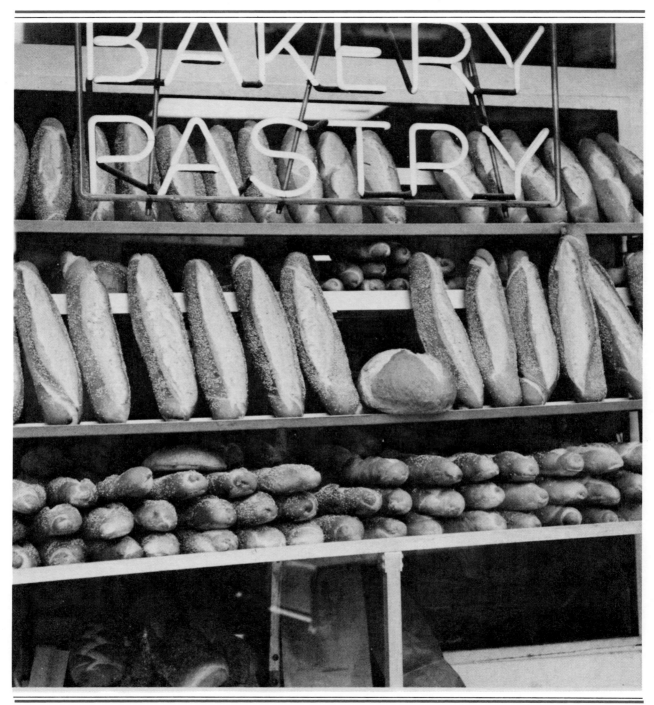

Bread, one of our most important sources of carbohydrate (and often called the "staff of life"), can offer a remarkable variety of taste, texture and eye appeal.

Chapter 4

Carbohydrates

Abbreviations

acetyl CoA: acetyl coenzyme A
ATP: adenosine triphosphate
CO_2: carbon dioxide
DNA: deoxyribonucleic acid
H_2O: water

NADP: nicotinamide adenine dinucleotide
    phosphate
O_2: oxygen
RNA: ribonucleic acid

Carbohydrates serve a significant function in nature because they are the chief source of energy for the animal kingdom. Through the process of *photosynthesis*—a series of complex chemical reactions—the chlorophyll of the plant is able to use the sun's energy to synthesize carbohydrates from carbon dioxide in the air and water from the soil. Thus plants provide animals with food. This nutrient is also the main source of food energy for people; it is found in rice, *cassava*, sugars, potatoes, corn, wheat, and other cereal grains that are used worldwide.

All carbohydrates contain carbon, hydrogen, and oxygen. An example of a simple carbohydrate molecule is one with six carbon atoms arranged in a chain with atoms of hydrogen and oxygen in a ratio of two to one—the same ratio as found in water. The chemical formula for glucose, a simple carbohydrate molecule with six carbon atoms, is presented in Figure 4.1. The energy value of carbohydrates is 4 kcal (17kJ) of energy per gram.

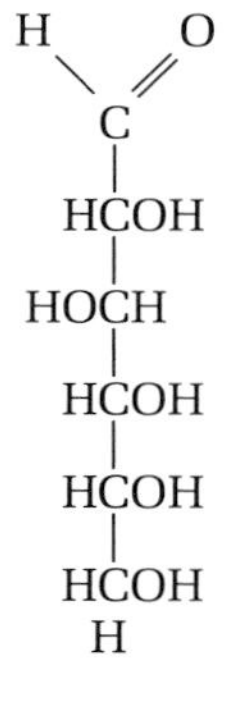

A simple classification of some of the carbohydrates that are important in nutrition, based on the number of single carbohydrate molecules found in each chemical structure, is presented in Figure 4.2.

Compounds with one carbohydrate molecule are called monosaccharides, those with two molecules are designated disaccharides, and those with more than two carbohydrate molecules are called polysaccharides. The three monosaccharides shown in Figure 4.2 are the carbohydrate molecules that make up the di- and polysaccharides. The mono- and disaccharides are soluble in water and have a crystalline structure and sweet taste; they are called sugars and all have the same suffix, -ose. By contrast, most polysaccharides are insoluble in water; they do not form crystals and do not taste sweet; they have no group name or characteristic suffix. The carbohydrate composition of several foods is presented in Table 4.1.

```
       H      O
        \    //
         C
         |
       HCOH
         |
       HOCH
         |
       HCOH
         |
       HCOH
         |
       HCOH
         H
```

Fig. 4.1. The chemical formula of glucose.

Certain Classes of Carbohydrate

The Monosaccharides

The three that are important in the study of nutrition are glucose, fructose, and galactose.

Glucose This monosaccharide, sometimes called dextrose or grape sugar, is widely distributed in nature. It is found in fruits, vegetables, and the

46

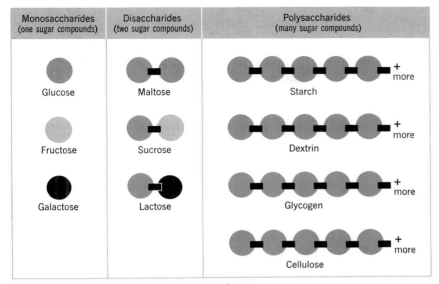

Monosaccharides (one sugar compounds)	Disaccharides (two sugar compounds)	Polysaccharides (many sugar compounds)
Glucose	Maltose	Starch + more
Fructose	Sucrose	Dextrin + more
Galactose	Lactose	Glycogen + more
		Cellulose + more

Fig. 4.2. A simple classification of carbohydrates.

sap of trees, as well as in honey, corn syrup, and molasses (Table 4.1). In animals and men it is an end product of the digestion of starch, sucrose, maltose, and lactose.

Fructose and Galactose Although these two monosaccharides have the same chemical formula as glucose ($C_6H_{12}O_6$), they differ in the arrangement of their chemical groups along the chemical chain.

Fructose, which is the sweetest of all the sugars, is also known as levulose or fruit sugar. It is found in the nectar of flowers, in honey and molasses, and in fruits and vegetables (Table 4.1). It is also produced during digestion in the hydrolysis of sucrose.

Galactose does not occur free in nature like glucose and fructose but is produced in the body during the digestion of the disaccharide lactose.

The Disaccharides

Sucrose, maltose, and lactose are the three disaccharides in foods.

Sucrose Sucrose is composed of one unit of glucose and one of fructose. White and brown sugars (whether produced from beet sugar or cane sugar) are almost 100 percent sucrose. Maple syrup and molasses contain more than 50 percent sucrose, whereas lesser amounts are found in *sorghum* and corn syrups (Table 4.1). Because of the added sugar, fruit jellies and jams are also high in sucrose.

Maltose and Lactose Unlike sucrose, maltose and lactose are not consumed in large amounts in the average diet.

Maltose (malt sugar) is found in sprouting grains, malted cereals, and malted milk. Of the commonly used sweetening agents, this disaccharide is found only in corn syrup (26 percent) and corn sugar (4 percent) (Table 4.1). Maltose is formed in the body as an intermediate product of starch digestion. When hydrolyzed, maltose yields two molecules of glucose.

Lactose (milk sugar) is found only in milk (Table 4.1). The amount of lactose in human and cows' milk is about 6.8 and 4.8 g per 100 ml,

47

Table 4.1. Common Carbohydrates of Various Foods

Food	Monosaccharides		Disaccharides			Polysaccharides		
	Glucose	Fructose	Sucrose	Maltose	Lactose	Starch	Dextrins	Cellulose
	g/100 g		g/100 g			g/100 g		
Apple	1.7	5.0	3.1	—	—	0.6	—	0.4
Beans, navy	—	—	—	—	—	35.2	3.7	3.1
Corn, fresh	0.5	—	0.3	—	—	14.5	0.1	0.6
Corn syrup	21.2	—	—	26.4	—	—	34.7	—
Grapes (Concord)	4.8	4.3	0.2	—	—	—	—	—
Honey	34.2	40.5	1.9	—	—	—	1.5	—
Jellies	—	—	40–65	—	—	—	—	—
Maple syrup	—	—	62.9	—	—	—	—	—
Milk, cows', whole	—	—	—	—	4.9	—	—	—
Molasses	8.8	8.0	53.6	—	—	—	—	—
Orange	2.5	1.8	4.6	—	—	—	—	0.3
Peas								
green	—	—	5.5	—	—	4.1	—	1.1
mature, dry	—	—	6.7	—	—	38.0	—	5.0
Potatoes (white)	0.1	0.1	0.1	—	—	17.0	—	0.4
Rice, polished, raw	2.0	—	0.4	—	—	72.9	0.9	0.3
Wheat flour, patent	—	—	0.2	0.1	—	68.8	5.5	—

From M. G. Hardinge, J. G. Swarner, and H. Crooks (1965). Carbohydrates in foods. *J. Am. Dietet. Assoc.*, **46**: 198–201.

respectively. Glucose and galactose are the two monosaccharides formed when lactose is hydrolyzed.

The Polysaccharides

These complex carbohydrates may contain as many as 60,000 simple carbohydrate molecules arranged in long chains in either a straight or a branched structure. The three that are important in nutrition are starch, glycogen, and cellulose.

Starch Throughout the world starch is the most abundant carbohydrate in man's diet. Roots, seeds, and tubers, which are easily and abundantly produced, all contain starch.

The seeds of plants are nature's richest storehouses of starch (Table 4.1). Corn, *millet*, rice, rye, and wheat—the important cereal grains—contain as much as 70 percent of this carbohydrate, whereas the dried seeds of *leguminous* plants (for example, beans and peas) average about 40 percent. Starch is found in the cells of plants in the form of granules that are visible under the microscope. These granules differ in size, shape, and markings according to the given plant. For example, wheat starch granules are oval-shaped, whereas cornstarch granules are small, rounded, and angular.

Starches are not soluble in cold water but when boiled with water they form pastes. As the temperature of the water rises, the starch granules begin to swell and the mixture becomes viscous; this change is called gelatinization. Cooking makes starch-containing foods more palatable and more easily digested. Glucose is the end product of all starch hydrolyzed in the body.

Partial breakdown products of starch are the dextrins. They are large molecules which, on further digestion (hydrolysis), yield maltose and finally glucose. Dextrins are formed both in the preparation of foods and the digestion of starch. An appreciable amount of dextrin is found in corn syrup; smaller amounts are found in wheat flour, honey, peanuts, corn, beans, and rice (Table 4.1).

Glycogen Glycogen is a polysaccharide composed of thousands of glucose units. It is found in the liver and muscles of animals and is the counterpart of starch in plants.

The body has a limited capacity to store glycogen—about 350 g (12 oz). Two-thirds of the total glycogen is stored in the muscles as muscle glycogen and can only be used for the energy needs within the muscle cells. In contrast, the glycogen stored in the liver (about one-third of the total) may be used as a source of energy for any body cell.

Cellulose Like starch and glycogen, the cellulose molecule is composed of many glucose units, as many as 12,000. This polysaccharide comprises 50 percent or more of all the carbon found in vegetation. In plants it is the structural constituent of the cell wall that makes up the skeletal part of the plant. Human beings and carnivores do not have the enzyme that is needed to digest cellulose. *Ruminant* animals (such as cows and sheep) have in their rumens (stomachs) bacteria whose enzyme systems break down the cellulose into molecules sufficiently small for the ruminant to use. Thus when man ingests products from these animals, he is indirectly using cellulose as a source of food. Otherwise cellulose in man's diet functions as a component of dietary fiber.

Digestion, Absorption, and Metabolism of Carbohydrates

Carbohydrate Digestion

The digestion of carbohydrate begins in the mouth where the enzyme salivary amylase (ptyalin) breaks down starch and dextrin by splitting off molecules of the disaccharide maltose from the long carbohydrate chain (Fig. 4.3). This action continues as the food passes into the stomach; here the salivary amylase becomes inactive by the acidity of the gastric juice.

Carbohydrate digestion is resumed in the first part of the small intestine, the duodenum, by the enzyme pancreatic amylase, which converts any remaining starch to maltose (Fig. 4.3). Even uncooked or raw starch may be digested by pancreatic amylase. However, raw starches are less digestible than cooked ones because of the nature of the starch granule. Raw potato starch, for example, is poorly digested and may pass through the digestive tract unchanged when large amounts are consumed.

Maltose, sucrose, and lactose found either in the original food consumed or as end products of amylase action are changed to simple sugars in the small intestine. The three enzymes—maltase, sucrase, and lactase called *carbohydrases*—complete the digestion to glucose, fructose, and galactose (Fig. 4.3).

Lactose Intolerance Many healthy persons, both children and adults, have the inability to use (an *intolerance* to) lactose, the sugar found in milk. The defect, either inherited or acquired, results in an inadequate secretion of lactase, the sugar-splitting enzyme of the small intestine, needed to break down lactose to its simple sugars. The undigested lactose in the intestinal tract produces symptoms including abdominal pain, *diarrhea,* and *flatulence.* Milk to which the enzyme lactase is added (27, 37) and fermented dairy products

49

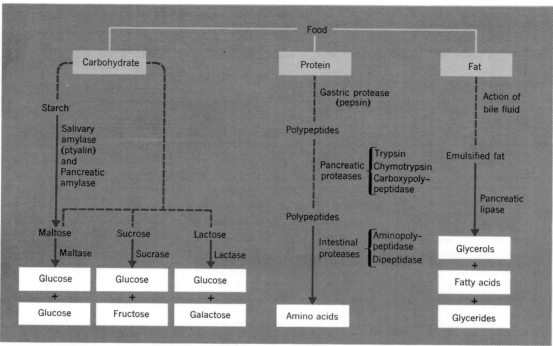

Fig. 4.3 Carbohydrate, fat, and protein digestion.

such as yogurt, cottage cheese, and buttermilk (17) may be used by the lactose intolerant person without adverse affects.

Lactose intolerance is not common among individuals of European background. However, it is found among blacks in North America (72 to 77 percent) and in Africa and among Chinese, Thais, Malays, and Indians (as high as 100 percent) (34). A high incidence of the intolerance has been observed among South Americans in Columbia (37); Alaskan Indians and Eskimos, United States Indians, and Canadian Indians (13); Jamaican children (46); Mexicans (28); and Mexican Americans (45).

The intolerance to lactose begins early in life and becomes more prevalent with age (18, 46). It has been found to occur in over one-half of a group of Jamaican rural children under 4 years of age. A group of nonwhite children living in Boston showed an increased lactose intolerance with age: 11 percent among 4- to 5-year-olds and 72 percent among those 8 to 9 years of age.

Because of the high probability of nonwhite children being lactose malabsorbers, should all the world's children be given milk to drink? Studies show that lactose intolerant children appear to have sufficient lactase to digest small amounts of milk (33, 18). In the Boston study no child was intolerant to 240 ml (8 oz) milk and only mild to moderate symptoms were encountered when 480 ml of milk was ingested. The Protein Advisory Group of the United Nations (39), the Food

50

and Nutrition Board of the NAS–NRC, and the Committee on Nutrition of the American Academy of Pediatrics agree that "... it would be inappropriate to discourage programs for increasing milk supplies and consumption because of a fear of milk intolerance" (2).

Absorption of End Products of Carbohydrate Digestion

Essentially all carbohydrates are absorbed as monosaccharides, and the absorption takes place in the small intestine's duodenum and jejunum (Fig. 2.4). Glucose and galactose pass through the brush border cells of the microvilli into the blood stream by active transport and fructose by diffusion (Fig. 2.5).

It was once thought that carbohydrates other than monosaccharides were not absorbed through the intestinal wall. However, new evidence indicates that very small amounts of maltose, sucrose, and lactose may be absorbed as two-sugar compounds. Maltose, sucrose, and lactose so absorbed appear in the urine, not as simple sugars but as disaccharides. This may occur after eating a meal rich in sugars.

Carbohydrate Metabolism

Carbohydrates, together with fat, are the main energy sources of the body cells and the energy-rich compound ATP. The body's immediate needs determine whether digested and absorbed carbohydrate is used for energy, converted and stored as glycogen, or changed to fat and stored in adipose tissue. Because glucose is the principal sugar used by the body cells and tissues, it is important to summarize the sources of the nutrient.

Sources of Glucose   Glucose comes from several carbohydrate and noncarbohydrate sources (Fig. 4.4).

From the digestion of dietary carbohydrate. Much of the food an individual eats is a potential source of glucose. Glucose is formed from the

digestion of starch, dextrin, maltose, sucrose, and lactose in foods.

From the conversion of fructose and galactose. The three simple sugars have the same chemical formula but differ in the arrangement of the hydrogen and oxygen units along the carbon chain. During metabolism, the liver cells are able to change the absorbed fructose and galactose molecules to molecules of glucose. The lack of an enzyme to convert galactose to glucose produces an unusual hereditary disorder in infants known as galactosemia, in which galactose appears in the urine and there is an abnormal amount of galactose in the blood. The infant fails to thrive, the liver and spleen become enlarged, cataracts develop, and the infant becomes mentally retarded. The condition can be prevented by giving the baby a galactose-free (milk-free) diet.

From the breakdown of liver glycogen. Glycogen stores in the liver are broken down when the need for glucose exceeds the available supply in the blood. The normal liver contains only about 100 g of glycogen, which is equivalent to about 400

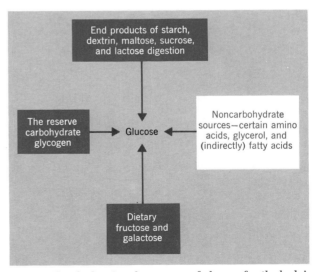

Fig. 4.4 Sketch showing the sources of glucose for the body's use.

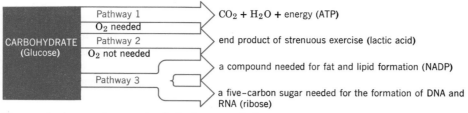

Fig. 4.5 The three pathways of carbohydrate metabolism.

kcal (1674 kJ) of energy. This amount would supply the energy needs of a college man and woman (19 to 22 years old) for only about 3.2 and 4.6 hours, respectively.

Glucose cannot be formed directly from muscle glycogen because muscle tissue lacks the necessary enzymes for this conversion. Indirectly, however, muscle glycogen can furnish glucose. When the muscle contracts, glycogen is converted to a compound called lactic acid, which is changed by the liver to glucose.

From noncarbohydrate sources. If the need for energy by the body cells is greater than the available supplies of glucose and the glycogen stores, noncarbohydrate sources are used to supply glucose. These include certain amino acids from protein, the glycerol from fat, and indirectly, the fatty acids from fat.

Pathways of Carbohydrate Metabolism There are three ways that glucose is metabolized in the body (Fig. 4.5). Most of the glucose is broken down or oxidized (in a series of reactions in the cells that require O_2) to supply energy for body work and heat (Pathway 1). At times when individuals perform strenuous exercise, such as participation in certain sports or jogging, some glucose is metabolized (in the absence of O_2) to lactic acid (Pathway 2). Some glucose must be used to form new compounds—a substance called NADP needed for the formation of fats and lipids and a five-carbon sugar (ribose) required for the formation of DNA and RNA (Pathway 3).

When more carbohydrates are consumed than the body requires to meet its energy need, the excess is converted to fat and stored in the tissues. This has been demonstrated in experiments with animals and human beings. Figure 2.6 shows how a fat may be formed from a carbohydrate by way of acetyl CoA.

Certain amino acids (the unessential ones) also may be formed from carbohydrates and are called *glycogenic* amino acids. Fig. 2.6 shows how amino acids may be formed from carbohydrates by way of either pyruvic acid or acetyl CoA.

Hormones that Control Carbohydrate Metabolism The hormone insulin, secreted by the cells of the pancreas, is important in the body's use of carbohydrates. Not only is insulin necessary for the entry of glucose into the cells and for its oxidation to supply energy, but it is needed in the formation of glycogen from molecules of glucose.

Two other hormones—another from the pancreas (glucagon) and one from the adrenal glands (epinephrine)—are involved in the release of the body's glycogen stores to provide glucose.

Blood Glucose Glucose is the carbohydrate found in the bloodstream to provide an immediate source of energy for the cells and tissues. The normal level in man is within the narrow range of 80 to 100 mg glucose per 100 ml of blood. Blood glucose originates from dietary sources, from stores of glycogen, and from noncarbohydrate sources (Fig. 4.4).

A rise in the blood glucose above its normal level is referred to as hyperglycemia. *Diabetes mellitus* ("sugar" diabetes) is a disorder in which the cells are unable to use glucose because of insufficient body supplies of the hormone insulin. In this disorder the blood glucose may be elevated to levels as high as 1200 mg per 100 ml. When diabetes is stabilized by diet and regular injections of insulin, the blood glucose may be maintained within normal levels.

Less common is the condition hypoglycemia (the term used to describe blood sugar levels below the normal range). Overproduction of insulin by the pancreas or overinjections of insulin result in the removal of glucose from the blood and the lowering of the blood glucose level. Normal individuals may tolerate hypoglycemia for brief periods of time without harm to the body. When the blood sugar remains low for an extended period of time, however, injections of glucose must be administered to replenish the supply of the nutrient for the normal function of the brain and nervous tissue.

ficient. This has been shown to occur during periods of weight reduction and periods of semistarvation. The explanation for this metabolic effect is that the first physiological demand of the body—the energy need—must be satisfied before nutrients are used for other purposes.

Certain carbohydrates serve special functions in the body. Lactose, for example, aids the absorption of calcium, and the five-carbon sugar ribose is a constituent in the important compounds DNA and RNA. Cellulose and other indigestible polysaccharides are components of dietary fiber. Dietary fiber is a new term coined to describe the indigestible polysaccharides found inside the plant cell and in the plant cell wall; it includes cellulose, *hemicelluloses, lignin,* and *pectin* (44, 47).

At present there is no RDA for carbohydrate because the nutrient can be produced in the body. It is desirable, however, to include 50 to 100 g of carbohydrate in the diet daily ". . . to avoid *ketosis,* excessive breakdown of body protein, loss of *cations* especially sodium and involuntary dehydration" (40).

Functions of Carbohydrate

The main function of carbohydrate is to supply energy for the body. Some of this is used as glucose to meet immediate energy needs, some is stored as glycogen in the liver and muscles, and the rest is converted to fat and stored as adipose tissue. The central nervous system is entirely dependent on glucose for energy. Little glycogen is stored in the nerve tissue, and even that appears not be be utilizable; in other tissues, however, there is some glycogen that can be utilized when the blood sugar is low.

Another important function of dietary carbohydrate is its protein-sparing action. At the expense of tissue building and maintenance, relatively more protein is used for energy when the carbohydrate and fat content of the diet is below the desirable caloric level than when it is suf-

Dietary Fiber

Cellulose, a component of dietary fiber, has long been known to aid intestinal elimination by providing bulk to the diet. The present theories by British scientists that low intakes of dietary fiber are related to certain noninfectious diseases and disorders have their origins in *epidemiological* studies among people of Africa. It was found that tribes ingesting primitive diets high in fiber were less likely to develop certain diseases of the colon and metabolic disorders than were their kinsmen who lived in urban areas and consumed low-fiber diets similar to those in western countries. The Africans ingesting the western-type diets had hard and formed feces that only weighed about 100 g per day whereas the stools of those ingesting the native diet were soft, formless, and weighed about 400 g per day (6, 7).

Diverticulosis

The hypothesis that there is a high correlation between low-fiber diets and human gastrointestinal diseases (12, 36, 41) has been accepted by hospitals and clinics as the basis for change in the dietary management of diverticular disease of the colon (diverticulosis). This disease is described as the presence of a sac or pouch formed by protusion of the mucous membrane through a defect in the muscular lining of the intestine. Diverticulosis is regarded as ". . . an acquired disease *endemic* in western civilization on low fiber diet . . ." (35). It is now treated with a high-fiber diet rather than a low-fiber prescription once used for conditions of colonic irritation. The high-fiber diet appears to relieve the pain and bowel irregularities of the disorder and allows the person with diverticulosis to have a normal food intake (19, 38, 42). After the diverticulosis is corrected, it is suggested that the high-fiber intake should become a routine dietary pattern. The role of dietary fiber in the relief of this disorder is not known.

Role of Dietary Fiber

It is generally agreed that dietary fiber increases the bulk of the feces; other roles given to it are only speculative at this time (8, 31). One theory is that dietary fiber causes the fecal matter to pass quickly through the intestinal tract, thus shortening the time for bacterial action; another is that dietary fiber combines with *bile acids* and other substances and prevents their absorption into the body.

Dietary Fiber in the American Diet

The shift to a more refined diet in western countries and the fact that many of the cereal foods and starchy foods are now eaten in their refined form (for example, white flour and white rice) is evident in data from the U. S. Department of Agriculture. Early in the century more than two-thirds (68 percent) of the food energy came from fiber-containing starchy foods as compared to 47 percent in 1976 (Fig 4.6). This 1976 value is lower than data cited from other parts of the western world that is, about 60 percent in the United Kingdom (32) and 55 to 60 percent for high-income countries from a FAO/WHO survey (14).

Data on the fiber content of the American diet are difficult to obtain, but estimates show that the crude fiber intake was about one-third less in 1974 (4 g per capita per day) than in 1909–1913 (6 g per capita per day). This decline is attributed

Food Energy and Energy-Yielding Nutrients Available Per Capita, Per Day

	1909–1913	1965	1970	1975	1976[1]
Food energy (calories)	3480	3140	3300	3210	3290
Protein	102	96	100	99	102
Fat	125	144	156	152	157
Carbohydrate (grams)	492	372	379	370	376

[1]Preliminary

Fig. 4.6 Carbohydrate and food energy available per capita per day and the percentage supplied by starches and sugars.

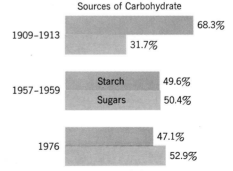

Sources of Carbohydrate

1909–1913 — 68.3% / 31.7%

1957–1959 — Starch 49.6% / Sugars 50.4%

1976 — 47.1% / 52.9%

Per Capita Per Day. 1976 preliminary

(From 1977 Handbook of Agricultural Charts, Agr. Handbook No. 524 Washington, D.C.: U.S. Dept. Agr., 1977, p. 53.)

Table 4.2. Crude Fiber Content of 100 g Portions of Some Foods

Almonds	2.6	Cheese, cottage	0	Mashed	.4
Apples[a], raw	1.0	Chicken[b]	0	Prunes[b]	.8
dried	3.1	Collards[b]	1.0	Raisins	.9
Applesauce	.6	Corn[b]	.7	Rice[b]	
Apricots, raw	.6	Corn flakes	.7	Brown	.3
dried	3.0	Cornmeal		White	.1
Beans[b]		Whole ground	1.6	Spinach[b]	.6
Green	1.0	Degermed	.6	Squash[b]	
Lima	1.8	Egg	0	Summer	.6
Beef[b], ground	0	Grapefruit	.2	Winter	1.4
Beets[b]	0.8	Grapes	.6	Strawberries	1.3
Bran	7.8	Lettuce	.7	Sugar	0
Bread		Milk	0	Tomatoes	.5
Rye	.4	Orange	.5	Tuna fish	0
White	.2	Peanut butter	1.9	Turnip greens[b]	.7
Whole wheat	1.6	Peanuts	2.4	Wheat bran	9.1
Butter	0	Pears[a]	1.4	Wheat germ	2.5
Cabbage	.8	Peas[b]	2.0	Wheat flour	
Carrots	.6	Pecans	2.3	White	.3
Celery	.6	Potatoes[b]		Whole-grain	2.3
		Baked	.6		

[a] Including skin.
[b] Cooked.
From *Composition of Foods: Raw, Processed, Prepared.* Agr. Handbook No. 8 (Washington, D. C.: U.S. Dept. Agr., 1963).

to the decreased use of grain products and potatoes (16).

There are some data on the intake of fiber by individuals in the United States. *Nonvegan* subjects in California ingested between 8.4 and 12.2 g of fiber per day (21) whereas the diets of subjects in Connecticut contained smaller amounts (mean = 3.5 g; range = 1.6–11.0 g) (11). The 3.5 g mean value of the Connecticut group is below the adult fiber intake level of 5 to 6 g per day suggested by Cowgill (9).

Food Sources of Dietary Fiber

Dried fruits, whole-grain cereals, nuts, and fruits and vegetables are the best sources of dietary fiber (Table 4.2). It is evident that whole-grain cereals have considerably more fiber than do refined ones; wheat bran is the richest fiber food; *legumes* (peas and beans) and nuts are fiber rich; and dairy products, meat, fish, poultry, eggs, fats and oils, and sugars and syrups are devoid of fiber.

New findings indicate that two components of dietary fiber, the hemicelluloses and lignin, are lost or destroyed in the crude fiber analysis (49). Therefore the crude fiber values in Table 4.2 are lower than the actual dietary fiber values.

As a means of adding extra fiber to the diet, "high-fiber breads" have been developed and marketed under various brand names, for example, "Fresh Horizons," "Vim," and "Contour." They contain about 7 percent fiber in the form of powdered cellulose, about four to five times as much as whole wheat bread, and are lower in

Table 4.3. Carbohydrate Content of Various Foods as Served

	Per 100 g of food	Per average serving	
	---	---	---
	Carbohydrate, g	Size of serving, g	Carbohydrate, g
Sugar (white)	100	12	1 tbsp	12
Honey	81	21	1 tbsp	17
Crackers (saltines)	73	11	4 crackers	8
Jellies	72	18	1 tbsp	13
Angel food cake	60	53	$^1/_{12}$ of cake	32
Chocolate (milk, plain)	57	28	1 oz	16
Bread (white, enriched)	50	28	1 sl	14
Pie (cherry)	39	135	$^1/_7$ of pie	52
Ice cream	24	67	$^1/_2$ c	16
Rice (white, cooked)	24	103	$^1/_2$ c	25
Potato (white, baked)	21	156	1 med	33
Orange juice (frozen, diluted)	11	124	$^1/_2$ c	13
Carbonated beverage (cola-type)	10	369	12 oz	37
Oatmeal (cooked)	10	240	1 c	23
Green beans (frozen, cooked)	6	68	$^1/_2$ c	4
Liver (beef, fried)	6	85	3 oz	5
Milk (white, whole)	5	244	1 c	11
Egg	2	50	1 lg	1
Butter	tr	14	1 tbsp	tr
Ground beef (broiled)	0	82	2.9 oz patty	0

From *Nutritive Value of Foods* (1977). Home and Garden Bull., No. 72, revised. Washington, D.C.: U.S. Dept. Agr.

kilocalories than regular bread. The use of cellulose as a replacement for part of the white flour in cakes and biscuits has also been recommended (5).

Food Sources of Carbohydrate

Sugars and syrups, cereal grains, legumes, and dried fruits are the richest food sources of carbohydrate (Table 4.3). Processed foods that contain appreciable quantities of carbohydrate include pasta products (noodles, spaghetti, etc.), nonfat dry milk solids, crackers, pretzels, jams, jellies, pastries, breads, breakfast cereals, and candies. Although most fresh fruits and vegetables are generally low in carbohydrate, bananas, dates, and white and sweet potatoes are quite high. Eggs, fish, poultry, cheese, fresh milk, and meats (with the exception of liver) contain little carbohydrate, and animal and vegetable fats contain none. The carbohydrate content of a variety of foods is presented in Table 4.3.

Carbohydrate In College Meals

For seven consecutive days in 1969, four breakfasts and four noon and evening meals (84 in all) were collected at 50 colleges located in 31 states for nutrient analyses by the U. S. Department of Agriculture. They were coeducational except for two men's colleges and five women's colleges.

The carbohydrate content of the meals averaged

288 g per person per day (range, 205 to 342 g). Carbohydrate was present in the largest amounts of any nutrient studied (50).

Carbohydrate in the United States' Food Supply

Since 1910 there has been a steady decline in the quantity of carbohydrate food in the American food supply (Fig. 4.6). The amount of carbohydrate available per capita per day averaged about 492 g for the period 1909–1913 but was 376 g in 1976 (1, 16). About 57 percent of the total energy intake came from carbohydrates at this earlier period, but it dropped to 46 percent in 1976.

During this century there has also been a shift in the proportion of dietary carbohydrate that comes from starches and sugars. The percentage of the total carbohydrate derived from high-starch foods (flour, cereals, potatoes) has been progressively decreasing since 1909–1913, whereas the percentage from sugars has been increasing (Fig. 4.6). In the period 1957–1959 the amount of carbohydrate available for consumption per capita from both sources was about equal, but since then sugars have accounted for more than starches. An estimate of the 1974 total sugar consumption from refined cane, beet, or corn sugar and occurring naturally in foods was 126 g sucrose, 25 g lactose, 16 g glucose, 7 g maltose, 6 g fructose, and 8 g from other sugars per capita per day (16).

Carbohydrate and Dental Caries

The precise role of carbohydrates in the development of dental caries is that of interaction with microorganisms on the tooth surface, causing an increase in dental plaque (a soft, tenacious bacterial deposit on the surface of a tooth). The plaque is composed of microorganisms embedded in a matrix of protein, carbohydrate, and a small amount of lipid; the water content is about 80 percent (3). The microorganisms in the plaque have the capacity of producing polysaccharides from other sugars, forming a hard surface on the tooth (4).

The mere physical presence of plaque will not of itself cause dental caries. However, the microorganisms in the plaque form acid from a number of sugars. After the ingestion of sugar (sweets), the pH values in the region of the teeth may go as low as 4.5. (Enamel begins to dissolve at around pH 5.5.) The pH usually remains low for about 20 minutes and then slowly approaches neutrality. Repeated consumption of sugar causes repeated production of acid and the maintenance of a low pH in the mouth.

Frequency of Eating

In one phase of a long-term study of the relationship between sugar consumption and the incidence of dental caries (carried out among patients in a mental institution in Vipeholm, Sweden), a 300 g supplement of sucrose was given daily to two experimental groups; one group took the supplement with meals (in solution or added to bread), the other took it between meals (in the form of toffee, chocolate, or caramels). The incidence of dental caries was much higher among those taking the sugar between meals than among those taking it with their meals (20). That between-meal consumption of candy produces more dental caries than the same amount of sugar taken with meals was confirmed by King and his co-workers (26) in England.

Brushing the teeth thoroughly within ten minutes after eating (or at least rinsing out the mouth) helped to reduce the incidence of dental caries in a study of college students. The 429 students either brushed their teeth or rinsed out their mouths after eating, and 276 controls did not. At the end of two years the control group had developed an average of 3.87 new carious surfaces (as determined by clinical and radiographic examinations), whereas the experimental group had developed only 2.02 carious surfaces (15).

57

Form of Carbohydrate

In addition to time of eating sugar (whether with meals or between meals), the form of the sugar also makes a difference in its harmfulness to teeth. Sucrose in solution was found to be less harmful than when taken in granular form. King and his co-workers (26) found the type of candy that produced the greatest incidence of caries was toffee, which is sticky.

Kinds of Carbohydrate

Whether sucrose is uniquely cariogenic or if it is incriminated because it is the predominant sugar in human diets remains to be evaluated. There is no firm evidence demonstrating that other sugars (glucose, fructose, or corn syrup) are any less cariogenic than sucrose (3, 43).

Starches or dextrins as the sole source of carbohydrate in purified diets usually cause a lower incidence of dental caries in experimental animals than do the same quantities of sugars (43). One of the few studies done with humans was with Guatemalan children; one group was given a diet that included candy, cake, and other sweets, the other group consumed a high starch diet. Those who consumed the sweets had more caries and more bacteria in their dental plaque than did the children on the high starch diet (29).

Alcohol consumption

Man has used carbohydrates for centuries to make alcoholic beverages. Because ethyl alcohol (ethanol) yields energy when it is metabolized in the body, the intake of alcoholic beverages must be accounted for in calculating an individual's food intake (14). Alcohol requires no prior digestion in the body, and about one-third of the intake is absorbed directly from the stomach, the remainder from the small intestine. Most of the alcohol ingested is metabolized in the liver by the usual routes of carbohydrate metabolism and yields about 7 kcal (29 kJ) per g, or 5.6 kcal (23 kJ) per ml. Like some of the sugars and fats, alcohol is made up of "empty kilocalories," that is, rich in energy but poor in other nutrients.

According to the literature, the energy derived from alcohol metabolism may substitute in the body for carbohydrate, fat, and protein. However, in studies on the effect of wine and ethanol in human nutrition, the findings suggest that the kilocalories from alcohol may not be as efficiently used as those from carbohydrate and fat and that alcohol may adversely affect protein catabolism (30).

The intake of alcohol varies in a national diet. Some people consume none, whereas others have been reported to ingest as much as 1800 kcal (7531 kJ) per day in this form regularly (about 60 percent of the daily energy need) (30). The ingestion of moderate amounts of alcoholic beverages in addition to the recommended energy of the food intake may lead to obesity. Unlike traditional energy foods, alcohol depresses parts of the nervous system, and regular intake of excessive amounts of it leads to a deterioration of health (22).

Summary

Carbohydrates, the main source of food energy for animals and man, are manufactured in the green plant by the process of photosynthesis. The important classes of carbohydrates are the monosaccharides (glucose, fructose, and galactose), disaccharides (maltose, sucrose, and lactose), and polysaccharides (starch, glycogen, and cellulose).

Carbohydrate digestion begins in the mouth and continues in the small intestine to change food starch and the disaccharides to their respective monosaccharides.

The simple sugars then pass through the intestinal wall by either active transport (glucose and galactose) or by diffusion (fructose).

Carbohydrate may be used as an immediate

source of energy, converted to glycogen and stored in the body, or converted to fat and stored as adipose tissue. Most of the glucose formed from either carbohydrate or noncarbohydrate sources is oxidized to CO_2, H_2O, and energy-rich ATP; some may be converted to lactic acid during strenuous exercise; and some must be used to form NADP and the sugar ribose. The hormones insulin, epinephrine, and glucagon aid in carbohydrate metabolism. Glucose is the carbohydrate found in the blood.

The nutrient functions in several ways: to supply energy for the body, to spare protein for tissue building and maintenance, and to provide dietary fiber. There is no RDA for carbohydrate, but it is desirable to include 50 to 100 g of the nutrient in the daily diet.

The richest food sources of carbohydrate are found in sugar and syrups, cereal grains, legumes, and dried fruits.

The amount of carbohydrate foods ingested by Americans has decreased throughout this century, and the proportion of the nutrient derived from starches and sugars has shifted with a greater intake of sugars than starches at this time.

Carbohydrates interacting with microorganisms on the tooth surface cause an increase in dental plaque. The microorganisms in the plaque form acids from sugars (and from starch, too, but to a lesser extent), which lowers the pH on the tooth surface, causing dissolution of the enamel and initiation of caries when the pH is sufficiently low. Between-meal eating of candy and sweets is conducive to caries formation.

The intake of alcohol provides kilocalories and must be included in the daily energy count.

Among today's most controversial nutritional topics are the hypotheses that dietary fiber serves as a protective agent against certain noninfectious diseases and disorders, for example, diseases of the colon (cancer, diverticulosis) and metabolic diseases (*ischemic heart disease,* diabetes mellitus, obesity) (31).

Critics point out that there are many unanswered questions related to the possible role that dietary fiber may have in the health and well-being of humans. Some of these are: Exactly what is dietary fiber? How is dietary fiber measured? Do deficiencies or excesses of dietary fiber exist throughout the world? Is there evidence that metabolic or colonic diseases are related to dietary fiber? (41).

There have been several studies reporting the effect or lack of effect of dietary fiber.

1. A high-carbohydrate diet with 15 g of dietary fiber was effective in controlling blood glucose levels in mildly diabetic subjects who required either oral hypoglycemic agents or less than 30 units of insulin per day (25).

2. When the daily food intakes of normal subjects and subjects with either diverticulosis or cancer of the colon were compared, there were no significant differences in fiber intakes among the subjects (11).

3. Cooked bran has less effect on stool size and *transit* time in the human intestine than does uncooked bran (51).

4. Wheat bran did not substantially reduce either *serum cholesterol* or *triglyceride* levels in human subjects (24, 48), but the supplementation of the diet with 140 g of rolled oats (10) or 100 g of brown beans (23) resulted in a decrease in serum cholesterol levels.

At this time (1978) there has been much speculation about the role of dietary fiber in health and disease but very little research to prove or disprove the theories. Nevertheless, hospitals and clinics are now using high-fiber diets for the treatment of diverticulosis and other disorders of the colon, and some individuals, upon their own initiative, have increased their daily intake of dietary fiber.

Glossary

bile acids: glycocholic and taurocholic acid, formed in the liver and secreted in the bile.

carbohydrases: a group of enzymes that digest disaccharides.

59

cassava: a tropical plant of the spurge family with edible starchy roots.

cation: an ion having a positive charge; sodium, potassium, iron, calcium.

diabetes mellitus: a disorder of carbohydrate metabolism in which the ability to oxidize and use carbohydrate is lost as a result of disturbances in the normal insulin mechanism; an elevated blood sugar and sugar in the urine are among the symptoms.

diarrhea: rapid movement of fecal matter through the intestine producing a frequent, watery stool.

endemic: a disease of low morbidity that is constantly present in a human community.

epidemiology: the scientific study of factors that influence the frequency and distribution of infectious diseases in man.

flatulence: excessive formation of gas in the stomach or intestines.

glycogenic: pertaining to glycogen or sugars.

hemicellulose: a polysaccharide that is more soluble than cellulose.

intolerance: a sensitivity or allergy to certain foods.

ischemic heart disease: deficiency of blood supply to the heart muscle due to obstruction or constriction of the coronary arteries.

ketosis: the accumulation of large amounts of ketone bodies (substances synthesized by the liver as a step in the combustion of fats) in the body tissues and fluids.

legume: the pod or fruit of peas and beans.

leguminous: adjective form of legume.

lignin: a substance, along with cellulose, that makes up the woody structure of plants; it is not a carbohydrate.

millet: the white seeds of the grass *Panicum miliaceum* used in parts of the world as food.

nonvegan: a person who includes all proteins of animal origin in the diet, a nonvegetarian.

pectin: a class of soluble carbohydrates resistant to animal enzymes; apples are rich in pectin.

photosynthesis: the complex chemical reaction of CO_2, H_2O, and sunlight in the chlorophyll tissues of plants to form carbohydrates.

ruminant: an animal that has a stomach with four complete cavities and that characteristically regurgitates undigested food from the rumen, the first stomach, and masticates it when at rest.

serum cholesterol: the level of the sterol cholesterol in the blood.

serum triglyceride: the level of fat in the blood.

sorghum: syrup from the juice of the grass plant *Sorghum vulgare*; it resembles cane syrup and contains considerable fructose and some starch and dextrin.

transit: the act of passing through.

Study Questions and Activities

1. Identify the following: lactose, chlorophyll, polysaccharide, glycogen, levulose, photosynthesis, and blood sugar.

2. Compare the prices of the following foods at a local grocery store: honey, white sugar, brown sugar, white potatoes, white rice, white flour, and whole wheat flour. What is the cost per pound of each? As food sources of carbohydrate, which ones are the most expensive and which are the cheapest?

3. What monosaccharides, disaccharides, and polysaccharides are important in nutrition? List a good food source for each.

4. Describe three functions of carbohydrate in the body.

5. Describe briefly the kind and proportion of carbohydrates consumed in the United States.

6. How does the caloric value of alcohol compare with that of a carbohydrate such as white sugar?

7. Define dental plaque. What is its relationship to dental caries?

8. Trace the digestion, absorption, and metabolism (via the glycolytic pathway) of food starch.

9. How does the body's use of muscle glycogen differ from that of liver glycogen?

10. In order to minimize the incidence of dental caries, what are some practical suggestions in regard to eating foods that contain sugar?

11. Write a brief paragraph on dietary fiber. Tell what it is, how high-fiber diets are now used in hospitals and clinics, and the foods that are rich in fiber.

60

References

1. *Agricultural Statistics* (1977). Washington, D.C.: U.S. Dept. Agr., p. 561.

2. American Academy of Pediatrics, Committee on Nutrition (1974). Should milk drinking by children be discouraged? *Pediatrics*, **53**: 576.

3. Bowen, W. H. (1977). Role of carbohydrates in dental caries. In *Carbohydrates and Health*, edited by L. F. Hood, E. K. Wardrip, and G. N. Bollenback. Westport, Conn.: Avi Publ. Co., Inc., p. 109.

4. Brown, A. T. (1975). The role of dietary carbohydrates in plaque formation and oral disease. *Nutrition Rev.*, **33**: 353.

5. Brys, K. D., and M. E. Zabik (1976). Microcrystalline cellulose replacement in cakes and biscuits. *J. Am. Dietet. Assoc.*, **69**: 50.

6. Burkitt, D., and N. Painter (1975). Gastrointestinal transit times; stool weights and consistency; intraluminal pressures. In *Refined Carbohydrate Foods and Disease: Some Implication of Dietary Fibre*, edited by D. P. Burkitt and H. Trowell. New York: Academic Press, pp. 69–84.

7. Burkitt, D. P., A. R. P. Walker, and N. S. Painter (1974). Dietary fiber and disease. *J. Am. Med. Assoc.*, **229**: 1068.

8. Connell, A. M. (1976). Natural fiber and bowel dysfunction. *Am. J. Clin. Nutrition*, **29**: 1427.

9. Cowgill, G. R., and W. E. Andersen (1932). Laxative effects of wheat bran and "washed" bran in healthy man: a comparative study. *J. Am. Med. Assoc.*, **98**: 1966.

10. DeGroot, A. P., R. Luyken, and N. A. Pikaar (1963). Cholesterol-lowering effect of rolled oats. *Lancet*, **2**: 303.

11. Dorfman, S. H., M. Ali, and M. H. Floch (1976). Low fiber content of Connecticut diets. *Am. J. Clin. Nutrition*, **29**: 87.

12. Eastwood, M. A. et al. (1970). Perspectives on the bran theory. *Lancet*, **1**: 1029.

13. Ellestad-Sayed, J. J., and J. C. Haworth (1977). Disaccharide consumption and malabsorption in Canadian Indians. *Am. J. Clin. Nutrition*, **30**: 698.

14. *Energy and Protein Requirements* (1973). FAO Nutrition Meetings Rept. Series 52 and WHO Tech. Rept. Series 522. Rome: Food and Agr. Organ.

15. Fosdick, L. S. (1950). The reduction of the incidence of dental caries. I. Immediate toothbrushing with a neutral dentifrice. *J. Am. Dental Assoc.*, **40**: 133.

16. Friend, B., and R. Marston (1974). Nutritional review. *National Food Situation*. Nov. Washington, D.C.: U.S. Dept. Agr., p. 20.

17. Gallagher, C. R., A. L. Molleson, and J. H. Caldwell (1974). Lactose intolerance and fermented dairy products. *J. Am. Dietet. Assoc.*, **65**: 418.

18. Garza, C., and N. S. Scrimshaw (1976). Relationship of lactose intolerance to milk intolerance in young children. *Am. J. Clin. Nutrition*, **29**: 192.

19. Goldstein, F. (1972). Diet and colonic disease. *J. Am. Dietet. Assoc.*, **60**: 499.

20. Gustaffson, B. E. et al. (1954). The Vipeholm dental caries study. The effect of different levels of carbohydrate intake on caries activity in 436 individuals observed for five years. *Acta Odontol. Scand.*, **11**: 232.

21. Hardinge, M. G., A. C. Chambers, H. Crooks, and F. J. Stare (1958). Nutritional studies of vegetarians. III. Dietary level of fiber. *Am. J. Clin. Nutrition*, **6**: 523.

22. Hartroft, W. S. (1967). Alcohol metabolism and liver disease. *Federation Proc.*, **26**: 1432.

23. Hellendoorn, E. W. (1976). Beneficial physiologic action of beans. *J. Am. Dietet. Assoc.*, **69**: 248.

24. Jenkins, D. J. A., M. S. Hill, and J. H. Cummings (1975). Effect of wheat bran on blood lipids, fecal steroid excretion, and serum iron. *Am. J. Clin. Nutrition*, **28**: 1408.

25. Kiehm, T. G., J. W. Anderson, and K. Ward (1976). Beneficial effects of a high-carbohydrate, high-fiber diet on hyperglycemic diabetic men. *Am. J. Clin. Nutrition*, **29**: 895.

26. King, J. D., M. Mellanby, H. H. Stones, and H. N. Green (1955). *Effect of Sugar Supplements on Dental Caries in Children*. Medical Research Council Special Rept. Series 288. London: H. M. Stationery Office.

27. Kobayashi, A., S. Kawai, Y. Ohbe, and Y. Nagashima (1975). Effect of dietary lactose and a lactase preparation on the intestinal absorption of calcium and magnesium in normal infants. *Am. J. Clin. Nutrition*, **29:** 681.

28. Lisker, R., G. Lopez-Habib, M. Daltabuit, I. Rostenberg, and P. Arroyo (1974). Lactase deficiency in a rural area of Mexico. *Am. J. Clin. Nutrition*, **27:** 756.

29. Loesche, W. J., and C. A. Henry (1967). Intracellular microbial polysaccharide production and dental caries in a Guatemalan Indian village. *Arch. Oral Biol.*, **12:** 189.

30. McDonald, J. T., and S. Margen (1976). Wine versus ethanol in human nutrition. I. Nitrogen and calorie balance. *Am. J. Clin. Nutrition*, **29:** 1093.

31. Mendeloff, A. I. (1976). Dietary fiber. In *Nutrition Reviews' Present Knowledge of Nutrition*. 4th ed. New York: The Nutrition Foundation, Inc., pp. 392–401.

32. Ministry of Agriculture, Fisheries, and Food (1976). *Manual of Nutrition*. London: H. M. Stationery Office.

33. Paige, D. M., T. M. Bayless, and W. S. Dellinger, Jr. (1975). Relationship of milk consumption to blood rise in lactose intolerant individuals. *Am. J. Clin. Nutrition*, **28:** 677.

34. Paige, D. M., T. M. Bayless, G. D. Ferry, and G. G. Graham (1971). Lactose malabsorption and milk rejection in Negro children. *The Johns Hopkins Med. J.*, **129:** 163.

35. Painter, N. S., and D. P. Burkitt (1971). Diverticular disease of the colon. A disease of this century. *British Med. J.*, **2:** 450.

36. Painter, N. S., A. Z. Almeida, and K. W. Colebourne (1972). Unprocessed bran in treatment of diverticular disease of colon. *British Med. J.*, **2:** 137.

37. Payne-Bose, D., J. D. Welsh, H. L. Gearhart, and R. D. Morrison (1977). Milk and lactose-hydrolyzed milk. *Am. J. Clin. Nutrition*, **30:** 695.

38. Plumley, P. F., and B. Francis (1973). Dietary management of diverticular disease. *J. Am. Dietet. Assoc.*, **63:** 527.

39. Protein Advisory Group of the United Nations System (1972). *Report on the PAG Ad Hoc Working Group Meeting on Milk Intolerance—Nutritional Implications*. New York: United Nations.

40. *Recommended Dietary Allowances, Eighth Edition* (1974). Washington, D.C.: Natl. Research Council.

41. Reilly, R. W., and J. B. Kirsner (1975). Fiber deficiency and colonic disorders. *Am. J. Clin. Nutrition*, **28:** 293.

42. Robinson, C. R. (1976). Thirteenth Annual Lenna Frances Cooper Memorial Lecture: Nutrition education—what comes next? *J. Am. Dietet. Assoc.*, **69:** 126.

43. Shaw, J. H., and E. A. Sweeney (1973). Nutrition in relation to dental medicine. In *Modern Nutrition in Health and Disease*, edited by R. S. Goodhart and M. E. Shils. 5th ed. Philadelphia: Lea and Febiger, p. 733.

44. Southgate, D. A. T. (1977). The definition and analysis of dietary fibre. *Nutrition Rev.*, **35:** 31.

45. Sowers, M. F., and E. Winterfeldt (1975). Lactose intolerance among Mexican-Americans. *Am. J. Clin. Nutrition*, **28:** 704.

46. Stoopler, M., W. Frayer, and M. H. Alderman (1974). Prevalence and persistence of lactose malabsorption among young Jamaican children. *Am. J. Clin. Nutrition*, **27:** 728.

47. Trowell, H. (1977). Food and dietary fibre. *Nutrition Rev.*, **35:** 6.

48. Truswell, A. S., and R. M. Kay (1976). Bran and blood lipids. *Lancet*, **1:** 367.

49. Van Soest, P. J., and J. B. Robertson (1977). What is fibre and fibre in food? *Nutrition Rev.*, **35:** 12.

50. Walker, M. A., and L. Page (1975). Nutritive content of college meals. Proximate composition and vitamins. *J. Am. Dietet. Assoc.*, **68:** 34.

51. Wyman, J. B., K. W. Heaton, A. P. Manning, and A. C. B. Wicks (1976). The effect on intestinal transit and the feces of raw and cooked bran at different doses. *Am. J. Clin. Nutrition*, **29:** 1474.

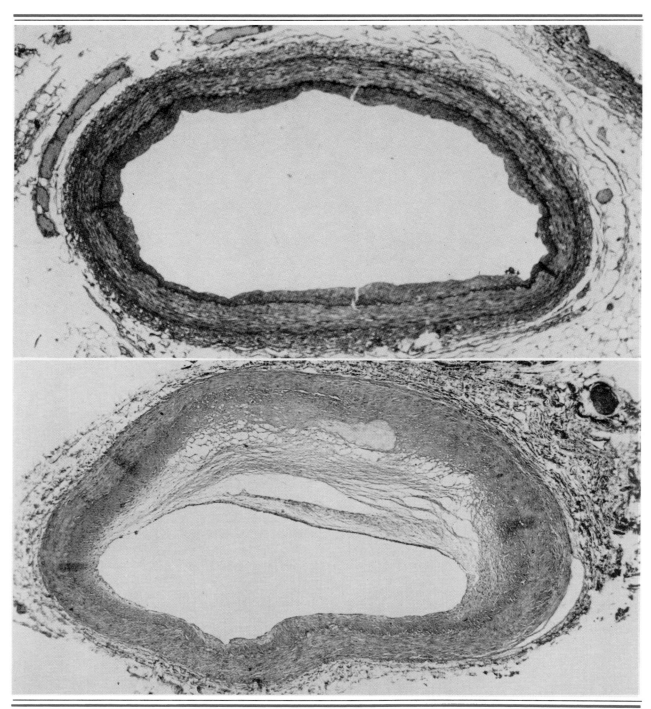

Above, a normal artery. Below, an artery with atherosclerotic deposits (plaques of cholesterol and other fatty substances).

Chapter 5

Fats and other Lipids

Abbreviations

acetyl CoA: acetyl coenzyme A
ATP: adenosine triphosphate
CHD: coronary heart disease
CHOL: cholesterol
CO_2: carbon dioxide
CoA: coenzyme A
EFA: essential fatty acid

HDL: high density lipoprotein
H_2O: water
LDL: low density lipoprotein
LRC: Lipid Research Clinic
RDA: Recommended Dietary Allowances
TRG: triglyceride
VLDL: very low density lipoproteins

Fats are the best-known members of a chemical group called the *lipids*. Like carbohydrates, lipids contain carbon, hydrogen, and oxygen, and some also have phosphorus and nitrogen. Lipids, found widespread in nature, are insoluble in water but will dissolve in ether, chloroform, benzene, or other fat solvents. *Fatty acids*, fats and oils, *phospholipids*, *sterols*, and *lipoproteins* are several groups of compounds among the lipids that are important in the study of nutrition.

Lipids are classified into three groups according to their chemical structure: *simple lipids* (fats and oils), *compound lipids* (phospholipids and lipoproteins), and *derived lipids* (fatty acids and sterols).

Fatty Acids

Fatty acids, which are composed entirely of carbon, hydrogen, and oxygen, are found in all the simple and compound lipids. Some of the common fatty acids are palmitic, *stearic*, oleic, and *linoleic* (Table 5.1). There are short-chain (10 or fewer carbon atoms), long-chain (12 to 18 carbon atoms), and extra-long-chain (20 or more carbon atoms) fatty acids. Fatty acids of 10 carbon atoms or less are seldom found in animal products except for milk fat. Long-chain fatty acids occur in animal fats and most vegetable oils; the extra-long-chain ones are found in fish oils (Table 5.1).

Table 5.1 Some of the Fatty Acids Found in Fats

Name	Number of carbon atoms	Length of carbon chain	Type	Occurrence in food
Acetic	2	short	saturated	vinegar
Butyric	4	short	saturated	butter
Caproic	6	short	saturated	butter
Caprylic	8	short	saturated	coconut
Myristic	14	long	saturated	nutmeg and mace
Palmitic	16	long	saturated	lard and palm oil
Stearic	18	long	saturated	beef tallow
Oleic	18	long	monounsaturated	olive oil
Linoleic	18	long	polyunsaturated	corn oil
Clupanadonic	22	extra long	polyunsaturated	fish oils

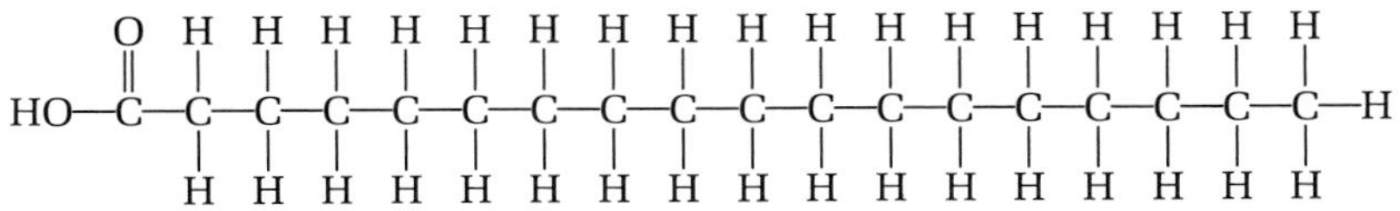

Stearic acid (saturated) $C_{18}H_{36}O_2$

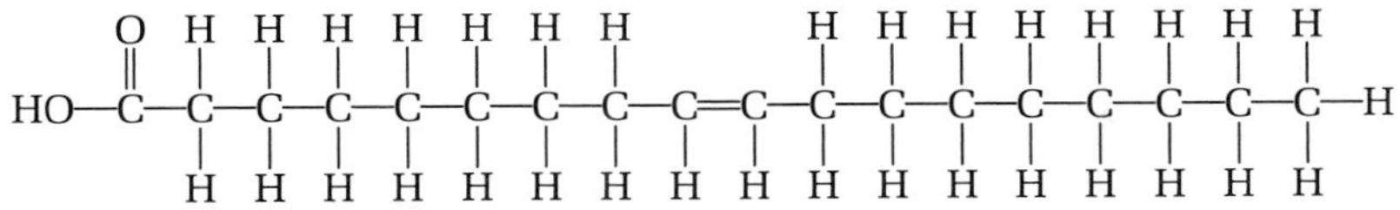

Oleic acid (monounsaturated) $C_{18}H_{34}O_2$

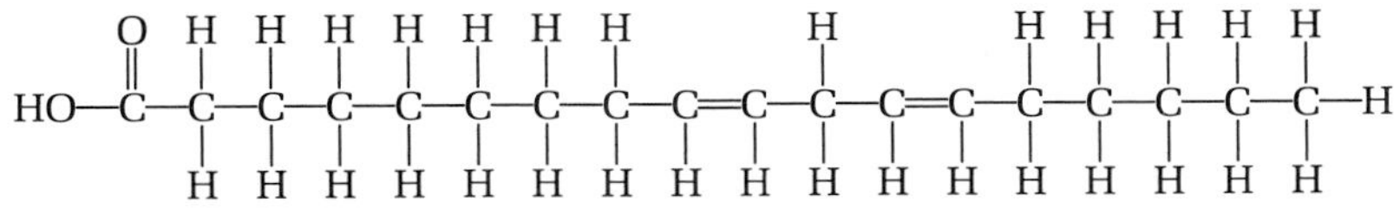

Linoleic acid (polyunsaturated) $C_{18}H_{32}O_2$

KEY:

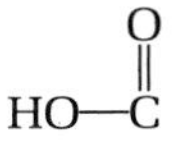 = acid group

(═) = "double bond" linkage

Fig. 5.1 The chemical structure of a saturated, monosaturated, and polyunsaturated fatty acid.

Fatty acids are also classified according to their degree of saturation or unsaturation (Table 5.1). Certain fatty acids, such as stearic acid, contain as many hydrogen atoms as the carbon chain can hold: they are called saturated fatty acids (Fig. 5.1). Others have only one "double-bond" linkage (two hydrogen atoms missing) in the carbon chain; they are referred to as monounsaturated fatty acids (Fig. 5.1). A third group, the *polyunsaturated* fatty acids, may have two, three, four, or more double-bond linkages in the carbon chain with four, six, eight, or more hydrogen atoms missing (Fig. 5.1).

Saturated fatty acids (largely animal fats) comprise about 35 percent of the total fat in the American diet (10). The most common saturated fatty acids are stearic acid and palmitic acid. The fat of butter and cows' milk contains about 60 percent saturated fatty acids; those of meat vary from about 46 percent for lamb to 28 percent for chicken and beef liver (Table 5.2).

Monounsaturated fatty acids constitute about 40 percent of the total fat in the diet of most Americans. An example of a long-chain monounsaturated fatty acid is oleic acid, which is found in appreciable amounts in many foods (Table 5.2). It comprises nearly one-third of the fat content of chicken and about 47 percent of the fat content of margarine (Table 5.2).

Polyunsaturated fatty acids are long-chain and extra-long-chain fatty acids. Most Americans consume far less of these acids than of either the saturated or monounsaturated ones. However, their intake is increasing. In 1947–1949, linoleic acid constituted 10.7 percent of the total fat consumed and in 1973, 15.4 percent (10). Although

Table 5.2 Percentage of Saturated, Monounsaturated (Oleic Acid), and Polyunsaturated (Linoleic Acid) Fatty Acids in Some Foods[a]

Food	Fat content, percent	Type of fatty acid		
		Saturated, percent	Monounsaturated (Oleic acid), percent	Polyunsaturated (Linoleic acid), percent
Beef, ground[b]	21	41	39	2
Butter	86	60	24	3
Cheese, American	25	62	23	2
Chicken leg[c]	11	28	33	23
Corn oil	100	13	25	57
Egg yolk	35	28	35	10
Fats, cooking[d]	100	24	44	24
Ice cream, regular	11	62	25	2
Lamb chops[b]	36	46	38	4
Lard	100	40	41	10
Liver, beef[c]	11	28	39	11
Lowfat milk[e]	2	58	24	2
Margarine	81	18	47	27
Nonfat (skim milk)[e]	1	40	10	tr
Milk, whole	3	64	26	3
Peanut butter	50	19	46	29
Pork chop[b]	32	36	42	9
Safflower oil	100	9	12	73
Veal cutlet[b]	11	44	38	4

[a] Values do not add up to 100 because not all the monounsaturated and polyunsaturated fatty acid values are included.
[b] Broiled.
[c] Fried.
[d] Vegetable fat.
[e] Milk solids added.
Calculated from *Nutritive Value of Foods*, Home and Garden Bull. No. 72, revised. Washington, D.C.: U.S. Dept. Agr., 1977.

safflower oil (about 73 percent) and corn oil (about 57 percent) are among the richest sources of linoleic acid, other good sources include nuts, fish, poultry, and other vegetable oils (Table 5.2).

Fats and Oils

Every fat molecule has essentially four parts. The core of the molecule is *glycerol,* a three-carbon compound that is related to the alcohols. Three fatty acids combine with the glycerol molecule to form a fat, as illustrated in Figure 5.2.

The nature of a fat depends on what kinds of fatty acids are linked to the glycerol core, the number of carbon atoms of the fatty acids, and the degree of saturation or unsaturation of the fatty acids. The three fatty acids in the fat tristearin (Fig. 5.2) are stearic acids, long-chain, and saturated.

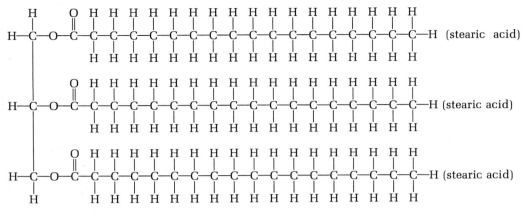

Glycerol

Fig. 5.2 The chemical formula of tristearin (a fat found in beef): $C_{57}H_{110}O_6$.

A fat molecule may be composed of three identical fatty acids, three different ones, or a combination of two alike and one different. When all the fatty acids in a fat are identical, the molecule is called a simple *triglyceride* (TRG); a fat with different fatty acids is called a mixed TRG. The fat tristearin (Fig. 5.2) is a simple TRG. The mixed TRGs are found both in animal and vegetable foods.

TRGs that are solid at room temperature are called fats and those that are liquid are called oils. Whether the TRGs are solid or liquid depends upon the kind of fatty acids in their structure (Table 5.1). Fats contain a higher proportion of saturated fatty acids than do oils, whereas oils contain more unsaturated fatty acids than do fats. Fats (butter, lard, and animal fats) are the predominant TRGs in animals; oils (corn and safflower) are the main TRGs in plants.

Antioxidants

Chemical substances known as antioxidants delay the oxidation of double-bond linkages in TRGs, thus prolonging the shelf life of a fat or oil by retarding the development of objectionable odors and flavors (rancidity). The chemical changes that take place with rancidity are oxidation at the double bonds and hydrolysis (partial breakdown of the fat, with the addition of water).

There are both natural and synthetic antioxidants. Vitamins C and E are natural antioxidants. Vitamin E, for example, is one of the body's antioxidants that prevents damage to living tissue from the harmful end products of fat oxidation. There are many types of synthetic antioxidants used in food processing; sodium benzoate, for example, is used in corn oil margarine to prevent rancidity and preserve flavor. Antioxidants apparently inhibit oxidation because they are more easily oxidized than the TRGs they protect.

Hydrogenation of Fats and Oils

The oils from plants can be hardened to form solid TRGs, and soft fats can be hardened to increase their melting point by a chemical process known as *hydrogenation*. In this commercial procedure, hydrogen is added to some (not all) of the double bonds of the unsaturated fatty acids to increase the firmness of the glyceride mixture; some of the polyunsaturated fatty acids are changed to monounsaturated ones. Liquid corn

69

oil, for example, is hydrogenated in the manufacture of solid corn oil margarine (Table 5.2).

Phospholipids, Sterols, and Lipoproteins

Phospholipids are found in every living cell and are formed primarily in the liver from the alcohol glycerol, fatty acids, phosphoric acid, and a nitrogenous base. (Choline, a compound related to the B-complex vitamins, is one of the nitrogenous bases found in these complex lipids.)

The sterols have a common basic structure but their physiologic functions are widely diversified. Three with functions associated with nutrition are ergosterol (a plant sterol), 7-dehydrocholesterol (an animal sterol), and *cholesterol* (an animal sterol). Ergosterol and 7-dehydrocholesterol are two preforms of vitamin D. Cholesterol (CHOL), the best known of the sterols, has attracted attention in scientific circles throughout the world because of the association of elevated blood CHOL levels with *atherosclerosis* and *coronary heart disease.*

The lipoproteins, synthesized in the liver, are composed of about one-fourth to one-third protein and the remainder lipids (13). The four groups that have been identified are *chylomicrons, very low density lipoproteins* (VLDL), *low density lipoproteins* (LDL), and *high density lipoproteins* (HDL). Like CHOL, there is much interest now in certain lipoproteins because their concentration in the blood plasma may or may not be a "risk factor" in coronary heart disease (9).

Digestion, Absorption, and Metabolism of Fats and Cholesterol

Fat Digestion

The digestion of fats begins in the small intestine. Two secretions important in splitting fat molecules are bile (a secretion of the liver) and the

enzyme pancreatic lipase (Table 2.1). Bile neutralizes the acidity of the food mass (called chyme) as it passes into the small intestine. Then a fraction of the bile fluid—bile salts—helps emulsify the fat globules. Emulsification breaks up fat into small globules which are hydrolyzed by pancreatic lipase partially to glycerol and fatty acids and partially to mono- and *diglycerides* (Table 2.1).

Absorption of End Products of Fat Digestion

The end products of fat digestion appear to be absorbed in two forms: 20 to 45 percent as fatty acids and glycerol and the remainder as mono- and diglycerides. Bile salts play an important role in fat absorption by dispersing the fatty acids and glycerides into tiny units called micelles for passage through the intestinal membrane. In the mucosal cells of the small intestine, the digestion of the mono- and diglycerides may be completed by the action of the enzyme intestinal lipase (13). The fatty acids and glycerol are resynthesized and again form TRGs in the intestinal cells. (This breakdown and reformation of fats are necessary for their passage through the cell membranes.) The TRGs are carried by lipoproteins to the adipose tissue (fat cells) by way of the *lymph* and the venous blood. The lipoprotein-encased lipids are called chylomicrons (7). (Any free glycerol, short-chain fatty acids, or synthetic *medium-chain TRGs* are absorbed directly into the capillaries.)

Fat Metabolism

The oxidation of glycerol and fatty acids in the body cells to release energy occurs in two ways. The glycerol portion is metabolized like a carbohydrate to form pyruvic acid (Fig. 5.3). The fatty acids require the compound coenzyme A (CoA) to split off two-carbon units from the fatty acid forming acetyl CoA. This reaction, called beta oxidation, is repeated until the chains of fatty

70

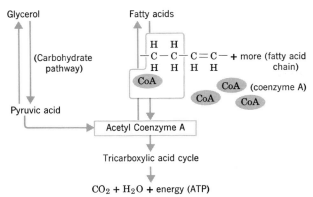

Fig. 5.3 A simple sketch depicting several steps in fat metabolism.

acids are broken down to acetyl CoA (Fig. 5.3). Pyruvic acid and acetyl CoA enter the tricarboxylic acid cycle where they are oxidized to CO_2, H_2O, and energy (ATP).

When fat is oxidized in the body to release energy, more oxygen is required than when an equal amount of carbohydrate is oxidized. The ratio of carbon and hydrogen to oxygen in the fat molecule is greater than that in a carbohydrate molecule. In tristearin, for example, there are 57 atoms of carbon and 110 atoms of hydrogen to only six atoms of oxygen. In glucose, which also has six atoms of oxygen, there are only 12 atoms of hydrogen and six of carbon. The average energy value of 1 gram of fat is 9 kcal (38 kJ) and of 1 gram of carbohydrate, 4 kcal (17 kJ).

Absorption and Metabolism of Cholesterol

CHOL from food, called exogenous CHOL, is slowly absorbed from the intestinal tract and enters the body via the *lymphatic system*. Much of the sterol combines with fatty acids and circulates in the plasma as CHOL esters (11). There is a maximum amount of CHOL that can be absorbed by the intestines; the excess is excreted in the feces.

The liver cells synthesize CHOL from acetyl CoA. The body manufactures about 1500 mg daily and more than three-fourths of this is excreted in the feces, mostly as bile acids (2). When people increase their intake of dietary CHOL, the higher intake does not affect their CHOL synthesis or the rate at which CHOL is converted to bile acids (6).

Functions of Fats and Other Lipids

Functions of Fats and Oils

Fats and oils are sources of energy in the diet. They are the most concentrated form of energy in foods, 9 kcal (38 kJ) per gram, yielding more than twice as much energy per gram as either carbohydrates or proteins. In the body, fats are deposited under the skin where they function as nonconductors of heat, helping to insulate the body and prevent rapid loss of heat. Also, cushions of fat support the viscera and certain body organs. Moreover, the greatest supply of reserve energy in animals and man is found in the fat stores of the body. These stores result from the consumption of an excessive quantity of energy from any one or a combination of the energy-yielding nutrients—carbohydrate, fat, and protein. Of the estimated fuel reserves of adult man, 1000 kcal (4184 kJ) are in the form of carbohydrate, 141,000 kcal (589,944 kJ) are in the form of fat, and 24,000 kcal (100,416 kJ) are in the form of protein (3).

No RDA for fat has been established, but it has been suggested that fat should not comprise more than 35 percent of one's daily total kilocalories (less than 10 percent should come from saturated fatty acids and up to 10 percent from polyunsaturated ones) (15).

Essential Fatty Acid Although some fatty acids can be synthesized from extra amounts of energy in the body, one fatty acid that is essential for growth and the maintenance of normal skin cannot thus be synthesized. This essential fatty acid (EFA) is linoleic acid (12).

71

Another fatty acid, *arachidonic acid,* was formerly considered essential. However, in studies with children and animals, it was found that there is no dietary requirement for arachidonic acid when linoleic is supplied in sufficient amounts. Thus it was established that arachidonic acid is not a true dietary essential because it can be formed in the body from linoleic acid.

Little is known about the EFA requirements of human beings. Infants who were given a low-fat diet failed to grow satisfactorily (12) and tended to develop skin disorders. When linoleic acid was added to their diets in amounts to provide at least 1 percent of their total energy intake, there was a distinct improvement. The symptoms of an EFA deficiency in adults appear to be less well defined than in infants. The commonly described symptoms of eczematous dermatitis has (8) and has not (16) been observed in EFA-deficient studies.

Functions of Phospholipids, Cholesterol, and Lipoproteins

Phospholipids The main function of phospholipids and other lipids (like CHOL) is the formation of structural membranes within the body to prevent the absorption of water-soluble substances and water evaporation from the skin (11). And, they aid in the transport of fatty acids through the intestinal wall into the *lymph.* One phospholipid (a cephalin) is a component of thromboplastin, a substance that initiates blood clotting, and another (a sphingomyelin) acts as an insulator around nerve fibers.

Cholesterol About 80 percent of the body's CHOL is used by the liver to form the bile acid, cholic acid, a constituent of bile salts, which are necessary in the digestion and absorption of fats. Most of the hormones of the adrenal cortex and certain ones of the ovaries (progesterone and estrogen) and testes (testosterone) are derivatives of CHOL (11).

Lipoproteins Little is known about the function of lipoproteins except that they transport lipid material in the plasma throughout the body (7, 9).

Food Sources of Fats and Cholesterol

Food Sources of Fats and Oils

The most abundant sources of fat in the diet are vegetable oils (corn oil, peanut oil, olive oil), vegetable shortenings, and animal fats (beef fat, lard, and butter). Nuts also rank high, with pecans containing the most fat and cashews the least (Appendix, Table A-3). Meat, poultry, and fish vary in their fat content; bacon contains more than beef or salmon (a fatty fish). All cheeses, with the exception of cottage and other skim-milk cheeses, contain appreciable amounts. In eggs fat is found only in the yolk. Processed and prepared foods made with fats and oils (potato chips, cakes, pastries, cookies, and candy bars) often contain significant amounts of fat. Vegetables and fruits (with the exception of avocados) contain little. The fat content of certain foods is shown in Table 5.3.

The Effect of Cooking on Fats and Oils

There is little change in the EFA content of meat and poultry when they are roasted or fried (4). However, there are slight losses of linoleic acid in vegetable oils that are used for deep-fat frying during several hours (5). After heating corn oil, cottonseed oil, and shortening (soft fat) for 7½ hours to fry 4.5 kg (10 lb) of potatoes, about 11 percent of the original linoleic acid content was lost; safflower oil lost only about 4 percent (14).

High heat decomposes the glycerol of the fat molecule to the chemical substance *acrolein,* which has a disagreeable choking odor and is intensely irritating to the eyes and nose. Acrolein is

72

Table 5.3 Fat Content of Various Foods as Served

Food	Per 100 g of food	Per average serving		
	Fat, g	Size of serving, g		Fat, g
Oils (salad and cooking)	100.0	14	1 tbsp	14
Butter	85.7	14	1 tbsp	12
Margarine	85.7	14	1 tbsp	12
Mayonnaise	78.6	14	1 tbsp	11
Bacon (cooked)	53.3	15	2 sl	8
Potato chips	40.0	20	10 chips	8
Cheese (American)	32.1	28	1 oz	9
Ground beef (broiled)	20.7	82	2.9 oz patty	17
Egg	12.0	50	1 large	6
Pie (apple)	11.1	135	$\frac{1}{7}$ of pie	15
Fish sticks	10.7	28	1 stick	3
Liver (beef, fried)	10.6	85	3 oz	9
Pizza (cheese)	6.7	60	4¾-in. sector	4
Salmon (pink, canned)	5.9	85	3 oz	5
Milk (whole)	3.3	244	1 c	8
Yogurt (from lowfat milk)[a]	1.8	227	1 c	4
Bread (white, enriched)	0.4	28	1 sl	1
Milk (nonfat, skim)	tr	245	1 c	1
Peas (green, frozen)	tr	160	½ c	tr

[a] With added milk solids.

From *Nutritive Value of Foods*, Home and Garden Bull. No. 72, revised. Washington, D.C.: U.S. Dept. Agr., 1977.

produced when foods are fried at a high temperature. To reduce the formation of acrolein when frying in deep fat, discard the fat if it foams a great deal when the food is added, discard the fat if it has become substantially darker in color, use a large amount of fat (around 1.4 kg or 3 lb), and add fresh fat to maintain the volume each time the fat is reused (17).

Food Sources of Cholesterol

The CHOL values of various foods are presented in Table 5.4. Note that eggs, butter, lard, and meat are all high in CHOL, whereas foods from plant sources have none.

Fats and Oils in College Meals

Analyses for fat and fatty acids were made by the U.S. Department of Agriculture on meals served for one week at 50 American colleges in 31 states (see p. 56) (18). The meals contained, per person per day, an average of 125.6 g fat (range, 97.0 to 163.7 g), which was about 42 percent (range, 37 to 47 percent) of the total kilocalories. The saturated, monounsaturated, and polyunsaturated content of the meals averaged 46.3 g (range, 34.8 to 62.5 g), 49.0 (range, 35.8 to 71.8 g), and 18.3 g (range, 11.2 to 35.0 g) per person per day, respectively. About 92 percent of the total fatty acids came from palmitic, stearic, oleic, and linoleic

73

Table 5.4 Cholesterol Content of Various Foods

Food	Per 100 g of food Cholesterol, mg	Per average serving Size of serving	Per average serving Cholesterol, mg
Egg yolk			
dried	2630	—	—
fresh	1480	1 yolk	252
frozen	1270	—	—
Kidney (all kinds), cooked	(804)[a]	½ c	(563)
Egg, whole	504	1 med	252
Sweetbreads (thymus), cooked	(466)	3 oz	(396)
Liver (beef, calf, hog, lamb), cooked	(438)	3 oz	(372)
Heart (beef), cooked	(274)	½ c	(199)
Butter	250	1 tbsp	35
Shrimp, canned, drained solids	150	11 large	96
Cheese (cream)	111	1 tbsp	16
Milk, dried, whole	109	1¾ c[b]	131
Crab, canned, meat only	(101)	½ c	(80)
Veal, cooked, bone removed	(101)	3 oz	(86)
Cheese (Cheddar)	99	1 oz	28
Lamb, cooked, bone removed	(98)	3 oz	(83)
Lard and other animal fats	95	1 tbsp	12
Beef, cooked, bone removed	(94)	3 oz	(80)
Chicken, cooked, drumstick, meat only	91	2¾ oz	73
Pork, cooked, bone removed	(89)	3 oz	(76)
Lobster, cooked, meat only	85	½ c	61
Chicken, cooked, breast, meat only	79	2¾ oz	63
Halibut	(60)	4½ oz	(75)
Margarine (⅔ animal fat, ⅓ vegetable fat)	50	1 tbsp	7
Ice cream, regular (approx. 10% butterfat)	40	½ c	26
Cheese (cottage, creamed, 4% butterfat)	19	½ c	24
Milk, fluid, whole	14	1 c	34
Milk, fluid, skim	2	1 c	5
Margarine (all vegetable)	0	—	—
Egg, white	0	—	—

[a] Numbers in parentheses denote imputed values.
[b] Amount needed for reconstitution to 1 quart.
From Feeley, R. M., P. E. Criner, and B. K. Watt (1972). Cholesterol content of foods. *J. Am. Dietet. Assoc.*, **61:** 134–149. Used by permission.

acids; the average linoleic acid content was 17.2 g (range, 10.6 to 29.7 g) per person per day.

Fats and Oils in the United States' Food Supply

The amount of fat in the American food supply increased almost steadily from 1909–1913 to 1972 and has since dropped slightly (1, 10) (Fig. 5.4). The amount of nutrient fat available per person per day was 125 g (1909–1913), 140 g (1947–1949), 144 g (1965), 159 g (1972), and 157 g (1976).

During the past half-century, the kinds of fats available in the national food supply have changed. Animal fats and oils (butter and lard) are used less often, whereas the use of vegetable fats and oils has increased sharply (Fig. 5.4). This change is partly due to the increased availability of soybean oil, the changing tastes and preferences of American consumers, and education programs to reduce the intake of saturated fats in the diet. The U.S. Department of Agriculture reported that during 1976 the total consumption of fats and oils, including butter, was 27.1 kg (59.6 lb) per capita (1).

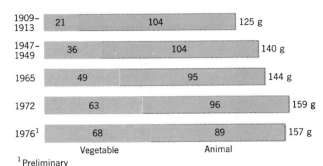

1909–1913	21	104	125 g
1947–1949	36	104	140 g
1965	49	95	144 g
1972	63	96	159 g
1976[1]	68	89	157 g

Vegetable   Animal

[1] Preliminary

Fig. 5.4 Sources of nutrient fat in the United States, grams per capita per day. (From 1976 *Handbook of Agricultural Charts*, Agr. Handbook No. 504. Washington, D.C.: U.S. Dept. Agr., 1976, p. 68.)

Diet and Coronary Heart Disease

Coronary heart disease (CHD) is a leading cause of death in the United States. In 1974 about 665,000 persons died from CHD (34 percent of all causes of death) and about 24 percent of them were under 65 years of age (22) (Fig. 5.5).

There are a number of factors ("risk factors") associated with susceptibility to CHD that can be

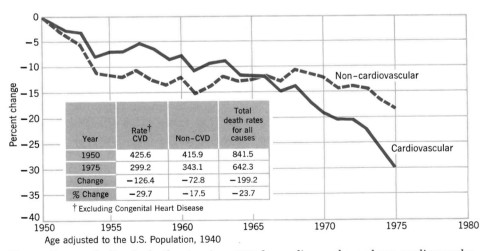

Year	Rate[†] CVD	Non–CVD	Total death rates for all causes
1950	425.6	415.9	841.5
1975	299.2	343.1	642.3
Change	−126.4	−72.8	−199.2
% Change	−29.7	−17.5	−23.7

[†] Excluding Congenital Heart Disease

Age adjusted to the U.S. Population, 1940

Fig. 5.5 Percent decline in death rates since 1950 for cardiovascular and non-cardiovascular diseases. (From *The National Heart, Lung, and Blood Institute's Fact Book for Fiscal Year 1976*, DHEW Publ. No. NIH 77-1172. Bethesda, Md.: U.S. Dept. Health, Education, and Welfare, 1976, p. 31.)

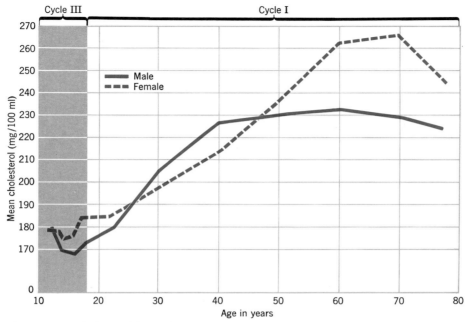

Fig. 5.6 Mean cholesterol levels for adults in the Health Examination Survey Cycle I (1960–1962) and youths in the Health Examination Survey Cycle III (1966–1970): United States. (From *Total Serum Cholesterol Values of Youths 12–17 Years, United States*, DHEW Publ. No. HRA 76-1638. Rockville, Md.: U.S. Dept. Health, Education, and Welfare, Public Health Service 1976, p. 9.)

controlled to a large extent. These include an elevation in plasma lipids (especially plasma CHOL), high blood pressure (hypertension), heavy cigarette smoking, obesity, and physical inactivity. The risk factors related to diet will be considered here.

Effect of Diet on Blood Lipids

Plasma Cholesterol　Human blood CHOL values vary at different ages. Figure 5.6 shows the change in average blood CHOL values of individuals from age 12 to 79 years in the Health Examination Surveys of the Public Health Service (20). The mean CHOL levels, expressed as mg per 100 ml or mg per dl (deciliter is one-tenth liter or 100 ml), are about 180 at age 12 and rise gradually with age. The gradual rise in CHOL levels does not begin until the mid-twenties for women; in males

it begins earlier and is steeper (Fig. 5.6). The mean CHOL values for men and women 19 to 24 years is 178.1 and 184.7 mg per 100 ml, respectively (20).

It is believed that the average individual ingests between 500 and 800 mg CHOL per day. It has been proposed that for each 100 mg CHOL ingested per 1000 kcal (4184 kJ), there is an increase of about 12 mg CHOL per 100 ml serum (15).

The optimal CHOL level for the retardation of CHD is probably under 200 mg per 100 ml (15), but this level is unobtainable by many adult Americans unless they markedly change their eating patterns. For some population groups, including vegetarians in the United States, low CHOL values are common: some Japanese have levels of 150 to 170 mg per 100 ml. An average CHOL blood level of about 126 ± 30 mg per 100 ml

76

was found in over 100 American vegetarians, most of them between the ages of 16 and 29 years, as compared to 184 ± 37 mg per 100 ml for the control subjects who ate the more traditional American diet (18). The "normal" or "average" CHOL blood levels found in healthy American adults range from 170 to 240 mg per 100 ml (19).

The dietary prescription given to lower blood CHOL is the partial replacement of the dietary sources of saturated fat with those of unsaturated fat (especially those rich in polyunsaturated fatty acids) and a reduction in the consumption of foods rich in CHOL. Newer findings from human feeding studies indicate that elevation of blood CHOL levels is not due to higher dietary intakes of the sterol (1, 11). Nevertheless, there is evidence from studies with middle-aged men to suggest that the faithful and continued consumption of a low CHOL diet over a period of years can reduce the coronary attack rate (13). Modifying the diet before CHD occurs seems to be more effective than after it becomes evident.

Caloric restriction also lowers blood CHOL levels (10). In coronary prevention programs, caloric control or restriction is one of the dietary prescriptions (13).

Whether or not insufficient dietary fiber (21), low intake levels of ascorbic acid (vitamin C) (16), or high animal protein content of the diet (17) are causative agents for high blood CHOL and CHD remains to be proven.

Plasma Triglycerides   Elevation of serum TRGs (hypertriglyceridemia) is also associated with increased risk of CHD. The level of carbohydrate in the diet and obesity significantly affect the serum TRG concentration.

Alaskan Artic Eskimo teenagers eating a diet supplemented with large amounts of candy and soft drinks showed significantly higher blood TRGs than a comparable group eating the native diet (5). Obese adults (10) and obese children (6) are reported to have high TRG blood levels. However, with caloric restriction, plasma TRGs were decreased by 41 ± 12 percent in the

adults and by about 42 percent (to normal levels) in the children.

Effect of Factors Other than Diet on Blood Lipids

Some researchers believe that physical activity is more important than either the amount or kind of fat in the diet in controlling CHOL levels. The very physically active Samburu tribe of Africa has a high-fat diet but extremely low CHOL blood levels that do not appear to increase with age. In Switzerland it was found that active farm families with a high intake of fat have the same plasma CHOL levels as less active city families who consumed less fat. Exercise in human beings also lowers fasting plasma TRG levels even during periods of increased caloric intake (7).

Research findings suggest that feeding or meal patterns may influence the level of blood CHOL; however, the results are more clear-cut with animals than with human beings. In a study of college men on one, three, and six meals a day (where the nutrient intake was the same for all), the mean CHOL values were found to be significantly higher for those eating one meal a day than for the other two groups; the mean CHOL level was lowest for those eating six meals a day (23).

Trace element imbalance as a cause of cardiovascular diseases is now under study by the WHO (14); the United States is one of the nine participating countries. Of particular interest is the study of cadmium, chromium, copper, selenium, and zinc levels in autopsy tissues.

New Survey Data

Belgians, particularly in the north, have shifted their food intake to one of lower saturated fat and food CHOL and higher polyunsaturated fat by doubling their intakes of margarine and decreasing their intakes of butter (four to five times smaller than that in the south). Data from the last ten years show a significantly higher serum

CHOL with higher coronary morbidity and mortality among Belgians in the south and decreasing serum CHOL and increased life expectancy (2.2 years higher in males age 30) among the northern Belgians (9).

Preliminary findings from the ongoing collaborative US–USSR study (begun in 1972) on the prevalence of plasma lipids and other risk factors to atherosclerotic disease have been reported for men aged 40 to 59 years (3). The Soviet men have higher plasma CHOL and HDL levels but lower plasma TRG levels than the American men.

The Lipid Research Clinics (LRCs) Program of the National Heart, Lung, and Blood Institute (National Institutes of Health) has been underway since 1971 in 12 sites (11 in the United States and one in Canada) and has screened about 70,000 subjects and studied in more detail about 15,000 of them. Its goal is to prevent "premature atherosclerosis through the diagnosis and treatment of hyperlipidemia (disorders in which the blood fats are elevated)" (19). Some of the findings in the 1977 status report of the LRC are a drop in the average daily CHOL intake, a decrease in the ratio of saturated to unsaturated fat in the diet, a slight reduction in the average level of plasma CHOL, and the finding that slightly, but significantly, lower blood lipids are observed in subjects of higher educational or socioeconomic groups. (Future studies in the program will involve the relationship of plasma lipoproteins to diet and CHD.)

Screening for Hyperlipidemia in Childhood, Adolescence, and Early Adulthood

The development of CHD in human beings is believed to begin early in life (4). Support for this hypothesis comes from the Muscatine study of nearly 5000 children, ages one through 12, where a considerable number of children were found to have serum lipid levels and relative body weights (obesity) indicative of early CHD in adults (12). Twenty-nine percent of the children of victims of early heart attacks have been shown to have elevated blood lipids (2). Therefore children, adolescents, and college students with any of these "risk factors" and offspring of early heart attack victims should be screened and preventative measures begun in childhood, adolescence, or early adulthood.

Summary

Lipids, a group of organic compounds soluble in fat solvents, occur in both plants and animals. The lipids important in nutrition are fatty acids, fats and oils, phospholipids, sterols, and lipoproteins.

Fatty acids are classified according to their degree of saturation or unsaturation. There are saturated, monounsaturated, and polyunsaturated ones.

Fats and oils (triglycerides [TRGs]) are made up of glycerol and three fatty acids. Their shelf life is prolonged by antioxidants, and they can be hardened to solid TRGs by hydrogenation. Fats and oils supply energy (9 kcal per gm), insulate the body to prevent rapid heat loss, support certain body organs, and provide the EFA, linoleic acid. There is no RDA for fat. Rich sources of fats and oils are vegetable oils, vegetable shortening, animal fats, and nuts. High temperature frying decomposes them.

Phospholipids function as structural materials in every cell to prevent the absorption and the loss of water from the body and aid in the transport of fatty acids.

Cholesterol (found in the food intake and synthesized in the body) is necessary to form bile salts needed in fat digestion and absorption. The hormones of the adrenal glands and certain sex hormones are derivatives of CHOL. Eggs, butter, lard, and meats are rich in the sterol.

Lipoproteins, composed of protein and lipids, serve in the transport of lipids. There are four types: chylomicrons, VLDL, LDL, and HDL.

Blood CHOL, blood TRGs, and certain lipoproteins have been identified as "risk factors" in CHD, a leading cause of death among Americans. The partial replacement of dietary fat with unsaturated fat and a reduction in dietary CHOL is the prescription followed by many to reduce the risk of CHD. Exercise is also beneficial in lowering the blood lipid "risk factors." Because CHD is believed to develop early in life, there is interest in the screening of children, adolescents, and young adults for signs of "risk factors."

Is the plasma CHOL level the best indicator of the rate of coronary attack?

For nearly two decades many studies have been reported relating serum lipids, particularly CHOL, to CHD. New findings show, however, that total CHOL levels may be a good indicator for individuals under 50 years of age but not for individuals in older age groups (8). A more sensitive measure for all age groups appears to be the fractions of the serum lipoproteins (VLDL, LDL, and HDL). The higher the levels of VLDL and LDL, the greater the risk of CHD. In contrast, the higher the level of HDL, the less risk of CHD (8, 19). (HDL appears to remove excess CHOL from the body cells and carries it to the intestines for disposal.)

Some interesting facts about HDLs follow (8). The average serum HDL is 45 mg per 100 ml (men) and 55 mg per 100 ml (women). Newborn babies have about one-half their total CHOL as HDL. Members of long-lived families have been found to have high HDL levels (about 75 mg per 100 ml or more). Long-distance runners have higher HDLs (about 66 mg per 100 ml) than the normal population. The vitamin niacin increases the HDL level and decreases the LDL level. A change in diet that emphasizes vegetables, cereals, fish, little if any meat, and no foods rich in saturated fats will decrease the LDL and increase the HDL levels (18).

Glossary

acrolein: a volatile, irritating liquid that results from overheating fat.

arachidonic acid: a 20-carbon atom fatty acid with four double bonds; in the body it is synthesized from the essential fatty acid linoleic acid.

atherosclerosis: a condition in which the inner walls of the arteries have been thickened by deposits of material, including cholesterol.

cholesterol: a sterol found chiefly in animal tissues; distributed widely in all cells of the body.

chylomicron: a lipoprotein composed of about 1 percent protein and 99 percent total lipids.

compound lipids: compounds (esters) of fatty acids containing groups in addition to an alcohol and fatty acid; for example, a phospholipid.

coronary heart disease: a cardiac disability arising from a reduction or arrest of blood supply to part of the heart muscle either by a narrowing or complete obstruction of a blood vessel.

derived lipids: compounds (esters) formed from the breakdown (hydrolysis) of lipids; examples are fatty acids, glycerol, cholesterol.

fatty acids: see page 28.

glyceride: see page 28

glycerol: see page 28

high density lipoprotein (HDL): a lipoprotein composed of about 50 percent protein and the rest total lipids; also called alpha-cholesterol.

hydrogenation: the addition of hydrogen to a compound, especially to an unsaturated fat or fatty acid; adding hydrogen at the double bond will solidify soft fats or oils.

linoleic acid: the essential fatty acid; it is unsaturated and occurs widely in plant glycerides.

lipids: see page 11

lipoprotein: a compound composed of a lipid and a protein.

low density lipoprotein (LDL): a lipoprotein composed of about 11 percent protein and 89 percent total lipids; also called beta-cholesterol.

lymph: see page 28

lymphatic system: see page 28.

medium-chain triglycerides (MCT): manufactured triglycerides containing fatty acids of eight to ten carbon atoms; for individuals with a fat malabsorption disorder.

phospholipid: see page 11.

polyunsaturated fatty acids: fatty acids containing two or more double bonds, such as linoleic, linolenic, and arachidonic acids.

simple lipids: compounds (esters) of fatty acids with various alcohols; fats and waxes are examples.

stearic acid: a saturated fatty acid composed of 18 carbon atoms.

sterol: an alcohol of high molecular weight, such as cholesterol and ergosterol.

triglyceride (fat): an ester composed of glycerol and three fatty acids.

very low density lipoprotein (VLDL): a lipoprotein composed of 7 percent protein and 93 percent total lipids; also called pre-beta cholesterol.

Study Questions and Activities

1. Identify the following: 7-dehydrocholesterol, stearic acid, antioxidant, endogenous cholesterol, linoleic acid, monounsaturated fatty acid, hydrogenated fat, triglyceride, phospholipid, double-bond linkage, and lipase.

2. Describe the kind and amount of fat that has been available in the American food supply since 1909–1913.

3. How does a saturated fatty acid differ from a polyunsaturated one?

4. What are the functions of fat in the body?

5. Explain what an essential fatty acid is and what human experiments have shown about such acid deprivation.

6. About how much cholesterol does the average American adult consume each day? About how much does his body synthesize? What is the role of cholesterol in the body? Why is high serum cholesterol considered undesirable?

7. What recommendations have been made to reduce the formation of acrolein when food is fried in deep fat?

8. What are the four kinds of lipoproteins and what is their significance in the body?

9. Trace the digestion of fat in the gastrointestinal tract.

References

Fatty Acids, Fats and Oils, Phospholipids, Sterols, and Lipoproteins

1. *Agricultural Statistics* (1977). Washington, D.C.: U.S. Dept. Agr., pp. 561–564.

2. Anderson, J. T., F. Grande, and A. Keys (1973). Cholesterol-lowering diets. *J. Am. Dietet. Assoc.,* **62:** 133.

3. Cahill, G. E., Jr. (1970). Starvation in man. *New Engl. J. Med.,* **282:** 668.

4. Chang, I. C. L., and B. M. Watts (1952). The fatty acid content of meat and poultry before and after cooking. *J. Am. Oil Chemists' Soc.,* **29:** 334.

5. Chang, I. C. L., L. I. Y. Tchen, and B. M. Watts (1952). The fatty acid content of selected foods before and after cooking. *J. Am. Oil Chemists' Soc.,* **29:** 378.

6. Cholesterol absorption versus cholesterol synthesis in man (1970). *Nutrition Rev.,* **28:** 11.

7. Eisenberg, S., and R. I. Levy (1975). Lipoprotein metabolism. *Advances Lipid Res.,* **13:** 1.

8. Fleming, C. R., L. M. Smith, and R. E. Hodges (1976). Essential fatty acid deficiency in adults receiving total parenteral nutrition. *Am. J. Clin. Nutrition,* **29:** 976.

9. Frederickson, D. S., R. I. Levy, and R. S. Lees (1967). Fat transport lipoproteins — an integrated approach to mechanisms and disorders. *New Engl. J. Med.,* **276:** 34–44, 94–103, 148–156, 215–225, 273–281.

10. Friend, B. (1973). Nutritional review. *National Food Situation,* Nov. NFS-146. Washington, D.C.: U.S. Dept. Agr., p. 23.

11. Guyton, A. C. (1976). *Textbook of Medical Physiology.* 5th ed. Philadelphia: W. B. Saunders Co., Chapter 68.

12. Hansen, A. E., H. F. Wiese, A. N. Boelsche, M. E. Haggard, D. J. D. Adam, and H. Davis (1963). Role of linoleic acid in infant nutrition. *Pediatrics,* **31:** 171.

13. Harper, H. A., ed. (1975). *Review of Physiological Chemistry.* 15th ed. Los Altos, Calif. Lange Medical Publications, pp. 279–281.

14. Kilgore, L., and M. Bailey (1970). Degradation of linoleic acid during potato frying. *J. Am. Dietet. Assoc.,* **56:** 130.

15. *Recommended Dietary Allowances, Eighth Edition* (1974). Natl. Acad. Sci.-Natl. Research Council. Washington, D.C.: Natl. Research Council.

16. Richardson, T. J., and D. Szontas (1975). Essential fatty acid deficiency in four adult patients during parenteral nutrition. *Am. J. Clin. Nutrition,* **28:** 258.

17. Stasch, A. R., and L. Kilgore (1963). *Influences of Repeated Use for Cooking on Some Changes in Composition of Frying Fats.* Agr. Expt. Sta. Bull. No. 662. State College, Miss.: Mississippi State College.

18. Walker, M. A., and L. Page (1975). Nutritive content of college meals. II. Lipids. *J. Am. Dietet. Assoc.,* **68:** 34.

Diet and Coronary Heart Disease

1. Anderson, J. T., F. Grande, and A. Keys (1976). Independence of the effects of cholesterol and degree of saturation of the fat in the diet of serum cholesterol in man. *Am. J. Clin. Nutrition,* **29:** 1184.

2. Chase, H. P., R. J. O'Quinn, and D. O'Brien (1974). Screening for hyperlipidemia in childhood. *J. Am. Med. Assoc.,* **230:** 1535.

3. Collaborative US–USSR study on the prevalence of dyslipoproteinemias and ischemic heart disease in American and Soviet populations. Prepared by the US–USSR Steering Committee for Problem Area 1: the pathogenesis of atherosclerosis (1977). *Am. J. Cardiology,* **40:** 260.

4. Danilevicius, Z. (1974). When does CHD start? *J. Am. Med. Assoc.,* **230:** 1565.

5. Feldman, S. A., A. H. Rubenstein, K. Ho, C. B. Taylor, L. A. Lewis, and B. Mikkelson (1975). Carbohydrate and lipid metabolism in the Alaskan Artic Eskimo. *Am. J. Clin. Nutrition,* **28:** 588.

6. Forget, P. P., J. Fernandes, and P. H. Begemann (1975). Plasma triglyceride clearing in obese children. *Am. J. Clin. Nutrition,* **28:** 858.

7. Gyntelberg, F., R. Brennan, J. O. Holloszy, G. Schonfeld, M. J. Rennie, and S. W. Weidman (1977). Plasma triglyceride lowering by exercise despite increased food intake in patients with type IV hyperlipoproteinemia. *Am. J. Clin. Nutrition,* **30:** 716.

8. High blood lipid levels can be good or bad — depending on the lipid (1977). *J. Am. Med. Assoc.,* **237:** 1066.

9. Joossens, J. V., E. Brems-Heyns, J. H. Claes, M. Graffar, M. Kornitzer, R. Pannier, O. Van Houte, K. Vuylsteek, J. Carlier, G. De Backer, H. Kesteloot, J. Lequime, A. Raes, M. Vastesaeger, and G. Verdonk (1977). The pattern of food and mortality in Belgium. *Lancet,* **I:** 1069.

10. Kudchodkar, B. J., H. S. Sodhi, D. T. Mason, and N. O. Bohani (1977). Effects of acute caloric restriction on cholesterol metabolism in man. *Am. J. Clin. Nutrition,* **30:** 1135.

11. Kummerow, F. A., Y. Kim, M. D. Hull, J. Pollard, P. Ilinov, D. L. Dorossiev, and J. Valek (1977). The influence of egg consumption on the serum cholesterol level in human subjects. *Am. J. Clin. Nutrition,* **30:** 664.

12. Laurer, R. M., W. E. Connor, P. E. Leaverton, M. A. Reeter, and W. R. Clarke (1975). Coronary heart disease risk factors in school children. Muscatine study. *J. Pediatrics,* **86:** 697.

13. Long-term effects of diets prescribed in coronary prevention programs (1977). *Nutrition Rev.,* **35:** 140.

14. Masironi, R., ed. (1974). *Trace Elements in Relation to Cardiovascular Diseases.* WHO Offset Publ. No. 5. Geneva: World Health Organ.

15. Mattson, F. H., B. A. Erickson, and A. M. Kligman (1972). Effect of dietary cholesterol on serum cholesterol in man. *Am. J. Clin. Nutrition,* **25:** 589.

16. Pauling, L. (1976). *Vitamin C, the Common Cold and the Flu.* San Francisco: W. H. Freeman and Co.

17. Plant foods and atherosclerosis (1977). *Nutrition Rev.,* **35:** 148.

18. Sacks, F. M., W. P. Castelli, A. Donner, and E. H. Kass (1975). Plasma lipids and lipoproteins in vegetarians and controls. *New Engl. J. Med.,* **292:** 1148.

19. *Status Report: Current Findings of the Lipid Research Clinic Programs* (1977). LRC Press Briefing, July 13, 1977. Bethesda, Md.: National Institutes of Health, National Heart, Lung, and Blood Institute, 65 pp.

20. *Total Serum Cholesterol Values of Youths 12–17 Years United States* (1976). DHEW Publ. No. HRA 76-1638. Rockville, Md., U.S. Dept. Health, Education, and Welfare, Public Health Service.

21. Tuswell, A. S. (1977). Food fibre and blood lipids. *Nutrition Rev.,* **35:** 51.

22. *Vital Statistics of the United States 1974* (1976). Vol. II—Mortality, Part B. Rockville, Md.: U.S. Dept. Health, Education, and Welfare, Public Health Service.

23. Young, C. M., L. F. Hutter, S. S. Scanlan, C. E. Rand, L. Lutwak, and V. Simko (1972). Metabolic effect of meal frequency on normal young men. *J. Am. Dietet. Assoc.,* **61:** 391.

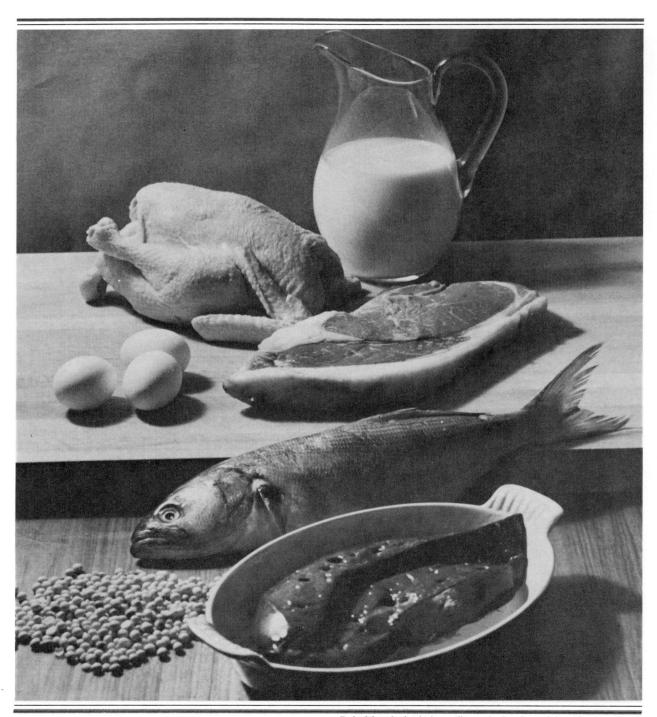

Each of these foods (chicken, milk, eggs, beef, soybeans, fish and liver) contains all of the essential amino acids, making them good sources of protein.

Chapter 6

Amino Acids

Abbreviations

Acetyl CoA: acetyl coenzyme A
$-NH_2$: amino or basic group
$-COOH$: carboxyl or acid group
DNA: deoxyribonucleic acid
FAO: Food and Agriculture Organization
m-RNA: messenger RNA
PKU: phenylketonuria

RDA: Recommended Dietary Allowances
RNA: ribonucleic acid
TAC: tricarboxylic acid cycle
t-RNA: transfer RNA
For amino acid abbreviations, see Appendix Table A-11

Amino acids are the building blocks of proteins. The chemical elements that make up the amino acids are carbon, hydrogen, oxygen, nitrogen, and sometimes sulfur. As the name suggests, an amino acid is a compound that contains an amino group ($-NH_2$) and a carboxyl or acid group ($-COOH$). Amino acids have the following general formula:

$$R-\underset{\underset{H}{|}}{\overset{\overset{NH_2\ (amino\ group)}{|}}{C}}-COOH\ (carboxyl\ group)$$

The chemical structure of the simplest amino acid—glycine—is given in Figure 6.2. All of the common amino acids except one—proline—have the same general formula.

Table 6.1. Common Amino Acids

alanine	lysine
arginine	methionine
asparagine	phenylalanine
aspartic acid	proline
cysteine	serine
cystine	threonine
glutamic acid	tryptophan
glycine	tyrosine
histidine	valine
isoleucine	
leucine	

Twenty different amino acids have been isolated and identified in body and food proteins (Table 6.1). The kinds of amino acids, the number of *molecules* of each, and their order of sequence vary in different proteins. Amino acids are white crystalline substances, and each has its own structure. They differ in taste: some are sweet (glycine, alanine, and serine), and others are sour (aspartic acid and glutamic acid). Their solubilities in water vary greatly depending on the structure of the *R* group.

Metabolism of Amino Acids

Absorption of Amino Acids

The digestion of protein takes place in the stomach and small intestine (see p. 102). Of the total amino acid content of the small intestine available for absorption, only a part of it comes from ingested food; the remainder is from digestive secretions and desquamated cells from the lining of the intestine. The amino acids are absorbed into the *portal blood* by *active transport*.

General Pathways of Metabolism

The amino acids are carried by the portal blood to the liver (Fig. 6.1). There the destination of the amino acids is determined: the liver synthesizes some of them into plasma proteins, some are retained in the liver, and some enter the circulation

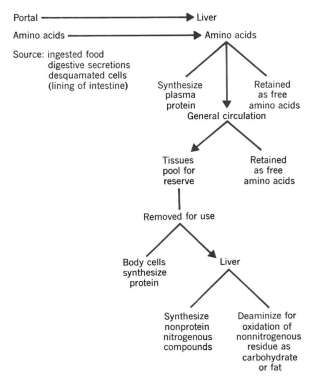

Fig. 6.1 Source and use of amino acids.

as free amino acids. Removal of amino acids from the general circulation by the tissues is controlled by need and by other factors. An increase in insulin level in the blood accelerates the removal of amino acids by the muscle and may reduce muscle protein breakdown. Carbohydrate in the diet favors a higher insulin level in the plasma and a greater uptake of amino acid by the muscle (7). The tissues take up amino acids from the general circulation forming pools of free amino acids (uncombined with other amino acids or molecules) available for use by the tissue cells for protein synthesis.

Surplus amino acids that are not used in syntheses and those needed for energy are *deaminized* (the amino group removed); the nonnitrogenous carbon residues of most amino acids are oxidized by the carbohydrate pathway (*glycogenic*), a few are oxidized by the fatty acid pathway (*ketogenic*), and for some the pathway may be either glycogenic or ketogenic. The pathways of oxidation of carbohydrates and fat are discussed on page 27. The removed amino group may be excreted by way of the kidney as ammonia or *urea* (urea is synthesized in the liver), or it may be transferred to an appropriate acid to form a new amino acid; this process (*transamination*) takes place in the liver.

Interconversion of Carbohydrates, Fats, and Proteins

Cells have the remarkable capacity for converting one type of molecule into another. Some amino acids, after the amino group is removed, are converted to carbohydrate and some to fats; the determining factor is whether or not the appropriate intermediary compounds can be formed. Glucose can be converted into fat or into amino acids (utilizing available amino groups) by means of common intermediates such as pyruvic acid, and acetyl coenzyme A (CoA). Fatty acids generally are not converted to glucose because the pathway between pyruvic acid and acetyl CoA is one-directional; however, under special circumstances, such conversion may occur in plants and microorganisms. Glycerol (two molecules required) is convertible to glucose by reverse glycolysis (Fig. 4.4); also, one molecule of glycerol can form one molecule of pyruvic acid and continue on into the tricarboxylic acid cycle (TAC) where most of the compounds (carbon skeletons) for amino acid *synthesis* are formed.

In this discussion of the metabolism of the energy nutrients, only a few key points of the complex processes have been presented. The enzymes that are essential, the intermediate compounds formed, the interconversion of nutrients, and the pathways of synthesis were only touched upon as an overview of the essential metabolic processes.

87

Disorders of Amino Acid Metabolism

Phenylketonuria (PKU) is the most common inherited metabolic disorder in which the central nervous system is susceptible to damage; the incidence is approximately one in 11,000 births. Since 1952 PKU has been successfully treated with a phenylalanine-restricted diet; mental retardation results in untreated PKU (4, 5).

The defect in phenylketonuria is congenital lack of the enzyme (phenylalanine hydroxylase) necessary for the conversion of phenylalanine to tyrosine, the normal metabolic pathway. As a result, phenylalanine accumulates in excess in the blood plasma and tissues and is excreted in the urine. By-products of alternate metabolic pathways also accumulate and account for the characteristic odor of the urine; one of these metabolites—phenylpyruvic acid—reacts with ferric chloride, giving a vivid green color that is the basis for the commonly used diaper test.

Affected children are usually fair-skinned even though their parents may be dark-complexioned. The production of pigments is reduced because of the block in tyrosine formation, an amino acid involved in the formation of melanin, a skin pigment.

The successful treatment of PKU depends on early diagnosis. An estimated 90 percent of babies born in the United States are screened for PKU before they leave the hospital (8). Early detection is important; if treatment is not initiated before three years of age, little improvement in mental development can be expected. A diet restricted in phenylalanine content is essential. Phenylalanine is an essential amino acid, so some of it must be provided in the diet. A commercial product (Lofenalac®)[1] from which 95 percent of the phenylalanine content has been removed is used as a source of protein. The restricted diet is continued throughout early childhood. Usually, when the child is around six years of age, the dietary restrictions are discontinued. In follow-up studies, no notable lowering of the I.Q. was found upon discontinuing the low phenylalanine diet around age six (16).

Functions of Amino Acids

Protein Synthesis

When the amino group of one acid links with the carboxyl group of another, eliminating a molecule of water, a *peptide* linkage is formed between the two (Fig. 6.2). A dipeptide results when two amino acids are joined by the peptide linkage; a tripeptide is formed when three amino acids are joined by two peptide linkages; and polypeptides are produced when a large number of amino acids are joined together. Proteins are polypeptides.

---

[1] Lofenalac®, Mead Johnson and Company, Evansville, Indiana.

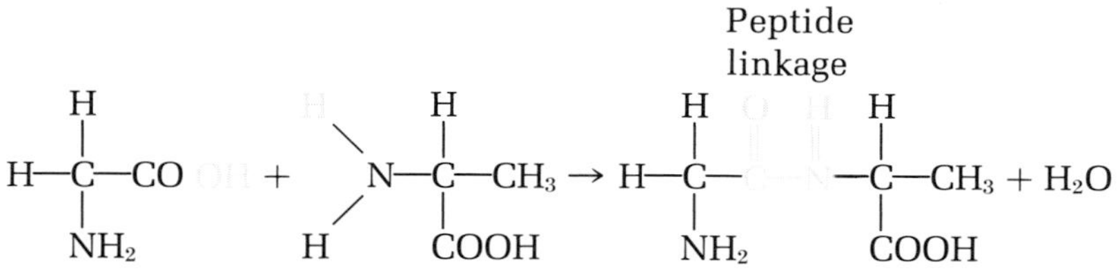

Fig. 6.2 Chemical formulas of two amino acids, glycine and alanine, showing the formation of a dipeptide by the peptide linkage.

88

Within living organisms, each cell is capable of *synthesizing* the proteins needed for its functions. The synthesis of proteins is directed by *deoxyribonucleic acid* (DNA). DNA, located in the nucleus of the cell, serves as the "information center" for the synthesis of the *ribonucleic acids (RNAs)* (see p. 16). Three kinds of RNA function in protein synthesis:

1. Messenger RNAs (m-RNAs), to which DNA transcribes specific genetic information for protein synthesis; m-RNAs are lined up on the *ribosomes.*

2. Transfer or soluble RNAs (t-RNAs), which carry the *activated amino acids* to the proper site for coupling on the messenger RNA.

3. Ribosomal RNAs (r-RNAs), which are in the ribosomes (their function is not known).

The first step in protein synthesis is the formation of the three RNAs in the granular area of the cell nucleus, the nucleolus. Messenger RNA is the *template* of DNA, which embodies the code specifying the order in which the amino acids are to be assembled to produce a specific protein. The RNAs travel from the nucleus to the cytoplasm of the cell, where the synthesis of the protein takes place.

The t-RNAs pick up specific activated amino acids from the cell cytoplasm and carry them to the m-RNA on the ribosomes where the peptide linkage is formed (Fig. 6.3). Multiple ribosomes (polysomes) are attached to a single m-RNA. There is a specific t-RNA for each amino acid. When the t-RNA has added the last amino acid to the m-RNA ribosome complex, the newly synthesized protein and ribosomes are released from the m-RNA. The freed ribosomes attach themselves to a new starting point on the m-RNA to initiate the protein synthesis circuit again. A great deal of energy is used in the synthesis process. Protein synthesis apparently proceeds rapidly: for example, a polypeptide chain the size of one of the chains of hemoglobin (141 amino acids) can be synthesized in about 1 minute.

Experimental work with animals shows that

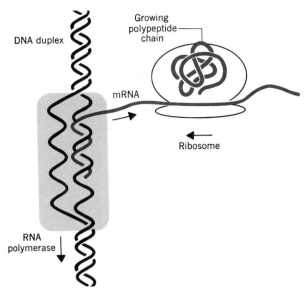

Fig. 6.3 Diagrammatic representation of a growing peptide chain, a step in protein synthesis. RNA polymerase, an enzyme that functions in a process whereby the genetic information of DNA is copied in the form of RNA (transcription), DNA, m-RNA, and a ribosome form the functional complex. Transfer RNA, not shown, moves amino acids to m-RNA. (From Lehninger, A. L., *Biochemistry*, 2nd ed., Worth Publishers, 1975, p. 948.)

for a particular protein to be synthesized, all of the amino acids required for its formation must be available simultaneously and in the correct proportions (9). If even one of the needed amino acids is either missing in the diet or available in insufficient quantity, there will be growth retardation.

Building Substances for Enzymes, Hormones, Antibodies, and Other Compounds

Amino acids are required for the synthesis of all enzymes, including digestive enzymes and those that are required for oxidation, reduction, and all chemical processes in the cells; certain *hormones*, including insulin, thyroxine, *epine-*

89

Lys-Glu-Thr-Ala-Ala-Ala-Lys-Phe-Glu-Arg-Gln-His-Met-Asp-Ser-Ser-Thr-Ser-Ala-Ala-Ser-Ser-Ser-Asn-
Tyr-Cys-Asn-Gln-Met-Met-Lys-Ser-Arg-Asn-Leu-Thr-Lys-Asp-Arg-Cys-Lys-Pro-Val-Asn-Thr-Phe-Val-
His-Glu-Ser-Leu-Ala-Asp-Val-Gln-Ala-Val-Cys-Ser-Gln-Lys-Asn-Val-Ala-Cys-Lys-Asn-Gly-Gln-Thr-
Asn-Cys-Tyr-Gln-Ser-Tyr-Ser-Thr-Met-Ser-Ile-Thr-Asp-Cys-Arg-Glu-Thr-Gly-Ser-Ser-Lys-Tyr-Pro-Asn-
Cys-Ala-Tyr-Lys-Thr-Thr-Gln-Ala-Asn-Lys-His-Ile-Ile-Val-Ala-Cys-Glu-Gly-Asn-Pro-Tyr-Val-Pro-Val-
His-Phe-Asp-Ala-Ser-Val$_{124}$

Fig. 6.4 The amino acid sequence of bovine ribonuclease. For amino acid abbreviations see Appendix Table A-11 (From Lehninger, A. L., *Biochemistry*, 2nd ed., Worth Publishers, 1975, p. 110.)

phrine, *parathyroid hormone, calcitonin,* and some of the secretions of the *pituitary gland;* and all antibodies in the blood. Amino acids are also precursors of some vitamins.

Enzymes are catalysts for chemical reactions in living cells. Essentially all biochemical reactions are enzyme catalyzed and each by a specific enzyme; each cell contains many different enzymes. Most chemical reactions in cells would occur too slowly to support life were it not for catalysis by enzymes. Ribonuclease, the enzyme that breaks down ribonucleic acid, is made up of a chain of 124 amino acids, one of the shortest enzyme chains. In 1963, the complete sequence of the amino acids in ribonuclease was identified and its partial synthesis accomplished (24) (Fig. 6.4). Six years later the synthesis was announced by two teams of investigators, one from Rockefeller University and the other from Merck, Sharp, and Dohme Research Laboratories (20). Ribonuclease, with a molecular weight of 13,700, was the first true protein to be synthesized—a milestone in protein chemistry.

Hormones are regulatory substances secreted principally by *endocrine glands.* They are transported in the blood to the specific organ or tissue where the special effect of the hormone is produced. The majority of hormones are proteins, polypeptides, or derived from amino acids. Thyroxine, composed of two molecules of the amino acid tyrosine plus the mineral iodine, has a rather simple structure (see chapter 14). Sanger (22) won the Nobel Prize in 1958 for his determination analytically of the sequence of amino acids in insulin. He showed that this hormone (which is produced in the pancreas) consists of

two parts—one fraction containing 21 *amino acid residues* and the other 30.

The *antibodies* in the blood belong to a class of proteins called *immunoglobulins.* Antibodies appear in the blood in response to the introduction of a foreign protein; such a foreign substance is called an *antigen.* The antibodies produced combine with the antigen, which stimulated their formation, forming an antigen–antibody complex; the reaction is called the immune response. A greater incidence of bacteria or viruses in the body fluids leads to a higher level of immunoglobulins in the blood and a greater capacity to protect the body against the invading agents.

Source of Energy

The nonnitrogenous residues of amino acids can be used as a source of energy (as indicated in the section on General Pathways of Metabolism, p. 86).

Nutritional Differences in Amino Acids

Essential Amino Acids

In 1931 a new type of protein study became possible using a mixture of chemically pure amino acids. This kind of study was possible only after the amino acids had been isolated. Between 1924 and 1938, nine new amino acids were identified. William Rose of the University of Illinois pioneered in studies of amino acid mixtures using young albino rats. One by one each amino acid was eliminated from the rats' diet, and the effect on their growth was observed. When certain amino acids were removed the growth of the animals was impaired, but the elimination of others had no effect. It was found that ten different amino acids were required in the diet of the rat; the body could not synthesize them, at least at a sufficiently rapid rate to meet the animals' need for growth. These amino acids, designated as "essential" or "indispensable," are listed in Table 6.2. Those that can be synthesized in amounts sufficient to meet the body's need for them are called "nonessential" and "dispensable".

Rose then conducted studies to determine the need of human adults for specific amino acids (21). The experimental diet consisted of the amino acids found to be essential for the rat, cornstarch, sucrose, corn oil, inorganic salts, and vitamin concentrates. One by one each amino acid was removed from the diet (as in the rat studies), and the effect on the nitrogen balance (for explanation of nitrogen balance, see p. 92) was observed. If the removal of an amino acid from the diet resulted in a greater excretion than intake of nitrogen, this indicated that the amino acid was essential in the diet for adults, since the body could not synthesize it at the rate needed. If the balance was unchanged by the removal of an amino acid, that particular amino acid was considered non-essential. Eight amino acids in the original work were found to be necessary in the diet for tissue maintenance in adults. These same eight amino acids, with the addition of histidine, were required for the growth of young children. It had been believed that the amino acid arginine was also essential for growth until Holt (12) conducted a study with infants and found that it was not.

Histidine — An Essential Amino Acid for Adults?

Histidine is an essential amino acid for the normal growth of infants. Recent research indicates that it may be essential for adults also (3, 6, 25). The earlier studies (1951) showing that histidine was not required to maintain nitrogen equilibrium were of shorter duration than a more recent one (1973), indicating that it may be needed (21, 25). During 35 days on a histidine-deficient diet, the nitrogen balance of four adults gradually became negative, and the level of *plasma* histidine fell by 82 percent. With the return of histidine to the diet, the nitrogen balance became positive,

Table 6.2. Amino Acids Essential for Growth in Young Rats, Growth in Children, and Maintenance in Adults

Amino acid	Essential for growth in young rats	Essential for growth in children	Essential for maintenance in adults
Arginine	x		
Histidine	x	x	
Isoleucine	x	x	x
Leucine	x	x	x
Lysine	x	x	x
Methionine	x	x	x
Phenylalanine	x	x	x
Threonine	x	x	x
Tryptophan	x	x	x
Valine	x	x	x

91

and the level of plasma histidine rose (17, 25). In another investigation (1977) a histidine-free *parenteral* diet was fed intravenously to an adult for 27 days; among the numerous observations made was the nitrogen balance, which approached zero (but was not negative) and the histidine plasma level, which decreased (27).

Nonessential Amino Acids

The term "nonessential amino acids" may be confusing; it simply means that these amino acids do not have to be provided "ready-made" in the diet—the body can synthesize them as needed, using nitrogen that is already available in the body. The nonessential amino acids function in *metabolic reactions* that are important to the cell and in the synthesis of many essential body constituents. When the food intake provides enough nonessential amino acids, lesser amounts of the essential amino acids are needed than when it provides only essential amino acids. In addition, certain specific nonessential amino acids spare the need for certain essential amino acids. For example, although tyrosine is a nonessential amino acid, its synthesis in the body requires the essential amino acid phenylalanine. Thus if there is enough tyrosine in the diet, less phenylalanine is needed. In mammals cystine is formed from methionine. In experimental studies with rats, it was found that the dietary requirement for methionine was reduced by one-half when sufficient cystine was provided in their food.

Quantitative Need for Essential Amino Acids

Methods for Determining Quantitative Need

Nitrogen Balance The usual method for determining the amino acid and protein requirements of human beings is nitrogen balance; measurement of nitrogen is the preferred analytical technique because nearly all dietary nitrogen comes from protein (a small, but insignificant, amount is furnished by a few vitamins). Nitrogen values can be converted to grams of protein by multiplying by the factor 6.25 (100/16); most proteins contain about 16 percent nitrogen. The following data from a nitrogen balance study of college women illustrate the use of the conversion factor. The intake of nitrogen was 6.99 g, which is equivalent to 43.7 g of protein (6.99 x 6.25); the total excretion (urine and feces) was 6.40 g of nitrogen; and the retention was 0.59 g of nitrogen, which is equivalent to 3.69 g of protein (0.59 x 6.25) (19).

The study of nitrogen balance is based on the principle that the amount of nitrogen consumed minus the amount excreted in the urine and feces and the skin losses, which include hair, desquamated cells of the skin surface, nails, *insensible perspiration,* and sweating, indicates the amount of protein needed by the body under the conditions of the study. All food eaten by each person in the study is weighed, and a daily sample is analyzed for nitrogen. Each person's daily urinary and fecal excretions are separately collected and separately analyzed. The skin losses are usually not determined. The level of urinary nitrogen excretion is usually about 70 percent of the dietary intake; fecal excretion is 10 to 20 percent and skin losses, 5 to 10 percent of the intake (2). In tropical climates, the skin losses may be twice as high as in temperate zones.

Most of the urinary nitrogen comes from the amino acids of the food not needed for the synthesis of protein and other compounds (see p. 87). And some urinary nitrogen arises from amino acids released in the breakdown of body tissue. Fecal nitrogen is comprised chiefly of undigested food protein and desquamated cells from the intestinal wall plus some bacteria.

The nitrogen balance method enables researchers to determine an individual's minimum protein requirement and the requirement for essential amino acids (10). When the individual is in nitrogen equilibrium the intake and the excretion are the same. To determine the minimum protein or amino acid requirement, the intake is gradually reduced until the balance becomes negative (the excretion exceeds the intake). The minimum requirement is the lowest level of intake at which nitrogen equilibrium can be maintained.

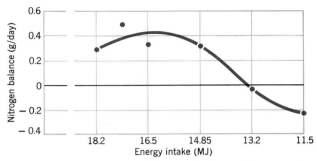

Fig. 6.5 Effect of energy intake on N balance of human subjects at constant N and lysine intakes. (Data from Clark, H. E., S. P. Yang, L. L. Reitz, and E. T. Mertz 1960. J. Nutrition, 72: 87.)

Conditions that Influence Nitrogen Balance The physiological state of an individual influences the nitrogen balance. It is positive during growth, during pregnancy, following depletion of protein reserves such as occurs after a period of low nitrogen intake, febrile condition, or injury. Emotional stress lowers the retention of nitrogen (23), as does prolonged bed rest. An adult under normal conditions is in nitrogen equilibrium, retaining only enough nitrogen to restore that loss from the body.

The level of energy intake influences the nitrogen balance. As the energy intake decreases below a certain critical level, nitrogen retention decreases, indicating that some amino acids are being deaminated and used as energy. Excess dietary energy with a low protein intake spares the loss of *labile protein* (13). An example of the influence of energy intake on nitrogen balance is shown in Fig. 6.5. The nitrogen intake of the human adults remained constant, but the energy intake was reduced from 18.2 megajoules (MJ) (4368 kcal) to 11.5 MJ (2760 kcal) daily. Reduction below 14.9 MJ (3576 kcal) daily caused a negative nitrogen balance.

The amount and proportion of essential amino acids in the diet and the level of total nitrogen in the diet each influence the nitrogen balance when the energy intake is adequate. For the balance to be positive all essential amino acids must be present in adequate amounts and in the proper pattern. The relative amount of each amino acid in relation to the total nitrogen content is considered to be near ideal in whole egg. Deviations from the pattern, causing an imbalance, result in

a less efficient use of nitrogen and a lowered nitrogen balance, especially when the diet is low protein.

Providing the total amino acid needs accounts for only 15 percent of the total protein (nitrogen) need in an adult (50 percent in an infant). The additional nitrogen can be provided from a variety of sources, such as nonessential amino acids or simple nitrogen-containing compounds, such as urea (18).

It should be pointed out, however, that nitrogen balance is an algebraic sum of the gains and losses of nitrogen in all body tissues, so that some tissues may be gaining while others are losing even though there is overall equilibrium. Table 6.3 shows nitrogen balance data.

Table 6.3. Nitrogen Balance Data (grams per day)

Nitrogen intake	Nitrogen excretion	Nitrogen balance
8	8.85	−0.85[a]
8	6.35	+1.65[b]
8	8.00	0.00[c]

[a] Negative balance.
[b] Positive balance.
[c] Equilibrium.

93

Table 6.4. Estimated Amino Acid Requirements

Amino acid	Requirement (per kg. body wt.), mg/day		
	Infant (3–6 mo.)	Child (10–12 yr.)	Adult
Histidine	33	?	?
Isoleucine	80	28	12
Leucine	128	42	16
Lysine	97	44	12
Total S-containing amino acids methionine, cystine, cysteine	45	22	10
Total aromatic amino acids phenylalanine, tyrosine	132	22	16
Threonine	63	28	8
Tryptophan	19	4	3
Valine	89	25	14

From National Academy Sciences (1974). *Recommended Dietary Allowances.* 8th revised ed. Washington, D.C.: National Academy Sciences, p. 44.

Growth Rate For infants and children, growth rate together with nitrogen retention provides a good criterion for adequate amino acid intake (10).

Plasma Amino Acid Levels The relationship between plasma level and intake of the amino acid is a rather recent method for determining amino acid requirement. With reduction of intake, the plasma concentration of the amino acid lowers until a level is reached which remains fairly constant; the intake at that constant level is the minimum requirement for the amino acid (26).

Estimated Amino Acid Requirements

It is useful to know how much of each essential amino acid is needed in order to assess the adequacy of a diet and to estimate the protein needs of people throughout the world. Studies to determine the minimum amounts of essential amino acids needed have produced different results, even for the same age and sex groups. There are some differences in methodology; also the

data for specific individuals suggest that there may be large inherent differences in individual requirements (11, 14). The RDA for the essential amino acids are presented in Table 6.4.

Food Sources of the Amino Acids

The amino acid content of more than 300 foods has been compiled by the Nutrition Division of FAO for world use (1). Values from the table for 74 foods commonly used in the United States are presented in Appendix Table A-1 (values expressed in mg/100 g food). Appendix Table A-2 presents values for some foods in terms of mg/g total nitrogen, which shows the relative amount of total nitrogen provided by each amino acid.

The amino acid whose content in a food meets least well the amount necessary for protein synthesis is the limiting amino acid of that food. Lysine is the limiting amino acid of cereals, methionine of beans. (For effects of the addition of lysine to cereals and methionine to beans in human feeding studies, see Chapter 7, [15].) Egg provides all of the essential amino acids in sufficient amounts for protein synthesis and without excess. The ideal amino acid composition of egg has led to its use as a reference pattern against which the amino acid composition of other foods can be compared to recognize their sufficiencies and lacks.

Summary

Amino acids are the building blocks of proteins. Twenty different ones have been isolated and identified in body and food proteins. The kinds of amino acids, the number of molecules of each, and their order of sequence vary in different proteins.

Amino acids are absorbed from the small intestine into the portal blood by active transport and carried to the liver. There some of the amino acids are synthesized into plasma proteins, some are retained in the liver, and some enter the general circulation as free amino acids. Removal of amino acids from the general circulation by the tissues is controlled by need and other factors.

Functions of the amino acids include the synthesis of proteins and of other essential body substances: enzymes, hormones, and antibodies. The synthesis of protein takes place within the cell directed by deoxyribonucleic acid (DNA) and with three ribonucleic acids functioning in the process: messenger RNA (m-RNA), transfer RNA (t-RNA), and ribosomal RNA (r-RNA).

Amino acids differ in nutritional quality. Some cannot be synthesized at least fast enough to satisfy the body's needs; they are designated "essential" or "indispensable." Some can be synthesized adequately; they are designated "dispensable." The eight amino acids essential for the adult human are: isoleucine, leucine, lysine, methionine, phenylalanine, threonine, tryptophan, and valine. Histidine is an essential amino acid for the normal growth of infants; research indicates that it may be essential for adults also.

The quantitative requirement for amino acids is usually determined by nitrogen balance; in the young the capacity for growth may also be used. The relationship between plasma level and intake of the amino acid is a much simpler method than the nitrogen balance procedure; some investigators are beginning to use it. With reduction of intake, the plasma concentration of the amino acid lowers until a level is reached that remains fairly constant; the intake at that constant level is considered the minimum requirement for that amino acid.

The amino acid content of more than 300 foods has been compiled by the Nutrition Division of FAO for world use.

Glossary

activated amino acid: an amino acid which is to be attached to molecules of transfer RNA; the transfer is an energy-requiring process that is carried out by a set of spontaneous reactions during which the amino acid becomes linked to intermediate products.

active transport: see page 27.

amino acid residues: that portion of an amino acid that is present in a peptide; the amino acid minus the atoms that are removed from it in the process of linking it to other amino acids by means of peptide bonds.

antibody: a protein of the globulin type that is formed in an animal organism in response to the administration of an antigen and is capable of combining specifically with that antigen.

antigen: any substance not normally present in the body, which when introduced into it stimulates the production of a protein (antibody) that reacts specifically with it.

calcitonin: one of two hormones responsible for fine regulation of blood calcium level; the other is the parathyroid hormone. Calcitonin, secreted by the thyroid gland, inhibits bone reabsorption and release of calcium to the blood, thereby lowering blood calcium.

deamination: removal of an amino group from a compound.

deoxyribonucleic acid (DNA): see page 28.

95

endocrine gland: a ductless gland that produces one or more hormones and secretes them directly into the blood.

epinephrine: a hormone secreted by the adrenal gland; causes an increase in blood pressure, heart rate, and elevates the blood sugar level by increasing the breakdown of liver glycogen.

glycogenic: see page 60.

hormone: substance secreted by endocrine glands and transported in the bloodstream to the targets of its action.

immunoglobulin: a protein of animal origin that has a known antibody activity.

insensible perspiration: perspiration that evaporates before it is perceived as fluid on the skin.

ketogenic: conducive to the production of ketones, products of fatty acid oxidation which eventually are broken down to carbon dioxide and water.

labile protein: reserve protein available in most tissues.

metabolic reactions: chemical changes that occur in a living organism; some are synthetic (the formation of new compounds) and some are degradative (the breakdown of compounds).

molecule: the smallest unit of a compound; for example, a molecule of water is H_2O.

parathyroid hormone: the hormone secreted by the parathyroid glands, which stimulates the release of calcium from bone and leads to an increase in the level of calcium in the blood.

parenteral: administered other than by mouth; may be subcutaneously (beneath the skin), or intramuscularly (into the muscle), or intravenously (into a vein).

peptide: see page 88.

pituitary gland: an endocrine gland, located below the brain, that regulates a large portion of the endocrine activity of vertebrates.

plasma: the fluid portion of the blood; contains the clotting factor fibrinogen, which serum does not have.

portal blood: see page 28.

R group: the side chain of an amino acid. Each amino acid has in common an amino group and a carboxyl group but has one group that is different in each amino acid; this group is designated the R group.

ribonucleic acid (RNA): see page 28.

ribosomes: see page 28.

synthesis: the process whereby a more complex substance is produced from simpler substances by a reaction or a series of reactions.

template: a molecule that functions as a mold or pattern for the synthesis of another molecule.

transamination: the transfer of an amino group of an amino acid to another acid, forming an amino acid.

urea: one of the final products of nitrogen metabolism, a waste product excreted in the urine; when fed the nitrogen is utilizable, contributing to the total nitrogen need.

Study Questions and Activities

1. Define or explain the following terms: amino acid, essential amino acid, positive nitrogen balance, and polypeptides.

2. What method was used to determine the amino acids essential for young rats? For adult men?

3. What is the value of nonessential amino acids in the diet?

4. A diet that contains 4 g of nitrogen would contain approximately how much protein?

5. What is the meaning of "limiting amino acid?" Of what useful importance might this information be?

6. How can PKU be controlled when phenylalanine in the diet worsens the condition and phenylalanine is an essential amino acid?

References

1. Amino Acid Content of Foods and Biological Data on Proteins (1970). FAO Nutritional Studies No. 24. Rome: Food and Agr. Organ. pp. 36 to 162.

2. Anderson, C. F., R. A. Nelson, J. D. Margie, W. J. Johnson, and J. C. Hunt (1976). Nutritional therapy for adults with renal disease. In Present Knowledge in Nutrition. 4th ed. D. M. Hegsted, Chm. and Editorial Com. Washington, D.C.: The Nutrition Foundation Inc., p. 402.

3. Anderson, H. W., E. S. Cho, P. A. Krause, K. C. Hanson, G. F. Krause, and R. L. Wixom (1977). Effect of dietary histidine and arginine on nitrogen retention of men. *J. Nutrition,* **107:** 2067.

4. Bender, D. A. (1975). *Amino Acid Metabolism.* New York: John Wiley and Sons, Inc., p. 164.

5. Brady, R. O. (1976). Inherited metabolic diseases of the nervous system. *Science,* **193:** 733.

6. Cho, E. S., G. F. Krause, and H. W. Anderson (1977). Effects of dietary histidine and arginine on plasma amino acid and urea concentrations of men fed a low nitrogen diet. *J. Nutrition,* **107:** 2078.

7. Crim, M. C., and H. N. Munro (1976). Protein. In *Present Knowledge in Nutrition.* 4th ed. D. M. Hegsted, Chm. and Editorial Com. Washington, D.C.: The Nutrition Foundation Inc., p. 45.

8. Culliton, B. (1976). Genetic screening: States may be writing the wrong kind of laws. *Science,* **191:** 926.

9. Dalgliesh, C. E. (1957). Time factors in protein biosynthesis. *Science,* **125:** 271.

10. *Energy and Protein Requirements* (1973). FAO Nutrition Report Series No. 52; WHO Technical Report Series No. 522. Rome: Food and Agr. Organ., p. 48.

11. Hegsted, D. M. (1973). The amino acid requirements of rats and human beings. In *Proteins and Human Nutrition,* edited by J. W. G. Porter and B. A. Rolls. New York: Academic Press, p. 275.

12. Holt, L. E., and S. E. Snyderman (1961). The amino acid requirements of infants. *J. Am. Med. Assoc.,* **175:** 100.

13. Inoue, G., Y. Fujita, and Y. Niiyama (1973). Studies on protein requirements of young men fed egg protein and rice protein with excess and maintenance energy intakes. *J. Nutrition,* **103:** 1673.

14. Irwin, M. A., and D. M. Hegsted (1971). A conspectus of research on amino acid requirements of man. *J. Nutrition,* **101:** 539.

15. Jansen, G. R. (1977). Amino acid fortification. In *Evaluation of Proteins for Humans,* edited by C. E. Bodwell. Westport, Conn.: Avi Publ. Co., p. 177.

16. Johnson, C. F. (1972). What is the best age to discontinue the low phenylalanine diet in phenylketonuria? *Clin. Pediatrics,* **11:** 148.

17. Kopple, J. D., and M. E. Swendseid (1975). Evidence that histidine is an essential amino acid in normal and chronically uremic man. *J. Clin. Invest.,* **55:** 881.

18. Korslund, M. K., C. Kies, and H. M. Fox (1977). Protein nutrition value of urea supplementation of opaque-2 corn for adolescent boys. *Am. J. Clin. Nutrition,* **30:** 371.

19. Leverton, R. M., M. R. Gram, and M. Chaloupka (1951). Effect of the time factor and calorie level on nitrogen utilization of young women. *J. Nutrition,* **44:** 537.

20. A medical look at RNase synthesis (1969). *J. Am. Med. Assoc.,* **207:** 849.

21. Rose, W. C., R. L. Wixom, H. B. Lockhart, and G. F. Lambert (1955). The amino acid requirements of man. XV. The valine requirement; summary and final observations. *J. Biol. Chem.,* **216:** 225.

22. Sanger, F. (1955). The chemistry of insulin. *Science,* **129:** 1343.

23. Scrimshaw, N. S., J.-P. Habicht, M. L. Piche, B. Cholakos, and G. Arroyave (1966). Protein metabolism of young men during university examinations. *Am. J. Clin. Nutrition,* **18:** 321.

24. Smyth, D. G., H. H. Stein, and S. Moore (1963). The sequence of amino acid residues in bovine pancreatic ribonuclease: Revisions and confirmations. *J. Biol. Chem.,* **238:** 227.

25. Swendseid, M. E., and J. D. Kopple (1973). Nitrogen balance, plasma amino acid levels, and amino acid requirements. *Trans. New York Acad. Sci.,* **35:** 471.

26. Tontisirin, K., V. R. Young, W. M. Rand, and N. S. Scrimshaw (1974). Plasma threonine response curve and threonine requirements of young men and elderly women. *J. Nutrition,* **104:** 495.

27. Wixom, R. L., H. L. Anderson, B. E. Terry, and Y-B Sheng (1977). Total parenteral nutrition with selective histidine depletion in man. I. Responses in nitrogen metabolism and related areas. *Am. J. Clin. Nutrition,* **30:** 887.

97

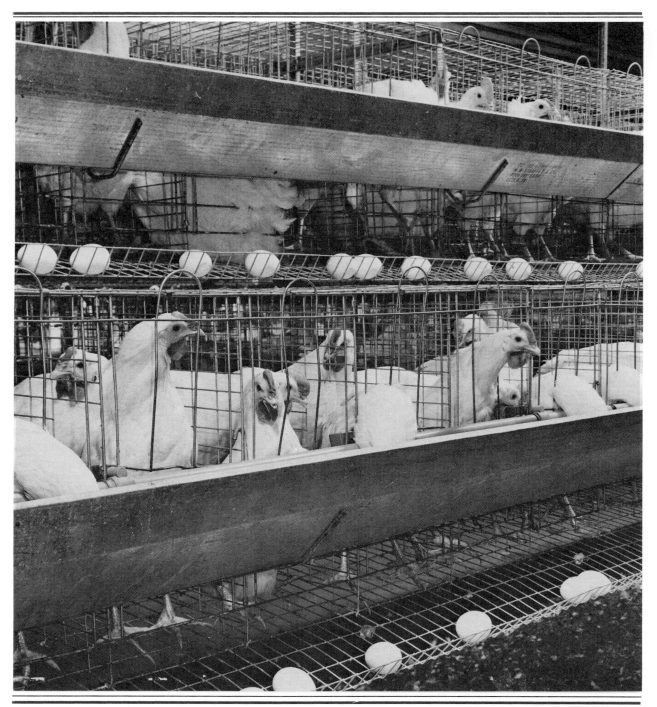

The hen's egg is used as a standard of protein quality worldwide.

Chapter 7

Proteins

Abbreviations

ADA: American Dietetic Association
—NH₂: amino or basic group
—COOH: carboxyl or acid group
FAO: Food and Agriculture Organization
INCAP: Institute of Nutrition of Central
   America and Panama
LPC: leaf protein concentrate
NPU: net protein utilization

PCM: protein–calorie malnutrition
PER: protein efficiency ratio
RDA: Recommended Dietary Allowances
SCP: single cell protein
SPC: soy protein concentrate
UNICEF: United Nations International Children's
   Emergency Fund
WHO: World Health Organization

The word "protein," derived from Greek, means "to come first." It was Gerardus Mulder, a Dutch chemist (1802–1880), who proposed the use of the term in 1838 because he believed that proteins were the most important of all known substances in the *organic kingdom.*

Protein is one of the most abundant components of the body; it is exceeded only by water. One-half of the dry weight of the body is protein, and it is distributed in the following manner: one-third in the muscles, one-fifth in the bones and cartilage, one-tenth in the skin, and the remainder in other tissues and body fluids. Urine and bile are the only fluids of the body that do not normally contain protein.

Composition of Proteins

The chemical elements that make up protein are carbon, hydrogen, oxygen, and nitrogen. Sulfur is found in some protein molecules, as are phosphorus, iron, iodine, and cobalt. Nitrogen is especially significant because it is always present in protein but does not occur in fat or carbohydrate. The building blocks of proteins are the amino acids (p. 86).

Proteins are more complex than either carbohydrates or lipids in terms of both size (molecular weight) and variety of constituent units. A polysaccharide, for example, is made up of repeated units of glucose, whereas a polypeptide is constituted of a variety of different amino acids.

There is an enormous number of different proteins (possibly as high as 10^{10} or 10^{12}). The combinations of different numbers and kinds of amino acids (there are about 20 different ones found commonly in proteins, see p. 86) and different sequential arrangements of the amino acids in the molecule make possible the astronomical number of different proteins that exist.

Classifications of Proteins

Because of the great number of proteins, attempts have been made to classify them. One simple procedure divides all proteins into two general classes based on chemical composition: simple proteins and compound or conjugated proteins. Simple proteins are substances that yield amino acids upon complete *hydrolysis.* Examples include the albumin of egg, zein of corn, keratin of hair, and globin of hemoglobin. Compound or conjugated proteins are compounds of a protein with some other nonprotein molecule. Examples include the hemoglobin (protein + *heme*) of blood, casein (protein + phosphoric acid) of milk, mucin (protein + carbohydrate) of saliva, and lipoprotein (protein + lipid) of blood.

100

Another classification is based on nutritional value, which is determined by content of the essential amino acids (p. 90) in the protein. This classification is discussed on page 105.

Still another classification is by conformation of the protein. Conformation refers to the three-dimensional shape of *native proteins;* conformation of a protein is determined by its amino acid sequence. The two major classes are fibrous proteins and globular proteins. The polypeptide chains of fibrous proteins are arranged in a parallel manner along an axis yielding long fibers (Fig. 7.1). Fibrous proteins are tough and are insoluble in ordinary solvents (water, dilute salt solutions). The following proteins are fibrous: the collagen of tendons and *bone matrix* (see Chapter 13); the α-keratin of hair, skin, nails, and feathers; and the elastin of elastic connective tissue, such as in the arteries of the *blood vascular system.* The polypeptide chains of globular proteins are, on the other hand, tightly folded into compact spherical or globular shapes (Fig. 7.1).

Most globular proteins are soluble in water and salt solutions. Almost all known enzymes and antibodies, many of the hormones, and many proteins with a transport function, such as hemoglobin (see Chapter 14), are globular proteins. There are also some proteins that have characteristics of both the fibrous and globular types. For example, myosin, a muscle protein, and fibrinogen (see Chapter 13), essential in blood clotting, have the structure of fibrous proteins and the solubility of globular proteins.

The architecture of proteins is classified as primary, secondary, tertiary, and quarternary structures. The primary structure is simply the sequence of amino acid residues in a polypeptide chain and its energy bonds; the secondary structure is the regular, recurring arrangement in space along one dimension as is characteristic of the fibrous proteins; the tertiary structure refers to the manner in which the polypeptide chain is bent into three dimensions to form the compact, tightly folded structure of globular proteins;

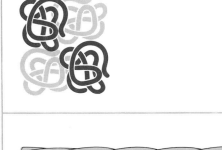

Globular proteins

The polypeptide chain is folded into a compact globular shape, called the tertiary structure. Short lengths of the polypeptide chain of globular proteins may also have regular coiled or zigzag secondary structure. In oligomeric proteins the three-dimensional packing arrangement of the polypeptide chains is referred to as the quaternary structure.

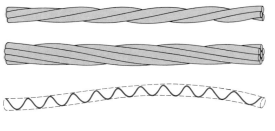

Fibrous proteins

The backbone of the polypeptide chain in a typical fibrous protein, α- keratin. The term secondary structure refers to regularly coiled or zigzag arrangements of polypeptide chains along one dimension.

Fig. 7.1 Fibrous and globular proteins. (From Lehninger, A. L., *Biochemistry,* 2nd edition. New York: Worth Publ., Inc. 1975, p. 61.)

and the quartenary structure refers to the manner in which individual polypeptide chains of a protein with two or more chains are arranged in relation to each other (Fig. 7.1; see ribonuclease, Fig. 6.4).

Digestion of Protein

Proteins are digested in the stomach and the small intestine; the major part takes place in the small intestine (Table 2.1). Enzymes bring about the breakdown of proteins into their constituent amino acids by hydrolysis. There are two types of enzymes: the endopeptidases, which attack peptide bonds of the inner portion of the amino acid chain, and the exopeptidases, which break down the terminal bonds (Table 7.1). When the amino acids and small peptides (chiefly dipeptides) enter the cells of the intestinal mucosa for absorption, enzymes present in the cells, amino peptidases, and dipeptidases act specifically on

Table 7.1. **Proteolytic Enzymes**

Place of action	Proenzyme	Place of production	Activating agent	Active form	Action
Endopeptidases: attack peptide linkages in the interior of a peptide chain					
Stomach	Pepsinogen	Stomach	Hydrochloric acid	Pepsin	Breaks down peptide linkages involving phenylalanine, tyrosine, or tryptophan
Small intestine	Trypsinogen	Pancreas	Enterokinase	Trypsin	Breaks down peptide linkages involving arginine or lysine
	Chymotrypsinogen	Pancreas	Trypsin	Chymotrypsin	Breaks down peptide linkages involving tyrosine, phenylalanine, tryptophan, or methionine
Exopeptidases: attack terminal peptide linkages of a peptide chain					
Small intestine	Procarboxypeptidase A	Pancreas	Trypsin	Carboxypeptidase A	Breaks down peptide linkage of amino acids in the terminal position of polypeptide chains
	Procarboxypeptidase B	Pancreas	Trypsin	Carboxypeptidase B	Breaks down peptide linkage of lysine or arginine in the terminal position of a polypeptide chain
	Proaminopeptidase	Intestinal mucosa	Trypsin	Aminopeptidase	Breaks down certain dipeptides
	Prodipeptidase	Intestinal mucosa	Trypsin	Dipeptidase	Breaks down certain dipeptides

From A. L. Lehninger (1975). *Biochemistry.* 2nd ed. New York: Worth Publ. Inc., p. 560.

the dipeptides, converting most of them to amino acids (2, 9, 32). The amino acids are absorbed into the portal blood. Food proteins are from 90 to 97 percent digestible; very little escapes unchanged into the feces.

Sometimes proteins escape digestion for some reason, and the intact protein may be absorbed. This occurs more frequently in the very young; their intestinal mucosa is more permeable than that of older children or adults. The allergy that some babies have to milk may be due to the entry of unchanged protein into the circulation.

Absorption and metabolism of amino acids are discussed in Chapter 6, pages 86–87.

Dynamic State of Body Protein

Body proteins are being continuously synthesized and degraded (23). Since, in the adequately nourished adult, the amount of protein remains constant, the two processes apparently proceed at equal rates. Protein is necessary in the adult's diet in order to maintain equilibrium because of losses that continuously occur through the urine, feces, and skin (see p. 92). Even on a protein-free diet (with an adequate energy intake), losses by these routes continue; the urinary nitrogen excretion decreases as the body stores of protein become depleted; the fecal excretion, which comes primarily from the digestive juices and desquamated epithelial cells of the alimentary tract, remains fairly constant. Excretion through the skin occurs as losses of cells, hair, and nails, as well as the nitrogen excreted in perspiration.

It has been recognized for more than a century that the various body tissues respond differently to changes in nutrition—some gain or lose protein more rapidly than others. Thus arose the concept of labile protein—protein that is available for rapid use in an emergency. It is called storage protein, reserve protein, circulating protein, or labile protein. The liver, intestinal mucosa, and blood (tissues where the turnover rate of protein is relatively high) provide labile protein. Muscle also provides labile protein (even though the protein turnover rate is relatively low) because of the large mass of tissue. Well-nourished animals have this reserve; poorly nourished ones do not. The capacity of the human body to accumulate labile protein probably does not exceed 5 percent of the total body protein. Investigators agree that there are no special cells to store protein as in the case of fat, nor special storage compounds such as glycogen, the storage form of carbohydrates. However, there are blood and tissue proteins that increase or decrease in quantity as the dietary nitrogen is raised or lowered, respectively. During fasting or when consuming a protein-free diet, labile protein disappears from the body in a few days.

By feeding *isotopically labeled* amino acids, it is possible to determine the turnover time of proteins in a particular tissue. Turnover, which is the rate at which given amounts of tissue proteins and enzymes are replaced by newly synthesized proteins, varies substantially in different parts of the body. It is fairly rapid among the proteins of the liver and blood plasma (six days to replace one-half of the protein) and slow among muscle proteins (180 days to replace one-half of the protein).

What factors determine when a given protein molecule will undergo degradation? It seems that it is not the age of the molecule that determines its breakdown, but certain properties of the protein itself. For example, the iron-containing protein *ferritin* is less subject to degradation when the iron content is high than when it is low. One theory accounting for certain differences in stability is that proteins that are absolutely indispensable to the body have more stability, whereas those that are not indispensable have less (43).

Functions of Proteins

Dietary proteins provide amino acids to build and maintain tissues, and to form enzymes, some hormones, and antibodies. Proteins function in some body regulating processes and are a source of energy.

Body Building

Although protein is present in every body cell, its nature and behavior in the various tissue cells differ. The protein in muscle allows it to contract and to hold fluid, which gives the muscle firmness even though it is composed of at least 75 percent water; the protein in hair, skin, and nails is hard and insoluble, providing a protective covering for the body; in the walls of the blood vessels, protein contributes elasticity, which is essential for maintaining normal blood pressure; the mineral matter of bones and teeth is embedded in a framework composed of protein.

The need for protein to build new tissue and to maintain existing tissue continues throughout life. Although new tissues are largely formed in childhood, the process does continue in adulthood; hair and nails continue to grow, and the outer layer of skin is periodically replaced. The total quantity of protein needed for maintenance increases with age until a fairly constant level is reached at around 18 years; this level continues throughout adulthood and old age. Expressed as amount per kilogram of body weight, the protein required decreases with age until about 25 years, after which it remains fairly constant throughout the remaining years.

Proteins provide amino acids for the synthesis of all enzymes, certain hormones, all antibodies, and as precursors to some vitamins (see Chapter 6, p. 88). The process of protein synthesis is discussed on page 88.

Regulating Body Processes

Movement of Fluid Most of the interchange of fluid between the capillaries and the surrounding *interstitial fluid* is by simple *diffusion*. Fluid movement is affected by the relationship in the capillaries between the blood pressure (capillary pressure) and the *osmotic pressure* exerted by plasma proteins. When the capillary pressure exceeds the osmotic pressure, the fluid leaves the capillaries and enters the interstitial fluid (filtration); when the reverse situation prevails, the fluid moves from the interstitial fluid into the capillaries (absorption).

The capillary membrane is passive and *selectively permeable*, permitting rapid passage of small molecules and *electrolytes* but not large molecules, such as plasma proteins. Osmotic pressure varies with the protein concentration: low plasma protein levels lead to reduced osmotic pressure and possible *edema*.

Control of Acid-base Balance in the Tissues
During normal metabolism, both acids and bases are formed, but the acids predominate. The body has several mechanisms for maintaining the acid-base balance at a normal level; one is the use of proteins as buffers. (Other substances also function as buffers, but proteins are the most abundant.) It will be recalled that an amino acid has two characteristic groups—a carboxyl or acid group ($-COOH$) and an amino or basic group ($-NH_2$)—enabling proteins to be *amphoteric* (Greek, *amphi* means "both"), to act either as an acid or a base and to neutralize to a degree both stronger acids and stronger bases. (For a further discussion of acid-base balance, see Chapter 15.)

Providing Energy

One gram of protein supplies approximately 4 kcal (17 kJ). In the ordinary American diet, 10 to 15 percent of the total energy intake comes from protein.

Carbohydrates and fats in the diet have a sparing effect on the need for dietary protein because they provide energy. This is especially important because carbohydrate foods are more abundant and less expensive than protein foods. When the total energy intake is inadequate, more dietary protein is used to help meet the need for energy,

104

Table 7.2. Nitrogen Balance Data in Relation to Energy Intake in g/day[a]

Energy intake	N intake	Fecal N	Urinary N	N balance
Adequate	5.28 ± 0.71	0.92 ± 0.23	4.21 ± 0.90	0.14 ± 0.46
Restricted	5.28 ± 0.71	0.85 ± 0.20	5.12 ± 0.79	−0.68 ± 0.44
Adequate	4.58 ± 0.53	0.95 ± 0.12	4.02 ± 0.37	−0.39 ± 0.30
Restricted	4.58 ± 0.53	0.89 ± 0.15	5.09 ± 1.17	−1.40 ± 0.78

[a] Summary of findings on seven young men.
From Y. S. M. Taylor, V. R. Young, E. Murray, P. B. Pencharz, and N. S. Scrimshaw. (1973) Daily protein and meal patterns affecting young men fed adequate and restricted energy intakes. *Am. J. Clin. Nutrition,* **26:** 1216.

and therefore less is available to meet the needs specific to proteins. The data from a nitrogen balance study (see p. 92) done with seven young men show that on a restricted energy intake, protein (the carbon portion) is used for energy, and the nitrogen released from the protein is excreted in the urine. There is a loss of nitrogen from the body resulting in a negative nitrogen balance. When the amount of dietary protein is low, the restricted energy intake results in a greater loss of body protein than when the protein intake is adequate (50) (Table 7.2). (See also p. 93).

The Effect of Exercise It is generally believed that exercise does not increase the need for protein if the energy intake is sufficient to cover the increased energy output. This makes sense because glycogen, not protein, is used in muscle contraction. Prolonged exercise or short intensive bouts can deplete the glycogen of the skeletal muscle and of the liver. However, fat also is a major source of energy and is used during prolonged exercise. The source of the fat is the triglycerides stored in muscle cells and the free fatty acids, which come from adipose tissue (53).

Under special conditions—if the athlete is young or on a muscle building training program— some additional protein is recommended. Buskirk and Haymes (10) at Pennsylvania State University

advise for those with additional need, a dietary protein intake of 2g/kg body weight/day. However, as a general rule, the increased food intake that normally accompanies exercise supplies enough additional energy and protein from a regular diet without the need of any special supplements or alterations.

The Nutritional Value of Proteins

Complete and Incomplete Proteins

Proteins differ in nutritive value because of differences in the kinds and amounts of their constituent amino acids (see p. 90). In early studies on the nutritional value of proteins (1911–1924), whole proteins were fed to young rats; different proteins elicited different responses. Casein supported growth; gliadin of wheat and rye supported growth only with the addition of the amino acid lysine; and zein of corn required the supplementation of two amino acids—tryptophan and lysine. If a protein contains all of the essential amino acids and in the proportions needed by the body, it is a complete protein, one of high *biological value.* All animal proteins, except gelatin, are complete as is the protein of the soybean, a plant protein. If a protein lacks enough of any of the essential amino acids, it is an incomplete protein, one of low biological value. All vegetable proteins with the exception of the soybean are incomplete.

Methods of Evaluating Protein Quality

Proteins differ in their capacity to support growth and maintain the nitrogen-containing compounds of the body. The efficiency of a given protein to perform these functions depends upon the presence of relative amounts of the essential amino acids in that protein. To appraise protein quality, its relative efficiency in satisfying amino acid requirements is measured. Methods of appraisal are important because of the shortage of good quality protein in the world and the effort to develop new protein sources (each of which must be evaluated). With each method, the nitrogen retained is measured either directly by balance studies (see p. 92 for discussion of balance studies) or (in the case of experimental animals) by carcass analysis or indirectly by the growth of young animals. There is also a method in which the essential amino acid content of the protein is utilized in computing the quality. The following are some of the more common methods of appraisal (18, 24, 44).

Protein Efficiency Ratio (PER)   The following is a measure of weight gain in young animals per gram of protein eaten:

$$PER = \frac{\text{Weight gain (g)}}{\text{Protein intake (g)}}$$

It is generally used with laboratory rats but can be used with children as well. Certain standardized procedures have been established for studies with rats: the intake of energy and other nutrients must be adequate; the intake of protein must be at least 10 percent by weight of the diet; and the study must be carried out over a four-week period. It is assumed that the weight gain will be proportional to the body protein gain. PER is the simplest method of determining quality because it requires no chemical analyses.

Net Protein Utilization (NPU)   This is the most common procedure for determining protein quality. NPU is the proportion of food N that is retained in the body under specified conditions. This method entails doing a nitrogen balance study or carcass analysis. The higher the retention on a given intake, the better the quality of the protein (see Appendix, Table A-9).

Amino Acid Score (Chemical Score)   By this method the quality of a protein can be estimated from its amino acid composition as compared with a reference pattern. The protein of whole egg and of human milk have been used as reference patterns. The FAO/WHO Committee on Energy and Protein Requirements (18) has suggested, in addition, a provisional amino acid pattern and called it the amino acid scoring pattern (Appendix Table A-10). The pattern was based on estimates of amino acid requirements of infants, school children, and adults (the groups for whom research findings on amino acid needs were available). The Committee emphasizes the provisional nature of the reference pattern, pointing out that it will undoubtedly be modified as additional information becomes available. In addition to the FAO/WHO amino acid scoring pattern, the protein of whole egg and of human milk continue to be used as reference patterns.

The limiting amino acid of a food (see p. 94) is used in computing the amino acid score of that food. The amino acid score is the concentration of the limiting amino acid per gram of protein of the food being tested expressed as a percentage of the concentration of this amino acid in a gram of protein of the reference food or scoring pattern (see Appendix, A-9 for equation). It may be that the amino acid score is the logical method for predicting quality if digestibility of the protein and availability of the amino acid for absorption are not interfering factors. Data is insufficient but from that available, it appears that digestibility is not an interfering factor (24).

Table 7.3. Calculation of Recommended Dietary Allowance for Protein for Adults

	Protein g/kg body weight
Average maintenance requirement from nitrogen balance studies	0.47
Allowance for individual variability (30 percent)	0.14
Total requirement for high quality protein	0.60
Correction for protein less efficiently utilized (25 percent)	0.15
RDA for the mixed protein of U.S. diet	0.75
	0.8 (rounded value)
70 kg man: 56 g per day	
58 kg woman: 46 g per day	

From *Recommended Dietary Allowances* (1974). 8th ed. Washington, D.C.: National Academy of Sciences, p. 40.

Table 7.4. Recommended dietary allowances for protein

	Age, years	RDA g	RDA g (1000 kcal)
Infants	0.0–0.5	kg × 2.2	—
	0.5–1.0	kg × 2.0	—
Children	1–3	23	17.7
	4–6	30	16.7
	7–10	36	15.0
Male	11–14	44	15.7
	15–18	54	18.0
	19–22	54	18.0
	23–50	56	20.7
	51+	56	23.3
Female	11–14	44	18.3
	15–18	48	22.9
	19–22	46	21.9
	23–50	46	23.0
	51+	46	25.6
Pregnant		+30	—
Lactating		+20	—

From *Recommended Dietary Allowances.* (1974). 8th ed. Washington, D.C.: National Academy of Sciences.

Need for Protein

RDA for Protein

For the adult, the RDA for protein is 0.8 g (a rounded figure) per kg of body weight daily. The recommendation for a 70-kg (154 lb) male student and a 58-kg (128 lb) female student is 54 and 46 g per day, respectively. In establishing this recommendation, the Food and Nutrition Board estimated, from the results of nitrogen balance studies, that an average maintenance requirement for adults was 0.47 g per kilogram per day, which allowed for the losses through the urine, feces, and skin (sweat, loss of hair, nails, and desquamating skin). In addition an allowance was made for individual variability in protein metabolism (30 percent) and for the variations in biological value of dietary proteins (25 percent) (38). The computations are summarized in Table 7.3.

Protein needs for all age and sex groups expressed as RDA and grams per 1000 kcal are shown in Table 7.4.

107

Food Sources of Protein

Although protein is widely distributed in nature, few foods contain large amounts (Table 7.5). Animal foods, such as meat, poultry, fish, milk, cheese, and eggs, contain high-quality proteins and in sufficient quantity to make them first in order of importance. However, plants are also a significant source: soybean protein is a complete protein, equal in quality to most animal proteins, and soybeans are high in protein content. Other legumes provide a good quantity of protein but contain an insufficient amount of methionine (5). Although nuts contain a good amount of protein, the quality remains to be assessed (11). Grain products are low in protein, but because they are consumed in large amounts, they contribute a significant proportion of protein to the diet. Grains do not contain enough of the amino acid lysine. Fruits and vegetables provide little protein; sugars, syrups, pure fats, and oils have none.

Table 7.5 Protein Content of Various Foods as Served

| | Per 100 g of food | Per average serving | |
Food	Protein g	Size of serving	g	Protein g
Chicken breast, fried	33	½ breast	79	26
Beef, round, cooked	28	3 oz	85	24
Tunafish, canned	28	3 oz	85	24
Bacon, med. sl., fried crisp	27	2 sl	15	4
Lamb, leg, roasted	26	3 oz	85	22
Peanut butter	25	1 tbsp	16	4
Cheese, Cheddar	25	1 oz	28	7
Pork loin, oven-cooked	25	3 oz	85	21
Egg	12	1 med	50	6
Soybeans, dry, cooked[a]	11	½ c	90	10
Bread, white, enriched	7	1 sl	28	2
Beans, red, canned	6	½ c	128	8
Lima beans, frozen, cooked	6	½ c	85	5
Ice cream, vanilla	4	1 c	133	5
Milk, whole	3	1 c	244	8
Potato, baked	3	1	156	4
Broccoli, frozen, cooked	2	½ c	92	2
Oatmeal, cooked	2	½ c	120	2
Green beans, snap, cooked	2	½ c	62	1
Lettuce, head	1	¼ head	142	1
Orange juice, frozen, reconstituted	1	½ c	125	1

From: *Nutritive Value of Foods,* Home and Garden Bull. No. 72. Washington, D.C.: U.S. Dept. Agr. 1977.

[a] *Nutritive Value of American Foods,* Agr. Handbook No. 456. Washington, D.C.: U.S. Dept. Agr., 1975.

Protein available for consumption in 1977 was provided by the following sources: meat, poultry, fish, 42.6 percent; dairy products, 22.0 percent; flour and cereal products, 17.6 percent; vegetables, 5.9 percent; dry beans and peas, nuts, soy flour, and grits, 5.4 percent; eggs, 4.8 percent; fruits, 1.1 percent; and miscellaneous, 0.6 percent (33).

All protein-containing foods (with the exception of gelatin) contain more than one kind of protein. For example, corn contains glutelin (which is a complete protein) and zein (which is incomplete); wheat contains glutenin (which is complete) and gliadin (which is not); milk contains two complete proteins, lactalbumin and casein. If sufficient corn or wheat could be eaten to satisfy the needs for essential amino acids from the complete protein that each contains, those grains could be considered complete proteins. But it is not physically possible to eat that much of either grain. Gelatin is itself a protein—an incomplete one.

Complementary Value of Proteins

Proteins can complement each other: the amino acid deficits of one protein can be supplied by another protein, and the two together can provide a higher quality protein than either alone (16). For example, most legumes are deficient in the sulfur-containing amino acids methionine and cystine but are usually high in lysine content. Lysine is deficient in cereals. Combining the two foods gives an amino acid pattern much nearer the amino acid pattern of a complete protein than either one alone. Some plant food combinations, in amounts that might be consumed at one or two meals, are presented with their methionine, lysine, and threonine content in Table 7.6), along with the values for those amino acids in egg (which is considered to have an ideal amino acid composition). Most combinations compare well with egg in lysine and threonine content but not as well for methionine. The quantity of plant foods that must be eaten to provide the amino acid values

of one egg is large. How well the amino acids from these various food sources are absorbed and utilized enters into the quality of protein resulting from the plant food combinations. Little research on this question has been done.

In some parts of the world where animal proteins are in short supply, vegetable protein mixtures with a small supplement of complete protein, in some cases, are prepared for infant food and weaning mixtures.

Superamine is one of the precooked protein mixtures that was developed jointly by WHO, FAO, and UNICEF as infant food (Fig. 7.2). It has been marketed in Algeria since 1967 with acceptance rising slowly. It is composed of hard wheat (28 percent), chick peas (38 percent), lentils (18 percent), sugar (5 percent), skim milk (10 percent), and a vitamin and mineral mixture (1 percent).

Researchers at the Institute of Nutrition of Central America and Panama (INCAP) have been interested in the development of all-vegetable

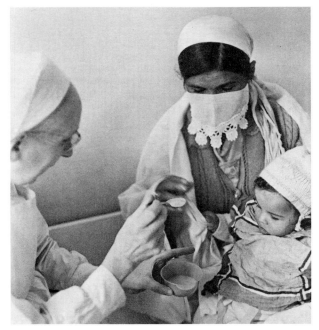

Fig. 7.2 An Algerian baby being fed Superamine. (F.A.O.)

109

Proteins

Table 7.6. Complementary Value of Proteins in Cereals, Legumes, and Nuts

Food combinations[a]	Dry[a] wt g	Cooked[b] Measure c	Cooked[b] Weight g	Protein g		Methionine[c] mg		Lysine[c] mg		Threonine[c] mg	
Beans, navy	62	1	180	14.8		145.1		987.7		468.7	
Rice	124	2	410	8.2	23.0	316.2	461.3	186.0	1173.7	290.2	758.9
Soybeans	58	1	180	19.8		304.5		1538.7		929.7	
Rice	62	1	205	4.1		158.1		93.0		145.1	
Wheat (whole meal)	32	1	245	4.4	28.3	62.7	525.3	119.7	1751.4	122.2	1297.0
Beans (navy)	62	1	180	14.8		145.1		987.7		468.7	
Wheat (whole meal)	64	2	490	8.8	23.6	125.4	270.5	239.4	1227.1	244.4	713.1
Soybeans	29	½	90	9.9		152.2		769.3		464.8	
Peanuts	36	¼	—	9.4		101.9		193.0		196.9	
Wheat (whole meal)	32	1	245	4.4		62.7		119.7		122.2	
Rice	62	1	205	4.1	27.8	158.1	474.9	93.0	1175.0	929.0	1175.0
Peanuts	72	½	—	18.7		243.4		745.9		550.1	
Sunflower seed	72	½	—	17.4	36.1	203.8	447.2	386.0	1131.9	393.8	943.9
Egg			50	5.7		580		696		464	
Recommended Allowance				kg/body wt		10 mg/kg		12 mg/kg		8 mg/kg	
Men 19/22 years				54		540		648		432	
Women 19/22 years				46		460		552		368	

[a] Combinations from *Manual of Clinical Dietetics* (1975). Chicago Dietetic Assoc. Inc., and S. Suburban Dietetic Assoc. of Chicago. Downers Grove, Ill.: Johnson Printers, Sec. 1, p. 3.

[b] Conversion of cooked to dry weights. Merrill, A. L., C. F. Adams, and L. J. Fincher. *Procedures for calculating nutritive values of home-prepared foods: As used in Handbook 8.* ARS62-13. Washington, D.C.: Agricultural Research Service, USDA, 1966.

[c] From *Amino Acid Content of Foods and Biological Data on Proteins.* FAO Nutritional Studies No. 24. Rome: Food and Agr. Organ., 1970.

mixtures that are high in protein. One of these, Incaparina, is now being produced commercially at low cost and requires little or no change in people's eating habits. Incaparina contains 29 percent whole ground corn, 29 percent whole ground sorghum, 38 percent cottonseed flour, 3 percent torula yeast (see p. 116), 1 percent calcium carbonate, and 4500 IU of vitamin A per 100 g. It can be made into a gruel or drunk as a beverage.

Such mixtures as Superamine and Incaparina are only available to those persons who buy their food in the market. Rural persons who consume chiefly home-grown food may have to rely upon mixtures of indigenous foods to supply their nutritional needs. In Haiti, a combination of 70 percent whole-grain cereal (rice, corn, or sorghum) and 30 percent beans *(phaseolus vulgaris)* was ground into a course flour and then enriched with minerals and vitamins. Groups of poorly nourished children (20 on the rice blend, 15 on the corn blend, and 21 on the sorghum blend) between one and five years of age were fed one of the enriched two-food mixtures three meals a day, six days a week for periods of six to eight weeks. The respective mixtures provided 90 percent of the

110

daily protein intake per child (23 g/rice blend, 32 g/corn blend, 39 g/sorghum blend) and 75 percent of the daily energy intake per child (637 kcal/rice blend, 738 kcal/corn blend, 874 kcal/sorghum blend). The children gained more weight during the experimental period than had been expected on the basis of other height–weight studies of Haitian children. The low serum protein concentrations (<6.0 mg/100 ml) and depressed serum albumin levels (<3.0 mg/100 ml) in about one-half the children rose to normal levels during this feeding program. The children who began with normal values maintained them (30). It is reasonable to assume that the improved condition of the children was due to the mixture because it made up such a large percentage of their diet.

A similar feeding experiment was carried out with four two-year-old children in Guatemala over a three-month period; 60 percent of the protein was from corn and 40 percent from beans, at a level of intake of 1.75 g/kg/day and 100 kcal/kg/day. Minerals and vitamins were added to make the diet completely adequate. The children were fed five meals daily; the excessive bulk limited the amount of food that could be eaten at one time. The children grew at a normal rate (3).

It can be concluded that a rational approach to providing adequate protein and energy is the use, in the majority of regions, of foods already available in the community. It is chiefly a problem of increasing the consumption of food and not providing special foods unavailable in the region (3).

Sources of Protein in Vegetarian Diets

Most people in the world subsist on foods that are largely of vegetable origin either because animal products are not available, or, if so, they are too expensive. Some people, however, are vegetarians by choice. In the United States, vegetarianism has long been practiced by certain religious groups. As part of its health and educational program, the Seventh-Day Adventist church practices vegetarianism. "To us, the whole matter of unclean food is primarily a question of health, for we believe that 'God is as truly the author of physical laws as He is the author of moral law' " (45). The Trappist monks, whose first monastery in the United States was established at Trappist, Kentucky, in 1848, are also vegetarians. The name of the order is "Order of Cistercians of the Strict Observance," which means complete renunciation not only of the world, its ambitions, and multiple concerns, but also of the monks' own judgment and taste. Writing about the life of these monks, one observer (52) said that a typical supper consisted of vegetables, bread, butter, and tea and that: "It would be very unappealing to the average person of the world, but it satisfies the monk who has nourished his soul throughout the day with the Bread of Life."

In recent years, there has been a trend, particularly among young adults, to become vegetarians (15). Their reasons for doing so are varied. For some it is health; they want a simpler diet and are opposed to the trend toward more convenience foods, which they feel are "removed from what is known to be safe and healthy" (54). Others are motivated by certain ethical or personal reasons. Among 100 American vegetarians, aged 21 to 35, 58 percent reported that their diets were the product of their spiritual, philosophical, or religious convictions (15).

Kinds of Vegetarian Diets Vegetarian diets are usually classified as: (a) lacto-ovo-vegetarian—an all-vegetable diet supplemented with milk, milk products, and eggs; (b) lacto-vegetarian—an all-vegetable diet supplemented only with milk and milk products; and (c) pure vegetarian (or vegan)—an all-vegetable diet containing no animal foods at all. In 1973 a study was made of 40 women and 60 men vegetarians (15 to 35 years of age) in a large city in the United States. It was found that 26 percent were lacto-ovo-vegetarian, 23 percent were vegans, 15 percent ate a vegetarian diet with either eggs or milk, 20 percent avoided only red meat and poultry, and 16 percent avoided only red meat (15).

111

Table 7.7 A One-Day Vegetarian Menu

Breakfast	Noon meal	Evening meal
Orange juice, 4 oz	Soy patties with tomato sauce, 2	Vegetable soup, 1 cup
Cooked oatmeal, 1 cup		Sandwich
Milk (LV),[a] 4 oz	Baked potato, 1	(whole wheat bread,
Soy milk (PV),[b] 4 oz	Margarine, 1 pat	2 slices, garbanzo-
Whole wheat toast, 1 slice	Peas, cooked, ²⁄₃ cup	egg filling) (LV)[a]
	Carrot salad, shredded ½ cup (scant)	Savory garbanzos (PV)[b]
Peanut butter, 1 tbsp	Dressing, ½ tbsp	Peaches, sliced, ½ cup
Clear hot cereal beverage, if desired	Wheat roll, 1	Walnut-stuffed dates, 4
	Margarine, 1 pat	Milk (LV),[a] 8 oz
	Strawberries, fresh or frozen (without sugar), ¾ cup	Soy milk (PV),[b] 8 oz
	Milk (LV),[a] 8 oz	
	Soy milk (PV),[b] 8 oz	

[a] Lacto-ovo-vegetarian (LV).
[b] Pure vegetarian (PV).
From U. D. Register and L. M. Sonnenberg (1973). The vegetarian diet. *J. Am. Dietet. Assoc.*, **62:** 253. Used by permission.

Table 7.8 Approximate Nutrient Composition of One-Day Vegetarian Diets.[a]

Nutrient	Lacto-ovo-vegetarian	Pure vegetarian	Recommended dietary allowances[b]
Energy, kcal	2030	2040	2000
Protein, g	78	75	46
Fat, g	76	77	—
Carbohydrate, g	260	265	—
Calcium, mg	1110	740	800
Iron, mg	18	24.8	18
Vitamin A value, IU	12,600	14,600	4000
Thiamin, mg	2.8	2.9	1.0
Riboflavin, mg	2.2	2.3	1.2
Niacin, mg	18.6	22.9	13.0
Vitamin C, mg	185	185	45

[a] For a woman 22–35 years of age.
From U. D. Register and L. M. Sonnenberg (1973). The vegetarian diet. *J. Am. Dietet. Assoc.*, **62:** 253. Used by permission.
[b] Recommended dietary allowances for a woman 23–50 years of age.
From *Recommended Dietary Allowances.* 8th ed. Washington, D.C.: Natl. Research Council, 1974.

Table 7.9 One-Day Vegetarian Menu with Variety Introduced by Use of ADA Food Exchange Lists for Meal Planning

Breakfast		Exchanges
Orange juice	½ c	1 fruit
Cooked oatmeal	1 c	2 bread
Milk (LV)[a]	½ c	½ milk
Soy milk (PV)[b]	½ c	
Whole wheat toast	1 slice	1 bread
Peanut butter	1 T	
Noon meal		
Soy patties	2	1 meat (nonmeat item)
Potato	1 small	1 bread
Margarine	2 tsp	2 fat
Peas, cooked	⅔ c	1⅓ bread
Carrot	½ c	1 vegetable
Salad dressing	2 tsp	1 fat
Wheat roll	1	1 bread
Strawberries (fresh or frozen)	¾ c	1 fruit
Milk (LA)[a]	1 c	1 milk
Soy milk (PV)[b]	1 c	
Evening meal		
Whole wheat bread	2 slices	2 bread
Egg	½	½ meat (nonmeat item)
Garbanzo (chick pea)	¼ c	½ meat (nonmeat item) (omit ½ bread exchange)
Peaches, sliced	½ c	⅔ fruit
Dates	4	2 fruit
Walnut halves	4	⅓ fat
Milk (LV)[a]	1 c	1 milk
Soy milk (PV)[b]	1 c	

[a] Lacto-ovo-vegetarian (LV).
[b] Pure vegetarian (PV).
Menu from U. D. Register and L. M. Sonnenberg (1973). The vegetarian diet. *J. Am. Dietet. Assoc.*, **62:** 253.

Planning Vegetarian Diets The chief departure of the lacto-ovo-vegetarian diet from the usual nonvegetarian diet is the replacement of meat by a variety of legumes, nuts, and products made from wheat and/or soy proteins. On the market are "meat analogs," simulated meat products made from vegetable proteins; some contain egg white or nonfat dry milk (35, 42).

A one-day menu planned for a lacto-ovo-vegetarian and a pure vegetarian is presented in Table 7.7. In Table 7.8 the approximate nutrient composition is presented along with the RDA (1974) for each of the nutrients. The diets as planned exceed the RDA for all of the nutrients. ADA Exchange Lists for Meal Planning (see Appendix Table A-12) can be used to introduce variety into the menu (Table 7.9).

Some planned vegetarian diets are not ade-

113

quate nutritionally; one of those is the Zen macrobiotic diet of the late George Ohsawa (39). Macrobiotics is also a philosophy: "Macrobiotics is a profound understanding of the orderliness of nature, the practical application of which enables us to prepare attractive, delicious meals, and achieve a happy and free life" (39). The diet has ten levels, progressively moving from a mixed diet of meat, vegetables, and cereals to the ultimate level to be achieved, a diet of brown rice alone. Brown rice does not provide an adequate diet. The protein of brown rice is not complete; it contains no vitamin A or vitamin C and insufficient amounts of other vitamins and of most minerals.

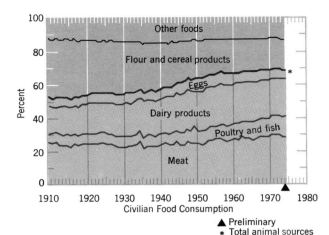

Fig. 7.3 Sources of protein. (*Handbook of Agricultural Charts,* Agr. Handbook No. 491. Washington, D.C.: U.S. Dept. of Agriculture, 1975, p. 66.)

Protein in College Meals

Meals served to college students were collected over a period of seven consecutive days at 50 colleges and analyzed for nutrient content in a U.S. Department of Agriculture study. The amount of protein in the meals exceeded the RDA at all colleges; the mean amount per person per day was 95.6 g with a range of 79.0 to 113.8 g (51).

Proteins in the Food Supply

In the United States

Since 1909 there have been generous amounts of protein available in the food supply of the United States. The USDA reported that the protein available for consumption in 1975 was 99 g daily per person; the estimate for 1977 is 103 g daily per person (33). There has been a gradual increase in the percentage of dietary protein from animal sources, from about 50 percent in 1909 to 70 percent in 1972. This means that, on the whole, people have been eating more meat, fish, poultry, dairy products, and eggs, but fewer grain products (Fig. 7.3).

Although protein foods are plentiful in the

United States as a whole, everyone does not consume enough to meet his nutritional needs. This is generally due either to poor food choices or to poverty.

In the World

The main concern is for enough food to feed the people of the world (17). A joint FAO/WHO committee on nutritional requirements came to the conclusion that it is quite likely that a dietary intake sufficient to cover the energy requirements would also be sufficient to meet the protein requirements (19). Findings from dietary studies done in India bear out the conclusions of the FAO/WHO committee (21). However, protein deficiency does occur where the staple foods are starchy roots, such as cassava and plantains, which are low in protein content. Consequently, a need for foods with a higher concentration of protein does exist; research has been in progress on developing such products. Some of the protein resources that have been investigated are improvement of cereals by genetic modification; isolation of proteins from oilseeds, nuts, and

114

leaves; production of single-cell proteins (such as algae, bacteria, yeast, and molds); fortification of foods with amino acids; and combinations of foods (especially vegetable plants) on the basis of amino acid content.

Genetic Improvement of Cereal Grains Through corn breeding experiments at the Purdue Agricultural Experiment Station, a special strain of corn, *Zea Mays* (which carries the gene designated *opaque-2*), was developed. In opaque-2 zein, the incomplete protein found in regular corn is reduced to one-half the usual concentration, while glutelin, a complete protein, is doubled. Both lysine and tryptophan are increased approximately 50 percent, and there is a better balance between leucine and isoleucine (less leucine and more isoleucine). The improved quality of opaque-2 corn has been demonstrated in feeding experiments with rats, infants, and young adults. The opaque-2 gene is now being introduced into the germ plasm of corn in other countries in an attempt to improve the quality of protein for the human population and for animal feed. Opaque-2 corn requires special treatment in milling and baking. A new corn with high quality protein, *sugary-2 opaque-2* has a harder kernel than opaque-2, a desired quality for culinary use (12). High lysine maize, sorghum, and barley have been developed; so have high protein rice and wheat. Mertz (34) believes that breeding for improved nutritional values in cereals has a bright future.

The cereal grain triticale, a cross between wheat and rye, produced by the International Maize and Wheat Improvement Center in Mexico in collaboration with the University of Manitoba (25), combines the yielding quality of wheat and the ruggedness of rye. The protein content of triticale is higher than that of common varieties of wheat; the lysine content is higher than that of wheat, approaching the level of rye. When triticale and wheat were fed to human adults at the same nitrogen level, the nitrogen balance was more favorable with triticale (29).

Seed, Nut, and Leaf Sources The isolation of protein from oilseeds and nuts is another means of increasing the supply of good quality protein. Some of these isolates are from soybeans. Soybeans have been eaten for thousands of years. They are prepared not only as cooked beans, but also as a milklike extract, as a precipitated curd of this extract (tofu), and as a variety of fermented products (such as tempeh). Soybeans are a source of food oil; the oil-free residue is high in protein content (50 percent). From this residue soy grits, soy flour, and the new soy protein concentrates (SPC) are made. These concentrates have a very high protein content (70 percent by one method of extraction; 90 to 98 percent by others). The SPC are used in baked goods, dairy-type products (whipped topping, beverage powder), ground meat preparations, and infant formulas (35, 36, 48). Research is being undertaken to develop protein isolates from cottonseed and peanuts.

Leaf protein concentrate (LPC) is being prepared and studied as a source of protein for human beings. Those who advocate its use do not claim that it is preferable to other sources of protein that might be developed, such as the increased production of legumes or the genetic improvement of cereals; they see LPC only as complementing other methods of obtaining protein. Methionine is the limiting amino acid in LPC. In experiments with malnourished infants, it was found that when LPC provided one-half of the nitrogen and milk the other half, the infants retained as much nitrogen as when they were given milk alone at the same level of nitrogen intake. LPC should only be used in conjunction with other sources of protein; when it has been the only source of protein, facial edema has been observed—possibly an allergic reaction. In regions where it is too rainy to dry seed crops, leaf protein production may be able to help alleviate the protein shortage (46).

Production of Single-cell Protein Single-cell protein (SCP) has come to be defined as protein whose source is either unicellular or simple multicellular organisms (yeast, bacteria, fungi, and algae) (48, 49). Yeast is the most popular SCP. Three types of food yeasts are available commercially: brewer's yeast, dried yeast, and dried torula yeast. Each differs in origin and method of cultivation. Brewer's yeast is recovered from the beer industry; molasses is the principal carbohydrate for cultivating dried yeast; and torula yeast uses sugar recovered from wood during the manufacture of wood pulp cellulose. Both brewer's and dried yeast have a somewhat higher quality protein than does torula yeast.

Yeast proteins are a good source of lysine and other essential amino acids, with the exception of methionine. Yeast also is high in total protein content, around 38 percent of the dry product. Therefore it is a good supplement for cereal grains, which are low in lysine and in total protein content (7).

The safety and acceptability of SCP from bacteria have not yet been determined. Unicellular algae are rich in protein, although deficient in the amino acids methionine and lysine. Studies with human beings show that algae are utilized more efficiently when they are eaten in small quantities or with other proteins. The digestibility of algae when eaten alone is low, 58 to 68 percent; mixing the algae with other foods improves its digestibility (31). There is a growing practice of using SCP in animal feeding. SCP is now produced commercially (41).

Fortification of Foods with Amino Acids and Proteins A question of international concern is the advisability of fortifying foods with amino acids, particularly the addition of lysine to cereal grains. Lysine is the essential amino acid that is least well supplied in cereals.

Research with animals shows that the addition of limited amounts of lysine to cereal diets improves their protein quality (13). In comparing young children who were fed wheat flour enriched with lysine as their source of protein with others who were fed unenriched flour, the former had a greater retention of nitrogen. This research was done in Peru (22) with children 11 to 24 months of age, and in Guatemala (8) with children 2 to 5 years of age. It was also found that girls from 7 to 12 years of age (observed in a boarding school) grew at a faster rate and stored more nitrogen when they ate kaffir corn enriched with lysine than when they ate the unenriched grain (14).

Regarding the feasibility of such fortification, the Joint FAO/WHO Expert Committee on Nutrition (19) concluded that fortification should be considered when the protein of a significant portion of a population is inadequate. However, insufficient protein is usually accompanied by an inadequate intake of energy. Therefore it is not clear whether much can be gained by additional amino acids or protein alone; it would be preferable to focus on increasing the food supply in general.

Protein Deficiency

Early symptoms of protein deficiency are nonspecific; they include loss of weight, fatigue, irritability, and lack of energy. In youngsters growth is retarded; this can readily be demonstrated in experimental animals by giving them a diet that is deficient in either quantity or quality of protein. Farmers and stock breeders are acutely aware of the need for adequate protein in order to ensure the best growth of their livestock.

Kwashiorkor is a severe clinical syndrome caused by a deficiency of protein; the condition may occur even though the intake of energy is adequate (40). Dr. Cecily Williams introduced the word "kwashiorkor" into the medical literature to describe a severe malnutrition *syndrome* that she had observed among young children in Ghana whose diet consisted of a maize gruel. Various definitions have been given for this word, which comes from the Ga tribe of Ghana. The most widely accepted definition is the disease of the "deposed child"—the one who has

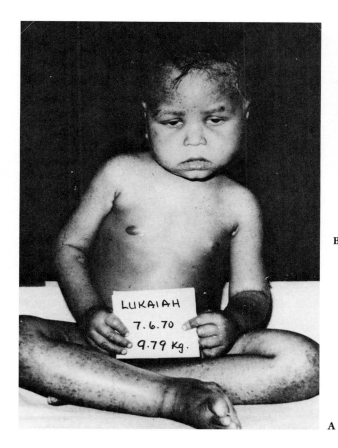

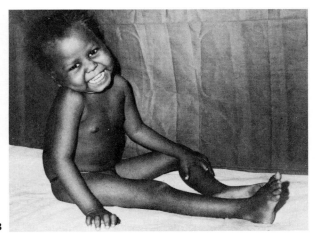

B

Fig. 7.4 (*A*) A child of 4½ years in a state of severe kwashiorkor showing edema; skin and hair changes; and misery. (*B*) The same child one month later following rehabilitation, edema-free; with normal skin, hair recovering; and happy. (W.H.O.)

A

been displaced by the birth of a new baby. Kwashiorkor occurs mainly among children between the ages of six months and three years. The second year of life is often the most vulnerable period. At that time the child may be weaned; he may make the transition from breast feeding to a diet that is high in carbohydrate and low in good quality protein just when he has an especially great need of protein for growth and the formation of muscle tissue.

Gopalan (21) noted in longitudinal studies of 300 Indian infants, 90 of whom were followed over a period of 3 years, that those who developed kwashiorkor and those who did not had essentially the same dietary pattern. Diarrhea or infections, such as chicken pox, were often the precipitating causes of kwashiorkor. At times, symptoms of

marasmus (wasting condition caused by insufficient food) and kwashiorkor exist in the same child. Some parts of the body are emaciated, but the face is moon-shaped (Fig. 7.4). Since one syndrome easily changes into the other, it was believed advisable to use one term for both conditions. In 1959, Jelliffe proposed the term "protein-calorie malnutrition" (PCM) for the whole spectrum of protein and calorie deficiencies, from distinct kwashiorkor at one end to distinct marasmus at the other. The Joint FAO/WHO Expert Committee on Nutrition accepted the term in 1970 (19, 28).

Exactly how prevalent PCM is on a worldwide basis is not known. Between 1966 and 1969, 80 surveys were made in 39 countries showing a prevalence of severe PCM between 0 and 7.6 percent in children below 5 years of age. Moderate PCM (second-degree malnutrition,[1] Gomez (20) classification) varied from 4.4 to 43.1 per-

---

[1] Second-degree malnutrition occurs when a child's weight is between 60 and 74 percent of the standard weight for his age.

117

cent in children under 5 years of age. The Joint FAO/WHO Expert Committee on Nutrition conceded that "existing knowledge is inadequate and that, from the available data, it is difficult to obtain even a rough estimate of the total number of malnourished children in the world." One of the difficulties in assessing the prevalence of PCM has been the lack of practical methods that are universally acceptable (19).

The characteristic symptoms of kwashiorkor are edema, lack of growth, muscle wasting with the retention of some subcutaneous fat, and psychomotor changes. Edema, according to Jelliffe (26), "is the cardinal sign of kwashiorkor and the syndrome should not be diagnosed in its absence." It gives children a deceptively plump appearance (Fig. 7.4). It is not known precisely how this fluid accumulation takes place. At one time it was believed that it was due to the fall in serum albumin that accompanies severe kwashiorkor. As the serum albumin drops, the osmotic pressure also drops, and so fluid passes from the blood into the tissues. However, observations of kwashiorkor do not confirm this explanation: children being treated for kwashiorkor lose their edema before their blood protein level rises (47).

The child with kwashiorkor is apathetic, inert, miserable, withdrawn, and without appetite. The hair may become a lighter color, straighter (if the normal hair is curly, as in Africa), more silky in texture, and loosely attached at the roots (as shown by its sparseness and easy pluckability) (26). Light-colored skin is a common characteristic of kwashiorkor, which can be more readily observed, of course, among darker-pigmented racial groups. The anemia of kwashiorkor results mainly from the lack of protein, although in some cases adding iron to the diet may hasten recovery (1). An occasional symptom of kwashiorkor is the flaky-paint rash, which resembles "dried paint that has long been exposed to sun, wind, and rain, and has commenced to flake off" (27), that appears on the buttocks, the backs of the thighs, and in the pelvic region.

A reduction in the prevalence of PCM can be obtained only by a comprehensive program involving both mother and child. Bengoa (6) points out that there must be surveillance of those at risk; there is no better tool than the growth chart. It detects deviation from the standard; it is a visual warning that the mother can comprehend. Education is essential and should place emphasis on breast feeding and should include introduction of supplementary feeding and weaning foods, food and personal hygiene, and family planning. Infection should be controlled chiefly through immunization programs and the early treatment of diarrhea. In some communities supplementary feeding programs may be advisable for the treatment and rehabilitation of malnourished children (4, 37, 54). (See Chapter 8 for a discussion of rehabilitation.) Food production activities at the community level may help considerably in the prevention of PCM.

Summary

Protein is one of the most abundant components of the body. The chemical elements present in all proteins are carbon, hydrogen, oxygen, and nitrogen. The building blocks of proteins are the amino acids.

Proteins are classified in various ways, one of which is on the basis of chemical composition, another by nutritional value, and also on the basis of conformation.

Digestion of protein takes place in the stomach and small intestine. The amino acids formed are absorbed from the small intestine into the portal vein.

Body proteins are continuously being synthesized and degraded and at equal rates. In the well-nourished, reserves of protein in the tissues are readily available.

Dietary proteins provide amino acids for building and maintaining tissues, and for the synthesis of enzymes, antibodies, and some hormones. Proteins function in some body-regulating processes and can serve as a source of energy.

Proteins differ in nutritive value because of differences in the kinds and amounts of their constituent amino acids. Animal proteins are of good quality; vegetable proteins are inferior, with the exception of soybean protein, which ranks well with animal proteins.

The RDA of 0.8 g per kilogram body weight daily for adults was established by adding to the maintenance requirement obtained from nitrogen balance studies a 30 percent allowance for individual variability and a 25 percent allowance for differences in the biological value of dietary proteins.

Some vegetarians are vegetarians by choice, others subsist on foods that are largely of vegetable origin because animal products are not available, or, if so, are too expensive. The protein content of vegetarian diets—whether they are lacto-ovo-vegetarian or pure vegetarian—can be adequate in both quantity and quality, if carefully planned.

There is a generous amount of protein available in the food supply of the United States. For 1977 it was 103 g daily per person, an amount that far exceeds the RDA for protein.

The main concern for the people of the world is that there be enough food to feed them. A joint FAO/WHO committee on nutritional requirements came to the conclusion that if the food consumed was enough to meet the energy needs, it would most likely meet the protein needs also. Even so, new protein resources are being sought through research.

Protein-calorie malnutrition occurs among the children of the world, particularly among those under five years of age.

Glossary

amphoteric: descriptive of a compound that has at least one group that can act as an acid and one group that can act as a base.

biological value: the relative nutritional value of a protein; the amino acid composition, digestibility, and availability of the products of digestion are taken into consideration.

blood vascular system: vessels that transport blood throughout the body.

bone matrix: the protein groundwork in which the minerals are deposited.

corn, opaque-2: genetically developed; lysine and tryptophan contents are significantly higher than that of common corn.

corn, sugary-2, opaque-2: corn with high quality protein; has harder kernel than opaque-2, a desired quality for culinary uses.

diffusion: the movement of molecules from a region of higher to one of lower concentration.

edema: an abnormal accumulation of fluid in the intercellular spaces of the body.

electrolyte: a substance that dissociates into two or more ions. Sodium chloride (table salt) dissociates into sodium (Na^+) and chloride (Cl^-) ions.

ferritin: an iron-containing protein; functions in the absorption of iron through the intestinal mucosa and serves as a storage form for iron in the liver, spleen, and other tissues.

heme: the nonprotein iron-containing constitutent of hemoglobin; it constitutes the pigment of the hemoglobin molecule.

hydrolysis: see page 19.

interstitial fluid: that portion of the body fluid between parts of or in the interspaces of a tissue.

isotopic label: marking a compound by introducing into it an isotope of one of its constituent elements, that is, using a form of the element with a different atomic mass. The atomic mass of carbon (C) is 12; an isotope of carbon has an atomic mass of 14, expressed in this manner ^{14}C.

native protein: a protein in its natural state.

organic kingdom: the animal and vegetable kingdoms.

osmotic pressure: the pressure that causes water or another solvent to move from a solution with a low concentration of solid (solute) to one having a high concentration of solute.

selective permeability: only certain substances are permitted to pass through the capillary membrane; others are rejected.

syndrome: a combination of symptoms resulting from a single cause.

Study Questions and Activities

1. Define or explain the following terms: complete protein, labile protein, simple protein, kwashiorkor, marasmus, single-cell protein (SCP).
2. What is the physiological significance of a situation in which all of the protein consumed by an individual must be used to meet his energy needs?
3. How many grams of protein did you consume yesterday? Did you meet your RDA for protein? What percentage of the protein consumed was of high biological value?
4. What is the approximate cost for one day of an inexpensive menu (adequate in protein content) for a college-age girl weighing 50 kg and for a young man weighing 80 kg?
5. Compare the cost of 10 g of protein from the following: eggs, rolled boneless roast, chicken; and milk. Obtain the local prices for these foods. Assume that each egg weighs 50 g; that cooking will reduce the weight of the boneless roast by one-third; that cooking and removing the bones from the chicken will reduce its weight by two-thirds. Use the food composition table (Appendix Table A-3) or Table 7.5 to determine the protein content of these foods.

References

1. Adam, E. B. (1969). Anemia associated with kwashiorkor. *Am. J. Clin. Nutrition,* **22:** 1634.
2. Adibi, S. A. (1976). Intestinal phase of protein assimilation in man. *Am. J. Clin. Nutrition,* **29:** 205.
3. Arroyave, G. (1975). Amino acid requirements and age. In *Protein-Calorie Malnutrition,* edited by R. E. Olson. New York: Academic Press, p. 1.
4. Ashworth, A. (1969). Growth rates in children recovering from protein–calorie malnutrition. *Brit. J. Nutrition,* **23:** 835

5. Aykroyd, W. R., and J. Doughty (1964). *Legumes in Human Nutrition.* FAO Nutritional Studies No. 19. Rome: Food and Agr. Organ., p. 75.
6. Bengoa, J. M. (1975). Prevention of protein–calorie malnutrition. In *Protein–Calorie Malnutrition,* edited by R. E. Olson. New York: Academic Press, p. 435.
7. Bressani, R. (1968). The use of yeast in human foods. In *Single-Cell Protein,* edited by R. I. Mateles and S. R. Tannenbaum. Cambridge, Mass.: M.I.T. Press, p. 90.
8. Bressani, R., O. W. Nilson, M. Behar, and N. S. Scrimshaw (1960). Supplementation of cereal proteins with amino acids. III. Effect of amino acid supplementation of wheat flour as measured by nitrogen retention of young children. *J. Nutrition,* **70:** 176.
9. Brobeck, J. R., ed. (1973). *Best and Taylor's Physiological Basis of Medical Practice.* 9th ed. Baltimore: Williams and Wilkins Co., pp. 2–51.
10. Buskirk, E., and E. Haymes (1972). Nutritional requirements for women in sports. In *Women and Sport: A National Research Council Conference,* edited by D. Harris. University Park: Pennsylvania State University.
11. Butler, L. C., V. T. Dawson, and Y. L. Adams (1970). Utilization by young women of peanut flour equalized to the FAO pattern. *Am. J. Clin.* **23:** 1169.
12. Clark, H. E., D. V. Glover, J. L. Betz, and L. B. Bailey (1977). Nitrogen retention of young men who consumed isonitrogenous diets containing normal, *Opaque-2* or *Sugary-2* corn. *J. Nutrition,* **107:** 404.
13. Daniel, V. A., B. L. M. Desai, D. Narayanaswamy, S. Kurien, M. Swaminathan, and H. A. B. Parpia (1970). Development of protein value of poor wheat diet by supplementation with limiting amino acids. *Nutrition Reports Int.,* **1:** 169.
14. Doraiswamy, T. R., T. S. Subramanya Raj Urs, S. Venkat Rao, M. Swaminathan, and H. A. B. Parpia (1968). Effect of supplementation of poor kaffir corn diet *(sorghum vulgare)* with L-lysine on nitrogen retention and growth of school children. *Indian J. Nutrition and Dietet.,* **5:** 191.

120

15. Dwyer, J. T., L. D. V. H. Mayer, K. Dowd, R. F. Kandel, and J. Mayer (1974). The new vegetarians: The natural high? *J. Am. Dietet. Assoc.*, **65:** 529.

16. Food and Agriculture Organization (1970). *Amino Acid Content of Foods and Biological Data on Proteins.* FAO Nutritional Studies No. 24. Rome: Food and Agr. Organ.

17. Food and Agriculture Organization (1976). *The State of Food and Agriculture 1975.* FAO Agriculture Series No. 1. Rome: Food and Agr. Organ., p. 75.

18. Food and Agriculture Organization/World Health Organization (1973). *Energy and Protein Requirements.* FAO Nutrition Meetings Rept. Series No. 52 and WHO Tech. Rept. Series No. 522. Rome: Food and Agr. Organ.

19. Food and Agriculture Organization/World Health Organization (1971). *FAO Nutrition Meetings Rept. Series No. 49. Eighth Report.* Rome: Food and Agr. Organ., p. 36.

20. Gomez, F., R. R. Galvan, J. Cravioto, and S. Frenk (1955). Malnutrition in infancy and childhood, with special reference to kwashiorkor. In *Advances in Pediatrics,* vol. 7, edited by S. Levine. Chicago: Year Book Medical Publishers, p. 131.

21. Gopalan, C. (1975). Protein versus calories in the treatment of protein–calorie malnutrition: Metabolic and population studies in India. In *Protein–Calorie Malnutrition,* edited by R. E. Olson. New York: Academic Press, p. 329.

22. Graham, G. G., R. P. Placko, G. Acevedo, E. Morales, and A. Cordano (1969). Lysine enrichment of wheat flour: evaluation in infants. *Am. J. Clin. Nutrition,* **22:** 1459.

23. Harper, A. E. (1974). Improvement of protein nutriture. In *Improvement of Protein Nutriture.* Washington, D.C.: National Academy of Sciences, p. 1.

24. Hegsted, D. M. (1974). Assessment of protein quality. In *Improvement of Protein Nutriture.* Washington, D.C.: National Academy of Sciences, p. 64.

25. Hulse, J. H., and D. Spurgeon (1974). Triticale. *Scientific American,* **231:** 72.

26. Jelliffe, D. B. (1966). *The Assessment of the Nutritional Status of the Community.* Geneva: World Health Organ., p. 182.

27. Jelliffe, D. B. (1968). *Infant Nutrition in the Subtropics and Tropics.* 2nd ed. Geneva: World Health Organ., p. 126.

28. Jelliffe, E. F. P. (1975). *Protein–Calorie Malnutrition of Early Childhood: Two Decades of Malnutrition.* Slough, England: Commonwealth Agricultural Bureaux.

29. Kies, C., and H. M. Fox (1970). Protein nutritive value of wheat and triticale grain for humans, studies at two levels of protein intake. *Cereal Chemistry,* **47:** 671.

30. King, K. W., W. Fougere, J. Foucald, G. Dominique, and I. D. Beghin (1966). Response of pre-school children to high intakes of Haitian cereal-bean mixtures. *Arch. Latinomericanos de Nutricion,* **16:** 53.

31. Lachance, P. A. (1968). Single-cell protein in space systems. In *Single-cell Proteins,* edited by R. I. Mateles and S. R. Tannenbaum. Cambridge, Mass.: M.I.T. Press, p. 145.

32. Latner, A. L. (1975). *Cantarow and Trumper Clinical Biochemistry.* 7th ed. Philadelphia: W. B. Saunders, p. 148.

33. Marston, R., and B. Friend (1978). Nutrient content of the national food supply. In *National Food Review.* NFR1, January. Washington, D.C.: Economic Research Service, USDA, p. 25.

34. Mertz, E. T. (1976). Genetic improvement of cereal proteins. In *Nutrition and Agricultural Development,* edited by N. S. Scrimshaw and M. Behar. New York: Plenum Press, p. 465.

35. Meyer, E. W. (1970). Soya protein isolates for food. In *Proteins as Human Food,* edited by R. A. Lawrie. Westport, Conn.: Avi Publishing Co., p. 355.

36. Milner, M. (1969). Status of development and use of some unconventional proteins. In *Protein-enriched Cereal Foods for World Needs,* edited by M. Milner. St. Paul: American Association of Cereal Chemists, p. 97.

37. Monckeberg, F. (1975). The effect of malnutrition on physical growth and brain development. In *Brain Function and Malnutrition,* edited by J. W.

121

Prescott, M. S. Read, and D. B. Coursin. New York: John Wiley and Sons, p. 15.

38. National Academy Sciences–National Research Council (1974). *Recommended Dietary Allowances*. 8th ed. Washington, D.C.: National Academy of Sciences.

39. Ohsawa, G. (1971). *Macrobiotics: An Invitation to Health and Happiness*. San Francisco: George Ohsawa Macrobiotic Foundation Inc.

40. Olson, R. E. (1975). The effect of variations in protein and calorie intake on the rate of recovery and selected physiological responses in Thai children with protein–caloric malnutrition. In *Protein–Calorie Malnutrition*, edited by R. E. Olson. New York: Academic Press, p. 275.

41. Protein–Calorie Advisory Group of the United Nations System (1976). Symposium on hydrocarbon-grown single cell protein products for animal feeding. *PAG Bulletin*, **6**(3): 1–50.

42. Raper, N. R. (1974). Vegetarian diets. *Family Econ. Rev.* Summer. Washington, D.C.: U.S. Dept. Agr.

43. Schimke, R. T. (1970). Regulation of protein degradation in mammalian tissues. In *Mammalian Protein Metabolism*, vol. 4, edited by H. N. Munro. New York: Academic Press, p. 212.

44. Scrimshaw, N. S., D. I. C. Wang, and M. Milner (1975). *Protein Resources and Technology: Status and Research Needs*. Washington, D.C.: National Science Foundation, p. 38.

45. *Seventh-day Adventists Answer Questions on Doctrine* (1957). Washington, D.C.: Review and Herald Publishing Assoc.

46. Singh, N. (1971). Feeding trials with children. In *Leaf Protein: Its Agronomy, Preparation, Quality and Use*, edited by N. W. Pirie. Oxford, England: Blackwell Scientific Publ., p. 131.

47. Srikantia, S. G. (1968). The causes of oedema in protein calorie malnutrition. In *Calorie Deficiencies and Protein Deficiencies*, edited by R. A. McCance and E. M. Widdowson. Boston: Little, Brown, p. 203.

48. Tannenbaum, S. R. (1971). Potential for new protein sources. In *Amino Acid Fortification of Protein Foods*, edited by N. S. Scrimshaw and A. M. Altschul. Cambridge, Mass.: M.I.T. Press, p. 139.

49. Tannenbaum, S. R., and D. I. C. Wang, ed. (1975). *Single-cell Protein II*. Cambridge, Mass.: M.I.T. Press.

50. Taylor, Y. S. M., V. R. Young, E. Murray, P. B. Pencharz, and N. S. Scrimshaw (1973). Daily protein and meal patterns affecting young men fed adequate and restricted energy intakes. *Am. J. Clin. Nutrition*, **26**: 1216.

51. Walker, M. A., and L. Page (1975). Proximate composition and vitamins of college meals. *J. Am. Dietet. Assoc.*, **66**: 146.

52. Whalen, C. W. (1945). *The Trappist Way*. Boston: Richard J. Cushing, Archbishop of Boston.

53. Williams, M. H. (1976). *Nutritional Aspects of Human Physical and Athletic Performance*. Springfield, Ill.: Charles C. Thomas, p. 73.

54. Winick, M. (1976). Early malnutrition brain structure and function. *Nutrition Notes*. American Institute of Nutrition, **12**: 1.

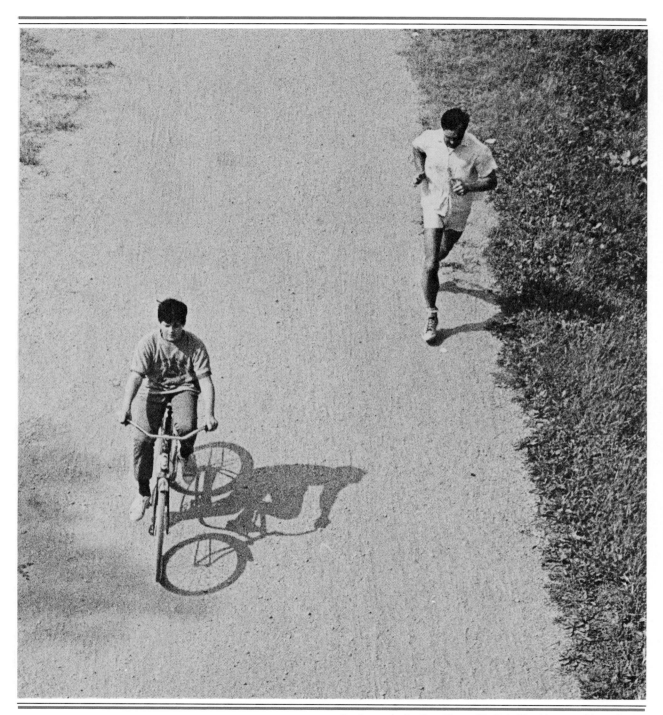

Regular exercise (together with a sensible diet) will enable one to achieve and maintain his ideal weight and good muscle tone.

Abbreviations

ATP: adenosine triphosphate
BMR: basal metabolic rate
C: Centigrade or Celsius
CO_2: Carbon dioxide
F: Fahrenheit
HANES: First Health and Nutrition Examination
 Survey

H_2O: water
kg: kilogram
min.: minute
MJ: megajoule
RDA: Recommended Dietary Allowances

Energy is needed by an individual to maintain life, to support growth, and to perform voluntary activities. The carbohydrates, fats, and proteins of the diet supply this energy. The desirable energy intake is one that matches the individual's energy need.

Weight control includes the problem of both those who weigh more and those who weigh less than their optimal weight. In the United States the greater problem is with those who weigh more than they should.

The Need for Energy

The amount of carbohydrate, fat, and protein in a food determines its energy value. The energy in these compounds comes from sunlight. The plant has a unique capacity to convert solar energy into the chemical energy of a variety of organic compounds (Fig. 8.1). Through the process of photosynthesis, water and carbon dioxide combine to form carbohydrate. Photosynthesis takes place because of the catalytic influence of the green pigment chlorophyll located in chloroplasts—small granules in the plant cell that are visible only with an electron miscroscope.

By means of radioactive carbon (isotopic carbon) and refined analytical methods, it has been possible to follow the pathway of carbon in photosynthesis. Radioactive carbon has been found not only in carbohydrate but also in the lipids and amino acids of the plant. The photosynthetic process takes place in the minute chloroplasts of the cell through many reactions and the formation of many intermediary compounds.

Because animals and man are dependent on food as a source of energy to do body work and maintain body temperature, it is obvious that photosynthesis is basic to life itself (Fig. 8.2). After food is ingested, digested, absorbed, and metabolized, the food energy is transferred to form the important compound adenosine triphosphate (ATP) (10). (ATP has been called an "energy currency" because it can be created and expended by the cells.) The energy from ATP is used by the cells as energy for the synthesis of body nutrients, proteins, nucleic acid, and other materials; for the contraction of muscles; for the conduction of nerve impulses; for glandular secretion; for the transport of substances through membranes (for example, sodium and potassium exchange in cells); and other functions (Fig. 8.2).

Only about 40 percent of the energy in food is transferred to create ATP (12); the rest becomes heat (Fig. 8.2). Of the total energy generated by working muscles, for example, only 20 percent of the energy is used for mechanical work (14). Because energy becomes heat both in the formation

126

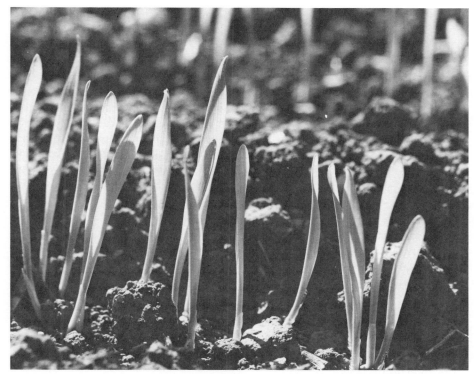

Fig. 8.1 Young wheat converting solar energy into chemical energy. (Grant Heilman.)

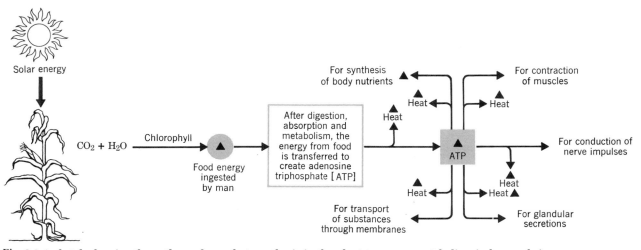

Fig. 8.2 A sketch showing the pathway from photosynthesis in the plant to energy metabolism in human beings.

127

of ATP and in the transfer of ATP energy to the cells, not more than 25 percent of all the energy from food is finally used by the cells for body work (10).

The process that food nutrients undergo in order to release energy for use by the cell is called energy metabolism.

Definition of Terms

A calorie is the standard unit for measuring food energy. The calorie used in nutrition is the kilocalorie (kcal) or large calorie (Cal). This unit is 1000 times larger than the small calorie (cal) used in chemistry and physics. The word "calorie," which is often used to describe the potential energy of food, is a unit of measure of heat (and not a nutrient).

A joule (pronounced "jool") is another unit for measuring work and energy. The kilojoule (kJ) is the unit used in nutrition and is 1000 times larger than the joule (J). Another unit that expresses human energy allowances is the megajoule (MJ); it is 1 million times larger than the joule and 1000 times larger than the kilojoule; it is sometimes used when presenting the energy content of diets that exceed 1000 kJ.

Calorimetry is the measurement of the amount of heat given off. The energy value of a particular food and the daily energy needs of a person are both determined by calorimetry and expressed in terms of kilocalories or kilojoules. If the actual heat produced is measured, it is called direct calorimetry; if heat production is measured indirectly, it is called indirect calorimetry.

A *calorimeter* is the instrument for measuring the kilocalories or kilojoules of heat produced. The energy value of foods is measured by either the oxycalorimeter or bomb calorimeter (Fig. 8.3). Two instruments that have been used to measure the heat production of man-directly or indirectly—are the Armsby Calorimeter (Fig. 8.6) and the Benedict-Roth apparatus.

The Kilocalorie and the Kilojoule About 90 percent of the world's population will soon be using the metric system of weights and measures. Because of this, the joule has been selected by international groups as the measuring unit for electrical work, heat, mechanical work, and energy in all sciences including nutrition (11). This means that the kilojoule will eventually replace the kilocalorie as the unit of energy in nutrition.

The Metric Conversion Act, passed by Congress in 1975, provides for the voluntary conversion to the metric system in the United States within ten years. The National Bureau of Standards, however, adopted the joule as the preferred unit of energy measurement in 1964. At the 1970 meeting of the American Institute of Nutrition, it was recommended "that replacement of the kilocalorie by the kilojoule (kJ) be effected in principal nutritional journals as soon as the mechanics of the transition can be established" (16). It has also been recommended that Canada adopt the kilojoule as the energy measurement unit for nutrition by 1980 (21). To introduce the student to the relationship between these two units of energy measurement, a conversion table is presented in Table 8.1.

Table 8.1. A Conversion Table for the Calorie and the Joule.

1 kilocalorie (kcal)	=	1000	cal
	=	1	Cal
	=	4.184	kJ
	=	4184	J
1 kilojoule (kJ)	=	240	cal
	=	0.24	Cal
	=	0.24	kcal
	=	1000	J
1 megajoule (MJ)	=	240	Cal
	=	240	kcal
	=	1000	kJ
	=	1,000,000	J

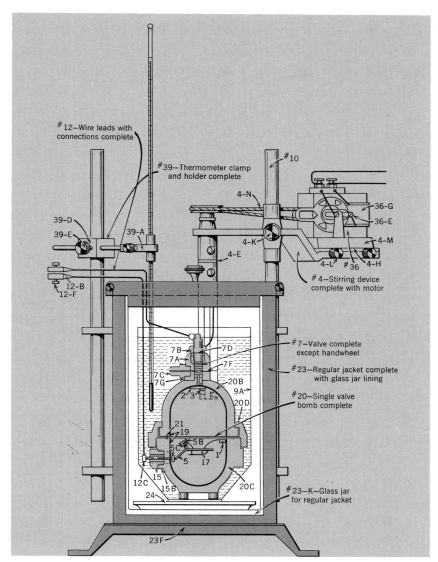

Fig. 8.3 A cross-section view of the Emerson oxygen bomb calorimeter. The apparatus consists of two parts: the bomb, in which the food is burned, and the water bath, in which the heat produced by the combustion is measured. (Courtesy Arthur H. Thomas Company, Philadelphia.)

129

Table 8.2. Data Used for Calculating Energy Values of Selected Foods.

Food	Protein			Fat			Carbohydrate		
	Coefficient of digestibility, %	Heat of combustion less 1.25,[a] kcal/g	Factor to be applied to ingested nutrients, kcal/g	Coefficient of digestibility, %	Heat of combustion, kcal/g	Factor to be applied to ingested nutrients, kcal/g	Coefficient of digestibility, %	Heat of combustion, kcal/g	Factor to be applied to ingested nutrients, kcal/g
Butter	97	4.40	4.27	95	9.25	8.79	98	3.95	3.87
Cane or beet sugar (sucrose)	—	—	—	—	—	—	98	3.95	3.87
Eggs	97	4.50	4.36	95	9.50	9.02	98	3.75	3.68
Fruits, All (except lemons, limes)	85	3.95	3.36	90	9.30	8.37	90	4.00	3.60
Immature lima beans, cowpeas, peas, other legumes	78	4.45	3.47	90	9.30	8.37	97	4.20	4.07
Macaroni, spaghetti	86	4.55	3.91	90	9.30	8.37	98	4.20	4.12
Margarine, vegetable	97	4.40	4.27	95	9.30	8.84	98	3.95	3.87
Mature dry beans, cowpeas, peas, other legumes, nuts	78	4.45	3.47	90	9.30	8.37	97	4.20	4.07
Meat, fish	97	4.40	4.27	95	9.50	9.02	—	—	[b]
Milk, milk products	97	4.40	4.27	95	9.25	8.79	98	3.95	3.87
Other cereals, refined	85	4.55	3.87	90	9.30	8.37	98	4.20	4.12
Other vegetable fats and oils	—	—	—	95	9.30	8.84	—	—	—
Potatoes and starchy roots	74	3.75	2.78	90	9.30	8.37	96	4.20	4.03
Rice, white or polished	84	4.55	3.82	90	9.30	8.37	99	4.20	4.16
Wheat, 97–100 percent extraction	79	4.55	3.59	90	9.30	8.37	90	4.20	3.78
Wheat, 85–93 percent extraction	83	4.55	3.78	90	9.30	8.37	94	4.20	3.95
Wheat, 70–74 percent extraction	89	4.55	4.05	90	9.30	8.37	98	4.20	4.12
Wheat, flaked, puffed, rolled, shredded, whole meal	79	4.55	3.59	90	9.30	8.37	90	4.20	3.78
Wheat bran (100 percent)	40	4.55	1.82	90	9.30	8.37	56	4.20	2.35

[a] The correction, 1.25 kilocalories, has been subtracted from the heat of combustion. This gives values applicable to grams of digested protein and identical with Atwater's factors per gram of available protein.

[b] Carbohydrate factor, 3.87 for brain, heart, kidney, and liver; 4.11 for tongue and shellfish.

From A. L. Merrill and B. K. Watt, *Energy Value of Foods*, Agr. Handbook No. 74 revised. Washington, D.C.: U.S. Dept. Agr., 1973, p. 25.

130

Table 8.3. **Calculating the Physiological Fuel Values of the Energy Nutrients**

	Carbohydrate	Fat	Protein
Fuel values (bomb calorimeter), kcal/g	4.10	9.45	5.65
Loss due to incomplete combustion of nitrogen, kcal/g	0	0	−1.25
Percentage of digestibility	98	95	92
Physiological fuel values, kcal/g	4 (17 kJ)	9 (38 kJ)	4 (17 kJ)

Physiological Fuel Value of Foods The energy obtained by man (as well as animals) from food ingested is less than that released from the same food when it is oxidized in the bomb calorimeter. In the calorimeter, foods are completely oxidized to carbon dioxide, water, and nitrous oxide. However, it is different with man: the energy available to the body is the gross energy of the diet minus the losses in the urine and feces. Foods eaten are not completely digested (resulting in energy loss in the feces), and the nitrogen of protein is not completely oxidized (resulting in energy loss in the nitrogen-containing compounds excreted in the urine). Digestibility varies from one food to another for each of the energy nutrients (protein, fat, and carbohydrate) (see Table 8.2). Digestibility is the percent of the ingested protein or fat or carbohydrate absorbed. In the case of protein, for example, digestibility is expressed as follows:

$$\frac{\text{Food nitrogen} - \text{feces nitrogen}}{\text{Food nitrogen}} \times 100 = \text{Percent of food nitrogen absorbed}$$

The value obtained indicates apparent absorption and is called the "coefficient of digestibility" or "percentage digestibility."

Urea and other nitrogenous compounds eliminated in the urine have energy value (an average of 1.25 kcal per gram of protein, corrected for digestibility, ingested). To compute the physiological fuel value of protein, the 1.25 kcal per gram of protein is subtracted from the heat of combustion and then corrected for incomplete digestibility; for carbohydrate and fat, it is only necessary to correct for incomplete digestibility. Data for calculating the energy values of foods or food groups are given in Table 8.2.

For making rapid estimates, an average figure for each of the energy nutrients was established to be used with all foods. The average physiological fuel values were determined by taking the means of the values for the heat of combustion and the coefficients of digestibility of various foods and food groups, weighted according to the prevalence of these foods in the U.S. diet (a sample of 185 diets) in 1897. The rounded figures are 4 kcal (17 kJ) per gram of protein, 9 kcal (38 kJ) per gram of fat, and 4 kcal (17 kJ) per gram of carbohydrate (Table 8.3).

Factors that Determine Total Energy Need

The total energy need of an adult depends upon his basal metabolism, his physical activity, and the specific dynamic effect of his food. The metabolism of food (which results in an increase in heat production)—the specific dynamic effect—requires the smallest percentage of energy expenditure. In childhood there is the additional factor of growth.

Energy Needed for Basal Metabolism Basal metabolism—the amount of heat given off by an individual during physical, digestive, and emotional rest—refers only to the amount of energy needed for vital life processes (the activities of the heart, kidneys, and other organs, as well as the metabolic processes within the cells).

The resting metabolism, a value used in formulating human caloric allowances and requirements, is the metabolism of an individual in a normal life situation during rest and thermal neutrality. It is about 10 percent higher than the basal rate and represents the average minimal metabolism of a person at any time during a 24-hour period when he is not physically active or exposed to unusual heat or cold; it includes the specific dynamic action of food (17).

Methods of Determining Basal Metabolism Measuring the basal metabolism of an individual may be done by indirect or direct calorimetry, although the former is more common. With this method, a measurement is made of the amount of oxygen consumed and/or the amount of carbon dioxide produced, thus indicating indirectly the amount of heat produced by oxidation in the cells of the body. A unit measure of oxygen is equivalent to a given number of kilocalories (or kilojoules) when certain foods are oxidized. It is assumed that when basal metabolism is being determined, the individual is oxidizing a mixed diet, that is, one that includes carbohydrates, fats, and proteins. The machine most widely used for indirect calorimetry is the Benedict-Roth apparatus, which measures oxygen consumption. Since it requires only a short time to take a measurement and is easy to operate, it is ideal for medical diagnosis.

Conditions Required for Measuring Basal Metabolism An individual's basal metabolism should be measured 12 to 18 hours after his last intake of food. Therefore morning is generally considered the best time. The individual should also be awake and lying quietly in a room at a comfortable temperature. (Metabolism is lowered approximately 10 percent during sleep. Any activity will increase the metabolic processes resulting in an energy expenditure above the basal metabolism.) The individual should be relaxed, because nervousness or tension may cause an increase in heat production.

A Method for Computing Basal Metabolism The rule of thumb for approximating basal metabolism under normal conditions is 1 kcal (4.2 kJ) per kilogram (kg) of body weight per hour for men, and 0.9 kcal (3.8 kJ) for women. For those over 50 years of age, the rate is reduced to 0.9 kcal (3.8 kJ) for men and 0.8 kcal (3.3 kJ) for women.

$$\text{Basal metabolism} = 1 \text{ kcal } (4.2 \text{ kJ}) \text{ or } 0.9 \text{ kcal } (3.8 \text{ kJ}) \times \text{body weight (kg)} \times 24 \text{ hr}$$

To determine the body weight in kilograms, divide the weight in pounds by 2.2. Thus the energy needed for basal metabolism by a college woman who weighs 132 lb would be:

$$\text{Basal metabolism} = 0.9 \times \frac{132}{2.2} \times 24 = 1296 \text{ kcal}$$
$$(5123 \text{ kJ})$$
$$\text{per 24 hr}$$

Factors that Affect Basal Metabolism Basal metabolism varies according to body size, body composition, age, status of health (fever, malnutrition, starvation), and secretions of the *endocrine glands*. At one time it was thought that race and climate might affect basal metabolism, but these factors have been ruled out.

Body Size *Basal metabolic rate* (BMR) varies according to body size. For a long time researchers had been seeking for a unit that would serve equally well for all species, whether small or large, and for variations within species; the unit that has been found that seems to meet this need is weight to the three-fourths power ($W^{3/4}$) (13).

132

The surface area had been accepted as the reference unit based on the assumption that heat loss from the body (and hence basal metabolism) is proportional to surface area (6).

Surface area has traditionally been used as a reference for expressing basal metabolism. It has been considered preferable to either height or weight alone because both height and weight are included in the surface area, thus correcting for body build. However, weight alone as a reference is almost as useful as surface area (9). Although surface area continues to serve as the unit of body size for clinical use (10, 20), weight (lb or kg) raised to the three-fourths power ($W^{3/4}$) has been found to relate more precisely to basal metabolism than does surface area. Expressed in terms of $W^{3/4}$ (called "metabolic size"), the BMR does not vary with the size of the animal, and it applies equally well to all species. Weight to the three-fourths power is the preferred unit for research studies (13).

Body Composition The kinds of tissue that make up the body directly affect basal metabolism. Because oxidative processes are constantly taking place in muscle tissue, more energy is expended there than in fatty tissue. It has been estimated that an athletic type of man with well-developed muscles will have a basal metabolism about 6 percent higher than a nonathlete of comparable body surface. Men generally have a basal metabolism that is 5 percent higher than women of comparable body size and age; this higher value, however, is not a sex difference, per se, but is due (at least in part) to the larger amount of lean body tissue that is usually found in men.

Research has shown that the human body may be divided into three parts: cell mass, extracellular supporting tissue, and energy reserve. The cell mass (the active cells) and the extracellular supporting tissue (the bone minerals and extracellular water, including the connective tissue [collagen] and blood plasma) together are called the lean body mass. The third part—the energy reserve—consists of the fat in the adipose tissue. Passmore (15) has given the following values for the proportion of the three parts in a healthy young man and woman:

	Man		Woman	
	kg	percent	kg	percent
Cell mass	36	55.5	26	47.5
Extracellular supporting tissue	21	32.0	15	27.5
Energy reserve	8	12.5	14	25.0
	65	100.0	55	100.0

Because the measurement of these parts is difficult to make, its usefulness in a routine assessment of body composition is quite limited at this time.

A simple technique for determining fatness is the skinfold measurement (see Chapter 18). Because about one-half of the total body fat is found in the subcutaneous tissue layer in young adults, estimating the amount there will give an approximation of the total amount of body fat. The skinfold (skin plus subcutaneous fat) is measured in several places by special calipers. For nutrition surveys, either one site (triceps) or two (the triceps and scapula) have been recommended.

Age Periods of rapid growth produce a high basal metabolism. The most rapid growth in childhood occurs in infancy: during the first 6 months of life a baby will double its birth weight; by the end of 12 months that weight will be tripled. At the end of the second year or the beginning of the third, the basal metabolic rate per square meter of body surface reaches the highest point in an individual's lifetime. Then there is a slight decrease in the rate from this time until adolescence, when both the growth rate and the basal metabolic rate increase significantly. After growth is completed, there is a gradual decline in basal metabolism from about age 20 onward. It has been estimated that the basal metabolism of a 75-year-old man is about 20 percent lower than that of a 20-year-old man.

133

Status of Health Basal metabolism by definition is a measurement of healthy persons. The metabolism of malnourished persons is lower than for normal persons of the same age and sex; the more severe the malnutrition, the lower the basal metabolism. This is due to two main factors: a decrease in the amount of active tissue and a decrease in the metabolic rate per unit of body weight. However, there may also be a lower than normal body temperature and decreased muscle tonicity.

Keys and his colleagues at the University of Minnesota have studied the effect of semistarvation on metabolism. Thirty-six healthy young men participated in a 14-month experiment. The time was divided as follows: a control period, in which the diet was adequate; a semistarvation period, in which the energy intake was one-half that of the control period; and a rehabilitation period, in which the men were fed the same diet as during the control period. At the end of six months on the semistarvation diet, the young men had lost about 25 percent of their body weight, and their basal metabolism had dropped 10 percent below that of the control period. After 20 weeks on an adequate diet during rehabilitation the basal metabolism per unit of body weight was about 13 percent above that of the control period. The metabolism of malnourished children, as in the case of adults, is lower than that of normal children.

An elevation in body temperature increases metabolism. Quantitatively, it is estimated that for each degree Fahrenheit (0.55°C) rise in body temperature above 98.6°F (37°C), metabolism is increased 7 percent. For example, a body temperature of 103.6°F (39.8°C), which is 5°F (2.8°C) above the accepted normal, increases metabolism 35 percent.

Secretions of the Endocrine Glands The secretion of the thyroid gland affects metabolism more than any other endocrine secretion. An undersecretion (hypothyroidism) may depress basal metabolism by 30 to 40 percent. An over-secretion (hyperthyroidism) may elevate metabolism as much as 80 percent.

Epinephrine (adrenalin), secreted by the adrenal glands, also increases metabolism. The sudden spurt of increased energy caused by fear, anger, and other emotional stresses is due to epinephrine. The modes of action of *thyroxine* and of epinephrine differ. When thyroxine is released, it is slow to take effect but continues for a relatively long time; by contrast, epinephrine acts immediately but its effect lasts only a short period.

The secretion of the thyroid-stimulating hormone of the pituitary gland affects metabolism by stimulating the thyroid to secrete thyroxine. The secretions of the other endocrine glands have little, if any, effect on metabolism.

Regulation of Body Temperature Man is classed as a homeotherm because he is able to maintain a near-constant internal body temperature. Both heat production through chemical reactions and heat loss through physical means are controlled physiologically. However, man does not depend only on his physiological responses; he tries to create for himself a comfortable microclimate (mean skin temperature of about 33°C [91°F]) by means of his clothing and the heating and cooling systems of his housing. If these adjustments are not possible, man tends to increase or reduce his physical activity according to his need for more or less heat production.

Body temperature normally varies, perhaps by as much as 1°C. It is lowest in the early morning and highest in the late evening. Normal body temperature varies from person to person somewhere around the accepted normal of 98.6°F (37°C).

Heat Production Heat is produced by metabolism; it is increased by involuntary and voluntary muscular activity. The body's first response to environmental cold is a general increase

134

in muscle tone by reflex action, which leads to shivering and thus to a marked increase in heat production. When he is cold, man voluntarily claps his hands and stamps his feet. In response to a warm environment, reflex muscle tone is diminished and this is followed by lower heat production.

For human beings and animals, metabolism is not affected within a given range of environmental temperatures. The range is rather narrow and differs for men and women; for men it is 81°F to 86°F (27°C to 30°C) and for women 81°F to 91°F (27°C to 33°C). As the environmental temperature is lowered, the body must produce extra heat to maintain normal body temperature.

Populations who have lived for generations in a cold climate have developed mechanisms for adjusting to the cold. The nomadic Lapps in northern Norway weather the cold by heavy clothing. The aborigines of central Australia, who are naked or scantily clad, withstand the cold because they have developed a physiological tolerance for low body temperature and a psychological tolerance for climate discomfort.

Extreme environmental temperature appears to have an effect on a person's energy requirements. Consolazio and others (5) recommend an increase in energy needs for men living and working in extremely hot environments. In a cold working environment, such as the polar regions, there might be a slight increase in energy need due to the "hobbling" effect of heavy clothing (3, 5).

Heat Loss Mechanisms Heat is lost from the body by means of radiation, convection, and water evaporation. Through radiation heat actually radiates from the body to the outside surface. Through convection the air next to the body is heated, moves away, and is replaced by cool air, which in turn is heated and moved away. Heat loss by these methods is effective when the environmental temperature is lower than that of the body surface. The temperature of the skin varies according to the blood flow to it; it is some-

where between the internal body temperature and the environment. The blood vessels to the skin are controlled by the vasoconstrictor nerves. Exposure to cold produces a constriction of the blood vessels to the skin, which increases skin insulation and lessens heat loss. Exposure to heat produces vasodilation, which enables heat to be lost.

Heat is also lost through evaporation of water from the skin and from the lining of the respiratory tract. On hot, humid days, when there is less evaporation, there is greater discomfort. Thus a low-humidity area such as Arizona with a temperature of 100°F (37.8°C) will not cause as much discomfort as a humid area with a temperature of 85°F (29.4°C). At normal room temperature a nude person loses 60 percent of his total heat loss by radiation, 12 percent by convection, 25 percent by evaporation, and about 3 percent by conduction to objects in the room (10).

Energy Needed for Physical Activity Any kind of physical activity increases the energy need above the basal metabolism. Persons expend more energy for physical activity than for basal metabolism when digging in the garden, walking rapidly, playing tennis, or engaging in other fairly strenuous activities. Table 8.4 gives energy costs of activities in kcal per kg per 10 min. By moving the decimal one point to the left, kcal per kg per min results. For example, running is 5.514 kcal/kg/10 min or 0.5514 kcal/kg/min.

Different activities require different amounts of energy (Table 8.4). For example, it takes almost three times as much energy to walk upstairs (2.540 kcal/kg/10 min) as it does to walk downstairs (0.976 kcal/kg/10 min); about twice as much to play tennis (1.014 kcal/kg/10 min) as to play Ping-Pong (0.566 kcal/kg/10 min); and about one and one-half times as much to write a theme (0.268 kcal/kg/10 min) as to sit and read a book (0.176 kcal/kg/10 min). The caloric expenditure for a given activity also depends upon the intensity with which it is performed. For example, a

Table 8.4. Energy Costs of Various Activities

Activity	kcal /kg/ 10 min	Activity	kcal /kg/ 10 min
Archery	0.754	Pick-and-shovel work	0.979
Bicycling on level roads	0.734	Pitching horseshoes	0.518
Bowling	0.975	Playing baseball	
Calisthenics	0.734	(except pitcher)	0.686
Canoeing, 2.5 mph	0.441	Playing football (American)	1.178
Canoeing, 4.0 mph	1.029	Playing football (association)	1.308
Carpentry	0.564	Playing Ping-Pong	0.566
Chopping wood	1.101	Playing pushball	1.122
Classwork, lecture	0.245	Playing squash	1.522
Cleaning windows	0.607	Playing tennis	1.014
Conversing	0.269	Repaving roads	0.734
Cross-country running	1.630	Resting in bed	0.174
Dancing, fox trot	0.650	Rowing for pleasure	0.734
Petronella	0.681	Running	5.514
Waltz	0.750	Running long distance	2.203
Rumba	1.014	Running on grade (treadmill)	
Eightsome reel	1.000	8.70 mph on 2.5% grade	2.652
Moderately	0.612	8.70 mph on 3.8% grade	2.803
Vigorously	0.831	Running on level (treadmill)	
Dressing	0.466	7.00 mph	2.045
Driving car	0.438	8.70 mph	2.273
Driving motorcycle	0.531	11.60 mph	2.879
Driving truck	0.342	Shining shoes	0.437
Farming, haying, plowing		Shooting pool	0.299
with horse	0.979	Showering	0.466
Farming, planting, hoeing,		Sitting, eating	0.204
raking	0.686	normally	0.176
Farming chores	0.564	playing cards	0.210
Gardening, digging	1.365	reading	0.176
Gardening, weeding	0.862	writing	0.268
Golfing	0.794	Sled pulling (87 lb) 2.27 mph	1.242
House painting	0.514	Sleeping	0.172
Ironing clothes	0.627	Snowshoeing 2.27 mph	0.835
Lying quietly	0.195	Sprinting	3.423
Making bed	0.572	Stacking lumber	0.856
Metal working	0.514	Standing, light activity	0.356
Mopping floors	0.665	normally	0.206
Mountain climbing	1.470	Stone masonry	0.930
Personal toilet	0.278	Sweeping floors	0.535

Table 8.4. Continued

Activity	kcal /kg/ 10 min	Activity	kcal /kg/ 10 min
Swimming (pleasure)	1.454	Walking on level (treadmill)	
Back stroke 25 yd per min	0.566	2.27 mph	0.513
Back stroke 30 yd per min	0.778	3.20 mph	0.690
Back stroke 35 yd per min	1.000	3.50 mph	0.733
Back stroke 40 yd per min	1.222	4.47 mph	0.969
Breast stroke 20 yd per min	0.704	4.60 mph	1.212
Breast stroke 30 yd per min	1.056	5.18 mph	1.382
Breast stroke 40 yd per min	1.408	5.80 mph	1.667
Crawl 45 yd per min	1.278	Walking downstairs	0.976
Crawl 55 yd per min	1.556	upstairs	2.540
Side stroke	1.222	Washing and dressing	0.382
Truck and automobile repair	0.612	Washing and shaving	0.419
Volleyball	0.505		

college man who walks on a level treadmill requires more than three times as much energy to go at a speed of 5.80 mph (1.667 kcal/kg/10 min) as at a speed of 2.27 mph (0.513 kcal/kg/10 min). The body size of the individual performing a task also affects his expenditure of energy. For example, to sit and take notes during a one-hour college lecture class would require 43 percent more energy for a 176-lb (80-kg) college football player (118 kcal) than for a 123-lb (56-kg) coed (82 kcal).

Figure 8.4 shows the continuous respiratory gas analyzer at the United States Army Medical Research and Nutrition Laboratory that was used to obtain the energy values in Table 8.4. Another compilation of energy expenditures is presented in the 1973 publication on energy requirements of the FAO/WHO (7).

Methods of Determing the Energy Expended for Physical Activities An early indirect way of measuring the energy used for a particular activity was the Douglas method. The expired air of the individual performing the activity was col-

lected in a large bag and then analyzed for carbon dioxide and oxygen. Although this method was accurate, its usefulness was limited because the collecting bag was cumbersome.

Around 1940 an apparatus called a respirometer was designed and constructed at the Max-Planck Institute in Germany (Fig. 8.5). It is a

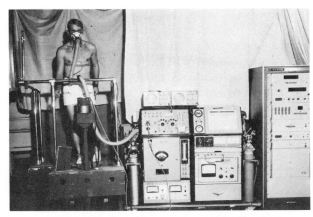

Fig. 8.4 Continuous respiratory gas analyzer. (Courtesy C. F. Consolazio, U.S. Army Medical Research and Nutrition Laboratory, Denver.)

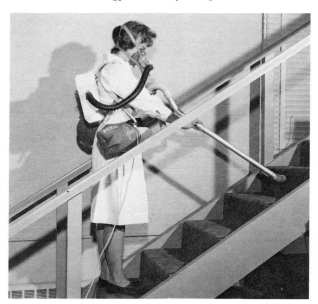

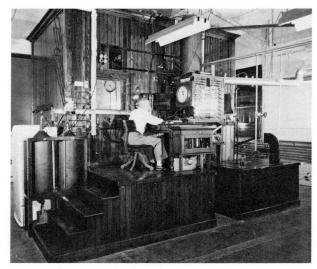

Fig. 8.6 The Armsby Calorimeter at The Pennsylvania State University. (Courtesy The Pennsylvania State University.)

Fig. 8.5 Kofranyi-Michaelis respirometer, which is shown measuring the amount of energy spent in vacuum cleaning. (Courtesy Doris E. Fulton, Professor Emeritus, Ohio Agricultural Research and Development Center, Department of Home Economics, The Ohio State University.)

lightweight box containing a meter to record the total volume of expired air and a bag for collecting a fractional part of it for analysis. The equipment, which weighs 8 lb (3.6 kg) or less, is strapped onto the back. This apparatus eliminates the cumbersomeness of the Douglas method and increases the length of time during which measurements can be made. After the sample of expired air has been analyzed for carbon dioxide and oxygen, the energy expenditure can be calculated.

Many of the early values for the energy cost of physical activities were obtained by direct calorimetry, using a respiration calorimeter. The calorimeters ranged in size from those that would only accommodate one man to those that would accommodate large farm animals. The Armsby Calorimeter (Fig. 8.6), the largest ever constructed, is now a museum piece at the College of Agriculture, Pennsylvania State University.

The respiration calorimeter combines both direct and indirect methods of energy determination. It consists of an airtight, well-insulated chamber for the experimental subject. With the direct method, the heat generated by the subject is absorbed by water circulating in metal coils near the ceiling of the chamber. The amount of heat given off during a certain period of time is computed from the water's rise in temperature during its passage through the chamber and the quantity of water circulating through the coils. The amount of water that evaporates from the skin and lungs also has to be taken into consideration; it is calculated by comparing the water content of the air entering and leaving the chamber. Indirectly, energy expenditure can be determined by analyzing the air entering and leaving the chamber for its oxygen and carbon dioxide content.

In the 1960s heart rate began to be used as an indicator of work cost (1, 4, 18). Parallel determinations using heart rate (recorded by telemetry or by counting the beats using a stethoscope with a long tube) and energy expenditure (by indirect calorimetry) as a measurement of work costs have been made with children and adults, both at rest

138

and while active, with close agreement in the findings. The heart rate in beats per minute and kilocalories of energy expended per minute varied in a parallel direction (Fig. 8.7). It was found that heart rate was a better predictor of oxygen consumption in those who are moving about than in those who are sitting or standing because of the tendency for blood to accumulate in the extremities during inactivity (4).

Energy Needed for the Specific Dynamic Effect of Food. The heat produced by the ingestion of food itself is called "specific dynamic effect" or "calorigenic effect." In the past, researchers estimated that the specific dynamic effect of food was larger than it is now known to be. They observed a dramatic increase in the heat metabolism of persons who had been fed meals consisting of only carbohydrate, or fat, or protein. These researchers assumed that the specific dynamic effect of a mixed meal would be the sum of the increases in heat production caused by each nutrient; thus they did not study the actual heat production of meals that combined carbohydrate, fat, and protein.

Now it is known that the energy spent for the specific dynamic effect of food is only a small fraction of the total energy expenditure of human beings. An experiment was conducted with college men to determine the dynamic effects of long-time intakes of both high-protein (about 122 g daily) and low-protein (about 34 g daily) diets of equal energy value (19). These mixed diets were composed of ordinary foods, and the two levels of protein intake represented two extremes that might be found in America. The Armsby Calorimeter measured the total heat production of the subjects at selected 48-hour periods. It was found that the specific dynamic effect on the high-protein diet was about 8 percent higher than that of the low-protein diet. In an ordinary mixed diet, the specific dynamic effect of food is about 6 percent of the energy value of the food ingested.

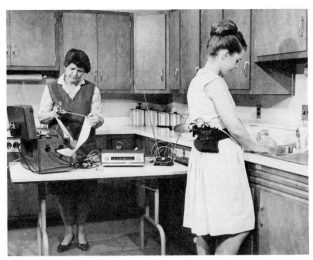

Fig. 8.7 Determining energy expenditure by measuring the heart rate. The subject is wearing a transmitter that transfers her heart signals to a recorder. The transmitter is in the packet of her cumberbund, and only the wires are visible. (Courtesy Doris E. Fulton, Professor Emeritus, Ohio Agricultural Research and Development Center, Department of Home Economics, The Ohio State University.)

A valid explanation for the increased heat production following the ingestion of food has been given by Hegsted (12). In the pathway of metabolism to create ATP (Fig. 8.2), only about 32 to 34 percent of the energy contained in food protein and 38 to 40 percent of that in food carbohydrate and fat is converted to ATP. The remainder, 66 to 68 percent of the protein energy and 60 to 62 percent of that from carbohydrate and fat, is lost as body heat. This would explain, for example, the increased heat production following an intake of protein alone. (Furthermore, if the food carbohydrate is first converted to fat before being used for energy, there is a net loss of 10.6 percent more.) More than 30 years ago, at the Pennsylvania State University, Forbes and Swift (8) demonstrated that there was a difference in the specific dynamic effect of carbohydrate, fat, and protein when measured separately as when mixed together.

139

Table 8.5 Activity Record and Energy Expended

Activity	Hours	Minutes	Total minutes	Energy cost of activity[a] (kcal/kg/min)	Energy expended (kcal/kg)
Sleep	8	0	480	0.0172	8.26
Washing and dressing	0	30	30	0.0382	1.15
Showering	0	10	10	0.0466	0.47
Making bed	0	5	5	0.0572	0.29
Eating meals and snacks	2	0	120	0.0204	2.45
Sitting in classes	4	0	240	0.0245	5.88
Sitting watching television	1	0	60	0.0176	1.06
Standing and working in lab	1	50	110	0.0356	3.92
Standing, normally	0	40	40	0.0206	0.82
Swimming (pleasure)	0	50	50	0.1454	7.27
Studying, sitting reading	2	10	130	0.0176	2.29
Studying, sitting writing	1	40	100	0.0268	2.68
Walking (about 2.27 mph)	0	55	55	0.0513	2.82
Walking downstairs	0	5	5	0.0976	0.49
Walking upstairs	0	5	5	0.2540	1.27
Totals	19	300	1440		41.12

[a] These figures are taken from Table 8.4

Total Energy Requirements It is possible to estimate one's total energy need using either the factorial method of calculation or tables of recommended energy allowances. Although both procedures have limitations, these can be taken into account and a satisfactory approximation obtained.

The Factorial Method By this procedure the energy expenditure for a 24-hour period is calculated using the energy cost factor for each activity engaged in (Table 8.4) and the time spent in each activity. Among the drawbacks to using this method is that it is difficult to determine exactly how much time was spent in any activity, and there are only limited data on the caloric costs of various activities. To illustrate the use of the factorial method, the energy required by a female college student (19 years old, weight 132 lb [60 kg], height 69 in [175 cm]) is presented. Table 8.5 lists the activities she participated in for one day, how long she spent in each one (in hours, minutes, and total number of minutes), the energy cost of each (in kcal per kg of body weight per minute), and the amount of energy she expended on each (in kcal per kg of body weight). To estimate the total energy required by this 60-kg young woman for one day, see the calculation below.

$$\text{Total energy expended} = 41.12 \text{ kcal/kg} \times 60 \text{ kg (body weight)} = 2467 \text{ kcal (10,321 kJ)}$$

Tables of Recommended Energy Allowances The Recommended Dietary Allowances for the United States were prepared by the Food and Nutrition Board of the National Academy of Sciences–National Research Council (17).

140

Recommended Dietary Allowances for Energy

The 1974 energy allowances recommended by the Food and Nutrition Board (17) are single average values for the activity pattern typical of most Americans (Table 8.6). College-age men and women (19 to 22 years) have energy allowances of 3000 kcal (12,522 kJ) and 2100 kcal (8786 kJ) per day, respectively. Individuals who gain weight on the recommended energy allowances because of a sedentary life should try to increase their physical activity rather than reduce their food (and thereby their caloric) intake. (See Appendix Tables A-14 and A-15 for suggested weights.)

Energy in College Meals The average energy value of meals served at 50 American colleges was 2665 kcal (11,150 kJ) with a range of 2145 to 3200 kcal (8975 to 13,389 kJ) per person per day (22). Further evaluation showed that the five women's colleges offered meals averaging more than 2300 kcal (9623 kJ) and the two men's colleges offered meals averaging less than 3000 kcal (12,522 kJ). The daily energy value of the meals served at the 43 coeducational institutions varied: three provided only 2200 kcal (9205 kJ), 11 provided less than 2600 kcal (10,878 kJ), 25 provided between 2600 and 3000 kcal (10,878 and 12,552 kJ), and four provided more than 3000 kcal (12,552 kJ).

Energy in the United States' Food Supply

The amount of food energy available for consumption per capita per day in the United States is greater than any of the caloric allowances recommended by the Food and Nutrition Board. The value for 1976 was 3290 kcal (13,765 kJ) per capita per day, a slightly higher value than for either 1974 or 1975 (2). (The food energy consumed per capita per day in 1976, however, was only about 5 percent less than in the early 1900s.)

Almost three-fourths of the kilocalories available in the 1976 food supply came from four major

Table 8.6. Recommended Dietary Allowances for Energy

	Age (year)	Energy (kcal)
Infants	0.0–0.5	kg × 117
	0.5–1.0	kg × 108
Children	1–3	1300
	4–6	1800
	7–10	2400
Males	11–14	2800
	15–18	3000
	19–22	3000
	23–50	2700
	51+	2400
Females	11–14	2400
	15–18	2100
	19–22	2100
	23–50	2000
	51+	1800
Pregnant		+300
Lactating		+500

From *Recommended Dietary Allowances, Eighth Edition,* Natl. Acad. Sci.-Natl. Research Council. Washington, D.C.: Natl. Research Council, 1974.

food groups: meats, poultry, and fish (20.0 percent); flour and cereal products (19.2 percent); fats and oils, including butter (18.6 percent); and sugars and other sweeteners (16.4 percent) (1). Dairy products (11.2 percent), vegetables (8.7 percent), fruits (3.4 percent), eggs (1.9 percent), and other foods (.6 percent) contributed the remainder of the food energy.

Food Sources of Energy

All foods contain some energy. As a general rule, foods with relatively large proportions of carbohydrate, fat, and protein per unit of weight are high in energy value, whereas those with smaller proportions are lower. A tablespoon of white sugar has an energy value of 45 kcal (188 kJ) be-

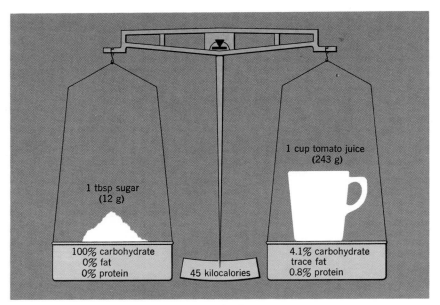

1 cup tomato juice
(243 g)

1 tbsp sugar
(12 g)

100% carbohydrate
0% fat
0% protein

45 kilocalories

4.1% carbohydrate
trace fat
0.8% protein

Fig. 8.8 An energy-rich and an energy-poor food.

cause of its high carbohydrate content. By contrast, a cup of tomato juice, which has the same energy value as the tablespoon of sugar, is 20 times heavier (Fig. 8.8.).

For a quick estimate of the energy value of a food, the protein, fat, and carbohydrate content of which is known, the 4-9-4 factors can be used (see p. 131). For example, the protein, fat, and the carbohydrate content of 100 g of whole milk is 3.3 g, 3.3 g, and 4.5 g, respectively. The kilocalories furnished by the protein of the milk total about 13 (3.3 × 4), by the fat 30 (3.3 × 9), and by the carbohydrate 18 (4.5 × 4), thus making a grand total of 61 (255 kJ).

Despite all that is known and that has been written about the energy value of foods, most people harbor a number of misconceptions. For example, some people believe that white bread is high in energy value and that cracked wheat, rye, and whole wheat bread are lower. Actually, identical weights of all four types have about the same energy value.

The energy value of various foods is listed in Table 8.7 (the energy content per average serving is listed in both kilocalories and kilojoules). A more extensive food list, given in kilocalories, is presented in Appendix Table A-3.

Food Calorie Equivalents of Physical Activity

How much time will it take a 154-lb (70 kg) college student to walk off (at 3.5 mph) the energy obtained by eating a hamburger sandwich or by drinking a glass of skim milk? To answer this question, one must know the energy value of the sandwich and the milk as well as the energy expenditure for walking. According to Table 8.8, it will take this student about 86 minutes to walk off the 450 kcal (1883 kJ) from the sandwich and 16 minutes for the 81 kcal (339 kJ) provided by the milk. The approximate times required to use up the same energy in swimming (40 minutes for the sandwich and 7 minutes for the milk) or

Table 8.7 Energy Content of Various Foods as Served

Food	Per 100 g of food, Energy, kcal	Per average serving Size of serving, g		Energy, kcal (kJ)[a]
Butter	714	14	1 tbsp	100 (418)
Peanut butter	594	16	1 tbsp	95 (398)
Chocolate (milk, plain)	518	28	1 oz	145 (607)
Salad dressing (French)	406	16	1 tbsp	65 (272)
Doughnuts (cake type)	400	25	1 doughnut	100 (418)
Beef steak (sirloin, broiled)	388	85	3 oz	330 (1381)
Cheese (American)	375	28	1 oz	105 (439)
Sugar (white)	375	12	1 tbsp	45 (188)
Cake (chocolate with chocolate icing)	341	69	1/16 of cake	235 (983)
Potatoes (French fried)	270	50	10 strips	135 (565)
Bread (white, enriched)	268	28	1 sl	75 (314)
Pie (lemon meringue)	254	120	1/7 of pie	305 (1276)
Pancakes (plain)	222	27	1 cake	60 (251)
Ice cream	202	67	1/2 c	135 (565)
Egg	160	50	1 lg	80 (335)
Beans, lima (frozen, cooked)	116	90	1/2 c	105 (439)
Fruit cocktail (canned)	77	128	1/2 c	98 (410)
Milk (whole)	62	244	1 c	150 (628)
Yogurt (whole milk)	62	227	8 oz	140 (586)
Milk (nonfat, skim)[b]	37	245	1 c	90 (377)
Strawberries	37	75	1/2 c	28 (117)
Lettuce (Iceberg)	15	135	1/4 head	20 (84)
Celery (raw)	13	40	1 stalk	5 (21)

[a] Calculated using 4.184 kJ = 1 kcal.
[b] Milk solids added.
From *Nutritive Value of Foods*, Home and Garden Bull. No. 72, revised. Washington, D.C.: U.S. Dept. Agr., 1977.

reclining (346 minutes for the sandwich and 62 minutes for the milk) are also shown in Table 8.8.

Overnutrition

When an individual's energy intake consistently exceeds expenditure, weight gain will occur and ultimately obesity results. The Law of Conservation of Energy, which states that energy can neither be created nor destroyed but can be changed from one form to another, explains this phenomenon. The excess energy consumed is stored in the tissues as potential energy in the form of fat.

There are many reasons why people eat more food than their bodies require, but the reasons are not always clear in any given case (26).

143

Table 8.8 Energy Equivalents of Food Calories Expressed in Minutes of Activity

Food	Energy, kcal	Activity for 70-kg individual		
		Walking,[a] min	Swimming,[b] min	Reclining,[c] min
Carbonated beverage, 1 glass	106	20	9	82
Cheese (cottage), 1 tbsp	27	5	2	21
Cookie (chocolate chip), 1	51	10	5	39
Hamburger sandwich (4 oz cooked meat, 1 roll)	450	86	40	346
Milk, skim, 1 glass	81	16	7	62
Milkshake, 1	421	81	38	324

[a] Energy cost = 5.2 kcal per minute at 3.5 mph.
[b] Energy cost = 11.2 kcal per minute.
[c] Energy cost = 1.3 kcal per minute.
From F. Konishi (1965) Food energy equivalents of various activities. *J. Am. Dietet. Assoc.*, **46**:187.

Fat Cells—Number and Size

Obese individuals may have a normal or an increased number of fat cells (25). (Fat cells, also called adipocytes, are connective tissue cells differentiated by the presence of fat in them and the function to store fat.) Some evidence suggests that persons who become obese as children (before age 15) have a higher number of fat cells than those who become obese as adults (8, 36). Although there is not complete agreement (48), the general belief is that the total number of fat cells reaches a maximum before the end of puberty. The amount of fat stored in the fat cells depends on the amount of excess energy consumed. When weight is being gained, the fat content of the adipocytes increases; when weight is being lost, it decreases.

The number of fat cells varies with location in the body and between the sexes. The upper middle abdominal region (*epigastric*) was found to have a greater number of cells in both men and women than the buttock (*gluteal*) or thigh (*femoral*) region. Women have more fat cells than men

and more fat (see Table 8.9). The proportion of fat in the body tends to increase with age in both sexes, and women tend to have a higher percentage of fat (in relation to total body weight) than do men. At age 25 the mean percentage of body weight that is fat is about 19 for men and 33 for women. For men at age 55, the mean percentage is 30, and for women at age 55, 44 (see Table 21.1).

Diagnosis of Obesity

The degree of obesity has usually been estimated by calculating the percentage by which the individual's weight exceeds the norm established for his height in a height–weight table (Appendix Table A-14 and Table A-15). Body density measurements enable one to estimate the lean body mass; from the body weight and the lean body mass, the amount of body fat can be calculated.

The relative amount of adipose tissue is determined by skinfold measurements (enabling one to estimate the amount of subcutaneous fat). Measurement of skinfold thickness appears to

Table 8.9. Comparison of Fat Cell Numbers in Men and Women

	Men	Women
Age	23	22
Fat cell number ($\times 10^{-10}$)	1.75	4.14
Regional fat cell number ($\times 10^{-3}$)		
Epigastric (upper middle abdominal region)	39	53
Femoral (thigh)	17	28
Gluteal (buttocks)	35	46

Adapted from L. Sjöström, J. Smith, M. Krotkiewski, and P. Björntorp (1972). Cellularity in different regions of adipose tissue in young men and women. *Metabolism,* **21:** 1146, 1147. Used by permission, Grune and Stratton, Inc., publishers.

be the most appropriate technique for use in epidemiology studies; it was used in the Ten State Survey (42) and in the First Health and Nutrition Examination Survey (1).

For further discussion of these methods, see Chap. 18

Prevalence of Obesity

Prevalence of obesity in the adult population (20 to 74 years) was assessed in the First Health and Nutrition survey, United States, 1971–1974 (1), using as the indicator the triceps skinfold measurement (Table 8.10 and Fig. 8.9). Since a large proportion of the body's adipose tissue is under the skin (about 50 percent in young adults), measuring the thickness of a fold of skin (with subcutaneous layer of fat) has been found to be a good index of overall fatness (9, 11). An individual of either sex and any age group was considered obese if the skinfold measurement was greater than the 85th percentile for men and women 20 to 29 years of age (1, 16, 39). Adults tend to accumulate fat with age; better health accrues to those who avoid this tendency. Hence it is for health reasons that the standard for determining obesity was set relative to the 20- to 29-year age group.

Results from the HANES report showed obesity to be more prevalent among women than men; the highest incidence of all age-sex groups was among Negro women, 45 to 64 years of age (43.0 percent). The lowest occurrence among all groups was among Negro men 65 to 74 years of age (5.7 percent). Income made a difference in the prevalence; women of low income showed a greater incidence of obesity than those above poverty level in most age groups. For men, it was the higher income group that had a greater incidence of obesity in all age groups (Table 8.10 and Fig. 8.9).

In an earlier study, the Ten-State Nutrition Survey, made to determine the status of nutrition of disadvantaged families using the same criteria for obesity as in the HANES study, obesity was more common among women than among men. The incidence was higher among white men than black men (42).

Health Implications of Obesity

A number of illnesses are closely related to obesity. For example, hypertension occurs more often among the obese than among the nonobese, and the mortality rate of those who are obese hypertensives is higher than for those who are only obese or only hypertensive (33).

There is also a close relationship between obesity and diabetes. The *Framingham Heart Study* of 5209 adult men and women over a 12-year period showed that overweight persons (those whose weight was 20 percent above the median weight for a given height) developed diabetes three times

145

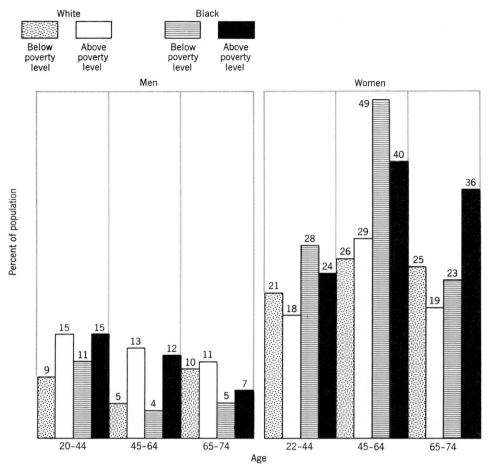

Fig. 8.9 Percent of adults obese by age, sex, race, and income levels: United States, 1971–1974 (Hanes). (From Health United States, 1976–1977, Chartbook. DHEW Publ. No. (HRA) 77-1233. Hyattsville, Md., U.S. Dept. Health, Educ. and Welfare; Natl. Center for Health Stat., p. 19.)

as often as those of normal weight (24). A questionnaire survey of 73,532 women who were all members of TOPS (Take Off Weight Sensibly) revealed that severe obesity in women 30 to 49 years of age increases the risk of diabetes 4.5 times (35).

Obese persons have abnormalities in blood and insulin levels, responsiveness to insulin, and *glucose tolerance*. Although obese persons have a high blood insulin level, which rises with each gain in body weight (3), the insulin does not function effectively. Consequently, in glucose tolerance tests, the blood glucose level of the obese persons remains elevated for a much longer period than that of normal persons. Although insulin promotes the uptake of glucose by the tissues, less glucose is taken up by the tissues of the obese. In vitro studies show that larger cells (fat

146

Table 8.10. Number and Percent of Obese Adults Aged 20 to 74 Years by Race, Sex, and Income Level in the United States, 1971–1974 (Hanes)

Age, race, sex	All incomes			Income below poverty level			Income above poverty level		
	n[a]	N[a]	per-cent	n	N	per-cent	n	N	per-cent
Male									
20–44 yr									
white	1,665	28,243	14.2	157	1,998	9.4	1,457	25,204	14.9
black	286	3,105	13.3	78	753	11.1	193	2,249	14.6
45–64 yr									
white	1,132	18,241	12.2	111	1,318	5.3	976	16,180	13.2
black	215	1,760	10.2	72	541	3.7	130	1,089	12.4
65–74 yr									
white	1,334	4,974	11.5	204	595	10.3	1,077	4,127	11.1
black	294	486	5.7	128	186	4.6	149	276	7.0
Female									
20–44 yr									
white	3,996	30,191	18.4	418	2,704	20.6	3,269	26,603	18.3
black	928	4,029	25.6	400	1,450	27.6	492	2,471	24.0
45–64 yr									
white	1,257	19,996	27.6	117	1,375	26.4	1,084	17,544	28.5
black	241	2,102	43.0	88	701	49.4	142	1,296	40.0
65–74 yr									
white	1,496	6,601	19.8	320	1,160	25.2	1,113	5,118	19.2
black	318	654	31.2	158	302	23.2	142	298	36.3

[a] n: number examined; N: estimated population in thousands. Persons with unknown income excluded.
From: S. Abraham, personal communication, unpublished data. Hyattsville, Md.: U.S. Dept. Health, Educ., and Welfare; Natl. Center for Health Stat.

cells) are less sensitive to insulin than smaller ones. This lack of sensitivity has been given as the reason for the carbohydrate intolerance of obese persons. When weight is lost and the size of fat cells is reduced, insulin sensitivity is regained (37).

The Framingham study also revealed that there was twice as much gallbladder disease among the obese as among those of normal weight or less (24).

Causes of Obesity

The causes of obesity (other than excessive consumption of energy) are speculative. Much has been investigated about causes in an effort to prevent or treat obesity more effectively by striking at the cause. The literature on the subject is extensive and will be discussed under behavioral factors, physiological factors, genetic factors, and environmental factors.

147

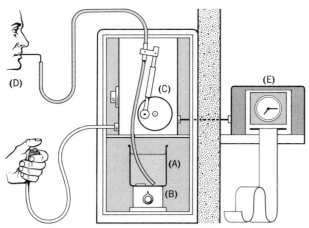

Fig. 8.10 Monitored Food-Dispensing Apparatus. The formula diet (A) is constantly mixed by a magnetic stirrer (B). Tubing from the reservoir leads to a dispensing syringe-type pump (C), which delivers a bolus of formula through the mouthpiece. The entire dispensing unit is contained within a refrigerator. The pump is adjusted to respond with a single delivery cycle to the signal of an actuating button (D). Whenever the button is pressed, a predetermined volume of homogenized formula is delivered directly into the subject's mouth by the pump. Each delivery is recorded by a printing timer (E) that prints out each event and the date and precise time at which the event occurred. The timer and recorder are in a room remote from the subject, who is kept unaware of their existence. When the apparatus is in use, the reservoir and pump remain covered. (From R. G. Campbell, S. A. Hashim and T. B. Van Itallie (1971). Studies of food-intake regulation in men: Responses to variations in nutritive density in lean and obese subjects. *New Engl. J. Med.* 285: 1402. Reprinted by permission.)

Behavioral Factors Eating offers comfort to some who suffer from feelings of inadequacy, inferiority, and failure. Some psychiatrists interpret excessive eating as a way of meeting emotional needs—"a compensation for basic personality problems." Therefore, as Forbes (15) explains, obesity is often very difficult to treat; it may require psychological counseling.

It appears that the obese are relatively insensitive to "internal" (physiologic) stimuli pertaining to hunger and satiety and more than normally responsive to "external" stimuli related to eating (38). To test this theory, ten grossly obese and eight normal-weight adults were given a nutritionally complete, bland liquid diet dispensed on demand from a feeding machine (Fig. 8.10) for 21 days or more. Each normal-weight person ate enough of the food to maintain his weight at its usual level, but each obese person ate far less than he needed and so he lost weight. It is speculated that the obese persons lost weight because their motivation to eat stems from external cues— taste, appearance, variety, aroma, and so forth— which were all absent from the bland liquid diet. The normal-weight people maintained their weight (despite the unappealing diet) because they were primarily motivated by the internal signals of hunger and satiety (44).

Observations made in a campus cafeteria revealed that the obese select more high-calorie, low-nutrient foods than do persons of normal weight (17). And the obese eat much more rapidly than do the nonobese (45).

As far as personality is concerned, there appears to be no single pattern characteristic of the obese as a group. The finding came from the use of a personality assessment instrument with 116 obese persons (23).

In the everyday life of some adults, certain factors tend to lower the energy need, whereas others tend to increase the energy intake, leading to a subtle, progressive weight gain. Insufficient exercise, for example, lowers the energy need. The widespread use of automobiles and the popularity of television and other passive forms of entertainment discourage healthful physical activity. Eating is an integral part of social life, but often the food given as gifts or served to guests is high in energy and low in nutritive value. Rather than offering cake or candy, there are many other possibilities, such as fresh fruit and cheese.

Some people overeat because of habit. They may eat a midnight snack because it is a custom and not because of hunger. Older persons may continue to eat the same quantities of food as when they were younger even though they are less active and their basal metabolic rate is lower. Women tend to gain excess weight following puberty, following their first pregnancy, and during the menopause. Men, on the other hand, tend to gain weight gradually after age 25.

Eating just a little bit more than the body needs each day will add weight gradually. For example, if a person consumes an extra 60 kcal (251 kJ) of energy each day (1 slice of bread, 1 small apple, or 2 Brazil nuts), this would amount to 21,900 kcal (91,630 kJ) at the end of a year and a gain of 2.7 kg (approximately 6 lb).

Physiological Factors Significant progress has been made in studying (through experiments with animals) the control of eating; even so, much more research is needed before any definitive statements can be made (8, 20). There is concurrence on the existence of a food intake regulation center located in the *hypothalamus* of the brain. Other influences, the gastrointestinal (absorption of nutrients) and hormonal (insulin, estrogens, growth hormone), appear to act through the hypothalmus (8).

The majority of persons are of normal weight; some physiological control on food intake would appear to be in operation. Few studies on mechanisms for control in the human have been done. In one controlled laboratory study, the investigators sought to determine if individuals could adjust to changes in caloric density of food eaten. Lean individuals, fed a formula (liquid) diet from a feeding machine (Fig. 8.10), adjusted their intake to the energy value of the formula to maintain a constant caloric intake; the obese did not adjust (10, 21).

In another type of experiment, normal weight medical students were fed a 1000 kcal (4184 kJ) snack at night over a 20-day period and the food intake measured the following day. The students did not diminish their usual food intake and gained weight (5). However, taking food immediately before a meal, or even up to two hours before, depresses the amount eaten at the meal (46).

There are other aspects of food intake control, such as the role of the gastrointestinal tract in signaling hunger or satiation, which upon further research may yield more definitive information (29, 41).

Genetic Factors Numerous investigations show a high incidence of obesity among the parents of the obese. In a study of 239 obese persons, 69 percent of them had obese parents (one or both) (8). In the case of adopted children, a lower correlation was observed between the weight of the children and their fathers or mothers than was observed between natural children and their fathers or mothers (49).

Environmental Factors Overfeeding in infancy may be a factor in the incidence of obesity later. Breast-fed infants rarely deposit an excess of body fat; formula-fed babies may if the formula is too concentrated and too much is fed. Early feeding of solids may also contribute to obesity in infants (47). Although there are differences of opinion, current evidence suggests that infants who gain excessive weight during the first six months of life have a greater liklihood of being obese later in childhood than do infants who gain normally (14, 22).

The prognosis of childhood obesity is poor. A convincing study was the 30-year later follow-up of 120 Hagerstown, Maryland, school children of ages 10 to 13 years (in 1937 to 1939). Fifty of the most overweight of each sex and 50 of average body weight were selected from the school records for follow-up. Only 120 persons out of the 200 were located. Over 80 percent of those who were overweight as children remained so as adults. However, a notable percentage who were of average weight as children also became overweight adults (2).

Prevention and Treatment of Obesity

It is easier to prevent obesity than to treat it. Such prevention should probably begin in early child-

Table 8.11 Daily Food Plan for Calorie Restricted Diets

			Number of exchanges*				
Diet	Vegetable[a] A	Vegetable[b] B	Skim milk	Fruit	Bread	Meat	Fat
800 kcal (3347 kJ)	as desired	—	2	2	2	5	3(2 teaspoon vegetable oil, 1 teaspoon margarine)
1000 kcal (4184 kJ)	as desired	1	2	2	3	5	5(4 teaspoon vegetable oil, 1 teaspoon margarine)
1200 kcal (5021 kJ)	as desired	1	2	3	4	6	6(5 teaspoon vegetable oil, 1 teaspoon margarine)
1500 kcal (6276 kJ)	as desired	1	2	4	6	6	9(8 teaspoon vegetable oil, 1 teaspoon margarine)

[a] Asparagus, broccoli, Brussel sprouts, cabbage, cauliflower, celery, chard (Swiss), chicory, collards, cucumber, escarole, eggplant, greens (spinach, turnip greens, etc.), kale, lettuce, mushrooms, okra, peppers, radishes, sauerkraut, string beans, squash (summer), tomatoes, watercress.
[b] Beets, carrots, onions, peas (green), pumpkin, rutabagas, squash (winter), turnips.
* For exchanges, see Appendix Table A-12.
Adapted from *Diet Manual*, The Commonwealth of Pennsylvania. (University Park, Pa.: The Institution Food Research and Services Project, 1976), pp. J–2, J–3, and J–4. Used with permission of M. C. McCann, Project Head.

hood and continue throughout adulthood. A gain of 2 kg (about 4 lb) above one's ideal weight should be a signal to begin curtailing one's energy intake or increasing one's energy expenditure. Minor variations in weight from day to day occur because of fluctuations in the body's water content.

An obese individual who wants to lose weight should first consult a physician. A physical examination and medical history can reveal if the obesity is caused in part by an endocrine problem (such as hypothyroidism) or if it is accompanied by diabetes or other health problems. The way in which obesity can be treated will vary from one person to another; it can include diet, dietary advice, psychological counseling, exercise, and drugs.

Diet In general, a diet should permit the gradual loss of weight—no more than 0.9 kg (2 lb) per week. If the daily deficit is 500 kcal (2092 kJ), the

Table 8.12. Approximate Composition of Low Calorie Diets

Energy (approximately)	800 kcal (3347 kJ)		1000 kcal (4184 kJ)		1200 kcal (5021 kJ)		1500 kcal (6276 kJ)	
		percent		percent		percent		percent
Nutrient	g	total kcal	g	total kcal	g	total kcal	g	total kcal
Protein	60	30	70	28	80	27	80	21
Fat	30	33	40	36	50	38	60	36
Carbohydrate	70	35	110	44	130	43	160	43

Adapted from *Diet Manual*, The Commonwealth of Pennsylvania. (University Park, Pa.: The Institution Food Research and Services Project, 1976), pp. J–2, J–3, and J–4. Used with permission of M. C. McCann, Project Head.

weekly loss will be about 0.5 kg (1 lb). One pound of fat is equivalent to about 3600 kcal (15,062 kJ). For moderate weight reduction, a diet for women should include between 1000 and 1500 kcal (4184 to 6276 kJ) and for men between 1500 and 2000 kcal (6276 to 8368 kJ). These levels supply the approximate amount of energy needed for basal metabolism per day. The first week or two there may be little weight loss due to water retention but later on the loss will be about what had been calculated.

To plan a moderate reducing diet for an adult, find the desired weight according to height and body build in Appendix Table A–14 or Table A–15; multiply this weight by the appropriate energy expenditure for maintenance, 15 kcal per lb (138 kJ/kg) if sedentary, and 20 kcal per lb (184 kJ/kg) if moderately active. From this amount, subtract the 500 kcal per day to lose an estimated 0.5 kg (1 lb) per week.

On the whole, a diet should be acceptable to the person who is reducing; it should consist of foods that he likes and provide a number of choices. This type of diet will more readily be adhered to and cause less of a feeling of deprivation. Such a diet, with some liberalization, should probably be followed even after the individual returns to normal weight.

Table 8.11 presents daily food allowances at four energy levels. In comparison with the food consumption of most persons in the United States, these diets provide for more energy from protein, less from carbohydrate and fat (Table 8.12). (The ordinary diet in the United States supplies about 12 percent of its energy from protein, 42 percent from fat, and 46 percent from carbohydrates [1976]). Table 8.13 presents model menus for the four energy levels: 800 kcal, 1000 kcal, 1200 kcal, and 1500 kcal (3347, 4184, 5021, and 6276 kJ). Even with different selections of food, the 800-kcal and 1000-kcal diet will not meet the RDA for iron, thiamin, and riboflavin and are borderline in other nutrients.

Quick-loss Diet Schemes The eagerness of many people for some type of panacea or quick weight loss often impels them to try an unbalanced or extremely limited eating pattern—one that they ought not to, and never could, adhere to for very long. No drastic regime should ever be adopted except under the guidance of a licensed physician.

One type of drastic regime is the liquid formula diets, which were first used experimentally in hospitals. It was found that, although these diets led to a loss of weight within two to four weeks, many people dropped out after that and returned to conventional foods, soon regaining their lost weight. However, formula diets can be used effectively at the beginning of a reduction regimen

151

Table 8.13. Low Calorie Diets: Sample Menus

	800 kcal	1000 kcal	1200 kcal	1500 kcal
Breakfast	Number of exchanges			
Fruit Exchange,[a] List 3	1	1	1	1
Meat Exchange, List 5	1	1	1	1
Bread Exchange, List 4	1	1	1	2
Fat Exchange, List 6	0	1	1	3
Milk Exchange, List 1	1	1	1	1
Coffee or tea, as desired (sugar substitute)				
Lunch				
Meat Exchange, List 5	1	1	2	2
Vegetable, List 2A[b]	as desired			
Vegetable, List 2B[c]	0	0	0	0
Bread Exchange, List 4	1	1	2	2
Fat Exchange, List 6	1	1	2	3
Fruit Exchange, List 3	1	1	1	2
Milk Exchange, List 1	½	½	½	½
Coffee or tea, as desired (sugar substitute)				
Dinner				
Meat Exchange, List 5	3	3	3	3
Vegetable, List 2A[b]	as desired			
Vegetable, List 2B[c]	0	1[d]	1[d]	1[d]
Bread Exchange, List 4	0	1	1	2
Fat Exchange, List 6	2	3	3	3
Fruit Exchange, List 3	0	0	1	1
Milk Exchange, List 1	½	½	½	½
Coffee or tea, as desired (sugar substitute)				

[a] For Exchange Lists see Appendix Table A-12.
[b] See Vegetables, A Table 8.11.
[c] See Vegetables, B Table 8.11
[d] number of vegetables.
Adapted from *Diet Manual*, the Commonwealth of Pennsylvania (University Park Pa.: the Institution Food Research and Services Project, 1976), pp. J–2, J–3, and J–4. Used with permission of M. C. McCann, Project Head.

or to replace one meal each day during a weight maintenance program.

The most popular diets have been those that are limited in carbohydrate content but unlimited in protein, fat, and kilocalories (4). In 1953 there was Pennington's *Treatment of Obesity with Calorically Unrestricted Diets,* in 1960 the "Air Force Diet" (for which the Air Force disclaimed any responsibility) (30), in 1961 Taller's *Calories Don't Count,* in 1965 Jameson and Williams *Drinking Man's Diet,* in 1967 Stillman's *Doctor's Quick Weight Loss Diet,* and in 1972 *Dr. Atkins' Diet Revolution: The High Calorie Way to Stay Thin Forever.*

The Council of Foods and Nutrition of the American Medical Association (4) reviewed the research on low-carbohydrate and unrestricted fat and protein intakes in relation to some of the claims made by the proponents of these regimes. Claims have been made that "an unlimited calorie intake [excluding carbohydrate] is associated with a consistent and physiologically advantageous loss of weight [which presumably continues as long as the diet is maintained]." Ultimately, however, the only way in which fat can be lost from the body is by expending more energy than is ingested. When experimental subjects consumed a 1000-kcal (4184 kJ), high-fat (90 percent of the kilocalories) diet for 8 to 10 days, they lost weight more rapidly than when they ingested a 1000-kcal (4184 kJ) diet with 90 percent of the kilocalories from carbohydrate. But when the experiment was repeated and continued for 18 to 24 days, the loss was the same for both diets. Because carbohydrate consumption affects the excretion of sodium and water, diets that contain very little carbohydrate tend to promote a temporary loss of these substances from the body. The ketone and uric acid levels in the blood are increased notably on a high-fat low-carbohydrate diet (40 percent–10 percent of the kilocalories) (28). See Table 8.14. Elevated blood uric acid levels appear to contribute to the development of gouty arthritis (19).

Because some people do lose weight on a low-carbohydrate, unrestricted-calorie diet, two English investigators (51) wanted to find out why. They studied six obese adults. These subjects were instructed to weigh and to record all of the

Table 8.14. Summary of Responses During Weight-Reduction Regimes

	High-fat diet	High-carbohydrate diet
Weight loss	5.2 kg	4.4 kg
Serum glucose	↓ 15%	↓ 7%
Plasma free fatty acid	↑ 350%	↑ 270%
Plasma ketones	↑ 2200%	↑ 300%
Serum uric acid	↑ 172%	↑ 11%
Serum triglyceride	↓ 45%	↓ 28%
Serum cholesterol	↓ 8%	↓ 3%

Adapted from S. B. Lewis, J. D. Wallin, J. P. Kane, and J. E. Gerick (1977). Effect of diet composition on metabolic adaptations to hypocaloric nutrition: comparision of high carbohydrate and high fat isocaloric diets. *Am. J. Clin. Nutrition*, **30:** 160.

food they ate for four weeks as follows: for the first two weeks they were to eat their usual diet, then for the next two weeks they were to decrease their carbohydrate intake to 50 g daily while eating all of the meat, fish, eggs, cheese, butter, margarine, and cream that they wanted. It was found that the subjects reduced their energy intake by 13 to 55 percent when they were on the low-carbohydrate diet; none ate more fat and some ate less during this period. Thus their weight loss was due to a lowered energy intake.

However, those who are accustomed to a low-carbohydrate diet are able to consume enough food to maintain their weight. Stephensson, the Arctic explorer who lived with the Eskimos for nine years, volunteered to continue his Arctic diet for another year after he returned to New York so that its metabolic effects could be studied. The caloric distribution of his diet was as follows: protein, 15 to 25 percent; fat, 75 to 85 percent; and carbohydrate, 1 to 2 percent. His diet consisted of beef, lamb, veal, pork, and chicken, and included muscle, liver, kidney, brain, bone marrow, bacon, and fat (31). Stephensson maintained his weight and apparent good health during this year; however, his blood cholesterol level was above normal (43).

Total fasting is sometimes used to treat obesity; for prolonged periods these persons must be hospitalized and closely supervised by a physician. Fasting may last anywhere from two days to two months (12). Protein, along with glycogen and fat, is lost from the bodies of those who fast (33). For extreme cases it appears that, in terms of maintaining a lower body weight for a prolonged period afterward, fasting produces better results than weight-reduction clinics (15, 30).

Predigested protein drinks have been promoted to the lay public as an aid in "modified fasting" diets. Although nutritionally inadequate products, they are promoted as the main item in the diet.

Dietary Advice and Nutrition Education Although these methods are not notably successful in treating obesity, they have sometimes been able to prevent it. Persons who tend to be overweight occasionally seek dietary advice on weight control, apply it, and thus prevent any further weight gain.

Whatever method is used to try to correct obesity, nutrition education is a valuable concomitant (32). Besides knowing the energy value of foods, one should know how to select an adequate diet totaling a fixed number of kilocalories per day. In order to control their weight, individuals must be able to plan a reasonable eating pattern that satisfies them personally and that they would be willing to follow every day, year in and year out, for the rest of their lives.

Behavior Therapy A relatively new approach to weight control is behavior modification. The premise of behavior therapy is that eating habits are learned behaviors. The focus is on eating habits, and the objective is to change them. A variety of techniques has been used in behavior modification programs to achieve weight loss, among them: self-monitoring and monitoring by others; stimulus control (limiting cues to eat, such as eating only at specified times and places); social reinforcement (receiving approval for constructive efforts to modify behavior); preventing

153

responses by using "road blocks" (avoiding eating cookies by having none on hand); and self-reward for successes (providing some nonfood reward). Nutritionists and dietitians, after some training with a psychologist and in cooperation with a psychologist (7, 34) and careful study of published works on behavior therapy, have carried out behavior modification programs for weight loss (40, 50). One of the more successful techniques is stimulus control. To illustrate the technique, a brief account of procedures used in one research study (34) follows. The participants (obese women) were made aware of their eating habits by keeping a daily food record and by using, for food eaten, a plate and bowl provided them by the investigators. There were *Dos* and *Don'ts* related to duties concerned with food, only two of which are given here: *Do* buy groceries from a shopping list after a full meal; *Do* store all foods, including refrigerated foods, in non-see-through containers. The program included 14 weekly meetings of one hour each; one portion of the program was concerned with behavior, another with nutrition. Each participant was encouraged

to develop a nutritionally sound meal pattern that would satisfy the nutritional needs and taste preferences of herself and her family. The women lost weight (8.4 kg or 18.5 lb) and at the 18-month follow-up were maintaining 80 percent of that loss, which is a better than usual record (34).

Exercise Exercise can be important in losing weight. Under controlled conditions of energy intake and exercise, it has been found that individuals will lose more weight when they exercise than when they do not (Table 8.15). In a study (13) made at Brigham Young University of 12 college women who were at least 40 percent overweight, a reduction of energy intake (1200 kcal [5021 kJ] per day) and an increase in energy expenditure (approximately 1400 to 1500 kcal [5858 to 6276 kJ]) on a treadmill and stationary bicycle (bicycle *ergometer*) four days a week resulted in a greater loss of weight than either method alone. At the end of six weeks, the mean weight losses were as follows: for the combined dietary restriction and exercise, 7.0 kg (15.3 lb);

Table 8.15 Body Weight Loss of Two Obese Women During Caloric Restriction with and Without Regular Exercise

Subject[a]	Regimen[b]	Days	Intake (kcal/day)	Weight loss (kg)	Weight loss (g/day)
1	No exercise	12	750	2.09	174
	1 hr exercise	13	750	2.77	213
	No exercise	24	650	2.07	86
	1 hr exercise	8	650	1.83	228
2	2 hr exercise	28	650	10.98	392
	No exercise	28	650	7.50	268
	2 hr exercise	27	650	7.41	275

[a] Subject 1: age 39, body weight 79 kg; Subject 2: age 35, body weight 130 kg.
[b] Exercise consisted of walking on the treadmill at 3 mph, 5 percent grade. The caloric equivalent of the walking was approximately 360 kcal per hour for Subject 1 and 400 kcal per hour for Subject 2.
From E. R. Buskirk, Increasing energy expenditure: the role of exercise. In N. L. Wilson, *Obesity*. Philadelphia: F. A. Davis Co., 1969, p. 169. Used by permission.

Table 8.16. Change in Appetite (Daily Caloric Intake) and the Composition of the Body Weight Loss in an Obese Young Woman[a] with and Without Regular Exercise

Period	Intake (kcal/day)	Days	Weight loss (kg)	Fat (kg)	Water (kg)	Fat-free water-free (kg)
No exercise (NE)	2170	14	−0.4	+1.4	−2.4	+0.6
Exercise[b] (E)	2900	28	−2.1	−0.7	−1.2	−0.2
Δ, E − NE	730	—	−1.7	−2.1	+1.2	−0.8

[a] Age 35, body weight 136 kg.
[b] Exercise level was approximately 1000 kcal per day.
From E. R. Buskirk, Increasing energy expenditure: the role of exercise. In N. L. Wilson, *Obesity*. Philadelphia: F. A. Davis Co., 1969, p. 170. Used by permission.

for dietary restriction alone, 6.4 kg (14.1 lb); and for exercise alone, 1.6 kg (3.5 lb). Those who neither dieted nor exercised did not lose any weight. A combination of diet and exercise was the most effective (27).

The common belief that exercise increases appetite was found to be true in a study of an obese woman whose food intake was voluntary but whose exercise was controlled. However, when she exercised, she expended more energy than she consumed so that she lost both total body weight and fat (Table 8.16). Several other obese women who imposed no dietary restrictions upon themselves and walked more than 30 minutes daily lost some weight (0.2 kg [0.5 lb] weekly) (18).

It has been found that obese men, women, boys, and girls all tend to be less active than the nonobese (8) (Table 8.17).

Drugs Most *anorexigenic* agents (appetite depressants) are *sympathomimetic* amines (compounds that produce effects similar to those of the sympathetic nervous system, that is, increases in heart rate, increases in the release of glucose from the liver, increases in the basal metabolic rate, decreases in the activity of the gastrointestinal tract, and so forth). How they work is not precisely understood. In most cases, after six

weeks of use, *amphetamines* no longer have the ability to depress the appetite. Furthermore, possible side effects include insomnia, irritability, restlessness, and tenseness. Any reducing drug should be used only under the direction of a physician.

One Explanation for Failure The number of fat cells plays a role in the capacity of an individual to lose weight. This was the finding from a Swedish study of obese women who were divided into two groups—those with an increase in fat cell number (hyperplastic) and those with an increase in the average fat cell size (hyperthrophic); a group of nonobese were controls. The obese were placed on a reducing diet of 1100 kcal (4232 kJ)/day. When no more weight was being lost, an examination showed that the enlarged fat cells in the two obese groups had decreased in size to that of the controls. Fat cell number remained unchanged, with the result that the obese with a normal number of cells ended up with a normal body fat, whereas those with a greater than normal number of cells remained obese even after some weight loss. Only under conditions of strictly controlled energy intake can fat cell size be reduced below the size of the fat cells of normal weight persons (6).

155

Table 8.17. Selected Comparisons from the Literature of Energy Expenditure Patterns in Nonobese and Obese Subjects

Measurement device and study	Type of subject	Number of subjects		+ (nonobese more active) 0 (nonobese and obese equal)
		Nonobese	Obese	
1. Timer: Bloom and Eidex	Men and women	6	7	+
2. Diary and indirect calorimetry: Durnin	Boys, girls, adults	—	—	+, +, 0
3. Activity records: Stefanik et al.	Boys	14	14	+
4. Motion pictures: Bullen et al.	Girls	108	52	+
5. Pedometer: Stunkard and Pestka	Girls	15	15	+
6. Pedometer: Chirico and Stunkard	Men	25	25	+
	Women	15	15	+
7. Pedometer: Dorris and Stunkard	Women	15	15	+
8. Diet and activity survey: McCarthy	Women	26	63	0

From E. R. Buskirk, Increasing energy expenditure: the role of exercise. In N. L. Wilson, *Obesity*. Philadelphia: F. A. Davis Co., 1969, p. 166. Used by permission.

Undernutrition

Undernutrition is the result of ingesting an insufficient quantity of food; malnutrition is the result of the consumption of food inadequate in quality. Deficiency of energy (undernutrition) is discussed in this section; deficiency of each essential nutrient is presented in the appropriate chapter.

Causes of Undernutrition

Individuals are underweight because their energy intake is less than their need. Their food consumption may be inadequate to meet their needs, or they may actually consume what normally would be enough food, but the body cannot properly utilize the food that is eaten, often due to digestive ailments and poor absorption. Intestinal parasites contribute to nutrient shortages by nourishing themselves on available nutrients and also by interfering with absorption of nutrients from the intestine (see chapts. 9 and 14); intestinal infestation by parasites is common in the tropics and subtropics, but much less so in the temperate regions.

The Underweight Person

Some slightly underweight persons want to maintain their weight for one reason or another—perhaps because of their appearance, because they feel better, or because it is required for their jobs (for example, fashion models and jockeys). They maintain this weight either by eating less, exercising more, or a combination of the two.

Others may be underweight because of poor health; they may have infections, poor digestion accompanied by diarrhea, or other ailments. Some may have poor food habits; they may eat to satisfy their appetite but not their nutrient needs. Some people live under extreme pressure or tension and have little opportunity to relax or to get away from disturbing problems; tension often contributes to poor appetite, faulty digestion, and underweight. If these people could slow down the tempo of their lives, relax before and after meals, and make mealtime an enjoyable occasion, they might be able to improve their digestion. And some people are undernourished because they do not have enough food available to them.

Anorexia Nervosa is a condition of self-induced severe weight loss. It occurs principally in adolescent girls who manifest a conscious and deliberate refusal of food. It is usually considered a disorder of psychological origin. Amenorrhea is a characteristic of the condition. Hospitalization and psychiatric therapy are usually necessary. The incidence of new cases was found to range from 0.6 to 1.6 per 100,000 (Britain); 40 percent of the cases recover completely, another 56 percent remain low in weight with some menstrual irregularities, and 5 percent fail to survive (13).

Prevalence of Undernutrition

Undernutrition is not an uncommon condition. The United Nations, in preparation for the World Food Conference in 1974, reassessed the world food situation, finding that "Millions of men, and even more women and children, simply do not have enough to eat. Definitions of undernourishment differ, and a wide variety of statistics can therefore be produced in support of this or that assertion. But, even on a cautious view, it is estimated that about a quarter of the population in the Far East, the Near East, and Africa do not have enough food to enable them to perform their ordinary human activities" (16).

The preliminary findings of the HANES (1) have not been analyzed to determine the incidence of undernutrition. Analyses have been made of the mean heights, weights, and triceps skinfold measurements of the children (1 to 17 years) according to income levels. The means for the group above the poverty level were greater; the differences were significant. The stunting effect observed in children of low-income families could almost be considered a universal truth, the finding has been confirmed so often (11).

Effects of Undernutrition

Growth With children, and the young of other species as well, an inadequate food intake limits growth. The young are endowed with the potential to grow; the capacity to do so is controlled by the environment, primarily by nutrition. In experimental animals that are fed at levels below their daily need, their stores of fat are utilized first to supply energy; protein is also taken from their muscle tissues. There is little loss of weight in the brain, bone, and kidney tissues during their deprivation; a greater loss occurs in the heart, liver, pancreas, and the organs of the alimentary tract.

Lack of Physical Well Being The body's normal resiliency to stresses is reduced in severely underweight persons. They are more susceptible to cold and manifest subnormal body temperatures. They may have a tendency toward subnormal blood pressure and edema.

Severely underweight persons are more likely to be ill, and their recovery from illness, surgery, or injury is apt to take longer than with normal persons. Infections that cause the undernourished to be acutely ill often have only a minor effect on the well-nourished (3, 14). The immune systems are less efficient in undernutrition: specific antibody synthesis is frequently impaired. Diarrhea, the primary cause of death for children under five years of age in less developed countries, occurs much more frequently among the undernourished than among the well-fed and worsens the condition; the rapid passage of material through the intestine allows for limited absorption of ·nutrients (15).

Undernutrition lessens the capacity for work; this has been observed under usual work conditions and in controlled laboratory experiments. During, and immediately following, World War II, Keller and Kraut (9) determined the work production of coal miners of the Ruhr district of Germany. In 1939, when the rations provided for an average daily energy intake per capita of 4500 kcal (18,828 kJ), the average amount of coal removed daily by each miner was 1.9 tons. In 1944, when the ration allowed only 1900 kcal (7950 kJ), 1.65 tons of coal were mined per man. In the experimental study of semistarvation carried out by Keys and his coworkers (10) at the University of Minnesota, the men suffered a marked loss of physical strength and endurance during the 24-week deprivation period. Voluntary exercise decreased; the men felt weak and tired.

Behavior Both children and adults who are slightly underfed tend to show an increase in motor restlessness. Those with a substantial loss of body weight manifest weakness and fatigue.

Those who are undernourished tend to be irritable, gloomy, and have an uneasy state of mind. Semistarved people are intensely preoccupied with thoughts of food. As a food shortage becomes worse, each person tends to fend for himself. Despite their unrest, semistarved persons are apathetic (8). The effects of hunger vary according to the severity of the deprivation and the capacity of the individual to adjust to his physical and mental stress.

Undernourished children behave differently from the well-nourished. Chavez and Martinez (5) noted this in their observations of two groups of children from birth to two years; one group was undernourished, the other well fed. One group of 17 mothers nursed their infants, giving them no supplementary food, as is the custom in the Mexican village where the study was done. The infants became undernourished; mother's milk alone was not sufficient. Another group of women, as sim-

ilar as possible to the first, socioeconomically and in other respects, was given from the 45th day of pregnancy on a supplement of minerals and vitamins, and 64 g of powdered milk. The infants born to the supplemented mothers were breast-fed and, in addition, were given supplements of milk and baby foods in amounts sufficient to maintain the infants at normal weight. As early as six months of life, differences in behavior between the children of the two groups had appeared. Those with supplements slept less during the day and played more. Those without supplements were sick more frequently and their illnesses were more severe and more prolonged; they were more passive, withdrawn, and timid, with greater dependence on their mothers. The children receiving supplements were more playful, bold, and mischievous—and they were demanding, disobedient, and aggressive with their mothers. The investigators expressed a desire to explore further a question raised by this study: "Did the supplement—that is to say, nutrition—only serve to accentuate the basic character of the child, or did his character change?"

Brain Structure and Function Undernutrition in early life may affect mental development and subsequent mental capacity. By the age of two years, the human brain has approached its adult size, weight, and cell number. The developing brain is notably more susceptible to injury during the period of most rapid growth than at any other time. That period, commonly called "growth spurt," begins in mid-pregnancy and continues to around 18 to 24 months after birth (7).

Few studies have been done on changes in the human brain due to malnutrition. At the Hospital Roberto Del Rio in Santiago, Chile, Winick and collaborators (17) observed that infants who die of malnutrition during the first year of life have fewer brain cells and a smaller head circumference. The functional implications of these changes are not known. The evidence that malnutrition causes mental retardation is not conclusive, only suggestive (6).

Rehabilitation from Undernutrition

Children undernourished when young are found able to catch up with the weight of their peers. In Jamaica, eight children ranging in age from ten months to three years who were recovering from protein–calorie malnutrition were studied. Because of their high food intake, they manifested a remarkable velocity in growth, frequently termed "catch-up growth." Their growth rate was 15 times that of normal children of similar age, and five times that of normal children of similar height and weight. When the children approached their expected weight for height, their food intake fell rather abruptly (30 percent) and their rate of growth dropped to a level comparable to that of normal children (2).

Rehabilitation from cerebral effects of undernutrition is less promising than from the physical effects. The vulnerability of the brain appears to be related to stage of development at the time of deprivation. Monckeberg (12) of Chile did a follow-up study on 14 infants who came to the hospital early in life with severe marasmic malnutrition (see p. 117), caused by adverse socioeconomic conditions in the home, to learn if the debilitating effects could be reversed. After discharge from the hospital, each child received free a total of 20 liters of milk each month with a similar amount for each other infant and preschool child in the family. The children were followed year after year. When they reached between four and seven years of age, their clinical examinations and blood analyses were normal. However, the average intelligence quotient of the group was significantly lower than the average Chilean preschool children of the lower socioeconomic class.

Adaptation to Inadequate Food Consumption

The body can adapt to many stresses imposed upon it. Cannon (4) used the term "homeostasis" to describe the ingenious body mechanisms that maintain normal conditions and that restore the physiological processes to a "steady state" after they have been disturbed.

The body adjusts to a certain level of undernutrition unusually well; the evidence for this can be seen in the remarkable ability of millions of undernourished people to survive. With inadequate food, the body loses weight, the basal metabolism is reduced, and activity is lessened. Obviously, therefore, less energy is needed. Of course, there is a level of energy intake for each person below which complete incapacitation occurs. Keys (10) pointed out that when the weight is reduced by around 20 percent from a previously normal weight, it is possible to maintain the body at the reduced weight on a diet of approximately 50 percent the energy value of the previous food intake, a fortunate physiological adjustment for the undernourished.

Diet for Gaining Weight

A diet for gaining weight should provide more energy than the body needs; there should be at least a normal amount (and possibly more) of protein, minerals, and vitamins. If the individual has no appetite, the diet should not include foods high in concentrated carbohydrates or fats. Concentrated carbohydrates cause the blood sugar level to rise quickly after eating and soon satisfy the appetite. Fat remains in the stomach a long time and gives a sensation of fullness. If the individual can eat a little more at each meal than he actually wants, and if he can eat snacks that are low in satiety value (such as fruit), his total energy intake can be increased.

Summary

Food energy is manufactured in the green plant using the raw materials CO_2 and H_2O in the presence of chlorophyll and solar energy. After the energy nutrients are ingested and metabolized, their energy is transferred by the cells to form the important compound adenosine triphosphate

159

(ATP). ATP provides energy for bodywork, for example, synthesis of important compounds and muscle contraction. (The process that food nutrients undergo to release energy for use by the cells is called energy metabolism.)

The unit used to measure energy is the kilocalorie (kcal), which is equal to 4.184 kilojoules (kJ).

The physiological fuel values of the energy nutrients are 9 kcal (38 kJ) for fat and 4 kcal (17 kJ) for both carbohydrates and protein.

The total energy need of an individual includes his basal metabolism, physical activity, and specific dynamic effect of his food. The basal metabolism is affected by body size, body composition, age, status of health, and secretions of the endocrine glands.

Man's body temperature is maintained by heat production and heat loss. Heat is produced by metabolism and increased muscular activity (voluntary and involuntary); heat is lost by radiation, convection, and water evaporation.

Any kind of physical activity increases the energy need above the basal metabolism. The energy cost of a physical activity depends upon the caloric expenditure for a given activity, the intensity with which it is performed, and body size of the individual performing the activity.

The specific dynamic effect is the heat produced by the ingestion of food itself and amounts to about 6 percent of the energy value of the food ingested.

One's total energy need can be estimated by the factorial method of calculation or by the table of recommended energy allowances. The RDAs for college-age men and women (19 to 22 years) are 3000 kcal (12,522 kJ) and 2100 kcal (8786 kJ) per day, respectively.

Foods with relatively large amounts of carbohydrates, fat, and protein per unit of weight are rich in kilocalories; those with smaller proportions are not. The energy value of foods may be found in food tables.

When an individual's energy intake consistently exceeds the energy expenditures, weight gain occurs and ultimately obesity results. The reason for overeating is an individual matter; it may be to compensate, or to conform to social practice, or it simply may be a habit of long standing. A physiological control does exist; a food intake regulation center has been identified in the brain in studies with experimental animals.

Children who are overweight are more apt to be obese adults than are normal-weight children. More women are obese than men, more black women than white, and more white men than black. The highest incidence (HANES data) for men was 14.2 percent, which was among white men, 20 to 44 years, and for women it was 43.0 percent, which was among black women, 45 to 64 years. Obese persons run a greater risk of diabetes, hypertension, and gall bladder disease than do persons of normal weight.

The best treatment for obesity is prevention. For those who are obese, caloric restriction, exercise, and behavior therapy have been found to be effective. Fasting should not be followed unless under the direct supervision of an accredited physician.

It appears that the number of fat cells may play a role in weight reduction. Those with an excessive number of fat cells lose weight until the fat content of the cells is reduced to the normal level (the same occurs with obese persons with a normal number of cells). But because of the greater than normal number of fat cells, obese persons remain somewhat overweight, whereas their normal-cell-number counterparts may attain normal weight.

Undernutrition results from the ingestion of an insufficient quantity of food or the inability of the body to utilize nutrients from the food eaten due to digestive ailments or poor absorption. Intestinal parasites nourish themselves on the nutrients available and interfere with absorption.

Undernutrition in children results in failure to grow normally, causes lack of physical and emotional well being, and appears to have a limiting effect on brain structure and function.

Within limits the body is able to adjust to an

inadequate energy intake by employing mechanisms for its conservation. Physical rehabilitation of undernourished children has been found possible; rehabilitation from cerebral effects is less certain.

Glossary

amphetamine: a drug (alpha-methylphenethylamine) used to reduce appetite; also reduces nasal congestion, increases blood pressure, stimulates central nervous system.

anorexigenic: an agent that diminishes appetite.

basal metabolic rate: the basal metabolism expressed as kilocalories per unit of body size (square meter of weight to the three-fourths power $W^{3/4}$).

calorimeter: the equipment used to measure the heat generated in a system. In nutrition it is an instrument for measuring the amount of heat produced by a food on oxidation or by an individual.

endocrine glands: those glands that produce one or more internal secretions (hormones) that enter directly into the blood and affect metabolic processes.

epigastric: region overlying the stomach.

epinephrine: a hormone produced by the medulla (inner part) of the adrenal gland; it helps to regulate the sympathetic branch of the autonomic nervous system.

ergometer: an instrument for measuring amount of work done under controlled conditions.

femoral: pertaining to the thigh.

Framingham Heart Study: a study initiated in 1949 in the town of Framingham, Massachusetts, with over 5000 healthy men and women, all over 30 years of age, participating. The purpose of the study was to identify factors in the lives of persons which are associated with coronary heart disease. At the beginning of the study the participants were examined clinically, certain laboratory (biochemical) tests were made, and the participants' life styles assessed. These observations are repeated every two years.

glucose tolerance: the body's reaction to ingested glucose; glucose tolerance can be determined quantitatively by the glucose tolerance test in which the in-

dividual ingests 100 g of glucose (12 hours after food), and later the blood glucose level is determined at intervals. Within 2 to 2½ hours after taking the sugar, the blood glucose level returns to normal unless an abnormality exists.

gluteal: pertaining to the buttocks.

hypothalamus: a portion of the brain lying at the base of the cerebrum.

sympathomimetic: an agent that produces effects similar to those of the sympathetic nervous system.

thyroxine: an iodine-containing hormone that is produced by the thyroid gland; it is a derivative of the amino acid tyrosine and has the chemical name tetra-iodothyronine.

Study Questions and Activities

1. Identify the following: calorimeter, specific dynamic effect of food, hyperthyroidism, Lavoisier, lean body mass, respirometer, and physiological fuel value.

2. Describe the ways in which heat is lost from the body.

3. How does basal metabolism differ from resting metabolism?

4. Compare the energy costs of walking (35 min at 2.27 mph), bicycling (45 min), driving a motorcycle (59 min), and driving a car (70 min) for a 121-ib (55 kg) college woman.

5. The energy costs of swimming and reclining for a 154-lb (70 kg) student are about 11.2 kcal and 1.3 kcal per minute, respectively. Using the values listed in Appendix Table A-3, calculate how long it would take that student to use up the energy value of 1 pint of vanilla ice cream, ½ cup peanuts, 20 pieces of French fried potatoes, 1 serving of apple pie, ¼ of a 14-in. pizza, a 12-oz can of beer, and an 8-oz cup of plain yogurt by both swimming and reclining.

6. List five factors that affect the basal metabolism of an individual. How does each affect the BMR?

7. How does food of high energy value differ from food of low energy value?

161

8. Calculate the energy cost of your basal metabolism for a 24-hour period. Use the following simple formula: 1 kcal per kilogram of body weight per hour.

9. Make a list of your activities for one day. Then estimate your total energy expenditure from the values presented in Table 8.4.

10. Three college women have recommended energy allowances of 1800 kcal, 2120 kcal, and 2600 kcal per day. What are their daily energy allowances in kilojoules and megajoules?

11. Have you any idea how many articles have appeared in women's magazines about weight control in the past year? How many this month? How many magazines did you examine?

12. Are there basic reasons for the incidence of obesity being greater among women than men? If so, explain.

13. Which do you consider the better method for determining obesity—height and weight or skinfold measurements? Justify your answer.

14. Why are there so many unsuccessful attempts to maintain the new weight attained after successful weight reduction?

15. Weigh yourself each day for a week after arising and going to the bathroom. Wear the same clothing at the weigh-in time each day. Plot the weights on graph paper. What was the maximum variation from one day to the next? How do you explain the variation?

References

The Need for Energy

1. Agan, T., S. Konz, and N. Tormey (1972). Extra heart beats as a measurement of work cost. *Home Economics Res. J.*, **1**: 28.

2. *Agricultural Statistics* (1977). Washington, D.C.: U.S. Dept. Agr., p. 561.

3. Boyd, J. J. (1975). The role of energy and fluid balance in weight changes found during field work in Antarctica. *Brit. J. Nutrition*, **34**: 191.

4. Bradfield, R. B., P. B. Huntzicher, and G. J. Fruehan (1969). Simultaneous comparison of respirometer and heart-rate telemetry techniques as measures of human energy expenditure. *Am. J. Clin. Nutrition*, **22**: 696.

5. Consolazio, C. F., and D. D. Schnakenberg (1977). Nutrition and the response to extreme environments. *Federation Proc.*, **36**: 1673.

6. Dubois, D., and E. F. Dubois (1916). Clinical calorimetry. A formula to estimate the approximate surface area if height and weight be known. *Arch. Int. Med.*, **17**: 863.

7. *Energy and Protein Requirements* (1973). FAO Nutrition Meetings Rept. Series 52, and WHO Tech. Rept. Series 522. Rome: Food and Agr. Organ.

8. Forbes, E. B., and R. W. Swift (1944). Associative dynamic effects of protein, carbohydrate, and fat. *J. Nutrition*, **27**: 453.

9. Garrow, J. S. (1974). *Energy Balance and Obesity in Man*. New York: American Elsevier Publishing Co., Chapter 5.

10. Guyton, A. C. (1976). Energetics and metabolic rate. In *Textbook of Medical Physiology*. 5th ed. Philadelphia: W. B. Saunders Co., Chapter 71.

11. Harper, A. E. (1970). Remarks on the joule. *J. Am. Dietet. Assoc.*, **57**: 416.

12. Hegsted, D. M. (1974). Energy needs and energy utilization. *Nutrition Rev.*, **32**: 33.

13. Kleiber, M. (1961). *The Fire of Life*. New York: John Wiley and Sons, p. 215.

14. Mitchell, J. W. (1977). Energy exchanges during exercise. In *Problems with Temperature Regulation during Exercise*, edited by E. R. Nadel. New York: Academic Press, Inc., pp. 11–26.

15. Passmore, R., and M. H. Draper (1964). The chemical anatomy of the human body. In *Biochemical Disorders in Human Disease*, 2nd ed., edited by R. H. Thompson and E. J. King. New York: Academic Press, pp. 8–10.

16. Proceedings. 32nd Annual Meeting. American Institute of Nutrition (1970). *J. Nutrition*, **100**: 1240.

17. *Recommended Dietary Allowances, Eighth Edi-*

tion (1974). Natl. Acad. Sci.-Natl. Research Council. Washington, D.C.: Natl. Research Council.

18. Richardson, R. H., D. E. Fulton, and F. E. Hunt. Columbus, Ohio: Ohio Agricultural Research and Development Center. Personal communication.

19. Swift, R. W., G. P. Barron, Jr. K. H. Fisher, N. D. Magruder, A. Black, J. W. Bratzler, C. E. French, E. W. Hartsock, T. J. Hershberger, E. Keck, and F. P. Stiles (1957). *Relative Dynamic Effects of High versus Low Protein Diets of Equicaloric Content.* Penn. State Univ. Agr. Expt. Sta. Bull. No. 618. University Park, Penn.: Pennsylvania State Univ.

20. Swift, R. W., and K. H. Fisher (1964). Energy metabolism. In *Nutrition: A Comprehensive Treatise*, vol. 1, edited by G. H. Beaton and E. W. McHenry. New York: Academic Press.

21. Thompson, K. (1977). Canada is adopting the joule. *J. Can. Dietet. Assoc.*, **66:** 146.

22. Walker, M. A., and L. Page (1975). Nutritive content of college meals. Proximate composition and vitamins. *J. Am. Dietet. Assoc.*, **66:** 146.

Overnutrition

1. Abraham, S., F. W. Lowenstein, and D. E. O'Connell (1975). *Anthropometric and Clinical Findings.* First Health and Nutrition Examination Survey, United States, 1971–72. DHEW Publ. No. (HRA) 75–1229. Rockville, Md.: U.S. Dept. Health, Educ. and Welfare, p. 25.

2. Abraham, S., and M. Nordsieck (1960). Relationship of excess weight in children and adults. *Public Health Repts.*, **75:** 263.

3. Albrink, M. J. (1968). Cultural and endocrine origins of obesity. *Am. J. Clin. Nutrition,* **21:** 1398.

4. American Medical Association, Council on Foods (1973). A critique of low-carbohydrate ketogenic weight reduction regimes. *J. Am. Med. Assoc.,* **224:** 1415.

5. Ashworth, N., S. Creedy, J. N. Hunt, S. Mahon, and P. Newland (1962). Effect of nightly food supplements on food intake in man. *Lancet*, **2:** 685.

6. Björntorp, P., G. Calgren, B. Isaksson, M. Krotkiewski, B. Larsson, and L. Sjöström (1975). Effect of an energy-reduced dietary regimen in relation to adipose tissue cellularity in obese women. *Am. J. Clin. Nutrition*, **28:** 445.

7. Blake, A. (1976). Group approach to weight control: behavior modification, nutrition, and health education. *J. Am. Dietet. Assoc.*, **69:** 645.

8. Bray, G. A. (1976). *The Obese Patient.* Philadelphia: W. B. Saunders Co.

9. Bray, G. A., ed. (1975). *Obesity in Perspective.* DHEW Publ. No. (NIH) 75–708. Washington, D.C.: U.S. Government Printing Office, p. 9.

10. Campbell, R. G., S. A. Hashim, and T. B. Van Itallie (1971). Studies of food-intake regulation in man: responses to variations in nutritive density in lean and obese subjects. *New Engl. J. Med.,* **285:** 1402.

11. Damon, A., and R. F. Goldman (1964). Predicting fat from body measurements: densitometric validation of ten anthropometric equations. *Human Biol.,* **36:** 32.

12. Drenick, E. J. (1969). Starvation in the management of obesity. In *Obesity*, edited by N. L. Wilson. Philadelphia: F. A. Davis Co., p. 191.

13. Dudleston, A. K., and M. Bennion (1970). Effect of diet and/or exercise on obese college women. *J. Am. Dietet. Assoc.,* **56:** 126.

14. Eid, E. E. (1970). Follow-up study of physical growth of children who had excessive weight gain in first six months of life. *Brit. Med. J.,* **2:** 74.

15. Forbes, G. B. (1967). The great denial. *Nutrition Rev.,* **25:** 353.

16. Garn, S. M. (1972). Commentary, the measurement of obesity. *Ecology of Food and Nutrition*, **1:** 333.

17. Gates, J. C., R. L. Huenemann, and R. J. Brand (1975). Food choices of obese and non-obese persons. *J. Am. Dietet. Assoc.,* **67:** 339.

18. Gwinup, G. (1975). Effect of exercise alone on the weight of obese women. *Arch. Int. Med.,* **135:** 676.

19. Hall, A. P., P. E. Barry, T. R. Dawber, and P. M. McNamara (1967). Epidemiology of gout and hyperuricemia. *Am. J. Med.,* **42:** 27.

20. Hamilton, C. L. (1973). Physiologic control of food intake. *J. Am. Dietet. Assoc.,* **62:** 35.

21. Hashim, S. A., and P. B. Van Itallie (1965). Studies in normal and obese subjects with a monitored food dispensing service. *An. New York Acad. Sci.*, **131**: 654.

22. Huenemann, R. L. (1974). Environmental factors associated with preschool obesity. I. Obesity in six-month-old children. *J. Am. Dietet. Assoc.*, **64**: 480.

23. Johnson, S. F., W. M. Swenson, and C. F. Gastineau (1976). Personality characteristics in obesity: relation of MMPI profile and age of onset of obesity to success in weight reduction. *Am. J. Clin. Nutrition*, **29**: 626.

24. Kannel, W. B., G. Pearson, and P. M. McNamara (1969). Obesity as a force of morbidity and mortality. In *Adolescent Nutrition and Growth*, edited by F. P. Heald. New York: Appleton-Century-Crofts, p. 51.

25. Knittle, J. L. (1972). Obesity in childhood: a problem in adipose tissue cellular development. *J. Pediatrics*, **81**: 1048.

26. Lepkovsky, S. (1973). Newer concepts in the regulation of food intake. *Am. J. Clin. Nutrition*, **26**: 271.

27. Lewis, S., W. L. Haskell, P. D. Wood, N. Manoogian, J. E. Bailey, and M. B. Pereira (1976). Effects of physical activity on weight reduction in obese middle-aged women. *Am. J. Clin. Nutrition*, **29**: 151.

28. Lewis, S. B., J. D. Wallin, J. P. Kane, and J. E. Gerich (1977). Effect of diet composition on metabolic adaptations to hypocaloric nutrition: comparison of high carbohydrate and high fat isocaloric diets. *Am. J. Clin. Nutrition*, **30**: 160.

29. Linton, P. H., M. Conley, C. Knechenmeister, and H. McClusky (1972). Statiety and obesity. *Am. J. Clin. Nutrition*, **25**: 368.

30. Long-term changes in body weight following complete fasting for obesity (1967). *Nutrition Rev.*, **25**: 168.

31. McClellan, W. S., and E. F. DuBois (1930). Prolonged meat diets with a study of kidney function and ketosis. *J. Biol. Chem.*, **87**: 651.

32. Orkow, B. M., and J. L. Ross (1975). Weight reduction through nutrition education and personal counseling. *J. Nutrition Educ.*, **7**: 65.

33. Overweight and hypertension (1969). *Nutrition Rev.*, **27**: 168.

34. Paulsen, B. K., R. N. Lutz, W. T. McReynolds, and M. B. Kohrs (1976). Behavior therapy for weight control: long-term results of two programs with nutritionists as therapists. *Am. J. Clin. Nutrition*, **29**: 880.

35. Rimm, A. A., L. H. Werner, B. Van Yserloo, and R. A. Bernstein (1975). Relationships of obesity and disease in 73,532 weight-conscious women. *Public Health Reports*, **90**: 44.

36. Salans, L. B., S. W. Cushman, and R. E. Weissman (1973). Studies of human adipose cell size and number in non-obese and obese patients. *J. Clin. Invest.*, **52**: 929.

37. Salans, L. B., J. L. Knittle, and J. Hirsch (1968). The role of adipose cell size and adipose tissue insulin sensitivity in the carbohydrate intolerance of human obesity. *J. Clin. Invest.*, **47**: 153.

38. Schachter, S. (1971). *Emotion, Obesity, and Crime*. New York: Academic Press, p. 72.

39. Seltzer, C. C., and J. Mayer (1965). A simple criterion of obesity. *Postgrad. Med.*, **38**: A101–A107.

40. Stuart, R. B., and B. Davis (1972). *Slim Chance in a Fat World: Behavioral Control of Obesity*. Champaign, Ill.: Research Press Co.

41. Stunkard, A. J., and S. Fox (1971). The relationship of gastric motility and hunger: A summary of the evidence. *Psychosom. Med.*, **33**: 123.

42. *Ten-State Survey, in the United States, 1968–1970* (1972). Washington, D.C.: U.S. Public Health Service, Dept. of Health, Educ. and Welfare.

43. Tolstoi, E. (1929). The effect of an exclusive meat diet on the chemical constituents of the blood. *J. Biol. Chem.*, **83**: 753.

44. Van Itallie, T. B., and R. G. Campbell (1972). Multidisciplinary approach to the problem of obesity. *J. Am. Dietet. Assoc.*, **61**: 385.

45. Wagner, M., and M. T. Hewitt (1975). Oral satiety in the obese and nonobese. *J. Am. Dietet. Assoc.*, **67**: 344.

46. Walike, B. C., H. A. Jordan, and E. Stellar (1969).

Preloading and the regulation of food intake in man. *J. Comp. Physiol. Psychol.,* **68:** 327.

47. Widdowson, E. M., and M. J. Dauncey (1976). Obesity. In *Present Knowledge in Nutrition.* D. M. Hegsted, Chm. Editorial Committee. Washington, D.C. Nutrition Foundation, Inc. p. 17.

48. Widdowson, E. M., and W. T. Shaw (1973). Full and empty fat cells. *Lancet,* **2:** 905.

49. Withers, R. F. J. (1964). Problems in the genetics of human obesity. *Eugen. Rev.,* **56:** 81.

50. Wollerscheim, J. P. (1970). The effectiveness of group therapy based upon learning principles in the treatment of overweight women. *J. Abnormal Psych.,* **76:** 462.

51. Yudkin, J., and M. Carey (1960). The treatment of obesity by the "high-fat" diet: The inevitability of calories. *Lancet,* **2:** 939.

Undernutrition

1. Abraham, S., F. W. Lowenstein, and D. E. O'Connell (1975). *Preliminary Findings of the First Health and Nutrition Examination Survey, United States, 1971–72.* DHEW Publ. No. (HRA) 75–1229. Rockville, Md.: U.S. Dept. Health, Educ. and Welfare.

2. Ashworth, A. (1969). Growth rates in children recovering from protein–calorie malnutrition. *Brit. J. Nutrition,* **23:** 835.

3. Awdeh, Z. L. (1976). Nutrition, infections, and immunity. In *Nutrition in the Community,* edited by D. S. McLaren. New York: John Wiley and Sons, p. 117.

4. Cannon, W. B. (1939). *The Wisdom of the Body.* New York: Norton, p. 19.

5. Chavez, A., and C. Martinez (1975). Nutrition and development of children from poor rural areas. V. Nutrition and behavioral development. *Nutrition Repts. Int.,* **11:** 477.

6. Cobos, F. (1972). Malnutrition and mental retardation: Conceptual issues. In *Lipids, Malnutrition and the Developing Brain.* New York: Associated Scientific Publishers, p. 227.

7. Dobbing, J. (1976). Nutrition and brain development. In *Present Knowledge in Nutrition.* 4th ed. D. M. Hegsted, Chm. Editorial Committee. New York: The Nutrition Foundation, Inc., p. 457.

8. Guetzkow, H. S., and P. H. Bowman (1946). *Men and Hunger.* Elgin, Ill.: Brethren Publishing House, p. 19.

9. Keller, W. D., and H. A. Kraut (1959). Work and Nutrition. In *World Review of Nutrition and Dietetics,* Vol. 3, edited by G. H. Bourne. New York: Hafner Publishing Co., p. 69.

10. Keys, A., J. Brožek, A. Henschel, O. Michelson, and H. L. Taylor (1950). *The Biology of Human Starvation.* Vol. 1. Minneapolis: The University of Minnesota Press.

11. Meredith, H. V. (1951). Relation between socio-economic status and body size in boys seven to ten years of age. *Am. J. Dis. Child.,* **22:** 702.

12. Monckeberg, F. (1975). The effect of malnutrition on physical growth and brain development. In *Brain Function and Malnutrition,* edited by J. W. Prescott, M. S. Read, and D. B. Coursin. New York: John Wiley and Sons, p. 15.

13. Russell, G. F. M. (1975). Anorexia nervosa. In *Textbook of Medicine,* edited by P. B. Beeson and W. McDermott. 14th ed. Philadelphia: W. B. Saunders Co., p. 1386.

14. Scrimshaw, N. S. (1975). Interactions of malnutrition and infection: Advances in understanding. In *Protein-Calorie Malnutrition,* edited by R. E. Olson. New York: Academic Press, pp. 353 and 360.

15. Scrimshaw, N. S., C. E. Taylor, and J. E. Gordon (1968). *Interactions of Nutrition and Infection.* Geneva: World Health Organization, p. 216.

16. United Nations (1974). *Things to Come. The United Nations World Food Conference.* New York: The United Nations.

17. Winick, M., P. Rosso, and J. A. Brasel (1972). Malnutrition and cellular growth in the brain: Existence of critical periods. In *Lipids, Malnutrition and the Developing Brain.* New York: Associated Scientific Publishers, p. 199.

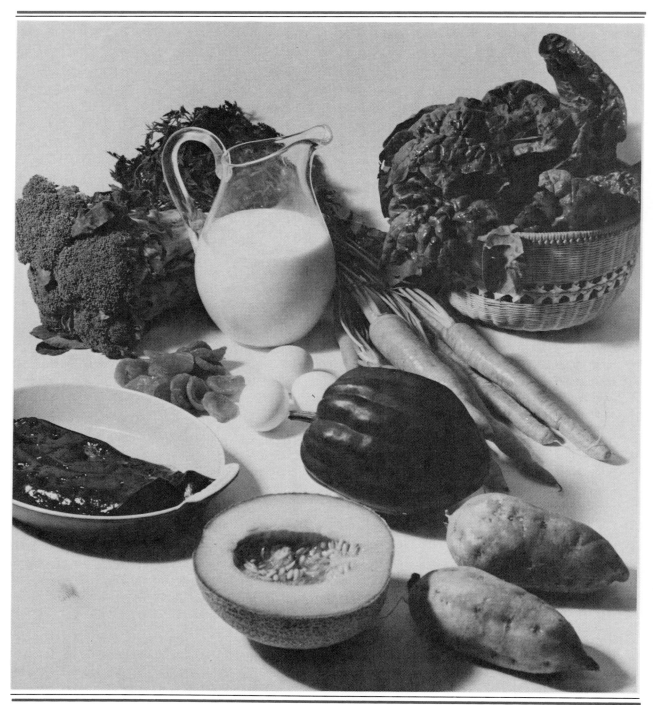

Liver, eggs, whole milk, spinach, carrots, sweet potatoes, winter squash, dried apricots, cantaloupe, and broccoli are excellent sources of vitamin A. Milk is fortified with vitamin D, making it a dependable year-round source of this vitamin.

Chapter 9

Introduction to the Vitamins and Fat-Soluble Vitamins

Abbreviations

HANES: Health and Nutrition Examination
  Survey
PUFA: polyunsaturated fatty acids
RBP: retinol-binding protein
RDA: Recommended Dietary Allowances
Vitamin D_2: activated provitamin, ergosterol
Vitamin D_3: activated provitamin
  7-dehydrocholesterol

Vitamin K_1: phylloquinone
Vitamin K_2: menaquinones
25-OH-D_3: 25-hydroxyvitamin D_3
1,25-$(OH)_2$-D_3: 1, 25-dihydroxyvitamin D_3
1 α-OH-D_3: 1 alpha-hydroxyvitamin D_3

Introduction to Vitamins

History

The discovery of vitamins ushered in a new era in nutrition. It was one in which minute substances in the diet assumed great importance. Although the percentage of body weight attributable to vitamins is almost negligible, they are indispensable for normal functioning.

The earliest evidence of the existence of vitamins came during the search for the treatment of certain diseases that had persistently plagued mankind. One of these diseases was scurvy—a hazard encountered by land explorers and sea voyagers. In 1747, some of the sailors in the British navy were cured of scurvy when they were given some of the limited supply of oranges and lemons that were aboard ship. It had not been known until then that a substance in these fruits could have such a remarkable effect. In another part of the world, a different disease, beriberi, was striking down Japanese sailors. Their diet had consisted mainly of white rice. With the addition of vegetables, meat, and fish (a change instituted in 1884), the incidence of beriberi decreased. However, it was not until the twentieth century that scientists and physicians recognized that beriberi was due to a dietary deficiency. Since it had been believed that disease could only be caused by microorganisms, it was difficult for scientists to accept the concept that certain diseases might be produced by deficiencies in the diet.

Another approach to the study of these diseases was by experimenting with animals in the laboratory. In the final analysis, it was the well-controlled laboratory experiments that eventually provided conclusive evidence that certain diseases were caused by the lack of given nutrients. In experimental studies, diets of a mixture of the following pure chemical compounds were used: pure protein (such as casein or albumin), pure fat (such as lard), pure carbohydrate (such as dextrin), and minerals. The purified diet was really the crux of the experiment: young animals on this diet failed to grow, and mature animals failed to maintain body weight. Something was missing in this mixture that was provided by foods (23). The first vitamin was discovered in 1913. Independently, Osborne and Mendel (the Connecticut Experiment Station) and McCollum and Davis (the University of Wisconsin) demonstrated that there was an essential dietary substance in fatty foods. Osborne and Mendel discovered it in cod liver oil; McCollum and Davis found it in butterfat and egg yolk. These researchers believed that only one factor was needed to supplement the purified diet, and they called it fat-soluble vitamin A. Three more fat-soluble vitamins were discovered and nine water-soluble vitamins (16) (see

168

Table 9.1 Dates of the Discovery, Chemical Isolation, and Synthesis of the Vitamins

Vitamin	Discovery	Isolation	Synthesis
Fat-soluble			
Vitamin A	1913	1937	1947
Vitamin D	1918	1931	1936
Vitamin E	1922	1936	1937
Vitamin K	1934	1939	1939
Water-soluble			
Vitamin C	1932	1932	1933
Thiamin (B_1)	1921	1926	1936
Riboflavin (B_2)	1932	1933	1935
Niacin	1867	1937 (as pellagra-preventing)	
Vitamin B-6	1934	1938	1939
Pantothenic acid	1933	1938	1940
Biotin	1924	1935	1942
Folacin	1945	1945	1945
Vitamin B-12	1948	1948	1973

Table 9.1). The designation "Vitamin B-17" has been used erroneously for the controversial compound amygdalin ("laetrile"), promoted for the cure of cancer. "Vitamin B-15" has been used, also erroneously, for the compound pangamic acid and promoted as a cure for certain diseases. No role in human nutrition has been found for this compound nor has its classification as a vitamin been established.

Definition of Vitamins

Vitamins are organic compounds that are required for growth and maintenance of life. They are regulatory substances (and sometimes structural), each performing (a) specific function(s). In general, the body cannot synthesize them, at least in large enough amounts to meet its needs. However, an exception is vitamin D; when an individual is exposed to ultraviolet rays, this vitamin is synthesized from its *precursor* found in the skin.

Vitamins needed varies among animal species; for example, man, monkeys, and guinea pigs need vitamin C, but rats, dogs, and rabbits are able to synthesize it.

Nomenclature of Vitamins

At first, naming the vitamins presented a problem since little was known about their structure or function. The word "vitamine" was coined in 1911 by Funk, a Polish biochemist, to designate the antiberiberi factor he was investigating at that time. He combined *vita* (meaning "essential for life") and *amine* (indicating its chemical structure). The term was accepted and used for all of the unknown factors. In 1919, the final "e" was dropped; by that time it was abundantly clear that there were several unknown essential factors, and that the known ones did not all have the amine structure. The change in spelling avoided any reference to chemical structure for the as yet unidentified essential factors.

169

The discovery of the first vitamin was facilitated by the finding that it was soluble in fat and fat solvents (alcohol and ether); it was called fat-soluble vitamin A. The discovery of the second was facilitated by the knowledge that it was soluble in water; it was called water-soluble B. A pattern was set and subsequent discoveries have fallen into either the fat-soluble or water-soluble category according to their properties. Also, there are some common characteristics of the fat-soluble vitamins that differ from those of the water-soluble group. Fat-soluble vitamins can be stored in the body; water-soluble vitamins cannot. The excretion of the fat-soluble group is chiefly by the fecal pathway; for the water-soluble vitamins, it is the urinary pathway.

Vitamins were generally designated by a letter of the alphabet, either by order of their discovery or by the initial letter of a word suggesting their role in nutrition. For example, in order of discovery, there were the fat-soluble vitamins A, D, and E and the water-soluble B_1, B_2, and C. Vitamin K, however, was named according to its antihemorrhagic function from the Danish term "Koagulation Faktor."

Later, as the chemical nature of vitamins was understood, names were introduced that pertained to their chemical structure. Then numerous compounds were identified that resembled the original vitamin in chemical structure and biological efficiency. Each compound, of course, required a specific name to identify it. The nomenclature, therefore, became more and more complex. Fortunately, the international bodies that determine nomenclature (the IUPAC—International Union of Pure and Applied Chemistry, the IUB—International Union of Biochemistry, and the IUNS—International Union of Nutritional Sciences) have recommended continuing the letter terminology for some vitamins (21). The terminology in general use is: vitamin A (retinol), vitamin D, vitamin E, vitamin K, thiamin, riboflavin, niacin, folacin, vitamin B-6, vitamin B-12, pantothenic acid, biotin, and vitamin C.

Measurement of Vitamins

Vitamins were discovered because of their effect on growth in young animals and their effect on the prevention and cure of specific deficiency diseases in both young and mature animals (for example, rats, chickens, pigeons, guinea pigs). Before the vitamins were isolated and their identities determined, the relative value of different foods as a source of these essential but unknown substances was measured; it was accomplished by measuring the effectiveness of the food being tested on the promotion of growth or the prevention and cure of deficiency disease. International units (IU) were established; they are under the surveillance of the World Health Organization. The animal procedure *(bioassay)* continues to be used for vitamins A, D, and E. Later microbiological assay methods were developed in which the vitamin source was given to a microorganism for which the vitamin was essential, and the rate of growth of the microorganism noted. With the identification of the chemical structure of the vitamins, chemical and physical methods of analysis were developed and used (5).

Functions of Vitamins

The failure of animals to grow on a ration of purified carbohydrate, fat, protein, and minerals equivalent in amounts to these nutrients in a food mixture led to the search for some substance essential for growth. The substance (soon to be learned, substances) found was called a vitamin. Thus one of the early recognized functions of vitamins was that they are essential for growth.

Chemical identification and refined research techniques led to the study of the basic function of each vitamin in the metabolic processes of the body: the building of body tissues (anabolic) and the breaking down processes (catabolic), the storage of energy and the release of energy for use—in fact, the functions of these substances, essential in the diet in small amounts, are basic to life itself. The further search for the basic functions of the vitamins is a continuing challenge to researchers.

A function of some of the vitamins is that of serving as a coenzyme. Certain enzymes function independently, whereas others require a cofactor. All enzymes are proteins, but the cofactor may be a metal or an organic molecule. The organic molecules are called coenzymes. The coenzymes are loosely bound to the enzyme; they facilitate reactions by donating or accepting chemical groups, such as amino ($-NH_2$) or aldehyde ($-CHO$) groups. Without the vitamin coenzyme, certain essential reactions cannot occur.

The specific functions of each vitamin will be discussed in later sections.

Vitamin A

Discovery of Vitamin A

McCollum and Davis (16, 17) and Osborne and Mendel (23) helped to establish the fact that 'one essential nutrient missing in purified diets of protein, fat, carbohydrate, and minerals was fat-soluble. This fact helped to speed the discovery of vitamin A, for it narrowed the range of compounds being considered (see p. 168). At the University of Wisconsin in 1919, Steenbock (32) found that yellow sweet potatoes and carrots would support normal growth and even supply enough of the unknown substances for reproduction. But rutabagas, beets, parsnips, potatoes, and sugar beets completely failed to provide the needed nutrient. It was noted that animals fed yellow corn as a supplement to the purified diet grew normally and were able to reproduce, whereas those fed white corn failed to grow and developed deficiency symptoms (32).

Thus, besides being soluble in fat, the nutrient was associated with yellow color in plant foods. But the relationship between the yellow plant materials and the fat substances, both of which

supplied the fat-soluble vitamin, was not yet understood. Ten years later (1929), German and English scientists demonstrated that crystalline carotene had vitamin A value. The exact chemical formula of the vitamin was determined in 1931, but it did not become available in synthetic form until 1947.

Nomenclature and Properties of Vitamin A and Carotene

Vitamin A is the general term used for several compounds, related chemically, that are effective sources of the vitamin. The major naturally occurring form is vitamin A alcohol (retinol); other forms are vitamin A aldehyde (retinal) and vitamin A acid (retinoic acid). In general, retinol is used synonymously with vitamin A, as it will be in this discussion. The chemical formula for vitamin A alcohol (retinol) is given in Fig. 9.1.

Vitamin A, an organic compound found only in the animal kingdom, is a very pale yellow (almost colorless) substance composed of carbon, hydrogen, and oxygen. The vitamin is soluble only in fat and fat solvents.

The plant kingdom provides a source of vitamin A for animals in the form of carotenoid pigments. The chief one in human nutrition is beta-carotene; in addition, there is alpha- and gamma-carotene and cryptoxanthin. The body converts these compounds into vitamin A in the intestinal mucosa during absorption. The conversion is not complete; some are absorbed unchanged. Actually all of the vitamin A in animal products originates directly or indirectly from the carotenoids of plants. Fish consume marine plankton, herbivorous land animals eat vegetable foods, and the carnivorous animals depend indirectly on herbivorous sources.

The carotenoid pigments are compounds composed of only carbon and hydrogen. The crystals of the pigments are a deep red color, but in solution they are intensely yellow. Their properties of solubility are like those of vitamin A. Beta-

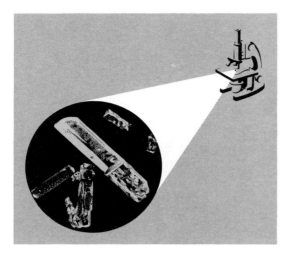

Fig. 9.1 Chemical formula of vitamin A alcohol (retinol) and photomicrograph of crystalline vitamin A acetate (retinylacetate). (Courtesy Hoffman-LaRoche, Inc.)

carotene is most prevalent in plants and is more efficiently converted to vitamin A than the other forms are. The term carotene will be used in this discussion when the carotenoid pigments are referred to.

Carotene is called provitamin A; that is, it is a substance that can be converted to vitamin A in the body. Precursor of vitamin A is also a designation for carotene (a precursor is a substance that precedes another, usually an inactive form convertible to an active form).

Measurements of Vitamin A and Carotene

Until recently vitamin A activity in foods has been expressed in International and *USP* (United States Pharmacopeia) Units (which are equal) with the following equivalencies:

1 IU = 0.3 μg retinol

1 IU = 0.6 μg beta-carotene

1 IU = 1.2 μg other provitamin A caroenoids

These relationships were derived from studies on the rat and are assumed to hold for man. The vitamin A values in most food tables are expressed in International Units.

The Food and Nutrition Board has recommended that Retinol Equivalents (RE) replace the International Unit. The maximum conversion of beta-carotene to vitamin A is about 50 percent and for the other carotenoids, about 25 percent. These values are from animal studies; no information is presently available for humans. In addition to the inefficiency of conversion, there is wide variability in intestinal absorption of carotenoids from different food sources. For man, absorption of the provitamins is estimated to be about one-third of the amount ingested; retinol is assumed to be completely absorbed. Taking into consideration both conversion and absorption, the overall utilization of beta-carotene is one-sixth that of retinol; for the other carotenoids, alpha-carotene and cryptoxanthin, it is one-twelfth (25).

Retinol Equivalents (RE) are derived with allowance made for efficiency of conversion and of absorption of the provitamins, giving the following equivalents:

1 RE = 1 μg retinol
1 RE = 6 μg beta-carotene
1 RE = 12 μg other provitamin A carotenoids

The relationship between retinol equivalents and the values for vitamin A and beta-carotene (in International Units) is as follows:

1 RE = 3.33 IU retinol
1 RE = 10 IU beta-carotene

Metabolism of Vitamin A and Carotene

Conversion of Carotene to Vitamin A   It was first believed that carotene was converted to vitamin A in the liver because of the high vitamin A content of that organ. However, this hypothesis was discarded when the provitamin administered intravenously was not converted to vitamin A. Then the intestinal wall was found to be the main site of the transformation, although the liver and other tissues are additional sites (11). Now there is evidence that when beta-carotene is injected into the blood, finely dispersed in an *emulsifying agent* (formerly an emulsifying agent was not used), vitamin A appears in the liver and kidneys.

The presence of enough protein of good quality helps the conversion of carotene to vitamin A. The factor of protein quality is important because in most developing countries carotene is the main source of vitamin A, and the people of these countries do not consume protein of high biological value (27).

Absorption   Vitamin A is absorbed from the small intestine into the *lymph* system (10, 31). It is assumed that vitamin A is absorbed efficiently because it is seldom found in the feces. However, certain factors affect the speed and completeness of its absorption. *Aqueous emulsions* of vitamin A are more rapidly, but no more completely, absorbed than oil solutions (4). Bile salts promote the absorption of vitamin A but are not essential (27). *Antioxidants* in the lumen of the intestine diminish the loss of vitamin A by oxidation (4).

Some of the carotene is absorbed as such into the lymphatic system; some is converted to vitamin A in the intestinal mucosa. The absorption of carotene depends upon other substances being present in the small intestine, including bile, dietary fat, and antioxidants. Because bile aids emulsification, it is necessary for carotene absorption. Fat must also be absorbed simultaneously. In Ruanda-Urandi (central Africa), Roels (28) traced the widespread vitamin A deficiency to the fact that less than 7 percent of the total energy value of the diet came from fat, although it contained an adequate amount of carotenoids; he found that the symptoms of vitamin A deficiency could be alleviated by administering small supplements of fat (28). When antioxidants such as alpha-tocopherol and lecithin are present in the small intestine, the loss of carotene by oxidation is decreased.

Effect of Intestinal Parasites on Absorption of Vitamin A and Carotene and the Conversion of Carotene to Vitamin A   In tropical regions where vitamin A deficiency is a serious health problem, intestinal parasite infections are common. In a study of children, the parasite *giardia lamblia* was found to interfere with the absorption of vitamin A and the conversion of carotene to vitamin A (8). The absorption of vitamin A was interfered with by the parasite *ascarias lumbricoides* in observations made on adults in India where the parasite is prevalent (14).

173

Transport   In the liver, vitamin A is bound to a specific retinol-binding protein (RBP). Vitamin A enters the blood bound to RBP and is transported to the tissues. RBP can leave the liver only when bound to vitamin A; in vitamin A deficiency, RBP accumulates in the liver (31).

Storage   The liver rapidly removes vitamin A from the blood and stores it; it also quickly releases vitamin A into the blood in order to maintain the blood level of the vitamin constant (12). About 90 percent of the vitamin A stored in the human body is found in the liver, but small amounts are also stored in the lungs, body fat, and kidneys. The amount of storage vitamin A tends to increase with age, but, of course, this depends on the quantity in the diet and the amount absorbed. It has been estimated that a normal adult liver could store as much as 600,000 IU of vitamin A, or enough to meet an adult's need for about four months. Carotene is stored in adipose tissue.

Excretion   Vitamin A is excreted chiefly by the fecal pathway; some is also excreted by way of the kidneys.

Functions of Vitamin A

Except for its role in vision, which has been clearly delineated by Wald, the basic functions of vitamin A are not well understood. (Wald was awarded the Nobel Prize for medicine in 1967 for his contributions to the understanding of the functioning of the human eye.) The differing physiological roles of the various chemical forms of vitamin A tend to complicate any determination of its functions. For example, vitamin A acid (retinoic acid) will promote growth but not vision in rats. If the only form of vitamin A they ingest is retinoic acid, they will become blind. Since many physiological functions are affected by vitamin A and a deficiency produces a large

number of pathological lesions, it appears that vitamin A plays an essential metabolic role in many biochemical systems and tissues in man.

Function in Vision   The retina of the eye has two kinds of photoreceptor cells: the rods, which are sensitive to light of low intensity and function in dim light; and the cones, which are sensitive to light of high intensity and function in bright light and provide color vision. The terms "rods" and "cones" are derived from the shape of the cells. Rhodopsin (visual purple) is the pigment in the rods that contains vitamin A; iodopsin is the main pigment in the cones that contains vitamin A. All of the visual pigments are composed of the same vitamin A fraction (retinal) but of different proteins. Opsin is the protein of rhodopsin.

The visual cycle proceeds in this manner: In the presence of light, opsin and retinal are liberated from rhodopsin. The atoms in the retinal molecule are rearranged with the formation of *trans*-retinal. In the dark, rhodopsin is regenerated; all *trans*-retinal is converted to another form (11-cis-retinal), which combines with opsin to form rhodopsin (27). Some vitamin A is used up (degraded) with each repetition of the visual cycle, which makes it necessary that additional amounts be available (see Fig. 9.2).

If a person remains in darkness for some time, practically all of the retinal and the opsin are converted to rhodopsin. Also large amounts of vitamin A are converted to retinal, which in turn is changed to rhodopsin. With all of this

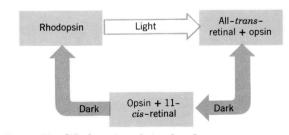

Fig. 9.2 Simplified version of visual cycle.

174

rhodopsin, the rods become sensitive to even a small amount of light. The person facing the lights of an oncoming car at night or the bright lights of the foyer on leaving the darkened theater is confronted with poor vision; with the eyes sensitive to even a small amount of light, sudden bright illumination has a blinding effect.

If, on the other hand, a person has been in bright light for a long time, large portions of the rhodopsin break down to retinal and opsin and much of the retinal changes to vitamin A. The sensitivity of the eye to light is reduced.

Night blindness is a condition that occurs in severe vitamin A deficiency; when the level of vitamin A in the blood becomes reduced, the quantities of vitamin A, retinal, and rhodopsin also become reduced. The condition is called night blindness because at night the amount of available light is far too little to permit adequate vision, whereas in the daytime it is sufficient even though the rhodopsin of the rods is notably reduced.

Growth Before vitamin A had been isolated and its chemical formula determined, its potency in food was measured by the growth rate. Since animals on a vitamin A-free diet stop growing when their bodies are depleted of its stores, foods to be assessed were fed to these animals in known amounts for a prescribed period of time and their growth response noted. Better growth meant a higher vitamin A content in the food.

If the intake of vitamin A is not sufficient for normal growth, the bones will stop growing before the soft tissues are affected. This cessation of bone growth may result in overcrowding the brain and central nervous system. It now seems clear that the paralysis that sometimes accompanies a vitamin A deficiency in very young animals is due to this failure of bone growth, which causes cranial pressure and consequent brain and nerve injury. In some instances the optic nerve is pinched, which results in blindness. However, a deficiency of vitamin A may cause degeneration of nervous tissue without causing bone malformation.

Health of the Epithelial Tissues The epithelial tissues cover the outer surface of the body and line the major cavities and all of the tubular systems within the body. These tissues are differentiated (specialized): the external covering is the resistant, protective *epidermis;* the internal tissue is a secretory mucous membrane. Insufficient vitamin A causes a suppression of the tissues' specialized functions and produces a keratinized (dry, horny) type of epithelium. The skin may become excessively dry and the mucous membranes may fail to secrete normally and thus become more prone to bacterial invasion. The exact role that vitamin A plays in maintaining the health of the epithelial tissues is not known (28).

Assessment of Vitamin A Status

Xerosis (dryness) of the conjunctiva (the delicate membrane that lines the eyelids and covers the exposed surface of the eyeball) is the best clinical indication of early vitamin A deficiency; xerosis of the cornea (the transparent membrane that coats the outer surface of the eye) and keratomalacia (softening of the cornea) characterize an advanced deficiency (1, 13).

Blood retinol determination is the only practical biochemical test currently available for assessing vitamin A status in population groups (5). Values less than 20 μg/100 ml are interpreted to indicate a low intake of vitamin A over a long period and a low reserve supply of the vitamin (29).

Vitamin A Deficiency

This deficiency may be due to a dietary lack of vitamin A, to a dietary lack of the provitamin, or to poor absorption. Among the various clinical manifestations, those of the eye and the skin are preeminent.

175

The Eye The earliest symptom is night blindness (nyctalopia), the inability to see normally in dim light. (See p. 175 for discussion.)

The next symptom to appear is usually dryness of the *conjunctiva* (Fig. 9.3a). The presence of one or both of these symptoms may be due to something other than vitamin A deficiency, but when there is conjunctival *xerosis*, night blindness, and a low blood level of vitamin A, inevitably there is a vitamin A deficiency.

Bitot's spots (named for the French physician who first discovered them) appear as small plaques of silvery gray, usually with a foamy surface, on the conjunctiva (Fig. 9.3b). When they are associated with generalized xerosis and occur in young children, the cause is usually a deficiency of vitamin A. However, in adults these spots may have another cause. McLaren (18), who has studied the relation of malnutrition to the eye in many parts of the world, found that Bitot's spots are definitely associated with malnutrition, although not necessarily with hypovitaminosis A.

A later stage of vitamin A deficiency is xerosis of the cornea. In the infant and preschool child this serious condition may develop before any other symptoms appear. The cornea becomes dry and loses its transparency, thus having a hazy appearance; it also becomes soft (Fig. 9.3c). Vision is obviously impaired, depending upon the extent of the corneal damage. Early treatment with vitamin A will restore full vision; however, if advanced changes have taken place, blindness is inevitable. The term "xerophthalmia" in the broad sense refers to all clinical conditions of the eye related to inadequate vitamin A.

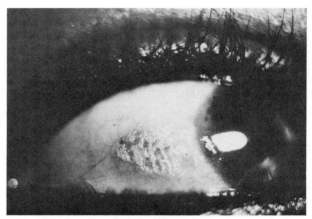

(b) A typical Bitot's spot, a warning sign of vitamin A deficiency.

Fig. 9.3 Signs of vitamin A deficiency. (Courtesy Professor D. S. McLaren, American University of Beirut, Lebanon.)

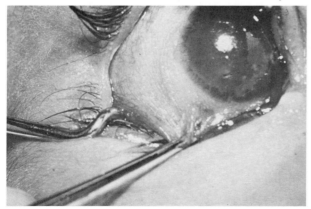

(a) Xerosis of the conjunctiva—an early clouding and infiltration of the cornea.

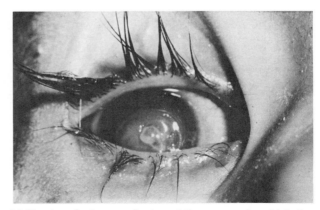

(c) Keratomalacia—a softening of the cornea, in which the cells weaken and are pushed out of shape.

The Skin Those with a prolonged and severe vitamin A deficiency may also experience changes in the skin, including dryness, wrinkling, slate-gray discoloration, and hyperkeratosis (thickening of the outer layer). The hair may lose its luster, and there may be a longitudinal furrowing of the fingernails and toenails.

World Prevalence of Vitamin A Deficiency Among the nutritional disorders affecting infants and young children, vitamin A deficiency ranks second after protein–calorie malnutrition. The most susceptible age group is nine months to four years; the severity of the eye lesion is usually inversely related to age.

Vitamin A deficiency is widely prevalent in the densely populated countries of southern and eastern Asia, in parts of Africa, the Middle East, and Latin America (34). Young children are being blinded by the deficiency (30).

Preventive Measures For the urgent prevention of blindness in a child, massive dosages of vitamin A (200,000 IU) by mouth at six-month intervals has been effective. Such programs have been underway in India, Indonesia, Bangladesh, and other places (22). Oomen (22) proposes that a continuing effective program would be to fortify a staple foodstuff eaten by children.

Vitamin A Consumption and Deficiency in the United States

Results from the Ten State Nutrition Survey (1968–1970) showed that of the 4455 individuals examined in the below-poverty group, 8.5 percent had low plasma vitamin A levels (less than 20 μg/100 ml); of the 7243 persons in the above-poverty group, 7.5 percent had low levels. The data for vitamin A intake show slight differences between the above- and below-poverty groups. Based on evidence from the biochemical measurements and the analysis of the dietary intake data, Spanish-Americans, mainly Mexican Americans,

have a low status of vitamin A nutriture. The sample for the Ten State Survey was representative of low-income families of the areas studied; those families from the area with higher incomes included in the sample were not representative of the middle- and high-income population (13).

Preliminary findings from the first Health and Nutrition Examination Survey, United States, 1971–1972 (HANES), revealed very few eye conditions characteristic of vitamin A deficiency among the 10,126 persons (1–74 years of age) examined (1). The highest prevalence of low serum vitamin A values (less than 20 μg/100 ml) was among Negro children 1–5 years of age (9.1 percent in the lower-income group; 10.3 percent in the income group above the poverty level). In all other age-sex-income and racial groups, the incidence was much less. The groups with the highest percentage of individuals not meeting the standard for daily vitamin A activity intake (see Appendix Table A–27 for standards), and the actual percentage were: 1–5 years, Negro and white, both income groups, 37 to 52 percent (standard = 2000 IU daily); males, 18–44 years, both income groups, 45 to 65 percent (standard = 3500 IU daily); females, white, 18–44 years, low-income group, about 73 percent (standard = 3500 IU daily); and adults 60 years of age and over, both income groups, 52 to 62 percent (standard = 3500 IU daily) (2). The dietary findings and serum vitamin A levels showed little correlation except for the 1–5-year-old Negro children, for whom both assessments were low.

Hypervitaminosis A

An excessive intake of vitamin A produces toxic symptoms in both humans and animals. A 51-year-old woman who had been taking 600,000 IU of vitamin A daily as a treatment for sinusitis (for the three years preceding her admission to the hospital) developed fatigue; severe pain in her knees, hips, and shoulders; loss of scalp and body hair; and coarse, yellowish skin, with prominent hair follicles (7). A 28-year-old woman who

177

had ingested 1,300,000 IU of vitamin A within a 27-hour period as a treatment for sunburn showed symptoms of nausea, vomiting, intense headache, and blurred vision (9). A 17-year-old boy who had been taking 200,000 IU of vitamin A daily for 18 months (for acne) developed discrete superficial hemorrhages in the retinae of both eyes. When the vitamin was discontinued, the symptoms began to regress in all three cases.

One of the most dangerous effects of the excessive use of vitamin A is increase in intracranial pressure. This symptom has been observed both in children and adults, with headache, nausea, vomiting, and lethargy (36).

Daily intakes of 25,000 to 50,000 IU of vitamin A can induce toxic symptoms in as short a time as 30 days in older children and adults. Infants manifest toxicity symptoms on lesser amounts, 14,000 to 20,000 IU daily (about ten times the RDA), in several weeks (36).

A beneficial Food and Drug Administration regulation limiting the dosage of vitamin A preparations to 10,000 IU without being classified as drugs, effective since October 1973 (20) was revoked. See Federal Register March 14, 1978.

Massive doses of carotene, on the other hand, are not harmful because it is not converted to vitamin A sufficiently rapidly to cause toxicity (19). The accumulation of excess carotene in the body produces a slightly yellow skin color, which disappears when the intake is reduced.

Recommended Dietary Allowances for Vitamin A

The daily RDA of vitamin A activity for men is 5000 IU (1000 RE) and for women 4000 IU (800 RE); recommendations in terms of RDA per 1000 kcal for young men (19 to 22 years) 1667 IU per 1000 kcal (4184 kJ) (333 RE per 1000 kcal [4184 kJ]) and for young women (19 to 22 years) 1905 IU per 1000 kcal (4184 kJ) (381 RE per 1000 kcal [4184 kJ]). These recommendations take into account the fact that the International Units of

the preformed vitamin A (retinol) and the provitamin (beta-carotene) in the United States' food supply are about equal (25, 26). The ordinary American diet in 1977 provided about 8200 IU of vitamin A value per day: 48.3% from fruits and vegetables; 21.3% from fats, oils, and dairy products; 27.9% from meat, fish, and eggs; and 2.2% from miscellaneous foods (15).

If the source of vitamin A activity should all be from the provitamin (as in the case of a completely vegetarian diet), the recommended intake would be 10,000 IU. The RDA of 5000 IU of vitamin A assumes that one-half of the vitamin activity is from the preformed vitamin (2500 IU or 750 μg) and one-half from the provitamin (2500 IU). The equivalent of 750 μg of vitamin A would be 4500 μg (7500 IU) of beta-carotene (the utilization of beta-carotene is one-sixth that of vitamin A. Adding together the 2500 IU (one-half the 5000 IU from carotene) and the 7500 IU (the equivalent in carotene of the 2500 IU from vitamin A) gives 10,000 IU (25).

The vitamin A activity needs for age and sex groups expressed as RDA and RDA per 1000 kcal are given in Table 9.2.

Samples of meals served in 50 colleges, analyzed for nutrient content, were found to have a vitamin A value more than double the 5000 IU recommended for men and about triple the 4000 IU allowance for women. The range was 6819 to 19,424 IU per person per day (35).

Food Sources of Vitamin A

Preformed vitamin A is found only in foods of animal origin, whereas carotene is found in both plant and animal products. Good food sources of vitamin A are whole milk, butter, egg yolk, liver, and kidney (Table 9.3). The amount of vitamin A in the liver increases with the age of the animal and varies with the species. The potency of the vitamin in butter fat and egg yolk depends upon the diet of the cow and the hen, respectively. If these animals are permitted to feed on green grass, the vitamin A content of milk and eggs is

178

Table 9.2 Recommended Dietary Allowances for Vitamin A Activity

	Age, years	RDA			
		RE	IU	RE/1000 kcal	IU/1000 kcal
Infants	0.0–0.5	420	1400	—	—
	0.5–1.0	400	2000	—	—
Children	1–3	400	2000	307.7	1538.6
	4–6	500	2500	277.8	1388.9
	7–10	700	3300	291.7	1375.0
Males	11–14	1000	5000	357.1	1785.7
	15–18	1000	5000	333.3	1666.7
	19–22	1000	5000	333.3	1666.7
	23–50	1000	5000	370.4	1851.9
	51+	1000	5000	416.7	2083.3
Females	11–14	800	4000	333.3	1666.7
	15–18	800	4000	381.0	1904.8
	19–22	800	4000	381.0	1904.8
	23–50	800	4000	400.0	2000.0
	51+	800	4000	444.4	2222.2
Pregnant		1000	5000	—	—
Lactating		1200	6000	—	—

From *Recommended Dietary Allowances* (1974). Eighth Ed. Washington, D.C.: Natl. Acad. Sciences.

likely to be higher. The synthetic forms of vitamin A (which are nutritively equivalent to the natural forms) are often used in food supplements.

The most important sources of carotene are generally the deep yellow, yellowish-red, and dark green fruits and vegetables. (The yellow carotene in green products is masked by the presence of chlorophyll.) Large amounts of carotene are provided by carrots, sweet potatoes, apricots, spinach, tomatoes, and kale. However, some fruits and vegetables (such as oranges, rutabagas, and wax beans) deviate from the general color rule because, although yellow, they contain *xanthophyll* or other pigments that do not have vitamin A activity. Head lettuce and avocados, two green-colored foods, contain small amounts of carotene. There is little vitamin A in nuts, grains, vegetable oils, muscle meats, and light-colored fruits and vegetables.

The term "vitamin A value of foods" is used instead of "vitamin A content" in Table 9.3. It would be incorrect to say that carrots, for example, have 10,400 units of vitamin A per 100 g, for actually they contain no vitamin A at all — only carotene.

In compiling the food composition tables for the U.S. Department of Agriculture Handbook No. 456 (1975), values for carotene in foods were converted to International Units of vitamin A activity on the assumption that 0.6 μg of beta-carotene, or 1.2 μg of the other carotenes with vitamin A activity and cryptoxanthin, was equivalent to 1 IU of vitamin A value (3). In Agriculture Handbook No. 8–1 being compiled currently, the vitamin A value of foods is expressed in both International Units and Retinol Equivalents (24).

Stability of Vitamin A and Carotene in Foods
Since both vitamin A and carotene are insoluble in water and stable under ordinary cooking temperatures, it was believed that little could be lost

179

Table 9.3 Vitamin A Value of Various Foods as Served

Food	Per 100 g of food Vitamin A value, IU	Per average serving Size of serving g	Vitamin A value IU
Liver			
beef, fried	53,400	3 oz 85	45,390
calf, fried*	32,700	3 oz 85	27,800
pork, fried*	14,900	3 oz 85	12,670
chicken, simmered*	12,320	3 oz 85	10,460
Carrots, boiled	10,440	½ c 78	8,140
Kale, boiled	8,300	½ c 55	4,565
Spinach, boiled	8,100	½ c 90	7,290
Sweet potato, baked in skin	8,100	1 med 114	9,230
Margarine, fortified	3,360	1 tbsp 14	470
Butter	3,100	1 tbsp 14	430
Apricots, canned	1,740	½ c 129	2,245
Peaches, raw	1,330	1 med 100	1,330
Cheese (Swiss)	860	1 oz 28	240
Green beans, boiled	550	½ c 62	340
Eggs (hard cooked)	520	1 whole 50	260
Orange juice, fresh	200	½ c 124	250
Milk, skim (with added vitamin A)	200	8 oz 245	500
Milk, whole	130	8 oz 244	310
Apple, raw	85	1 med 138	120
Beef, hamburger, cooked	25	3 oz 85	20
Potato (white), baked	tr	1 med 135	tr
Bread (white, enriched)	tr	1 sl 28	tr
Oatmeal, cooked	0	½ c 120	0

* *Nutritive Value of American Foods*, Agr. Handbook No. 456. Washington, D.C.: U.S. Dept. Agr., 1975.

From *Nutritive Value of Foods*, Home and Garden Bult. No. 72. Washington, D.C.: U.S. Dept. Agr., 1977.

in food preparation. However, a study in 1971 showed that there was a substantial loss in vitamin A value in cooking or canning vegetables; these processes produce a rearrangement of atoms in the carotene molecule, resulting in carotenes of lower vitamin A value. It is estimated that the vitamin A value of average cooked green vegetables is descreased by 15 to 20 percent and the

value of yellow vegetables 30 to 35 percent (33). Drying and dehydration also produce a considerable loss by oxidation. Freezing causes little loss.

Rancid fat destroys both vitamin A and carotene. When fat is stored in a cool, dry place, rancidity is delayed and so the vitamin is preserved. Margarines were found to lose less than 25 percent of the original vitamin A content when stored at −10°C (14°F) for up to two years, but when stored at 18°C (64°F), 75 percent of the original vitamin A content was lost in only 17 weeks (6).

Vitamin D

Discovery of Vitamin D

Vitamin D prevents and cures rickets, a disease in which the bones fail to calcify. Children had been afflicted with rickets for centuries before the relationship of the deforming disease to vitamin D (or sunshine) was understood. Rickets was prevalent in England (where it almost reached epidemic proportions during the Industrial Revolution), in most of the countries of Northern Europe, and in the larger cities of the United States (where it was still common even in the early 1930s).

The combined clinical observations of children with rickets and of experimental animals with induced rickets led to the identification of vitamin D as the antirachitic vitamin. As early as 1890, Palm (an English physician) observed that where sunshine was abundant, rickets was rare, but where the sun seldom shone, rickets prevailed. However, it was not until 1919 that Mellanby demonstrated that rickets was a nutritional deficiency disease. He produced rickets in puppies by using diets of mixed foods (such as whole milk, rice, and salt) and then cured it by giving them cod liver oil. But Mellanby incorrectly attributed the cure to the newly discovered fat-soluble vitamin A (17). In 1922, McCollum discovered that even when the vitamin A content of cod liver oil was destroyed by oxidation, it still retained its antirachitic potency. Obviously, cod liver oil contained two vitamins — vitamin A and the antirachitic factor, which McCollum named vitamin D (16).

By 1924, the mystery of how sunlight could prevent rickets had been partially solved. Steenbock (24) showed that antirachitic activity could be induced in foods and in animals by ultraviolet irradiation; research disclosed that it was the sterol that acquired antirachitic activity upon being irradiated. By the late 1920s, it had been established that rickets could be prevented and cured by exposure to direct sunlight, by irradiation with ultraviolet light, by feeding irradiated food, and by feeding cod liver oil. Later on, the natural vitamin D of fish liver oils was identified as the same substance as produced in the skin by irradiation.

Nomenclature and Properties of Vitamin D

The sterols that are potential sources of vitamin D are known as provitamins D; only two are important as provitamins D — 7-dehydrocholesterol (D_3) and ergosterol (D_2). The one found primarily in the skin and duodenal mucosa in higher animals and invertebrates is 7-dehydrocholesterol; ergosterol is found in large amounts in such lower plants as yeast and fungi.

Provitamin D can be converted to the vitamin

181

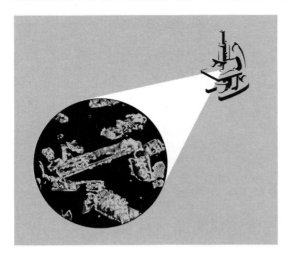

$$CH_3CH-CH=CH-CH-CH\genfrac{}{}{0pt}{}{CH_3}{CH_3}$$

Fig. 9.4 Chemical formula for vitamin D_2 and crystalline vitamin D_2 (ergocalciferol). (Courtesy Eastman Chemical Products, Inc., a subsidiary of Eastman Kodak Company.)

by exposure to ultraviolet light, cathode rays, X-rays, electric current of high frequency, and electrons; the compound is changed by opening the second ring in the provitamin D structure (see Fig. 9.4). In the laboratory it has been found that a series of intermediate products are formed before vitamin D is obtained, but further irradiation beyond vitamin D yields toxic products without antirachitic potency. The vitamin D produced from 7-dehydrocholesterol is called "cholecalciferol" and from ergosterol, "ergocalciferol."

The pure vitamins D are white, crystalline, odorless substances that are soluble in both fats and fat solvents (such as ether, chloroform, acetone, and alcohol). They are resistant to heat, oxidation, acid, and alkali. Crystals of ergocalciferol and its chemical formula are shown in Fig. 9.4. Since the relative antirachitic potency

of cholecalciferol and ergocalciferol are the same for human beings, the term "vitamin D" will be used in this discussion.

Metabolism of Vitamin D

Absorption Vitamin D taken by mouth is absorbed from the small intestine into the lymph system; the presence of bile is essential for absorption, and the presence of fat facilitates it. Vitamin D formed in the skin by irradiation of the provitamin present there is absorbed directly into the blood (14).

Utilization Vitamin D then enters the liver where it is *hydroxylated* to 25-hydroxyvitamin D_3 (25-OH-D_3) (4, 20). From the liver, 25-OH-D_3 is

182

transported to the kidney, where it is converted to 1,25-$(OH)_2$-D_3, the most active vitamin D *metabolite* in increasing calcium absorption, bone calcium mobilization, and increased intestinal phosphate absorption (6, 8, 9).

Storage Although significant amounts of vitamin D are found in liver, bone, blood, and kidneys, it is not known whether the vitamin is actually stored in any of these sites (7).

Excretion The main pathway of excretion of vitamin D is by way of the bile into the small intestine and the fecal excretion. Some of the vitamin is excreted by the urinary pathway (less than 4 percent of the intake) (3).

Functions of Vitamin D and Metabolites

Since the mid-1960s, remarkable progress has been made in solving the enigma of the metabolic action of vitamin D (15, 19). One of the characteristics of vitamin D action is the lag that occurs between time of administration of the vitamin and initiation of its actions (increase in absorption of calcium from the intestine and release of calcium from it storage place in bone [bone resorption] for use in other parts of the body). The lag led investigators to consider the possibility that some metabolic change needed to occur before the vitamin could function. The search led to a breakthrough, identifying 1,25-$(OH)_2$-D_3 as the most active naturally occurring metabolite as yet to be identified (1978) (12, 21). (See utilization, p. 182.) In addition, there are many active synthetic analogs (compounds synthesized introducing structural changes in the natural metabolite structure); an important one is 1 alpha-hydroxyvitamin D_3 (1 α-OH-D_3).

Calcium Transport It has been clearly established that vitamin D increases calcium absorption from the small intestine. A vitamin D deficiency produces large calcium losses in the feces. It is now known that vitamin D stimulates phosphate absorption separate from that of calcium. The increase in absorption of both minerals has been found to be related to the level of 1,25-$(OH)_2$-D_3 available. The ultimate result of the action of vitamin D on intestinal absorption is raising the serum calcium and phosphorus levels to permit normal mineralization of bone.

Bone Resorption The storage place for calcium is in the bones. To release this mineral for use in other parts of the body, vitamin D (1,25-$(OH)_2$-D_3) is required. Whether or not the parathyroid hormone (PTH) is necessary for release of the calcium is not clear as yet.

Measurements of Vitamin D and Metabolites

Vitamin D potency, like that of vitamin A, is expressed in International and USP (United States Pharmacopeia) Units (which are equal). One unit is equal to the activity of 0.25 μg of vitamin D_3 (irradiated 7-dehydrocholesterol). A bioassay method is used for measuring the content of vitamin D in foods and pharmaceutical products. The reference standard is USP reference vitamin D of known potency. The test material and the reference standard are fed to rachitic rats for a specified period of time. After sacrificing the animals, the degree of calcification in a leg bone is scored in both the test and reference standard (control) animals. The response of the animals fed the test material in comparison with that of the control animals enables one to determine the amount of vitamin D in the test material.

Methods employing chemical-physical techniques have been developed for determining vitamin D_3, 25-OH-D_3, and 1,25-$(OH)_2$-D_3 blood levels. Some values for the normal human adult are available for 1,25-$(OH)_2$-D_3: 2.6–5.8 ng (millimicrogram)/100 ml (5, 10).

183

Vitamin D Deficiency

This deficiency in children produces rickets, even though their diet may provide an ample intake of calcium and phosphorus. In rickets the bones are deformed when exposed to ordinary stresses. Ends of the long bones of the legs and arms may become enlarged. In rickets calcium and phosphorus are not deposited in developing bone cells, so the weight of the body causes the noncalcified portion to flatten and mushroom outward, giving the appearance of enlarged joints. Other bone changes include a row of beadlike protuberances on each side of the chest at the juncture of the rib bones and joining (costal) cartilage (rachitic rosary) (Fig. 9.5), bowed legs, knocked knees, and delayed closure of the fontanelle—all caused by failure of the bones to calcify normally.

Since the 1930s, the incidence of rickets has declined in the United States largely because of the addition of vitamin D to fluid and evaporated milk. Since 1968, nonfat dry milk has also been fortified with vitamins A and D for use in various food programs (23).

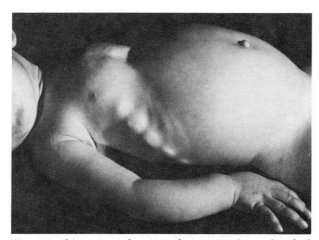

Fig. 9.5 Rachitic rosary showing enlargement of costochondral junctions. (From Wolbach, S. B., N. Jolliffe, F. F. Tisdall, and W. B. Cannon (1950). Clinical Nutrition. New York: Paul B. Hoeber, p. 113.)

Rickets may still be a serious public health problem in many tropical and semitropical countries (13). In 1965, WHO consultants surveyed the northern part of Africa to assess the prevalence and severity of rickets among children from birth to five years of age. Only 3 to 18 percent of the children examined had severe rickets, but as many as 45 to 60 percent showed mild signs of it. In these countries, rickets may be caused by the custom of not exposing babies to sunlight, little vitamin D or calcium in the diet, intestinal parasites, and recurrent diarrhea.

Hypervitaminosis D

Excessive amounts of vitamin D (above 2000 IU/day) are potentially dangerous and could lead to hypercalcemia and attendant complications (1, 22). Although the level of toxicity varies considerably from one person to another, the intake of vitamin D should not exceed a total of 400 IU per day.

Early symptoms of hypervitaminosis D include loss of appetite, thirst, and lassitude; these are followed by nausea, vomiting, diarrhea, abdominal discomfort, and loss of weight. The blood calcium level is elevated, leading to increased calcium excretion in the urine; calcium may be deposited in the kidney, resulting in damage to the organ and impaired function. In hypervitaminosis D, the cells in various organs of the body, as well as the arteries and arterioles, become prone to abnormal deposits of calcium. If massive dosages are continued, widespread calcification of the soft tissues may ultimately prove fatal.

Many parents think of vitamin supplements as tonics and do not realize the dangers of hypervitaminosis. Because of the vitamin D added to milk and infant foods, as well as the vitamin D produced by exposure to sunlight, parents should consider all of these sources before giving their children vitamin D supplements.

A beneficial Food and Drug Administration

regulation placed a 400 IU limit per dosage of vitamin D preparations (October 1973) (18); however, the regulation was revoked as published in the Federal Register, March 14, 1978.

Role of Vitamin D Metabolites in Bone Disorders

It is in the beginning stages, but very possible that 1,25-(OH)$_2$-D$_3$ and its *analogs* (some yet to be synthesized) will be effective in the treatment of a number of unexplained bone disorders: *renal osteodystrophy, osteoporosis, osteomalacia,* vitamin D-resistant rickets, and other bone disorders. Long-term administration of 1,25-(OH)$_2$-D$_3$ has been found to correct osteomalacia and general skeletal changes associated with renal disease (8, 10, 11, 21, 25).

Recommended Dietary Allowances for Vitamin D

The daily RDA for vitamin D for young men and women 19 to 22 years of age is 400 IU daily; recommendations in terms of RDA per 1000 kcal are for young men, 19 to 22 years, 133 IU per 1000 kcal (4184 kJ) and for young women, 19 to 22 years, 190 IU per 1000 kcal (4184 kJ). Adults over 22 years of age need only a small amount of vitamin D; in fact, under normal circumstances their need is met by the vitamin D contained in an ordinary mixed diet and by exposure to sunlight. Adults who work at night and those whose clothing or living customs shield them from sunlight need somewhat more vitamin D in their diet. The RDA for pregnant and lactating women is 400 IU per day (22).

For infants, 2.5 μg (100 IU) of vitamin D per day is sufficient to ensure adequate absorption of calcium and satisfactory growth rate, but 7.5 to 10 μg (300–400 IU) daily seemed to promote better calcium absorption and some increase in growth, so the RDA for infants, children, and adolescents is the higher level, 400 IU daily (22).

The vitamin D needs for age and sex groups ex-

Table 9.4 Vitamin D Needs Expressed as RDA and Nutrient Densities

Age, years		RDA	
		IU	IU/1000 kcal
Infants	0.0–0.5	400	—
	0.5–1.0	400	—
Children	1–3	400	307.7
	4–6	400	222.2
	7–10	400	166.7
Males	11–14	400	142.9
	15–18	400	133.3
	19–22	400	133.3
	23–50		
	51+		
Females	11–14	400	166.7
	15–18	400	190.5
	19–22	400	190.5
	23–50		
	51+		
Pregnant		400	—
Lactating		400	—

From *Recommended Dietary Allowances* (1974). 8th ed. Washington, D.C.: Natl. Acad. Sciences.

pressed as RDA and RDA per 1000 kcal are given in Table 9.4.

Sources of Vitamin D

Vitamin D can be obtained from food, vitamin supplements, and activation of the provitamin 7-dehydrocholesterol in the skin. Egg yolk, milk, butter, and liver are the main foods in the ordinary diet that contain vitamin D, but, without *fortification,* the amount is small and variable. It is estimated that a diet made up of the best (unfortified) food sources of vitamin D would supply only about 100 to 150 IU a day. Fish liver oils are an excellent source of the vitamin, but, of course, they are not part of the usual American diet.

Vitamin D is added to most commercial milk and infant formulas. Milk has been selected for such fortification because it is high in calcium and phosphorus content, the minerals that require vitamin D for absorption and use; 400 IU is added per quart. Milk is also consumed in larger quantities by the young, who especially need vitamin D for skeletal development. Although milk is the only food for which vitamin D fortification has been recommended by the Food and Nutrition Board of the National Research Council and the Council of Foods and Nutrition of the American Medical Association (2), other foods to which vitamin D is added include margarine, infant cereals, prepared breakfast cereals, chocolate beverage mixes, and cocoa.

Exposure to sunshine or ultraviolet irradiation will cause the provitamin 7-dehydrocholesterol, which occurs in the skin and in the blood, to be transformed into vitamin D. The amount that can be synthesized by this method is not known. Atmospheric smoke and fog, window glass, clothing, and skin pigmentation limit the skin's exposure to ultraviolet light. In the United States, exposure varies with the season; sunlight reaches its greatest intensity in the summer and is least in December.

Vitamin E

The Discovery of Vitamin E

In the early 1920s, Evans, Bishop, and Sure conducted research that eventually led to the discovery of vitamin E (12, 27). While investigating the effect of diet on the reproductive cycle of rats, they found that rats could not bear young when given a purified diet that contained all the then-known nutrients. However, when fresh green leaves or dried alfalfa was added to the diet, fertility was restored in the female but not in the male. This unknown fat-soluble factor was initially called substance X and later vitamin E. Unlike the xerophthalmia caused by a lack of vitamin A and rickets caused by a lack of vitamin D in experimental animals and in the human, the deficiency condition produced in rats on a vitamin E-deficient diet has not been produced in the human by lack of vitamin E.

Nomenclature and Properties of Vitamin E

The chemical name for vitamin E is tocopherol (from Greek *tokos*, childbirth; *pherein*, to bear; and chemical suffix -ol, signifying an alcohol). There are eight naturally occurring forms, which are collectively called vitamin E; they are alpha-, beta-, gamma-, delta-tocopherol, and alpha-, beta-, gamma-, delta-tocotrienol (26). Their biological activity varies, with alpha-tocopherol having by far the greatest potency (Fig. 9.6) (6).

Vitamin E is a yellow viscous oil that is insoluble in water but soluble in all of the fat solvents. Although it is quite stable to acids and heat (in the absence of oxygen), it is readily inactivated by ultraviolet light, alkalies, and oxygen. Alpha-*tocopheryl* acetate, a form stable to heat and

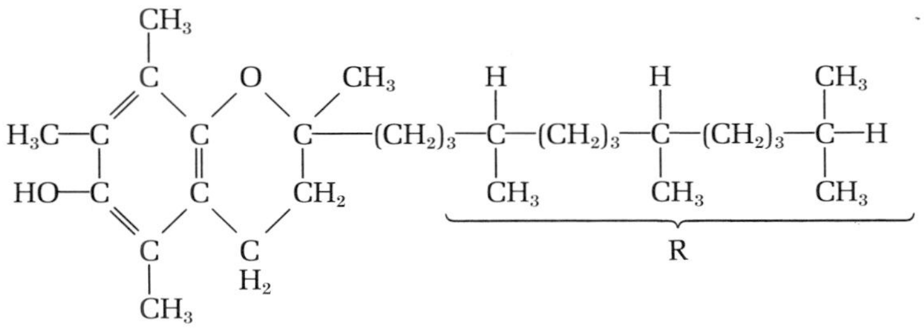

Fig. 9.6 Alpha-tocopherol.

oxidation, can be produced by condensing acetic acid with alpha-tocopherol. This stable form of natural alpha-tocopherol is added to animal feed, food, vitamin preparations, and various medicinal products.

Measurement of Vitamin E

Vitamin E is measured in terms of International Units. One IU of vitamin E is defined as the activity of 1 mg of dl-α-tocopheryl acetate. The activity of naturally occurring α-tocopherol is 1.49 IU per milligram.

In reference to diets, the term vitamin E activity is used indicating a mixture of the tocopherols and tocotrienols.

Metabolism of Vitamin E

Absorption   Vitamin E is absorbed from the small intestine into the lymphatic system; 20 to 30 percent of the intake is absorbed (3).

Utilization and Storage   In a normal adult population the total tocopherol content of the *plasma* was found to range from 0.5 to 1.2 mg/100 ml (7). The predominant form of vitamin E in both the plasma and red cells is alpha-tocopherol, accounting for 83 percent of the total blood tocopherol; the only other form present in more than a trace is gamma-tocopherol, occurring in plasma and in red cells as 13 percent of the total tocopherols (10).

A small amount of vitamin E is stored, primarily in body fat but also in most organs.

Excretion   The major pathway of excretion of vitamin E is by way of the feces (2). A small amount is excreted in the urine (19).

Functions of Vitamin E

The exact physiological function of vitamin E in man is not completely understood. It is difficult to determine the function(s) of this vitamin by using experimental animals because the early manifestations of a deficiency vary from one species to another. For example, a characteristic sign of vitamin E deficiency in the rat is reproductive failure; in the monkey, anemia; and in the rabbit, *muscular dystrophy*. But these are not the usual deficiency symptoms in man.

It has been postulated that the primary biological role of vitamin E is as a physiological antioxidant, inhibiting especially the oxidation of polyunsaturated fatty acids (PUFA) in tissue membranes (16, 17). The body contains many unsaturated fatty acids as constituents of phospholipids, for example, in the membranes that surround the cells, the subcellular particles (such as mitochondria, microsomes, and lysosomes), and the erythrocytes. Alpha-tocopherol is thought

187

to be an ideal antioxidant for body lipids because it is a normal constituent of the body.

Food processors have been using tocopherols for many years to retard rancidity in fats and high-fat foods. Adding tocopherols to foods helps to prevent oxidative changes in vitamin A, vitamin C, and PUFA.

Assessment of Vitamin E Status

Plasma tocopherol measurements and erythrocyte hemolysis tests are methods used for assessing vitamin E status (25). Tocopherol prevents *peroxidation* damage to cell membranes, which is the basis of the erythrocyte hemolysis test.

Vitamin E Deficiency

Deficiency symptoms have been produced in experimental animals fed a vitamin E-deficient diet; the symptoms are innumerable and vary with the species. Symptoms of deficiency in the human are limited almost exclusively to formula-fed premature infants (24, 28) and to individuals with a defect in lipid absorption (8). Newborn infants (especially the premature) have low plasma levels of vitamin E; transfer of the vitamin through the placenta to the fetus is limited. Premature infants fed a commercial formula were found to have a lower than normal serum vitamin E level, an increased number of blood platelets (thrombocytosis) and of young erythrocytes (reticulocytosis), and anemia (*hemolytic* in nature, caused by short survival time of erythrocytes). Vitamin E, given by mouth (75 to 100 IU daily), relieved the infants of all symptoms (23). The formula was high in PUFA content, necessitating a higher vitamin E concentration than was provided.

Individuals with a prolonged inability to absorb fat normally have low blood levels of vitamin E but no clinical symptoms which respond to the ingestion of vitamin E. A common finding in such individuals is the shortening of the life span of the red cells; anemia is not observed, however (8). In an experimental regime, adults consuming a diet low in vitamin E content for three years developed low plasma vitamin E levels and a slight decrease in red cell life span (18).

Megavitamin E Supplementation

Toxic Effects? Although toxic effects have been observed in experimental animals, there has been little evidence of high dosages causing toxicity in humans. Individuals ingesting from 100 to 800 IU of tocopherol daily over a period of three years were found to manifest no clinical or laboratory signs of vitamin excess (13). Bieri (3) states that "for most individuals daily doses below 300 IU are innocuous"; some complaints, nausea, and intestinal distress have been noted among persons ingesting more than that.

Beneficial Effects? The Committee on Nutritional Misinformation of the Food and Nutrition Board prepared a statement on vitamin E, which follows in part: "The list of ailments claimed to be relieved by this vitamin includes most noninfectious diseases, e.g., heart disease, sterility, muscular weakness, cancer, ulcers, skin disorders, burns, and shortness of breath. As for apparently healthy subjects, vitamin E has been claimed to promote physical endurance, enhance sexual potency, prevent heart attacks, protect against the health-related effects of air pollution, and slow the aging process and alleviate its accompanying ailments" (11).

How did these claims come about? To some extent they arose from a misinterpretation of the results of research on experimental animals.

Sterility and Male Impotency Vitamin E is required to prevent sterility in male rats and resorption of the fetus in the females. In the human there is no evidence to support the view "that supplemental vitamin E has any value in pre-

188

venting male impotency or sterility or in altering the outcome of pregnancy. Advocates of vitamin E supplementation in human beings overlook the fact that an effect on reproduction in animals can be demonstrated only when the animals have been fed on diets free of vitamin E. The widespread presence of the vitamin in human diets has prevented a deficiency, such as seen in animals under experimental conditions, from developing in man."

Muscle Wasting or Dystrophy "In most animal species that have been studied, severe vitamin E deficiency causes muscle wasting or dystrophy. Understandably, vitamin E has therefore been tested as a treatment for various muscle diseases of man, including hereditary muscular dystrophy." Results have been negative; vitamin E is present in the muscles of persons with dystrophy in normal amounts. There is no evidence that the condition in man is associated with insufficient dietary vitamin E.

Heart Disease In vitamin E-deficient animals, abnormalities in heart muscle are less severe than in skeletal muscle. However, in cattle and sheep heart-muscle abnormalities can be severe; in severely deficient monkeys with skeletal dystrophy and bone marrow failure, no cardiac involvement has appeared (11). "Similarly, there is no evidence that cardiac disease is a consequence of vitamin E deficiency in man and, to date, extensive tests have failed to demonstrate therapeutic benefit from supplemental vitamin E."

Aging There is no confirmed evidence that vitamin E is related to the aging process in experimental animals or in the human (21).

"Why has supplemental vitamin E been so ineffective in the treatment of disease? Clearly, it is because the reproductive failure, heart disease, and muscular dystrophy observed in man are not attributable to dietary deficiency of this vitamin. Similarly, there is no satisfactory scientific or clinical evidence that supplemental dietary vitamin E is beneficial in the treatment of such other conditions as burns, skin disorders, poor physical performance, and cancer" (11, 20). "Are there any special cases in which supplementary vitamin E is beneficial? Some physicians prescribe vitamin E for premature infants, who frequently have low blood levels of the vitamin because of limited transfer from the mother's blood before birth. Patients afflicted with conditions that interfere with normal digestion or absorption of fats and fat-soluble vitamins require supplements of these vitamins, one of which is vitamin E. Such individuals should be under the care of a physician; for others vitamin E supplements are unnecessary. Self-medication with vitamin E in the hope that a more or less serious condition will be alleviated may indeed be hazardous, especially when appropriate diagnosis and treatment may thereby be delayed or avoided" (11).

Interrelationships of Vitamin E with Other Nutrients

Vitamin A In experimental studies with the rat and the chick, vitamin E is found to increase both the utilization and storage of vitamin A (15). Combinations of vitamin A and vitamin E for the treatment of night blindness and prevention of xerophthalmia in children has shortened the period of treatment for night blindness from that with vitamin A alone (2). The explanation for this action has not been determined but may be due to antioxidant action in the intestine.

Selenium In many deficiency diseases, vitamin E and selenium are equally effective preventive agents (liver necrosis in the rat, exudative diathesis in the chick); in others, vitamin E is effective and selenium is not (muscle dystrophy and *encephalomalacia* in chicks and fetal re-

Table 9.5 Alpha-Tocopherol Content of Various Foods as Served

Food	Per 100 g of food α-tocopherol, mg	Per average serving Size of serving	α-tocopherol, mg
Mayonnaise	24.3	1 tbsp	3.6
Margarine (corn oil)	13.2	1 tbsp	1.8
Salmon steak, broiled	1.35	3 oz	1.15
Butter	1.0	1 tbsp	0.14
Liver, beef, broiled	0.63	3 oz	0.54
Peas, fresh, cooked	0.55	½ c	0.44
Egg, hard-cooked	0.46	1	0.23
Bread (whole wheat)	0.45	1 sl	0.11
Tomato, fresh	0.40	1 med	0.60
Beef, ground, pan fried	0.37	3 oz	0.31
Chicken breast, broiled	0.37	3 oz	0.31
Apple, fresh	0.31	1 med	0.46
Banana, fresh	0.22	1 med	0.33
Pork chop, pan fried	0.16	3 oz	0.14
Cornflakes	0.12	1 oz	0.03
Carrots, fresh	0.11	½ c	0.08
Orange juice, fresh	0.04	4 oz	0.05
Milk, whole	0.036	8 oz	0.09
Potato, whole	0.027	1 med	0.027

From R. H. Bunnell *et al.* (1965). Alpha-tocopherol content of foods. *Am. J. Clin. Nutrition*, **17:** 1. Used by permission.

sorption in pregnant rats). The postulated roles of vitamin E and selenium in preventing oxidation damage to cell membranes are: vitamin E prevents the formation of *hydroperoxide* and consequent cell damage; selenium, as a component of glutathionine peroxidase, converts hydroperoxides to alcohols, which are less damaging to the cell (16).

Recommended Dietary Allowances for Vitamin E

In considering the RDA for vitamin E, the Food and Nutrition Board concluded that the vitamin E content of diets consumed in the United States was adequate since no clinical or biochemical evidence of vitamin E deficiency has been detected in normal individuals on self-selected food intakes. Those consuming diets low in PUFA content will have lower intakes of vitamin E and also lower requirements for the vitamin than those on a higher PUFA intake. Diets supplying 1800 to 3000 kcal (7530–12,550 kJ) were found to contain 10–20 IU of vitamin E activity (80% α-tocopherol, 20% other tocopherols). The RDA for males 15 years of age and over is 15 IU of vitamin E activity daily, and for females 15 years of age and over, 12 IU of vitamin E activity daily (23).

The food of premature infants is important because of their susceptibility to vitamin E deficiency. For babies on formulas a concentration of 3 mg, or about 4.5 IU, of α-tocopherol per liter of formula containing 3.5 percent fat, a mixture of saturated and unsaturated fats, is recommended (23).

Food Sources of Vitamin E

Vitamin E (as alpha-tocopherol) occurs mainly in plant products, especially cold-pressed vegetable oils (such as wheat germ oil and cottonseed oil), leafy green vegetables, and whole-grain cereals. Although animal products contain little vitamin E, the best sources are liver, heart, kidney, and eggs (1, 9) (Table 9.5).

It has been customary to assess the vitamin E activity of foods solely on their alpha-tocopherol content; it is superior biologically and was believed to be present in foods in greater amounts than the other forms. However, in 1973, meals representative of a variety of eating habits were analyzed by Bieri and Evarts (5) for alpha-, gamma-, and delta-tocopherol content; the gamma-tocopherol content was two and one-half times that of alpha-tocopherol. The delta- and alpha-tocopherols were present in about equal amounts. In 1949, the ratio of alpha- and nonalpha-tocopherols in United States diets was 1:1 (22). The increased consumption of soybean oil and hydrogenated fats containing soybean oil are largely responsible for the increase in gamma-tocopherol consumption (4). Table 9.6 shows the shift to soybean oil in the United States between 1950 and 1971 (14); soybean oil is relatively high in gamma-tocopherol content (Table 9.7).

Table 9.6 Domestic Disappearance of Edible Fats and Oils in the United States

	Kilograms per person	
	1950	1971
Butter	4.0 (8.7 lb)	2.0 (4.3 lb)
Lard	6.1 (13.5 lb)	3.2 (7.1 lb)
Corn oil	0.7 (1.5 lb)	0.9 (2.0 lb)
Cottonseed oil	4.3 (9.5 lb)	2.2 (4.8 lb)
Soybean oil	4.3 (9.5 lb)	13.0 (28.5 lb)

From *U.S. Fats and Oils Statistics 1950–71*, Statistical Bulletin No. 489. Economics Res. Serv. Washington, D.C.: U.S. Dept. Agr., 1972.

Table 9.7 Alpha- and Gamma-Tocopherol Content of Edible Grade Soybean and Corn Oil

	alpha-tocopherol mg/100 g	gamma-tocopherol mg/100 g
Soybean oil	15	108
Corn oil	22	76
Safflower oil	26	2

From J. G. Bieri and R. P. Evarts (1975). Vitamin E adequacy of vegetable oils. *J. Am. Dietet. Assoc.*, **66**: 134.

Discovery of the unexpectedly large amount of gamma-tocopherol in meals consumed prompted Bieri and Evarts (4) to assess the comparative effectiveness of gamma- and alpha-tocopherol in preventing deficiency symptoms in experimental animals (liver *necrosis* in the rat; *exudative diathesis* and muscle dystrophy in the chick; and in the hamster, elevation of plasma *creatine phosphokinase*). The biological activity of gamma-tocopherol was an average of 10 percent that of alpha-tocopherol. The investigators (4) point out that gamma-tocopherol may contribute as much as 20 percent of the total vitamin E activity of the food consumed in the United States, and that calculations based only on alpha-tocopherol underestimate the amount of dietary vitamin E activity.

Commercially, tocopherols are usually isolated from vegetable oils, but they can also be prepared synthetically (17).

Vitamin K

Discovery of Vitamin K

In 1929, Dam, a Danish scientist, reported that chicks raised on a purified diet developed hemorrhages under the skin that could not be cured by adding vitamin C to their diet. However, this disorder, which was characterized by a prolonged blood clotting time, could be cleared up by giving the birds a mixture of cereals or other natural foods. Later Dam found that this antihemorrhagic factor appeared in the fat-soluble fraction of certain foods. He suggested calling it vitamin K, from the Danish term "Koagulation Faktor." By 1939, Dam had isolated and chemically identified the vitamin (2). In 1943, he received the Nobel prize in physiology and medicine for his work.

Nomenclature and Properties of Vitamin K

Vitamins K comprise a group of substances that exist in nature in two forms—vitamin K_1 (commonly called phylloquinone, now named phytylmenaquinone), which occurs in green leaves, and vitamin K_2 (formerly called the menaquinones, now referred to as multiprenylmenoquinone), which is produced by bacterial synthesis (6, 7). These yellow-colored vitamins are fat soluble and stable to heat, but unstable to alkalies, strong acids, oxidation, and light. There are also synthetic forms, one of which is menadione. The synthetic compounds are also yellow in color, stable to heat, but unstable to alkali and oxidation; salts of these compounds are soluble in water. (Formula of vitamin K,—Fig. 9.7).

Menadione, as well as several of its water-soluble derivatives, and vitamin K are available commercially.

Absorption and Storage of Vitamin K

Since the natural vitamins K are fat soluble, they require bile or bile salts in the intestine for optimal absorption. Anything that interferes with the normal absorption of fat, therefore, interferes with the absorption of natural vitamins K. By contrast, menadione and the simpler water-soluble forms are more easily absorbed. Absorption takes place mainly in the upper part of the small intestine into the lymph system. In omnivorous animals, such as man, both phylloquinone and the higher molecular weight menaquinones of bacterial origin (most likely derived from intestinal flora) are found in the liver (7). Vitamin K is apparently stored only in small amounts; no one tissue serves as a special depository.

Intestinal Synthesis of Vitamin K

Vitamin K is synthesized in both the small intestine and the colon by microorganisms present there. It appears that vitamin K synthesized in the intestine can be absorbed (3).

Functions of Vitamin K

Vitamin K is essential for the synthesis by the liver of blood clotting proteins (prothrombin factor II and factors VII, IX, and X). The exact way in which vitamin K functions in the synthesis of these vitamin K-dependent proteins is not known. Research (1, 10) indicates that vitamin K works with a regulatory protein helping to complete the structure of the blood clotting proteins and with their removal from the ribosomes, their site of synthesis. For more on blood clotting, see chap. 13.

Assessment of Vitamin K Status

The clinical manifestation of vitamin K deficiency is hemorrhage as a result of an increase in time required for blood to clot. With a deficiency in vitamin K, there is a deficiency in clotting factors: prothrombin and factor VII and, to a lesser extent, factors IX and X.

The laboratory test most commonly used to assess vitamin K status is the measurement in a plasma sample of the speed of conversion of prothrombin to thrombin. Another test used is

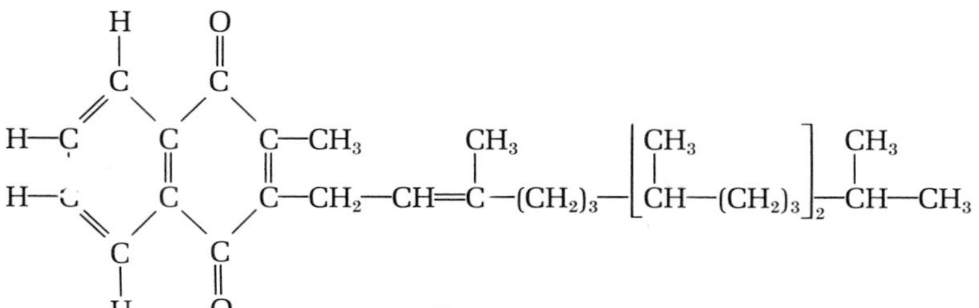

Fig. 9.7 Chemical formula for vitamin K_1.

clotting time; freshly drawn blood is placed in clean test tubes, which are tilted once each minute. The time required for the clot to form is the clotting time; for normal blood it is about ten minutes (9).

Vitamin K Deficiency

Few humans have demonstrated symptoms of a dietary lack of vitamin K. It is available in a variety of foods. And the microbiologic flora of the normal intestine synthesizes the menaquinones in amounts that may supply the bulk of the requirement for vitamin K (7). Antibiotics that sterilize the bowel, such as neomycin, reduce this source of vitamin K. Disorders of the liver or gall bladder that interfere with the secretion of bile sometimes produce a vitamin K deficiency due to malabsorption. In cases of obstructive jaundice, where a blockage of the bile duct prevents bile from entering the duodenum, the blood clotting time is increased. This can be alleviated by using water-soluble derivatives of menadione for oral administration; other forms of the vitamin are used for parenteral administration.

Newborn infants present a special case in regard to vitamin K nutrition because of the low level of clotting factors in the blood at birth and the possibility of hemorrhagic disease. In the first few days of life, intestinal bacteria are not well-established for the production of vitamin K. Because human milk provides less vitamin K than does cow milk, and because breast-fed infants usually consume less milk during the first few days of life than formula-fed babies, vitamin K deficiency in the newborn period is more common in breast-fed than in formula-fed babies. It is particularly important that a source of vitamin K be given to the breast-fed infant in the first few days of life. Supplements of vitamin K are not needed beyond the newborn period except for infants fed milk-free formulas; soy formulas have caused vitamin K deficiency. The soy formulas are now fortified with vitamin K (4, 5).

Need for Vitamin K

Although vitamin K is recognized as a dietary essential, allowances have not been established; apparently the amount needed by the body is quite small. Since this vitamin appears in a wide variety of commonly eaten plant foods, is synthesized by bacteria in the intestinal tract, is stable, and is insoluble in water, the normal person is not likely to suffer a deficiency (8).

It has been difficult to establish a quantitative recommendation because of the variable contribution of the intestinal flora to the amount of the vitamin available to the body. Antibiotic therapy suppresses bacterial growth and consequently the synthesis of vitamin K.

Another interfering factor is the action of vitamin K antagonists. Dicoumarol and hydrocoumarol are used therapeutically to relieve thrombosis (abnormal formation of blood clots in the

193

Table 9.8 Average Vitamin K Content of Some Ordinary Foods

Food	Vitamin K, mg/100 g	Food	Vitamin K, mg/100 g
Milk and Milk Products		Vegetables	
Milk (cows)	3	Asparagus	57
Cheese	35	Beans, green	14
Butter	30	Broccoli	200
		Cabbage	125
Eggs		Lettuce	129
Hens (whole)	11	Pear, green	19
		Spinach	89
Meat & Meat products		Turnip greens	650
Ground beef	7	Potato	3
Beef liver	92	Tomato	5
Ham	15	Watercress	57
Pork tenderloin	11		
Chicken liver	7	Fruits	
Pork liver	25	Applesauce	2
Bacon	46	Banana	2
		Orange	1
Fats		Peach	8
Corn oil	10	Raisins	6
Cereals & Grain Products		Beverages	
Maize	5	Coffee	38
Whole wheat	17	Cola	2
Wheat flour	4	Tea, green	712
Bread	4		
Oats	20		

From R. E. Olson (1973). Vitamin K. In *Modern Nutrition in Health and Disease*, 5th ed., edited by R. S. Goodhart and M. E. Shils. Philadelphia: Lea & Febiger, p. 168.

blood vessels). The chemical structure of these antivitamins (or antagonists) is similar to vitamin K; they act as anticoagulants by interfering with the synthesis of prothrombin and the other clotting factors.

Food Sources of Vitamin K

Vitamin K is found in vegetables; good sources are spinach, kale, cabbage, and cauliflower. The vitamin is associated especially with the chloroplasts of plants but is found in the nongreen areas as well. Meats and dairy products are intermediate in vitamin K content, and cereals and fruits are low (Table 9.8).

Summary

The discovery of the vitamins ushered in a new era in nutrition, one in which minute substances took on great importance. The vitamin discoveries began in 1913 with vitamin A and ended in 1948 with vitamin B-12. The use of experimental animals fed purified diets was the crux of the early vitamin discoveries.

The designation vitamin A continues to be used

as the generic name for several chemically related, naturally occurring compounds, each with a specific physiological function. Vitamin A is found only in the animal kingdom and is known as preformed vitamin A. The plant kingdom provides a source of the vitamin for animals in the form of carotenoid pigments, a portion of which can be converted to vitamin A in the intestinal mucosa of the animal (including the human). Beta-carotene is nutritionally the most important of the carotenoids.

The best understood function of vitamin A is its role in vision; retinal (vitamin A aldehyde) is a constituent of the visual pigments of the retina of the eye. Without sufficient vitamin A the eye's sensitivity to light can be reduced so much that vision is not possible. Vitamin A is essential for growth and for the health of epithelial tissue (the protective epidermis on the exterior of the body and the mucous-secreting membranes that line the interior cavities).

Vitamin A deficiency exists today (1978) in parts of the world, causing young children to be blind. Preventive measures are being studied and instituted, namely the administration of massive doses of the vitamin at six-month intervals. Because vitamin A can be stored in the body, the plan is workable. Negro children of preschool age, as judged by vitamin A blood serum levels, have the poorest state of vitamin A nutriture of all age-sex-race groups (1971–1972) in the United States.

Excessive dosages of vitamin A (25,000 to 50,000 IU daily) can produce toxic effects, the most serious of which is increased intracranial pressure. Symptoms of the pressure build-up are headache, nausea, and lethargy. Regression of the symptoms occurs when the vitamin is discontinued.

The best food sources of vitamin A activity are the animal products—liver, milk, and eggs. The best plant sources are deep yellow and dark green vegetables and fruits. The RDA for males 15 years of age and over is 5000 IU daily and for females 15 years of age and over, 4000 IU daily.

Vitamin D was originally recognized as the vitamin that could prevent and cure rickets, a disease in which bones fail to calcify. Vitamin D is different from most of the other vitamins in that the need for it can be satisfied without ingesting any of it. One of the sterols that is a provitamin D is present in the skin; on exposure to sunshine (or other source of ultraviolet rays), vitamin D is formed and absorbed directly into the blood.

It has long been known that vitamin D was essential for the absorption of calcium from the small intestine and for the release of calcium from bone (the storage place of the mineral) for use in other parts of the body, namely to maintain the blood calcium level at normal. However, there has been an enigma concerning the body's use of vitamin D. A delay occurs between the time of administration of the vitamin and the initiation of its physiological actions. Since the mid-1960s, this question has been under study with one lead following another, and it now appears that the breakthrough has occurred. All evidence indicates that the metabolite 1,25-dihydroxy-D_3 (1,25-$(OH)_2$-D_3) is the active one. The steps in its formation following the absorption of vitamin D_3 are a change in the liver (hydroxylation of vitamin D_3 to form 25-hydroxyvitamin D_3 [25-OH-D_3]) and in the kidney where the active metabolite, 1,25-$(OH)_2$-D_3, is formed from 25-OH-D_3. There are hopeful indications that many as yet unexplained bone diseases may be amenable to treatment with 1,25-$(OH)_2$-D_3.

The incidence of rickets in the United States has declined notably since the 1930s when the addition of vitamin D to fluid and evaporated milk became a common practice. Since 1968, nonfat dry milk has been fortified with vitamin D and vitamin A also. The ingestion of excessive amounts of vitamin D (above 2000 IU daily) can lead to elevated blood calcium levels and the danger of calcium deposits in organs of the body (namely, the kidney), the arteries and arterioles, and eventually soft tissues (such as muscle).

Foods providing vitamin D are egg yolk, milk, and liver; the potency of these sources depends on the food of the animal. Some foods on the market are fortified with vitamin D; milk has added 400 IU per quart. Among other foods to which vitamin D has been added are margarine and breakfast cereals. The RDA for young men and women (19 to 22 years) of 400 IU daily can be met under ordinary circumstances by the consumption of a mixed diet, plus that obtained from exposure to sunshine in the usual work-a-day life. Persons who work at night may need some additional vitamin D.

Vitamin E, which has no well-defined human function and for which deficiencies have not been observed, except in premature infants who are born with a low serum level due to limited placental transmission, appears to be widely used by the public and in large dosages. To some extent misapplications of the use of vitamin E have arisen from misinterpretation of results of research with experimental animals. It is fortunate that there is little evidence that high dosages of vitamin E cause toxicity in the human.

The primary function postulated for vitamin E is that of a physiological antioxidant, inhibiting especially the oxidation of polyunsaturated fatty acids in tissue membranes.

Vitamin E is the generic term for substances (tocopherols and tocotrienols) with vitamin E activity. The RDA, expressed in IU of vitamin E activity, is 15 IU for males over 15 years and 12 IU for females over 15 years. The recommendation is at the level of the average consumption of vitamin E activity by persons in the United States. Vitamin E (as alpha-tocopherol) occurs chiefly in plant products, wheat germ oil, cottonseed oil, leafy green vegetables, and whole-grain cereals.

Vitamin K is essential for the synthesis of blood clotting proteins. Few humans have demonstrated symptoms of a dietary lack of vitamin K; also the microbiologic flora of the normal intestine synthesize an amount sufficient to supply the bulk of the requirement for the vitamin. Antibiotics that sterilize the bowel, such as neomycin, reduce the intestinal source of vitamin K.

Disorders of the liver or gall bladder that interfere with the secretion of bile or conditions that block the bile duct preventing the entrance of bile in the duodenum are likely to cause a deficiency of vitamin K; bile is necessary for the absorption of vitamin K.

Newborn infants present a special case in regard to vitamin K nutrition because of the low level of clotting factors in the blood at birth and the possibility of hemorrhagic disease. It is important that a source of vitamin K be given to the breast-fed infant (human milk is lower in vitamin K than cow milk) in the first few days of life.

Vitamin K is the generic term for two forms of the vitamin that exist in nature, vitamin K_1 (phylloquinone), which occurs in green leaves, and vitamin K_2 (the menaquinones), which are produced by bacterial synthesis.

Although vitamin K is recognized as a dietary essential, allowances for it have not been established. Good food sources of vitamin K are spinach, kale, cabbage, and cauliflower; intermediate sources are meats and dairy products.

Glossary

amine: an organic compound containing nitrogen; derivative of ammonia (NH_3).

analog: a chemical compound with a structure similar to that of another but differing from it in some respect.

antioxidant: a substance that prevents or retards oxidation in another substance; for example, vitamin E prevents autoxidation of unsaturated fatty acids.

aqueous emulsion: solution of a liquid incapable of mixing with water (such as vitamin A) in water; the combination is made possible by use of an emulsifying agent (see below).

bioassay: also termed biological assay; the measurement of either the activity or the amount of a substance based on the use of living organisms; in the case of vitamin A, the rat is used.

conjunctiva: delicate membrane lining the eyelids and covering the eyeball.

creatine phosphokinase: the enzyme that catalyzes the

196

conversion of ADP (adenosine diphosphate, a high energy compound that functions in many reactions in the body) and phosphocreatine (a high energy phosphate compound occurring in muscle) to ATP (adenosine triphosphate; occurs in all cells where it represents energy storage) and creatine (a constituent of muscle).

emulsifying agent: a substance that aids the dispersion of one liquid in another, liquids that are naturally immiscible, such as oil and water.

encephalomalacia: softening of the brain; caused in chicks by a lack of vitamin E.

epidermis: the outermost layer of the skin.

exudative diathesis: accumulation of fluid in subcutaneous tissues, muscles, or connective tissues, caused by the escape of plasma from the capillaries.

fortified food: food to which nutrients have been added over and above those occurring naturally; may refer either to the increase in concentration of a naturally occurring nutrient, or to the addition of a different nutrient.

hemolysis: rupture of erythrocytes with release of hemoglobin into the plasma.

hydroperoxide: a strong oxidizing agent, with the general formula ROOH (in which R represents an organic group such as in C_2H_5OOH).

hydroxylation: introduction of a hydroxyl group (-OH) into an organic compound (a carbon-containing compound).

lymph system: see page 28.

metabolite: a substance that enters into a metabolic reaction as a reacting substance, an intermediate, or final product.

muscular dystrophy: a group of genetically determined muscle diseases that are progressively crippling because muscles are gradually weakened and become atrophied (shrunken).

necrosis: death of tissue, usually as individual cells, groups of cells, or in small localized areas.

osteodystrophy, renal: a bone condition resulting from chronic disease of the kidneys that has symptoms of several bone disorders: osteitis fibrosa cystica (rarefication of bone, with marked activity of the bone-destroying cells); osteomalacia (a condition marked by softening of the bones due to impaired mineralization with excess accumulation of organic matrix); and osteoporosis (abnormal rarefication of bone, seen most commonly in the elderly).

peroxidation: oxidation to the point of forming a peroxide, a compound (oxide) which contains an -O-O- group.

plasma: the fluid portion of blood in which the formed bodies (red blood cells, white blood cells, platelets) are suspended. Serum is plasma without fibrinogen; the fluid obtained from blood after it has been allowed to clot.

precursor: a compound from which another, usually more active, is formed.

tocopheryl: an ester form of tocopherol; alpha-tocopheryl acetate, for example, is the ester formed from the alcohol, alpha-tocopherol and acetic acid, splitting out a molecule of water.

USP: United States Pharmacopeia; a legally recognized compendium of standards for drugs published by the United States Pharmacopeial Convention, Inc.

xanthophyll: a yellow coloring matter of plants; a carotenoid which is not a provitamin A.

xerosis: abnormal dryness.

Study Questions and Activities

1. Discuss the function(s) of each of the fat-soluble vitamins.
2. What are some of the symptoms of excessive intakes of vitamins A and D?
3. Discuss the loss of fat-soluble vitamins in preparing food.
4. Why was milk selected as a food to be fortified with vitamin D?
5. Discuss the relationship between an appropriate fat-soluble vitamin and each of the following terms: beta-carotene, blood clotting, high polyunsaturated fatty acid diet, Bitot's spot, hypervitaminosis, ultraviolet rays, dicoumarol, International Unit, and retinol equivalent.
6. Considering your usual eating habits, what are your main sources of vitamin A?
7. Try to recall what you have eaten for the past 24 hours. Was your diet adequate in vitamin A? Ap-

197

proximately what percent of the vitamin A in your diet came from provitamin A?

References

Introduction to the Vitamins and Vitamin A

1. Abraham, S., F. W. Lowenstein, and D. E. O'Connele (1975). *Anthropometric and Clinical Findings.* Preliminary Findings of the First Health and Nutrition Examination Survey, U.S., 1971–1972. DHEW Publication No. (HRA)75–1229. Rockville, Md.: U.S. Dept. Health, Educ., and Welfare.

2. Abraham, S., F. W. Lowenstein, and C. L. Johnson (1974). *Dietary Intake and Biochemical Findings.* Preliminary Findings of the First Health and Nutrition Examination Survey, U.S., 1971–1972. DHEW Publication No. (HRA) 74-1219-1. Rockville, Md.: U.S. Dept. Health, Educ., and Welfare, p. 18.

3. Adams, C. F. (1975). *Nutritive Value of American Foods.* Agr. Handbook No. 456. Washington, D.C.: U.S. Dept. Agric.

4. Ames, S. R. (1969). Factors affecting absorption, transport and storage of vitamin A. *Am. J. Clin. Nutrition,* **22:** 934.

5. Baker, H., and O. Frank (1973). Vitamin analyses in medicine. In *Modern Nutrition in Health and Disease,* 5th ed., edited by R. S. Goodhart and M. E. Shils. Philadelphia: Lea and Febiger, p. 523.

6. Deuel, H. J., Jr., and S. M. Greenberg (1953). A comparison of the retention of vitamin A in margarines and in butters based upon bioassays. *Food Res.,* **18:** 497.

7. Di Benedetto, R. J. (1967). Chronic hypervitaminosis A in an adult. *J. Am. Med. Assoc.,* **201:** 700.

8. Ember, M., and L. Mindszenty (1967). Response of vitamin A serum levels to supplementary vitamin A. In *Proceedings of the Seventh International Congress of Nutrition, Hamburg 1966.* London, England: Pergamon Press, p. 625.

9. Furman, K. I. (1973). Acute hypervitaminosis A in an adult. *Am. J. Clin. Nutrition,* **26:** 575.

10. Ganguly, J. (1969). Absorption of vitamin A. *Am. J. Clin. Nutrition,* **22:** 923.

11. Glover, J. (1970). Biosynthesis of the fat-soluble vitamins. In *Fat-Soluble Vitamins,* edited by R. A. Morton. New York: Pergamon Press, p. 180.

12. Goodman, D. S. (1969). Retinol transport in human plasma. *Am. J. Clin. Nutrition,* **22:** 911.

13. *Highlights, Ten-State Nutrition Survey, 1968–1970* (1972). DHEW Publ. No. (HSM)72-8134. Atlanta, Ga.: Center for Disease Control, U.S. Dept. Health, Educ., and Welfare.

14. Mahalanbis, D., K. N. Jalan, T. K. Maitra, and S. K. Agarival (1976). Vitamin A absorption in ascaris. *Am. J. Clin. Nutrition,* **29:** 1372.

15. Marston, R., and B. Friend (1978). Nutrient content of national food supply. *National Food Situation.* NFR 1, January 13.

16. McCollum, E. V. (1957). *A History of Nutrition.* Boston: Houghton Mifflin, p. 202.

17. McCollum, E. V., and M. Davis (1913). The necessity of certain lipids in the diet during growth. *J. Biol. Chem.,* **15:** 167.

18. McLaren, D. (1963). *Malnutrition and the Eye.* New York: Academic Press, pp. 162, 177.

19. Moore, T. (1967). Pharmacology and toxicology of vitamin A. In *The Vitamins,* 2nd ed., vol. 1, edited by W. H. Sebrell, Jr., and R. S. Harris. New York: Academic Press, p. 289.

20. New regulations on vitamins A and D (1973). DHEW Publ. No. (FDA)74-2015. *FDA Consumer.*

21. Nomenclature policy: Generic descriptors and trivial names for vitamins and related compounds (1977). *J. Nutrition,* **107:** 7.

22. Oomen, H. A. P. C. (1976). Vitamin A deficiency, xerophthalmia and blindness. In *Present Knowledge in Nutrition,* 4th ed., edited by D. M. Hegsted, Chm., and Editorial Com. Washington, D.C.: The Nutrition Foundation, Inc., p. 73.

23. Osborne, T. B., and L. B. Mendel (1913). The relation of growth to the chemical constituents of the diet. *J. Biol. Chem.,* **15:** 311.

24. Posati, L. P. and M. L. Orr (1976). *Composition of Foods. Dairy and Egg Products. Raw-Processed-Prepared.* Agr. Handbook No. 8-1. Washington, D.C.: U.S. Dept. Agric.

25. *Recommended Dietary Allowances* (1974). 8th ed. Washington, D.C.: National Academy of Sciences.

26. Rodriguez, M. S., and M. I. Irwin (1972). A conspectus of research on vitamin A requirements of man. *J. Nutrition,* **102:** 911.

27. Roels, O. A. (1967). Biochemical systems. In *The Vitamins,* 2nd ed., vol. 1, edited by W. H. Sebrell, Jr., and R. S. Harris. New York: Academic Press, p. 167.

28. Roels, O. A. (1970). Vitamin A physiology. *J. Am. Med. Assoc.,* **214:** 1097.

29. Sauberlich, H. E., J. H. Skala, and R. P. Dowdy (1974). *Laboratory Tests for the Assessment of Nutritional Status.* Cleveland, Ohio: CRC Press, p. 4.

30. Simmons, W. K., and A. V. de Mello (1975). Blindness in the nine states of Northeast Brazil. *Am. J. Clin. Nutrition,* **28:** 202.

31. Smith, J. E., and D. S. Goodman (1976). Vitamin A metabolism and transport. In *Present Knowledge in Nutrition,* 4th ed., edited by D. M. Hegsted, Chm., and Editorial Com. Washington, D.C.: The Nutrition Foundation, Inc., p. 64.

32. Steenbock, H. (1919). White corn versus yellow corn and a probable relation between the fat soluble vitamin and yellow plant pigments. *Science,* **50:** 352.

33. Sweeney, J. P., and A. C. Marsh (1971). Effect of processing on provitamin A in vegetables. *J. Am. Dietet. Assoc.,* **59:** 238.

34. *Vitamin A Deficiency and Xerophthalmia* (1976). Technical Report Series 590. Geneva: World Health Organ.

35. Walker, M. A., and L. Page (1975). Nutritive content of college meals. *J. Am. Dietet. Assoc.,* **66:** 146.

36. Yaffe, S. J., and L. J. Filer, Jr. (1974). The use and abuse of vitamin A. *Nutrition Rev.,* **32** (suppl. 1): 41.

Vitamin D

1. American Academy of Pediatrics, Committee on Nutrition (1975). Hazards of overuse of vitamin D. *Am. J. Clin. Nutrition,* **28:** 512.

2. American Medical Association, Council on Foods and Nutrition (1968). Improvement of nutritive quality of foods. *J. Am. Med. Assoc.,* **205:** 160.

3. Avioli, L. V., S. W. Lee, J. E. McDonald, J. Lund, and H. F. DeLuca (1967). Metabolism of vitamin D_3-^3H in human subjects: Distribution in blood, bile, feces, and urine. *J. Clin. Invest.,* **46:** 983.

4. Blunt, J. W., H. F. DeLuca, and H. K. Schnoes (1968). 25-hydroxycholecalciferol: A biologically active metabolite of vitamin D_3. *Biochemistry,* **7:** 3317.

5. Brumbaugh, P. F., D. H. Haussler, R. Bressler, and M. R. Haussler (1974). Radioreceptor assay for 1 α,25-dihydroxy-vitamin D_3. *Science,* **183:** 1089.

6. Chen, T. C., L. Castillo, M. Korycka-Dahl, and H. F. DeLuca (1974). Role of vitamin D metabolites in phosphate transport of rat intestine. *J. Nutrition,* **104:** 1056.

7. DeLuca, H. F. (1967). Mechanism of action and metabolic fate of vitamin D. In *Vitamins and Hormones,* vol. 25, edited by R. S. Harris *et al.* New York: Academic Press, p. 315.

8. DeLuca, H. F. (1976). Metabolism of vitamin D: Current status. *Am. J. Clin. Nutrition,* **29:** 1258.

9. Garabedian, M., Y. Tanaka, M. F. Holick, and H. F. DeLuca (1974). Response of intestinal calcium transport and bone calcium mobilization to 1,25-dihydroxyvitamin D_3 in thyroparathyroidectomized rats. *Endocrinology,* **94:** 1022.

10. Haussler, M. R., and T. A. McCain (1977). Basic and clinical concepts related to vitamin D metabolism and action. *New Engl. J. Med.,* **297:** 974 and 1041.

11. Henderson, R. G., R. G. G. Russell, J. G. G. Ledingham, R. Smith, D. O. Oliver, R. J. Walton, D. G. Small, C. Preston, G. T. Warner, and A. W. Norman (1974). Effects of 1,25-dihydroxycholecalciferol on calcium absorption, muscle weakness, and bone disease in chronic renal failure. *Lancet,* **1:** 379.

12. Holick, M. F., H. K. Schnoes, H. F. DeLuca, T. Suda, and R. J. Cousins (1971). Isolation and identification of 1,25-dihydroxycholecalciferol. A

199

metabolite of vitamin D active in intestine. *Biochemistry*, **10**: 2799.

13. Joint FAO/WHO Expert Committee on Nutrition. *Seventh Report* FAO Nutrition Meetings Rept. Series 42. Rome: Food and Agr. Organ., p. 31.

14. Koehler, A. E., and E. Hill (1953). 7-dehydrocholesterol in human serum. *Federation Proc.*, **12**: 232.

15. Lawson, D. E. M. (1971). Vitamin D: New findings on its metabolism and its role in calcium nutrition. *Proc. Nutrition Soc.* (Cambridge), **30**: 47.

16. McCollum, E. V., N. Simmonds, P. G. Shipley, and E. A. Park (1922). Studies on experimental rickets. XII. Is there a substance other than fat-soluble A associated with certain fats which play an important role in bone development? *J. Biol. Chem.*, **50**: 5.

17. Mellanby, E. (1921). *Experimental Rickets*. Medical Research Council Special Rept. Series 61. London: H. M. Stationery Office.

18. New regulations on vitamins A and D (1973). DHEW Publ. No. (FDA)74-2015. *FDA Consumer.*

19. Norman, A. W., M. R. Haussler, T. H. Adams, J. R. Myrtle, P. Roberts, and K. A. Hibbard (1969). Basic studies on the mechanism of action of vitamin D. *Am. J. Clin. Nutrition*, **22**: 396.

20. Ponchon, G., and H. F. DeLuca (1969). The role of the liver in the metabolism of vitamin D. *J. Clin. Invest.*, **48**: 1273.

21. Procsal, D. A., W. H. Okamura, and A. W. Norman (1976). Vitamin D, its metabolites and analogs: A review of the structural requirements for biological activity. *Am. J. Clin. Nutrition*, **29**: 1271.

22. *Recommended Dietary Allowances* (1974). 8th ed. Washington, D.C.: National Academy of Sciences.

23. Schaefer, A. E. (1969). Statement before the United States Senate Select Committee on Nutrition and Related Human Needs. January 22, 1969. Washington, D.C.: U.S. Govt. Printing Office, p. 41.

24. Steenbock, H., and A. Black (1924). Fat-soluble vitamins. XVII. The induction of growth-promoting and calcifying properties in a ration by exposure to ultra-violet light. *J. Biol. Chem.*, **61**: 405.

25. Teitelbaum, S. L. (1976). Morphological effects of vitamin D and its analogs on bone. *Am. J. Clin. Nutrition*, **29**: 1309.

Vitamin E

1. Ames, S. R. (1972). Tocopherols. Occurrence in foods. In *The Vitamins*, 2nd ed., vol. 5, edited by W. H. Sebrell, Jr., and R. S. Harris. New York: Academic Press, p. 233.

2. Bauernfeind, J. C., H. Newmark, and M. Brin (1974). Vitamins A and E nutrition via intramuscular or oral route. *Am. J. Clin. Nutrition*, **27**: 234.

3. Bieri, J. G. (1976). Vitamin E. In *Present Knowledge in Nutrition*, 4th ed., edited by D. M. Hegsted, Chm., and Editorial Com. Washington, D.C.: The Nutrition Foundation, Inc., p. 98.

4. Bieri, J. G., and R. P. Evarts (1974). Gamma tocopherol: Metabolism, biological activity, and significance in human vitamin E nutrition. *Am. J. Clin. Nutrition*, **27**: 980.

5. Bieri, J. G., and R. P. Evarts (1973). Tocopherols and fatty acids in American diets. *J. Am. Dietet. Assoc.*, **62**: 147.

6. Bieri, J. G., R. P. Evarts, and J. J. Gart (1976). Relative activity of α-tocopherol and γ-tocopherol in preventing oxidative red cell hemolysis. *J. Nutrition*, **106**: 124.

7. Bieri, J. G., L. Teets, B. Belavady, and E. L. Andrews (1964). Serum vitamin E levels in a normal adult population in the Washington, D.C., area. *Proc. Soc. Exptl. Biol. & Med.*, **117**: 131.

8. Binder, H. J., and H. M. Spiro (1967). Tocopherol deficiency in man. *Am. J. Clin. Nutrition*, **20**: 594.

9. Bunnell, R. H., J. Keating, A. Quaresimo, and G. K. Parman (1965). Alpha-tocopherol content of foods. *Am. J. Clin. Nutrition*, **17**: 1.

10. Chow, C. K. (1975). Distribution of tocopherols in human plasma and red blood cells. *Am. J. Clin. Nutrition*, **28**: 756.

11. Committee on Nutritional Misinformation, Food and Nutrition Board (1973). *Supplementation of Human Diets with Vitamin E*. Washington, D.C.: National Academy of Sciences.

12. Evans, H. M., and K. S. Bishop (1922). On the existence of a hitherto unrecognized dietary factor essential for reproduction. *Science*, **56**: 650.

13. Farrell, P. M., and J. G. Bieri (1975). Megavitamin E supplementation in man. *Am. J. Clin. Nutrition*, **28**: 1381.

14. *Fats and Oils Statistics, 1950–1971 U.S.* (1972). Statistical Bull. No. 489. Washington, D.C.: U.S. Dept. Agric.

15. Green, J. (1972). Tocopherols IX. Biochemical systems. In *The Vitamins*, 2nd ed., vol. 5, edited by W. H. Sebrell, Jr., and R. S. Harris. New York: Academic Press, p. 261.

16. Hoekstra, W. G. (1975). Biochemical function of selenium and its relation to vitamin E. *Fed. Proceedings*, **34**: 2083.

17. Horwitt, M. K. (1976). Vitamin E: A reexamination. *Am. J. Clin. Nutrition*, **29**: 569.

18. Horwitt, M. K. (1960). Vitamin E and lipid metabolism in man. *Am. J. Clin. Nutrition*, **8**: 451.

19. Kelleher, J., and M. S. Losowsky (1970). The absorption of α-tocopherol in man. *Brit. J. Nutrition*, **24**: 1033.

20. Lawrence, J. D., R. C. Bower, W. P. Riehl, and J. L. Smith (1975). Effects of α-tocopherol acetate on the swimming endurance of trained swimmers. *Am. J. Clin. Nutrition*, **28**: 205.

21. Packer, L., and J. R. Smith (1977). Extension of the lifespan of cultured normal diploid cells by vitamin E: A reevaluation. *Proc. Natl. Acad. Science*, **74**: 1640.

22. Quaife, M. L., W. J. Swanson, M. Y. Dju, and P. L. Harris (1949). Vitamin E in foods and tissues. *Ann. N.Y. Acad. Sci.*, **52**: 300.

23. *Recommended Dietary Allowances* (1974). 8th ed. Washington, D.C.: National Research Council.

24. Ritchie, J. H., M. B. Fish, V. McMasters, and M. Grossman (1968). Edema and hemolytic anemia in premature infants. A vitamin E deficiency syndrome. *New Engl. J. Med.*, **279**: 1185.

25. Sauberlich, H. E., R. P. Dowdy, and J. H. Skala (1974). *Laboratory Tests for the Assessment of Nutritional Status*. Cleveland, Ohio: CRC Press, p. 77.

26. Slover, H. T. (1971). Tocopherols in foods and fats. *Lipids*, **6**: 291.

27. Sure, B. (1924). Dietary requirements for reproduction. II. The existence of a specific vitamin for reproduction. *J. Biol. Chem.*, **58**: 693.

28. Williams, M. L., R. J. Shott, P. L. O'Neal, and F. A. Oski (1975). Role of dietary iron and fat on vitamin E deficiency anemia of infancy. *New Engl. J. Med.*, **292**: 887.

Vitamin K

1. Almquist, H. J. (1971). Vitamin K group. IX. Biochemical systems. In *The Vitamins*, 2nd ed., vol. 3, edited by W. H. Sebrell, Jr., and R. S. Harris. New York: Academic Press, p. 466.

2. Dam, H. (1966). Historical survey and introduction. In *Vitamins and Hormones*, vol. 24. New York: Academic Press, p. 295.

3. Doisey, E. A., Jr., and J. T. Matschiner (1970). Biochemistry of vitamin K. In *Fat-Soluble Vitamins*, edited by R. A. Morton. New York: Pergamon Press.

4. Fomon, S. J. (1974). *Infant Nutrition*. Philadelphia: W. B. Saunders Co., p. 221.

5. Moss, H. H. (1969). Hypoprothrombinemic bleeding in a young infant. *Am. J. Dis. Child.*, **117**: 540.

6. Nomenclature policy: Generic descriptors and trivial names for vitamins and related compounds (1977). *J. Nutrition*, **107**: 7.

7. Olson, R. E. (1973). Vitamin K. In *Modern Nutrition in Health and Disease*, 5th ed., edited by R. S. Goodhart and M. E. Shils. Philadelphia: Lea and Febiger, p. 166.

8. *Recommended Dietary Allowances* (1974). 8th ed. Washington, D.C.: National Academy of Sciences.

9. Sauberlich, H. E., R. P. Dowdy, and J. H. Skala (1974). *Laboratory Tests for the Assessment of Nutritional Status*. Cleveland, Ohio: CRC Press, p. 83.

10. Suttie, J. W. (1976). Vitamin K. In *Present Knowledge in Nutrition*, 4th ed., edited by D. M. Hegsted, Chm., and Editorial Com. Washington, D.C.: The Nutrition Foundation, Inc., p. 111.

201

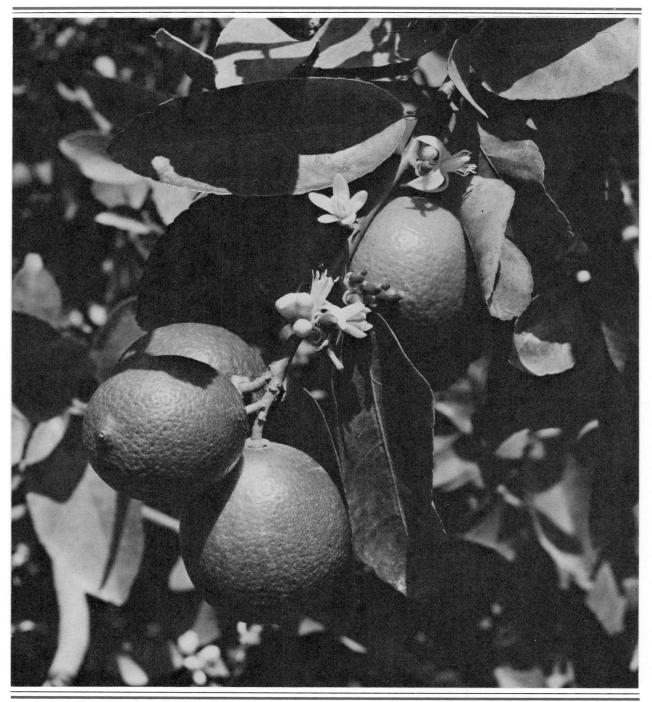

Limes were among the first fruits used to cure and prevent scurvy in the eighteenth century.

Chapter 10

Vitamin C

203

Abbreviations

ATP: adenosine triphosphate
CHOL: cholesterol
HANES: Health and Nutrition Examination
  Survey, United States

HIRS: high-income-ratio states
LIRS: low-income-ratio states
RDA: Recommended Dietary Allowance
USDA: U.S. Dept. Agriculture

Outbreaks of *scurvy* (now known to be caused by a severe deficiency of vitamin C) hampered the early explorations of the world. Not until 1750 was it shown that scurvy could be cured and prevented on shipboard by the intake of fresh or preserved juices of oranges and lemons (47). In 1795, the English Navy began to provide regular rations of lemon or lime juice to all of its men, and the word "limey" (which is still used to describe an English sailor) originated with this practice. Many years later (1933), the antiscorbutic factor was identified as vitamin C and since then has been produced in its synthetic form.

All animals need vitamin C, and most of them are able to synthesize the vitamin from the sugar glucose because they have the needed liver enzyme, L-gulonolactone oxidase (14). Besides man, primates (monkeys, apes, and chimpanzees), guinea pigs, Indian fruit bats, and red-vented bulbuls (birds native to India) lack this enzyme and need a dietary source of vitamin C. This defect has been referred to as an inborn error of ascorbic acid biosynthesis (39).

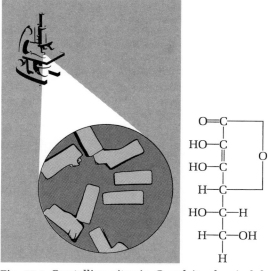

Fig. 10.1 Crystalline vitamin C and its chemical formula. (Courtesy Merck, Sharpe and Dohme Research Laboratories, Rahway, New Jersey.)

Properties of Vitamin C

Vitamin C appears as white crystals that readily dissolve in water (Fig. 10.1). When dry, vitamin C crystals are quite stable. In a water solution, the vitamin will undergo inactivation when exposed to air, heat, light, or metals such as copper and iron. The vitamin is unstable in an alkali medium but relatively stable in an acid one. (Vitamin C is often called the most labile vitamin.)

Chemical Forms of Vitamin C

Two forms of vitamin C are found in nature: the reduced form (ascorbic acid) and the oxidized form (dehydroascorbic acid). Because ascorbic acid is a strong reducing agent, it is easily converted to dehydroascorbic acid (by oxidation) and then changed back to ascorbic acid (by reduction) (see p. 19). Both forms exist in plant and animal tissues, and studies have shown that both are used by human subjects (18).

204

Certain derivatives of vitamin C (for example, erythrobic acid and ascorbyl palmitate) are used as antioxidants in food products to prevent rancidity, to prevent the browning of fruit, and to cure meat. One of these, erythrobic acid (D-araboascorbic acid), is only slightly antiscorbutic as compared with vitamin C (53).

Metabolism of Vitamin C

Vitamin C is absorbed from the upper part of the small intestine into the portal circulation. The tissues of the body contain various amounts of the vitamin. Except for muscle tissue, tissues of high metabolic activity have high concentrations of vitamin C, such as the eye, liver, and brain (24).

It has been shown that human beings are able to store some vitamin C; healthy, well-fed subjects store about 1500 mg. On vitamin C deprivation diets, these stores are used at an average rate of 3 percent of the existing reserve (pool) per day and supply the body with vitamin C for a period of about three months (9, 28).

Vitamin C is excreted by way of the kidneys. When the tissues are saturated a large amount is excreted (more than 50 percent of a 100-mg dose given intravenously), but when the tissue reserves are depleted only a small amount is excreted (less than 5 percent of a 100-mg dose given intravenously). Some vitamin C is always excreted by the kidneys even when the tissues are severely depleted.

Vitamin C status in people may be determined by clinical signs and blood levels of the vitamin. Evidence of capillary bleeding in the skin (perifolliculosis) and in the gums are clinical signs that may indicate a vitamin C deficiency (1). Serum vitamin C levels are the most widely used and practical measurement of vitamin C status, however (46). In the Iowa City–Denver human vitamin C studies, it was found that the earliest signs of vitamin C deficiency may appear after the blood serum levels fall below 0.20 mg per 100 ml (25).

Functions of Vitamin C

It is believed that vitamin C functions in *collagen* formation, in protein metabolism, and in fat and lipid metabolism. As new research findings become available, the precise action of the vitamin in these body processes may be known.

Collagen Formation and Vitamin C Reports of the role of vitamin C in collagen formation were published nearly 40 years after the relationship between the vitamin and collagen was first recognized. In 1933, it was observed that collagen material normally present in healthy tissue had disappeared from the cells of scorbutic guinea pigs (51). Later it was reported that vitamin C was important in wound healing (16). Using himself as a subject, Crandon demonstrated that after six months on a vitamin C-free diet, a wound would not heal completely until the vitamin was returned to his diet (Fig. 10.2). Newer data show that the complete healing of wounds in scorbutic men was managed with as little as 4 mg of vitamin C per day (25).

Collagen is one of the most abundant proteins in the body and is found in bone, cartilage, and connective tissue. Collagen contains the usual amino acids like other proteins and is synthesized like other proteins, except vitamin C is necessary for two chemical steps in its formation. Vitamin C aids in the addition of an −OH group (hydroxylation) to the amino acids proline and lysine to form hydroxyproline and hydroxylysine. These reactions take place only after the proline and lysine have been incorporated into the polypeptide chain during the biosynthesis of collagen (11). When vitamin C is missing, an underhydroxylated form of collagen is produced that has abnormal physical properties (36). (This finding could explain the unsatisfactory wound healing shown in Fig. 10.2.)

Protein Metabolism and Vitamin C The body's use of the amino acid tryptophan is related to vitamin C. One of the enzymes required for the conversion of tryptophan to a related compound needs both vitamin C and the mineral copper (15, 17).

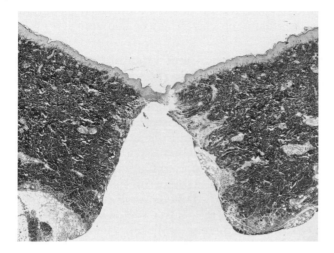

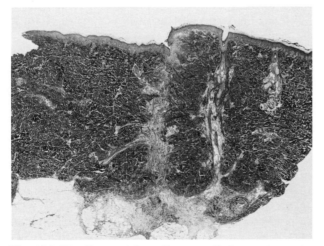

Fig. 10.2 The first satisfactorily controlled experiment in human scurvy was performed when Crandon placed himself on a vitamin C-free diet, supplemented by all other known vitamins. After six months on the diet, a wound was made in the midback region. A biopsy made ten days later (top) shows no healing except of epithelium (the gap in the tissue was filled with blood clot). After ten days of vitamin C treatment (bottom), another biopsy shows healing with abundant collagen formation. (Courtesy J. H. Crandon and The Upjohn Company, Kalamazoo, Michigan.)

When large amounts of the amino acid tyrosine are ingested, vitamin C is needed to reactivate an enzyme needed in tyrosine metabolism (35). This enzyme becomes inactive in the presence of high concentrations of one of the intermediary products formed during tyrosine metabolism, but vitamin C (or other reducing compounds) help to prevent this.

Another role given to vitamin C is that the nutrient accelerates the removal of ammonia (deamination) from certain unstable groups of peptides and proteins (45). It is thought that these deamination processes may permit ". . . the regulation of the lifetime and the role of protein in the development, function, and aging of living systems . . ." (38).

Fat and Lipid Metabolism and Vitamin C Vitamin C may have a role in the metabolism of cholesterol (CHOL). There appears to be a decrease in the liver's ability to convert CHOL to bile acids in a vitamin C deficiency (22).

Along with ATP and magnesium ions, vitamin C serves in fat metabolism as a cofactor in the inactivation of the enzyme adipose tissue lipase. (This enzyme mobilizes the free fatty acids from adipose tissue to meet the energy demands of the body.) Adipose tissue lipase requires vitamin C to reconvert it to its inactive form when the body's energy needs have been satisfied (49).

Other Functions of Vitamin C The body's use of the mineral iron is related to vitamin C. An intake of 200 mg or more daily of vitamin C helps the absorption of both the ferric and ferrous forms of iron; it facilitates the reduction of ferric to ferrous iron, the form that is more efficiently absorbed (see p. 19) (21, 37).

Vitamin C also helps to maintain the biological form of the vitamin folacin (tetrahydrofolacin) in its reduced state. When vitamin C is missing from the diet (scurvy), oxidation of tetrahydrofolacin occurs, and the activity of the folacin coenzymes is interferred with; the megaloblastic anemia of scurvy may result (48).

The discovery of a new form of vitamin C, ascorbic-2-sulfate, in the tissues and urine of man and animals has led to the speculation that the vitamin also may function in reactions involving S groups in the body (sulfation) (7, 34).

Vitamin C Deficiency

Scurvy is no longer an important disease in any part of the world (40). Sometimes it occurs in infants and children whose diets lack fruits and vegetables. Scurvy in adults is associated with poverty, alcoholism, famine, and nutritional ignorance (44).

Preclinical symptoms of scurvy include weakness, loss of weight, and fleeting pains in the arms and legs. Usually the first detectable clinical symptom is the formation of a horny growth in the hair follicles (follicular keratosis) which may occur on the legs, buttocks, arms, and back. This is followed by hemorrhages around the hair follicles. Soon there are scorbutic changes in the gums: at first they are red and swollen and then the swelling increases; there are hemorrhages, and the gum tissues become blue-red in color. (Fig. 10.3) If the condition persists, the teeth

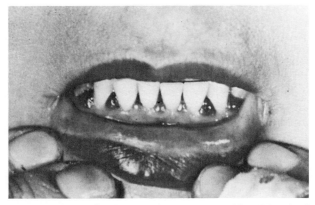

Fig. 10.3 Hemorrhagic gums in a woman with a Vitamin C deficiency. (Photo by Dr. William J. Darby. Reproduced with permission of NUTRITION TODAY Magazine, Annapolis, Maryland, © September 1966.)

may become loose. The failure of new wounds to heal and the tendency of old wounds to become red and break open are signs of scurvy that have been observed for centuries.

The Iowa City–Denver Experimental Scurvy Studies Using sophisticated biochemical and radioisotopic methods, a 210-day study was conducted by the University of Iowa and the Army Medical Research and Nutrition Laboratory in Denver in 1966–1967 using prisoners as subjects (8, 9, 27, 28). The plan was to give the subjects a liquid diet devoid of vitamin C for days 1–99 (the depletion period), a solid diet supplying 2.5 mg of the vitamin for days 100–197 (the repletion period), and a free-choice diet supplemented by 500 mg of vitamin C daily for days 198–210 (the saturation period). On day 23 and at prescribed times during the repletion period, the subjects were given varying amounts of ^{14}C-labeled ascorbic acid to label the body vitamin C pool during depletion and repletion. (The body pool includes all of the vitamin C in the body.)

The four subjects who completed the experiment developed clinical signs of scurvy, including follicular hyperkeratosis of the thighs, buttocks, calves, and arms with hemorrhages and congested follicles; swollen bleeding gums; and *conjunctival hemorrhages*. Although ocular vascular lesions are considered rare in human scurvy, they appeared among these subjects during days 74–95 of vitamin C deprivation (29).

This induced scurvy did not appear to affect other biological and physiological measurements of these subjects (27). No abnormalities were found in the hematologic measurements (blood counts, sedimentation rates), the battery of biochemical measurements (serum CHOL, plasma amino acids), the rate of wound healing, or physiological tests (basal metabolism, blood coagulation, electrocardiogram).

The Iowa City–Denver researchers conducted a second study of induced scurvy in which five men were fed a liquid diet devoid of vitamin C for 84 to 97 days (30, 31). In addition to the already-mentioned scurvy symptoms, four of the five subjects complained of joint pains (arthralgia) between days 67 and 96, with pain occurring in the knees of some; the ankles of others; and the elbows, shoulders, and wrists of one. There was an escape of fluid (effusion) in the knee joints of three of the subjects, and one man had a swelling of both ankle joints. The joint disorders appeared later than the other scurvy symptoms (30). This is only the second time that arthralgia and joint effusions have been reported in vitamin C-deprivation studies on human beings.

Recommended Dietary Allowances for Vitamin C

The RDA for vitamin C for adults of both sexes is 45 mg per day, which is less than the RDA of 1968. Canada, the United Kingdom, and the FAO/WHO established lower allowances for vitamin C because of the finding that the clinical symptoms of scurvy can be relieved by giving 10 mg of vitamin C daily (27, 50). Findings from the Iowa City–Denver human vitamin C studies indicate a mean use of only 9 mg (25). Although the lower RDAs of 1974 seem to be sufficiently generous to allow for individual variability and for potential losses of the vitamin in storing and preparing food, there are those who believe that the levels have been set too low (23). Table 10.1 shows the RDAs and the RDA per 1000 kcal (4184 kJ) for vitamin C for males and females of all age groups. (Vitamin C was not measured by the U.S. Department of Agriculture in the meals served at 50 American colleges [52].)

Cigarette Smoking and Vitamin C Requirement
It is well established that cigarette smokers have lower blood vitamin C levels than nonsmokers (43). Yet on high intakes of vitamin C (100 mg per day), these plasma vitamin C differences between smokers and nonsmokers are not evident (54). These findings suggest that a cigarette smoker's requirement for vitamin C is higher and

Table 10.1 Recommended Dietary Allowances for Vitamin C

	Age (years)	RDA (mg)	RDA (mg/1000 kcal[a])
Infants	0.0–0.5	35	—
	0.5–1.0	35	—
Children	1–3	40	31
	4–6	40	22
	7–10	40	17
Males	11–14	45	16
	15–18	45	15
	19–22	45	15
	23–50	45	17
	51+	45	19
Females	11–14	45	19
	15–18	45	21
	19–22	45	21
	23–50	45	23
	51+	45	25
Pregnant		60	—
Lactating		80	—

[a] Calculated.
From *Recommended Dietary Allowances* (1974). Washington, D.C.: National Academy of Sciences.

should be adjusted to compensate for the impaired bioavailability of the vitamin.

Food Sources of Vitamin C

Citrus fruits (oranges, grapefruit, lemons, and limes), berries, melons, tropical fruits (pineapples, guavas, and others), leafy green vegetables, broccoli, green peppers, cabbage, and tomatoes are all good sources of vitamin C (Table 10.2). The large quantity of potatoes used by those with a low income makes this vegetable an important source of vitamin C for many people.

The best natural sources of vitamin C are rose hips, the acerola fruit (West Indian cherry), and the *camu-camu* (a tropical fruit). Rose hips, which constitute the base of the rose bloom, are not eaten as such, but are either made into a syrup

208

Table 10.2 Vitamin C Content of Various Foods as Served

| Food | Per 100 g of food, vitamin C, mg | Per average serving | |
		Size of serving g	Vitamin C, mg
Acerola juice (raw)[a]	1600	121 ½ c	1936
Green pepper (raw)	127	74 1 pod	94
Brussel sprouts (frozen, cooked)	81	78 ½ c	63
Strawberries (raw)	59	75 ½ c	44
Broccoli (frozen, chopped, cooked)	57	93 ½ c	53
Orange	50	131 1 med	66
Mustard greens (cooked)	49	70 ½ c	34
Orange juice (frozen, reconstituted)	48	125 ½ c	60
Cabbage (raw, shredded)	47	45 ½ c	21
Lemon juice (raw)	46	122 ½ c	56
Kale (frozen, cooked)	39	65 ½ c	25
Grapefruit juice (canned, unsweetened)	34	124 ½ c	42
Lime juice (raw)	33	123 ½ c	40
Spinach (raw, cooked)	28	90 ½ c	25
Liver (beef, fried)	27	85 3 oz	23
Sweet potato (baked)	22	114 1 med	25
Tomato (raw)	21	135 1 med	28
Potato (white, baked)	20	156 1 med	31
Bean sprouts (Mung, raw)[a]	19	53 ½ c	10
Cantaloupe	19	477 ½ melon	90
Turnip greens (frozen, cooked)	19	83 ½ c	16
Grapefruit (raw)	18	241 ½ med	44
Tomato juice (canned)	16	122 ½ c	20
Peas, green (frozen, cooked)	14	80 ½ c	11
Pineapple (canned, chunks)	7	128 ½ c	9
Milk (whole)	1	244 1 c	2
Bread (white, enriched)	tr	28 1 sl	tr
Butter	0	14 1 tbsp	0
Egg	0	50 1 lg	0
Ground beef (broiled)	—	82 2.9 oz patty	—
Sugar (white)	0	12 1 tbsp	0

[a] From *Nutritive Value of American Foods in Common Units*, Agr. Handbook No. 456. Washington, D.C.: U.S. Dept. Agr., 1975.
From *Nutritive Value of Foods*, Home and Garden Bull. No. 72, revised. Washington, D.C.: U.S. Dept. Agr., 1977.

(or extract) or are brewed as tea. During the World War II food rationing in England, rose hip syrup was issued by the British Ministry of Food to help fortify the vitamin C intake of the English people.

Vitamin C Losses during Storage, Processing, and Cooking Food may lose much of its original vitamin C content from the time it is harvested until it is eaten. If fresh fruits and vegetables are

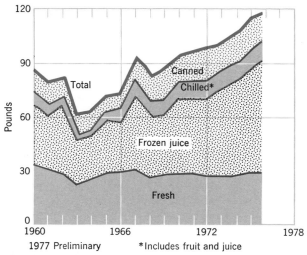

Pounds (y-axis)
1960 1966 1972 1978 (x-axis)
Total, Canned, Chilled*, Frozen juice, Fresh

1977 Preliminary   *Includes fruit and juice

Fig. 10.4 Citrus consumption per person (fresh equivalent basis) in the United States since 1960. (*From 1977 Handbook of Agricultural Charts,* Agr. Handbook No. 524, Washington, D.C.: U.S. Dept. Agr., 1977, p. 133.)

Vitamin C in the United States' Food Supply

The vitamin C available per capita per day amounted to about 123 mg in 1976 (3). There has been a gradual increase (about 20 percent) in the vitamin C content of the national food supply since 1964. Most of this rise is due to the increased per capita consumption of citrus products, particularly frozen concentrated orange juice (Fig. 10.4).

In 1976 nearly three-fourths of the vitamin C in the American food supply came from citrus fruit (28.2 percent), white and sweet potatoes (17.2 percent), and other vegetables, including tomatoes (26.4 percent). Other fruits contributed 11.8 percent, dark-green and yellow vegetables 8.3 percent, dairy products (excluding butter) 3.7 percent, meat 1.0 percent, and the remainder from other foods (3).

Vitamin C Consumption and Deficiency in the United States

Ten-State Nutrition Survey The standard used for evaluating vitamin C intake was the value 30 mg per day. The mean vitamin C intake exceeded the standard for all groups surveyed (infants and young children, adolescents, pregnant and lactating women, and persons 60 years of age and older). Among the infant and young children group and the adolescent group, however, there were large numbers who had vitamin C intakes below the standard (19).

The vitamin C status (measured by serum vitamin C levels) was less satisfactory in the low-income-ratio-states (LIRS) (Kentucky, Louisiana, South Carolina, Texas, and West Virginia) than in the high-income-ratio-states (HIRS) (California, Massachusetts, Michigan, New York, and Washington). Among the ethnic groups studied (white, black, and Spanish-American), the black subjects in the LIRS had the poorest vitamin C status.

stored for any length of time (especially in warm places), there is an appreciable loss of vitamin C. Citrus fruit juices stored in the refrigerator lose negligible amounts of the vitamin; the acid reaction of the juice helps preserve vitamin C. Frozen fruits and vegetables stored above −18°C (0°F) for 4 months and canned, nonacid vegetables stored above 18°C (65°F) for 6 months lose substantial amounts of vitamin C.

Vitamin C is lost during food preparation when fruits and vegetables are washed slowly, cut up into small pieces, soaked after peeling, cooked in copper or iron utensils (these ions inactivate the vitamin), cooked in large amounts of water, cooked and the cooking water discarded, and/or cooked and kept warm until served.

Whether a food is fresh, frozen, canned, or dehydrated significantly affects its vitamin C content. For example, an edible portion of lima beans weighing 100 g has an average vitamin C content of 29 mg (fresh, raw), 17 mg (fresh, cooked), 17 mg (frozen, cooked), 6 mg (canned, cooked), and none (dried, cooked).

210

Children had better vitamin C status than did adults; females (in all age groups) had better vitamin C status than did males. The data show that vitamin C was not a major problem in the populations studied (13).

First Health and Nutrition Examination Survey, United States (HANES) Preliminary findings from HANES show that the intake levels of vitamin C approached or were above the standard for the 10,126 persons, ages 1–74 years, examined (2) (Appendix Table A-27).

Bleeding and swollen gums (the clinical sign classified as "moderate risk") were found in 3.3 percent of those in the "income below poverty level" group and 2.5 in those in the "income above poverty level" group. The incidence of bleeding swollen gums was found almost twice as often among black than white subjects (1).

Results for the serum vitamin C tests will be presented in the final report of HANES (2).

Megavitamin C

Large daily intakes of vitamin C (megavitamin C) have been advocated for improvement of athletic performance, for the prevention and cure of the common cold, and for the cure of a variety of other disorders and diseases.

Athletic Performance and Vitamin C The use of large doses of vitamin C to improve performance in athletes has been a controversial issue for nearly 40 years. The present findings indicate that athletic performance does not increase with massive doses of the vitamin (26, 32). Scientists from the Research Institute of Federal School of Physical Education in Switzerland state that very high doses of vitamin C will never replace training and may have a ". . . negative effect on athletic performance by disturbing the equilibrium between oxygen transport and oxygen utilization" (32).

The Common Cold and Vitamin C Based on only limited evidence, the effectiveness of large doses of vitamin C in the prevention and treatment of the common cold is dealt with by L. Pauling in the 1970 book, *Vitamin C and the Common Cold* (41). In 1971, Pauling claimed that the regular intake of 1000 mg of vitamin C per day would lead to 45 percent fewer colds and 60 percent fewer days of sickness (42). (It should be noted that the common cold has never been observed as a sign of a vitamin C deficiency [12].)

Scientists at the University of Toronto were one of the groups who conducted studies of the effect of vitamin C on the common cold; their first report is considered to furnish the best evidence to support these claims. In the first study 1971–1972 (5), the findings suggest that 1000 mg of vitamin C per day may increase the number of persons who remained free from illness by about 7 percent and that 4000 mg of the vitamin daily, taken during a cold, reduce the number of days confined by one-half a day. In two further studies in 1972–1973 (6) and 1973–1974 (4), this group was unable to confirm the findings of their 1971–1972 study. They conclude that ". . . unless and until firm evidence is forthcoming that higher doses of vitamin C are more effective, we should . . . advise the public to limit their daily intake to 100 or 200 mg" (4).

At this time (1978), the following suggestions are made to the public concerning the effectiveness of large intakes of vitamin C and the common cold:

The Food and Nutrition Board (NAS–NRC) ". . . feels that many of these claims are not sufficiently substantiated, or the effects are not of significant magnitude, and that *routine consumption of large amounts of ascorbic acid is not advisable without medical advice*" (44).

The American Medical Association (Department of Drugs) — ". . . A review of the controlled studies of the efficacy of ascorbic acid in the prophylaxis and therapy of the common cold that meet some reasonable criteria of design reveals *little convincing evidence to support claims of clinically important efficacy*. . . . Until such time as pharmacologic doses of ascorbic acid have been shown to have obvious, important clinical value in the prevention and treatment of the common cold, and to be safe in a large varied population, *we cannot advocate its unrestricted use for such purposes*" (20).

Other Diseases and Disorders and Vitamin C It has been suggested that very large amounts of vitamin C exert a favorable effect on the prevention and treatment of cancer, mental retardation, atherosclerosis, and other diseases and disorders. There is no evidence whatsoever to support these claims (26, 33).

Summary

Most animals have the liver enzyme L-gulonolactone oxidase to synthesize vitamin C from glucose. Besides man, primates, guinea pigs, and several others lack the enzyme and need a daily source of the vitamin.

Vitamin C is very unstable; in a water solution it is inactivated by air, heat, light, and metals (iron and copper). The oxidized form (dehydroascorbic acid) and the reduced form (ascorbic acid) are found in nature and used by human beings.

The vitamin functions in the formation of collagen where it aids in the hydroxylation of proline and lysine to form hydroxyproline and hydroxylysine. In protein metabolism, vitamin C is required for the conversion of tryptophan to a related compound, for the reactivation of an enzyme needed in tyrosine metabolism, and for the removal of ammonia from certain groups in peptides and proteins. Vitamin C has a role in fat and lipid metabolism; it functions in CHOL metabolism, and along with ATP and magnesium ions acts as a cofactor in the inactivation of the enzyme adipose tissue lipase. Vitamin C enhances the absorption of iron and maintains the biological form of folacin (tetrahydrofolacin) in its reduced state. It is suggested that a new form of the vitamin, ascorbic-2-sulfate, may function in sulfation reactions of the body.

Weakness, loss of weight, and fleeting pains in the arms and legs followed by bleeding gums and failure of wounds to heal are some of the symptoms of scurvy.

The Iowa City–Denver human scurvy studies showed that well-nourished men have a body store of about 1500 mg vitamin C that will sustain them for over three months on a vitamin C-deficient diet. Serum vitamin C levels and bleeding gums are two measurements used to assess vitamin C status.

The RDA for vitamin C for adults is 45 mg per day. Cigarette smokers have a higher requirement for the vitamin than do nonsmokers.

Citrus fruit, berries, melons, tropical fruit, green leafy vegetables, and tomatoes are the best food sources of vitamin C. The vitamin is very labile and may be inactivated during food processing and preparation.

Findings from the Ten-State Nutrition Survey and First Health and Nutrition Examination Survey show that vitamin C is not a major nutritional problem among the populations studied.

Large daily intakes of vitamin C (greater than 1000 mg per day) do not increase athletic performance. There is no convincing evidence at this time (1978) to support the claim that large daily intakes of vitamin C should be ingested to prevent or cure the common cold.

What is a large intake of vitamin C and can it be toxic to human beings? Varying doses of vitamin C have been classified as follows: *physiologic dose*, 45 mg; *pharmacologic dose*, 100–2000 mg; and *toxic dose*, 2000–4000 mg (26).

The most significant hazards associated with toxic intakes of vitamin C are the development of kidney and bladder stones and alterations in carbohydrate metabolism (34). Other toxic effects (for example, CHOL disturbances, vitamin

212

B-12 destruction, and gastrointestinal disturbances) also have been reported (10).

Glossary

collagen: see page 28.

conjunctival hemorrhages: hemorrhages in the membranes that line the eyelids and cover the eyeball.

pharmacologic dose: usually ten times the physiologic dose used to treat an illness or condition quite unrelated to the deficiency signs or symptoms of a nutrient.

physiologic dose: the amount of a nutrient needed or recommended to prevent signs of a deficiency in practically all healthy persons; the RDA of a nutrient.

scurvy: a disease caused by vitamin C deficiency; weakness, loss of weight, and bleeding gums are among its symptoms.

toxic dose: very large intakes of a nutrient; 100 times or more the physiologic dose; may induce undesirable signs and symptoms.

Study Questions and Activities

1. Identify the following: collagen, acerola, dehydroascorbic acid, L-gulonolactose oxidase, pharmacologic dose of vitamin C, toxic dose of vitamin C.
2. What are the specific chemical properties of vitamin C, and how do they relate to the loss of this vitamin in cooking and processing food?
3. What are the functions of vitamin C?
4. In the late 1960s, a series of studies was conducted by researchers from Iowa City and Denver that produced experimental scurvy in adult men. What important findings from these investigations have been reported?
5. What harm is there in taking large daily doses of vitamin C?
6. List ten foods that are good sources of vitamin C.
7. What are some of the characteristic clinical and biochemical signs of a vitamin C deficiency?
8. If a person smokes cigarettes, what should he or she know about his or her vitamin C need?

References

1. Abraham, S., F. W. Lowenstein, and D. E. O'Connell (1975). *Anthropometric and Clinical Findings: Preliminary Findings of the First Health and Nutrition Examination Survey, United States, 1971–1972*, DHEW Publ. No. (HRA) 75-1229. Rockville, Md.: U.S. Dept. Health, Educ., and Welfare.
2. Abraham, S., F. W. Lowenstein, and C. L. Johnson (1974). *Dietary Intake and Biochemical Findings: Preliminary Findings of the First Health and Nutrition Examination Survey, United States, 1971–1972*, DHEW Publ. No. (HRA) 74-1219-1. Rockville, Md.: U.S. Dept. Health, Educ., and Welfare.
3. *Agricultural Statistics* (1977). Washington, D.C.: U.S. Dept. Agr., pp. 561–564.
4. Anderson, T. W. (1975). Large-scale trials of vitamin C. *Ann. New York Acad. Sci.*, **258:** 498.
5. Anderson, T. W., D. B. W. Reid, and G. H. Beaton (1972). Vitamin C and the common cold: a double blind trial. *Can. Med. Assoc. J.*, **107:** 503.
6. Anderson, T. W., G. Suranyi, and G. H. Beaton (1974). The effect on winter illnesses of large doses of vitamin C. *Can. Med. Assoc. J.*, **111:** 31.
7. Baker, E. M., J. E. Halver, D. O. Johnsen, B. E. Joyce, M. K. Knight, and B. M. Tolbert (1975). Metabolism of ascorbic acid and ascorbic-2-sulfate in man and the subhuman primate. *Ann. New York Acad. Sci.*, **258:** 72.
8. Baker, E. M., R. E. Hodges, J. Hood, H. E. Sauberlich, and S. C. March (1969). Metabolism of ascorbic-1-^{14}C acid in experimental human scurvy. *Am. J. Clin. Nutrition*, **22:** 549.
9. Baker, E. M., R. E. Hodges, J. Hood, H. E. Sauberlich, S. C. March, and J. E. Canham (1971). Metabolism of ^{14}C- and ^{3}H-labeled L-ascorbic acid in human scurvy. *Am. J. Clin. Nutrition*, **24:** 444.
10. Barnes, L. A. (1975). Safety consideration with high ascorbic acid dosage. *Ann. New York Acad. Sci.*, **358:** 523.
11. Barnes, M. J. (1975). Function of ascorbic acid in collagen metabolism. *Ann. New York Acad. Sci.*, **258:** 264.

213

12. Beaton, G. H., R. E. Hodges, W. J. Darby, and L. A. Barnes (1975). Panel discussion. *Ann. New York Acad. Sci.,* **258:** 546.

13. *Biochemical,* Ten-State Nutrition Survey, 1968–1970 (1972). DHEW Publ. No. (HSM) 72-8132. Atlanta, Ga.: Center for Disease Control, U.S. Dept. Health, Educ., and Welfare.

14. Burns, J. J. (1975). Introduction: Overview of ascorbic acid metabolism. *Ann. New York Acad. Sci.,* **258:** 5.

15. Chatterjee, I. B., N. C. Kar, N. C. Ghosh, and B. C. Guha (1961). Aspects of ascorbic acid biosynthesis in animals. *Ann. New York Acad. Sci.,* **92:** 36.

16. Crandon, J. H., C. Lund, and D. Dill (1940). Experimental human scurvy. *New Eng. J. Med.,* **223:** 353.

17. Cooper, J. R. (1961). The role of ascorbic acid in the oxidation of tryptophan to 5-hydroxytryptophan. *Ann. New York Acad. Sci.,* **92:** 208.

18. Davey, B. L., K. H. Fisher, and S. D. Chen (1956). Utilization of ascorbic acid in fruits and vegetables. II. Utilization of 24 fruits and vegetables. *J. Am. Dietet. Assoc.,* **32:** 1069.

19. *Dietary,* Ten-State Nutrition Survey, 1968–1970 (1972). DHEW Publ. No. (HSM) 72-8133. Atlanta, Ga.: Center for Disease Control, U.S. Dept. Health, Educ., and Welfare.

20. Dyke, H. M. and P. Meier (1975). Ascorbic acid and the common cold. Evaluation of its efficacy and toxicity. *J. Am. Med. Assoc.,* **231:** 1073.

21. Fairbanks, V. F., J. L. Fahey, and E. Beutler (1971). *Clinical Disorders of Iron Metabolism.* 2nd ed. New York: Grune and Stratton, p. 287.

22. Ginter, E. (1973). Cholesterol: Vitamin C controls at transformation to bile acids. *Science,* **179:** 702.

23. Harper, H. A. (1975). Recommended Dietary Allowances. *Ann. New York Acad. Sci.,* **258:** 495–497.

24. Harper, H. A. (1975). *Review of Physiological Chemistry.* 15th ed. Los Altos, Calif.: Lange Medical Publications, p. 99.

25. Hodges, R. E. (1971). What's new about scurvy? *Am J. Clin. Nutrition,* **24:** 383.

26. Hodges, R. E. (1976). Ascorbic acid. In *Nutrition Reviews' Present Knowledge in Nutrition.* 4th ed. New York: The Nutrition Foundation, Inc., p. 119.

27. Hodges, R. E., E. M. Baker, J. Hood, H. E. Sauberlich, and S. C. March (1969). Experimental scurvy in man. *Am. J. Clin. Nutrition,* **22:** 535.

28. Hodges, R. E., J. Hood, J. E. Canham, H. E. Sauberlich, and E. M. Baker (1971). Clinical manifestations of ascorbic acid deficiency in man. *Am. J. Clin. Nutrition,* **24:** 432.

29. Hood, J., and R. E. Hodges (1969). Ocular lesions in scurvy. *Am. J. Clin. Nutrition,* **22:** 559.

30. Hood, J., and R. E. Hodges (1970). Arthritis in experimental scurvy. *Am. J. Clin. Nutrition,* **23:** 664.

31. Hood, J., R. E. Hodges, J. E. Canham, H. E. Sauberlich, and E. M. Baker (1970). Manifestations of experimental scurvy. *Am. J. Clin. Nutrition,* **23:** 664.

32. Howard, H., B. Segesser, and W. F. Korner (1975). Ascorbic acid and athletic performance. *Ann. New York Acad. Sci.,* **258:** 459.

33. Jukes, T. H. (1975). Megavitamin therapy. *J. Am. Med. Assoc.,* **233:** 550.

34. King, C. G. (1975). Current status of vitamin C and future horizons. *Ann. New York Acad. Sci.,* **258:** 540.

35. LaDuc, B. N., and V. G. Zannoni (1961). The role of ascorbic acid in tyrosine metabolism. *Ann. New York Acad. Sci.,* **92:** 175.

36. Levine, C. I., and C. J. Bates (1975). Ascorbic acid and collagen synthesis in cultured fibroblasts. *Ann. New York Acad. Sci.,* **258:** 288.

37. Mazur, A. (1961). Role of ascorbic acid in the incorporation of plasma iron into ferritin. *Ann. New York Acad. Sci.,* **92:** 223.

38. New roles for ascorbic acid (1974). *Nutrition Rev.,* **32:** 53.

39. Nishikimi, M., and S. Undenfriend (1977). Scurvy as an inborn error of ascorbic acid biosynthesis. *Trends in Biochem. Sci.,* **2:** 111.

40. Passmore, R., B. M. Nicol, M. N. Rao, G. H. Beaton, and E. M. Demayer (1974). *Handbook on Human Nutritional Requirements.* Geneva: World Health Organ., p. 32.

41. Pauling L. (1970). *Vitamin C and the Common Cold.* San Francisco: W. H. Freeman and Co.

42. Pauling, L. (1971). Letter to editor. *Can. Med. Assoc. J.,* **105:** 448.

43. Pelletier, O. (1975). Vitamin C and cigarette smokers. *Ann. New York Acad. Sci.,* **258:** 156.

44. *Recommended Dietary Allowances, Eighth Edition* (1974). Natl. Acad. Sci.-Natl. Research Council Publ. Washington, D.C.: Natl. Research Council.

45. Robinson, A. B., K. Irving, and M. McCrea (1973). Acceleration of the rate of deamination of Gly Arg Asn Arg Gly and of human transferrin by addition of L-ascorbic acid. *Proc. Natl. Acad. Sci. U.S.,* **70:** 2122.

46. Sauberlich, H. E., J. H. Skala, and R. P. Dowdy (1974). *Laboratory Tests for the Assessment of Nutritional Status.* Cleveland, Ohio: CRC Press, p. 13.

47. Stewart, C. P., and D. Guthrie (1953). *Lind's Treatise on Scurvy: A Bicentenary Volume with Additional Notes.* Edinburgh, Scotland: Edinburgh University Press.

48. Stokes, P. L., V. Milikian, R. L. Leeming, H. Portman-Graham, J. A. Blair, and W. T. Cooke (1975). Folate metabolism in scurvy. *Am. J. Clin. Nutrition,* **28:** 126.

49. Tsai, S. C., H. M. Fales, and M. Vaughan (1973). Inactivation of hormone-sensitive lipase from adipose tissue with adenosine triphosphate, magnesium, and ascorbic acid. *J. Biol. Chem.,* **248:** 5278.

50. Vitamin C Subcommittee of the Accessory Food Factors Committee, A. E. Barnes, W. Bartley, I. M. Frankau, G. A. Higgins, J. Pemberton, G. L. Roberts, and H. R. Vichers (1953). *Vitamin C Requirements of Human Beings,* Medical Research Council Special Rept. Series 280. London: H. M. Stationery Office, p. 179.

51. Wolbach, S. B. (1933). Controlled formation of collagen and reticulum: A study of the source of intercellular substance in recovery from experimental scorbutus. *Am. J. Pathol.,* **9:** 689.

52. Walker, M. A. and L. Page (1975). Nutritive content of college meals. Proximate composition and vitamins. *J. Am. Dietet. Assoc.,* **66:** 146.

53. Wang, M. M., K. H. Fisher, and M. L. Dodds (1962). Comparative metabolic response to erythrobic acid and ascorbic acid by the human. *J. Nutrition,* **77:** 443.

54. Yeung, D. L. (1976). Relationship between cigarette smoking, oral contraceptives, and plasma vitamins A, E, C, and plasma triglycerides and cholesterol. *Am. J. Clin. Nutrition,* **29:** 1216.

215

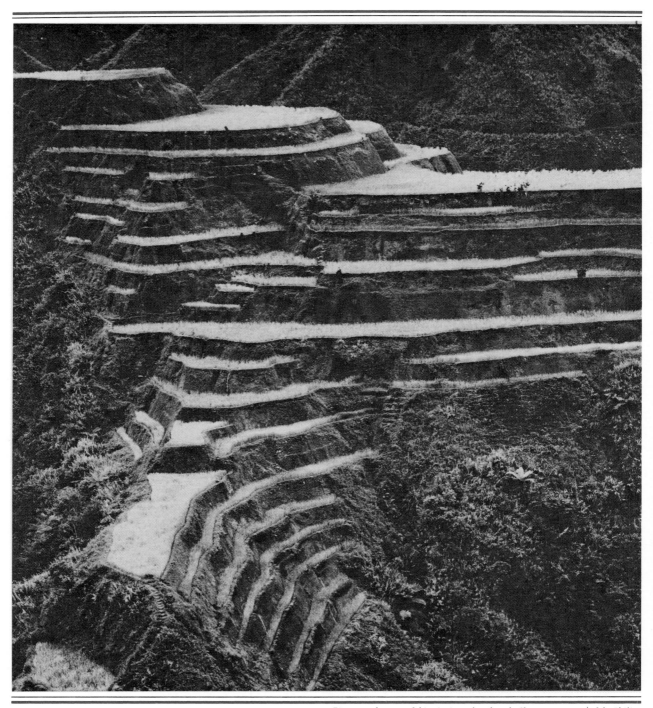

Rice, a good source of thiamin, is produced on the Ifugao rice terraces of the Philippines.

Chapter 11

The B-Complex Vitamins I

Abbreviations

Acetyl CoA: acetyl coenzyme A
ATP: adenosine triphosphate
CHOL: cholesterol
FAD: flavin adenine dinucleotide
FMN: flavin mononucleotide
HANES: Health and Nutrition Examination
  Survey, United States

NAD: nicotinamide adenine dinucleotide
NADP: nicotinamide adenine dinucleotide
  phosphate
RDA: Recommended Dietary Allowances
USP: United States Pharmacopeia

At one time (1915), "water-soluble B" was thought to be a single entity, the substance that cured pigeons of *polyneuritis*. Then it was demonstrated that rats also need a water-soluble factor in their diets. This factor seemed to differ from the original water-soluble B, for the food sources were not equally rich in both factors. At present (1978), there are eight well-defined B vitamins and several related compounds; collectively they are known as the vitamin B-complex. These vitamins differ in both chemical structure and specific functions, yet they are all water soluble and most of them are a part of a *coenzyme* molecule. The actions of many of them are interrelated; some of these interrelationships are shown in Table 11.1. There appears to be little capacity for the body to store the B vitamins, but certain organs, particularly the liver, contain higher concentrations of them than do others. These vitamins are excreted from the body by way of the kidney. (Para-

aminobenzoic acid, once listed as a B-complex vitamin, is now believed to be only a dietary precursor of the B vitamin folacin.)

Thiamin

Beriberi, a disease of the nervous system caused by the lack of thiamin in the diet, had a high morbidity and mortality rate in the Far East for centuries. In 1887, Takaki found that beriberi could be prevented by a good diet, and ten years later Eijkman began the work that led to the identification of thiamin as the antiberiberi vitamin. Funk (1911) called this substance "beriberi vitamine." In the years to follow, McCollum (1915) confirmed the existence of a single factor that not only cured polyneuritis but promoted growth, Donath (1926) demonstrated its curative effect on human beriberi, and R. R. Williams and

Table 11.1 Some Interrelationships Among the B-Complex Vitamins

Vitamin	Reaction and vitamin units involved
Thiamin	Conversion of pyruvic acid to acetyl CoA: Thiamin — thiamin diphosphate Niacin — nicotinamide-adenine dinucleotide (NAD) Pantothenic acid — coenzyme A
Niacin	Conversion of tryptophan to niacin: Vitamin B-6 — coenzyme pyridoxal phosphate

his group (1926) identified the chemical structure of thiamin and developed a method for synthesizing it.

Properties of Thiamin

The colorless crystals of thiamin (Fig. 11.1), which have a yeastlike smell and a salty taste, are very soluble in water. Thiamin is quite stable in acid solutions but is readily inactivated in a heated neutral or slightly alkaline solution. Commercially the vitamin is sold in the form of thiamin hydrochloride.

The amount of thiamin in foods or pharmaceutical products is determined by a chemical method. USP thiamin hydrochloride is the reference standard used.

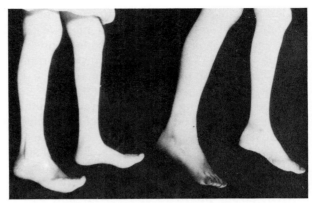

Fig. 11.2 The foot drop of beriberi. (left) Patient with peripheral neuritis of nutritional origin shows limit of flexion of ankles. (right) Moderate flexion is possible after 2½ weeks of thiamin therapy. (Courtesy H. Field, Jr. and The Upjohn Company, Kalamazoo, Michigan.)

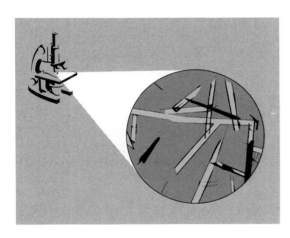

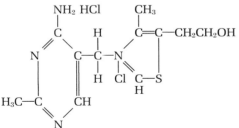

Fig. 11.1 Crystalline thiamin hydrochloride and its chemical formula. (Courtesy Merck, Sharpe and Dohme Research Laboratories, Rahway, New Jersey.)

Metabolism of Thiamin

As thiamin passes through the small intestine into the bloodstream, phosphate groups are added to it in the intestinal cells (the sodium ion and an enzyme are needed in the process). Of the 30 mg of thiamin found in the body (most of it as thiamin diphosphate), one-half is in the skeletal muscles and the remainder in the heart, liver, kidney, and brain.

The clinical signs used to measure thiamin deficiency in human beings are the prevalence of the decrease or absence in the reflex of the knee (knee jerks) and the drop in the muscles that support the foot (ankle jerk) (Fig. 11.2) (1).

The most widely used biochemical method to assess thiamin status in individuals is the measurement of the vitamin in the urine (17). The amount of thiamin excreted in the urine is related to its intake. With a well-balanced diet, approximately 0.1 mg is normally excreted every 24 hours.

Functions of Thiamin

Thiamin, like the other members of the B-complex group, functions as part of a *coenzyme* in mam-

219

malian physiology. A coenzyme (or cofactor) is a substance that combines with an inactive form of an enzyme to produce a new compound with enzyme activity. Thiamin diphosphate (formally called thiamin pyrophosphate) serves as a coenzyme in several enzyme systems (16).

In the metabolism of carbohydrates, thiamin diphosphate is needed in the conversion of pyruvic acid to the next chemical step (acetyl CoA) (see Fig. 2.6). For one of the chemical steps of the tricarboxylic acid cycle, the thiamin coenzyme is necessary to remove carboxyl groups (-COOH) from products of both fat and carbohydrate metabolism, thus continuing the chemical reactions to provide ATP. The activity of another enzyme (transketolase), which operates in the carbohydrate metabolic pathway to form the sugar ribose and NADP, also requires thiamin diphosphate (see Fig. 4.5).

Experimental studies on the role of thiamin in the nervous system (18) show that the vitamin is involved in the functioning of peripheral nerves. (There is some evidence that another phosphate form of thiamin, triphosphothiamin, may func-

tion in the normal mammalian nervous system [5].) The vitamin has value in the treatment of alcoholic *neuritis*, the neuritis of pregnancy, and beriberi.

Thiamin appears to have several indirect functions in the body because of its role in carbohydrate metabolism. The maintenance of normal appetite, the tone of the muscles, and a healthy mental attitude are all related to the status of thiamin nutrition.

Effects of a Thiamin Deficiency

The three general symptoms of beriberi are polyneuritis, either *edema* or *emaciation* of the tissues, and disturbances of the heart. Polyneuritis begins with a soreness in the muscles of the legs, followed by a decrease in the reflex of the knee and a drop in the muscles that support the toes and foot. This last symptom accounts for the high-stepping gait of beriberi patients (Fig. 11.2). As the disorder advances, however, the arms and other parts of the body are affected because there is a nerve degeneration and lack of muscle coordination. In cases of edema, the body tissues become swollen because fluid accumulates in the cells (Fig. 11.3). This condition is called "wet beriberi" and appears first in the legs and thighs of the patient. Emaciation, which may occur instead, is called "dry beriberi." Because the beriberi sufferer breathes with great difficulty and his heart beats rapidly and becomes enlarged (Fig. 11.4), death is usually caused by these cardiac impairments. In the United States beriberi heart disease occurs from time to time among elderly hospitalized persons (10). Some American POWs reported that they suffered from beriberi while in captivity during the Vietnam war.

Other symptoms of thiamin deprivation include changes in *electrocardiogram* measurement, low excretion of thiamin in the urine, reduced transketolase activity of the red blood cells, and an increase of pyruvic acid in the blood.

(a)   (b)

Fig. 11.3 Pitting edema. (a) Swelling of legs with pitting in ankle region marks beginning of so-called wet beriberi. (b) Same patient is shown four days after a single intravenous injection of 50 mg. of thiamin. During this period the patient's excretion of fluid exceeded intake by 10½ lb. (Courtesy T. Spies and The Upjohn Company, Kalamazoo, Michigan.)

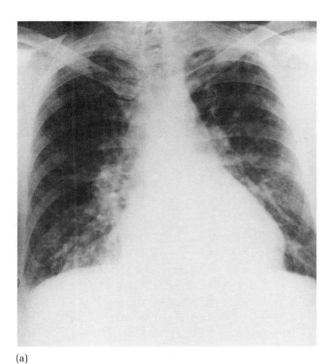

(a)

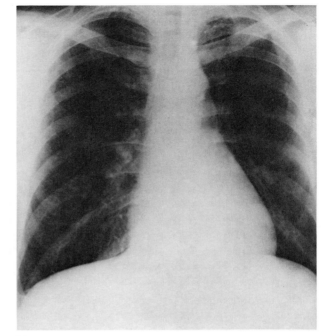

(b)

Fig. 11.4 Beriberi heart. (a) Thiamin deficiency leads to impaired function and enlargement of the heart, particularly of the right auricle and ventricle, as shown by X-ray. This patient was a chronic alcoholic whose diet had been poor for a long time. Polyneuritis and congestive heart failure accompanied the cardiac dilation. (b) After 1 week of thiamin therapy. (c) After 3 weeks of treatment (Courtesy H. Field, Jr. and The Upjohn Company, Kalamazoo, Michigan.)

(c)

Cases of mild thiamin deficiency are quite common (14). In countries prone to beriberi, a large number of people may suffer from loss of appetite *(anorexia), malaise,* and general weakness of the legs. This condition, which greatly reduces work capacity, after months or years may suddenly develop into "dry" or "wet" beriberi. The nutrition of Far Eastern infants and children has been improved by the use of thiamin-enriched commercial milk, but many still have marginal thiamin deficiencies (7).

One of the earliest symptoms of thiamin deficiency is the loss of appetite (or anorexia). In

221

Table 11.2 Recommended Dietary Allowances for Thiamin, Riboflavin, and Niacin

	Age, years	Thiamin		Riboflavin		Niacin	
		mg	mg/1000 kcal[a]	mg	mg/1000 kcal[a]	mg	mg/1000 kcal[a]
Infants	0.0–0.5	0.3	—	0.4	—	5	—
	0.5–1.0	0.5	—	0.6	—	8	—
Children	1–3	0.7	0.5	0.8	0.6	9	6.9
	4–6	0.9	0.5	1.1	0.6	12	6.7
	7–10	1.2	0.5	1.2	0.5	16	6.7
Males	11–14	1.4	0.5	1.5	0.5	18	6.4
	15–18	1.5	0.5	1.8	0.6	20	6.7
	19–22	1.5	0.5	1.8	0.6	20	6.7
	23–50	1.4	0.5	1.6	0.6	18	6.7
	51+	1.2	0.5	1.5	0.6	16	6.7
Females	11–14	1.2	0.5	1.3	0.5	16	6.7
	15–18	1.1	0.5	1.4	0.7	14	6.7
	19–22	1.1	0.5	1.4	0.7	14	6.7
	23–50	1.0	0.5	1.2	0.6	13	6.5
	51+	1.0	0.6	1.1	0.6	12	6.7
Pregnant		+0.3	—	+0.3	—	+2	—
Lactating		+0.3	—	+0.5	—	+4	—

[a] Calculated.

From *Recommended Dietary Allowances* eighth ed. (1974). Washington, D.C.: National Academy of Sciences.

studies of thiamin deprivation (12, 13), anorexia has been observed as early as the fourth day. Another symptom of the deficiency is a change in emotional stability. Williams et al. (20) found that their subjects (who were on restricted intakes of thiamin) became irritable, quarrelsome, and moody; they failed to cooperate; and they sometimes experienced periods of mental depression. Although thiamin is not a cure for mental disorders, it has been observed that mental patients whose intake is restricted may manifest an intensification of their psychiatric symptoms (11).

Recommended Dietary Allowances for Thiamin

The RDA for thiamin is based upon energy need (15). For men and women 19 to 22 years, the daily allowance for thiamin is 1.5 mg and 1.1 mg, respectively, or 0.5 mg per 1000 kcal (4184 kJ) (Table 11.2).

Thiamin in College Meals The thiamin content of the meals served to students at 50 American colleges averaged 1.37 mg per person per day, with a wide range of 0.48 to 2.78 mg (19). Seventeen colleges (including two women's colleges) had meals that provided less than 1.1 mg per person per day; 13 other colleges (including one men's college) offered meals with as much as 1.1 mg but less than 1.5 mg per person per day.

Food Sources of Thiamin

Nearly all foods except fats, oils, and refined sugars contain some thiamin, but none are exceptionally high in the vitamin. Brewer's yeast

Table 11.3 Thiamin Content of Various Foods as Served

Food	Per 100 g of food, Thiamin, mg	Size of serving g		Thiamin, mg
Brewer's yeast	15.63	8	1 tbsp	1.25
Wheat germ	1.83	6	1 tbsp	.11
Bran flakes, 40 percent	1.17	18	½ c	.21
Pork roast (cooked)	.92	85	3 oz	.78
Pecans	.86	59	½ c	.51
Ham (light cure, cooked)	.47	85	3 oz	.40
Bread (white, enriched)	.39	28	1 sl	.11
Walnuts (English)	.33	60	½ c	.20
Peas, green (frozen, cooked)	.28	80	½ c	.22
Liver (beef, fried)	.26	85	3 oz	.22
Potatoes (French fried)	.14	50	10 strips	.07
Peanut butter	.13	16	1 tbsp	.02
Rice (white, enriched, cooked)	.11	205	1 c	.23
Orange juice (frozen, reconstituted)	.10	124	½ c	.12
Beans, lima (frozen, cooked)	.09	90	½ c	.08
Egg	.08	50	1 lg	.04
Milk (whole)	.04	244	1 c	.09
Butter	tr	14	1 tbsp	tr
Sugar (white)	0	12	1 tbsp	0

From *Nutritive Value of Foods*, Home and Garden Bull. No. 72, revised. Washington, D.C.: U.S. Dept. Agr., 1977.

and wheat germ head the list of thiamin-rich foods (Table 11.3). The best sources of thiamin in the American diet are pork products, legumes, and whole-grain and enriched cereals. Nuts vary in their thiamin content but may be an important source when used in large amounts. A quart of milk each day contributes 0.36 mg to the thiamin intake.

Thiamin Losses during Processing and Cooking
Under ordinary conditions of home cooking, most of the thiamin that is lost is dissolved into the cooking water; it is not inactivated by heat. The least amount of thiamin will be lost if vegetables are cooked in the smallest amount of water possible. Pork products, excellent sources of

thiamin, retain about 70 percent of the original vitamin when they are roasted or broiled.

Thiamin in the United States' Food Supply

The thiamin content of the United States' food supply has increased since 1935–1939, when it was 1.43 mg per capita per day (9), to 2.06 mg per capita per day in 1976 (4.9). The 1974 enrichment standard for thiamin has increased the vitamin content by 50 percent in white flour and between 34 and 67 percent in breads and rolls (3). (The thiamin values of flour products shown in Tables 11.3 and Appendix A-3 include these increases.)

In 1976, 41.3 percent of the dietary thiamin

223

came from cereals; 25.0 percent from meats, poultry, and fish; 22.9 percent from vegetables, fruits, and legumes; 8.6 percent from dairy products; 2.1 percent from eggs; and 0.1 percent from other foods (4).

Thiamin Consumption and Deficiency in the United States

Ten-State Nutrition Survey The thiamin intake and thiamin status of individuals of all ages were measured in this study. The average intake of the vitamin for all groups surveyed approached or exceeded 0.4 mg thiamin per 1000 kcal (4184 kJ), the standard set for thiamin intake (8). Thiamin status of the survey participants, measured by urinary thiamin levels, was satisfactory both in the high- and low-income states; there were few individuals with "deficient" or "low" urinary thiamin values. It was concluded that thiamin nutriture was no apparent public health problem among the population surveyed (6).

First Health and Nutrition Examination Survey, United States (HANES) Dietary intake, urinary excretion, and clinical deficiency signs (the absence of knee and ankle jerks) were the measurements used in HANES to assess thiamin nutriture. Only the data on clinical signs have been published at this time (1978). They show a relatively high incidence of absent knee jerks (5.1 percent) and ankle jerks (13.6 percent) among Negro males age 60 years and older (1). Until the dietary data and urinary excretion levels for thiamin are examined, these findings are not considered to be significant (2).

Riboflavin

As early as 1920, some researchers began to doubt that water-soluble B was a single nutritive factor. Studies showed that after a food containing this nutrient had been autoclaved, it could still promote growth in animals even though its anti-neuritic powers had been destroyed. About 1928, it became definitely established that there were at least two different vitamins in this complex— an antineuritic factor (vitamin B_1, now called thiamin) and a growth-promoting factor (vitamin G or B_2, now called riboflavin).

The first steps in isolating riboflavin began about 1930, and since 1935 it has been produced synthetically.

Properties of Riboflavin

Riboflavin appears as yellow-orange crystals (Fig. 11.5), which are only slightly soluble in water; solutions of this vitamin have a yellowish-green fluorescence. Alkalies and light will inactivate riboflavin, but acids, air, and heat will not.

The amount of riboflavin in foods or pharmaceuticals is determined using a chemical method that measures the fluorescence (a characteristic of riboflavin) of a solution containing riboflavin. The standard used is USP riboflavin reference standard.

Metabolism of Riboflavin

Riboflavin is absorbed from the small intestine where phosphate groups are added to the vitamin (phosphorylation) in the mucosa during absorption (11). With a small intake, the amount absorbed is directly related to the quantity in the diet (19). The body has only small reserves of riboflavin. The amount in the liver (16 μg per g) and in the kidneys (20 to 25 μg per g) is comparatively larger than elsewhere; the blood serum level is around 3.2 μg per 100 ml in normal individuals.

Environmental and physiological factors may affect riboflavin metabolism. With respect to human beings, it has been found that sleep retarded the excretion of riboflavin, whereas enforced bed rest increased it. Short periods of hard physical work decreased the excretion, but both heat stress and acute starvation increased it (17).

224

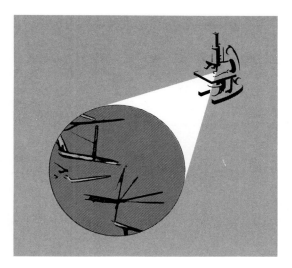

Fig. 11.5 Crystalline riboflavin and its chemical formula. (Courtesy Merck, Sharpe and Dohme Research Laboratories, Rahway, New Jersey.)

The chief pathway of excretion of riboflavin is through the urine; the amount excreted varies according to consumption. Low levels of excretion are associated with low intakes and increased intakes with increased excretion.

Clinical signs and urinary excretion levels are used to measure riboflavin nutriture in human beings (1, 14). A magenta-colored tongue, swollen and sore lips with cracks at the corners of the mouth (cheilosis), and an oily crust or scales on the skin (seborrhea) are clinical signs related to a riboflavin deficiency. One of the indicators of riboflavin insufficiency in a person is the ex-

cretion of less than 50 μg of the vitamin in a 24-hour period (8).

Functions of Riboflavin

Riboflavin forms part of the coenzymes flavin mononucleotide (FMN) and flavin adenine dinucleotide (FAD). (The vitamin is changed [phosphorylated] to FMN in the intestinal mucosa by the action of one enzyme; another enzyme then converts FMN to FAD [8].) These coenzymes (also called flavoproteins) act as hydrogen carriers in the transfer of the hydrogen ion from one

225

compound to another in the oxidation of carbohydrate, fat, and protein. FMN and FAD function as part of the enzyme system that helps to trap energy and transfer it to ATP.

Effects of a Riboflavin Deficiency

The first experimentally induced riboflavin deficiency in human beings was reported in 1938 by Sebrell and Butler (15). They found that their women subjects developed cheilosis and seborrhea, both of which disappeared when riboflavin was restored to their diet. (See Fig. 11.6 for cheilosis condition.) In a study of induced *ariboflavinosis* (9) in men (who were maintained on suboptimal intakes of the vitamin for 9 to 17 months), the same kind of skin lesions appeared, as well as scrotal dermatitis. It is believed that conjunctivitis as well as lacrimation (watering of the eye) may be attributed to ariboflavinosis.

Unlike thiamin and niacin, for example, riboflavin deficiency does not cause any serious disease in human beings, but clinical signs associated with it are found among persons of all ages in developing countries (12).

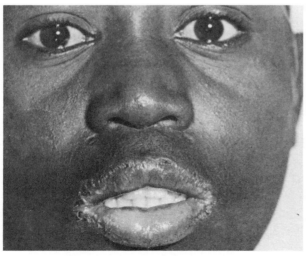

Fig. 11.6 Cheilosis in a boy suffering from a riboflavin deficiency. (F.A.O.)

Recommended Dietary Allowances for Riboflavin

College men and women, 19 to 22 years of age, have a recommended 1.8 mg and 1.4 mg riboflavin daily intake (13). The RDA per 1000 kcal (4184 kJ) is slightly higher for the female (0.7 mg) than for the male student (0.6 mg) (Table 11.2).

Riboflavin in College Meals The meals served at 50 American colleges provided adequate amounts of riboflavin for all students—2.53 mg per person per day with a range from 1.79 to 3.03 mg (18).

Food Sources of Riboflavin

Because the best food sources of riboflavin—brewer's yeast and glandular meats—are not extensively used in the ordinary American diet, they do not make a large over-all contribution (10) (Table 11.4). However, because milk is widely used, it is probably the chief source of riboflavin for most Americans. Three cups of whole milk per day contribute approximately 1.20 mg of the vitamin, which is about 70 percent and 90 percent, respectively, of the daily riboflavin requirement of college-age men and women. Cheese, eggs, veal, beef, leafy green vegetables, and salmon are also good sources, and the use of whole-grain or enriched cereal products will increase the vitamin intake.

Students sometimes wonder why, according to a food composition table, a 100-g portion of whole wheat bread has less riboflavin (0.11 mg) than an equal portion of enriched white bread (0.25 mg). The answer is that a larger quantity of synthetic riboflavin is added to white flour during enrichment to more than make up for the natural riboflavin lost in milling whole wheat grain.

Riboflavin Losses during Storage, Processing, and Cooking The two factors that may produce

Table 11.4 Riboflavin Content of Various Foods as Served

Food	Per 100 g of food, Riboflavin, mg	Per average serving		
		Size of serving		Riboflavin, mg
		g		
Brewer's yeast	4.25	8	1 tbsp	.34
Liver (beef, fried)	4.19	85	3 oz	3.56
Heart (beef, braised)	1.22	85	3 oz	1.04
Cheese (Cheddar)	.39	28	1 oz	.11
Egg	.30	50	1 lg	.15
Bread (white, enriched)	.25	28	1 sl	.07
Veal cutlet (broiled)	.24	85	3 oz	.21
Ground beef (broiled)	.21	82	2.9 oz patty	.17
Salmon (pink, canned)	.19	85	3 oz	.16
Asparagus (raw, cooked)	.18	73	½ c	.13
Milk (whole)	.16	244	1 c	.40
Spinach (raw, cooked)	.14	90	½ c	.13
Broccoli (frozen, chopped, cooked)	.12	93	½ c	.11
Bread (whole wheat)	.11	28	1 sl	.03
Orange juice (frozen, reconstituted)	.02	124	½ c	.02
Butter	tr	14	1 tbsp	tr
Sugar (white)	0	12	1 tbsp	0

From *Nutritive Value of Foods*, Home and Garden Bull. No. 72, revised. Washington, D.C.: U.S. Dept. Agr., 1977.

a loss of riboflavin are that it dissolves in water and that it is inactivated by light. In home cooking or commercial canning the extraction of the vitamin by the water is usually less than 20 percent (10).

The inactivation of riboflavin in milk by light was a serious problem when milk was generally distributed in glass bottles. Now most milk is packaged and sold in paper or opaque containers (16).

Riboflavin in the United States' Food Supply

The increased amount of riboflavin in the United States' food supply is attributed to several factors —the enrichment of cereal grains and the increased use of meats, fish, poultry, and dairy products. The 1976 value (2.47 mg per capita per day) is about 0.66 mg more than was available in 1935–1939 (4, 7).

The 1974 enrichment standard for riboflavin has increased the vitamin content by 50 percent in white flour and between 0 and 34 percent in breads and rolls (3). (The riboflavin values given in Tables 11.4 and A-3 include these increases.)

In 1976, dairy products accounted for 38.6 percent of all riboflavin in the American food supply; meat, poultry, and fish, 24.4 percent; cereals, 20.8 percent; vegetables, fruits, dry beans and peas, 10.8 percent; eggs, 4.7 percent; and all other foods, 0.7 percent (4).

227

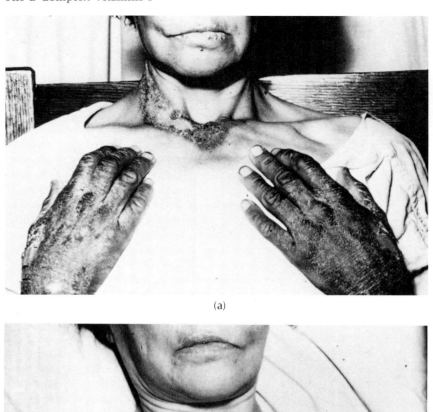

(a)

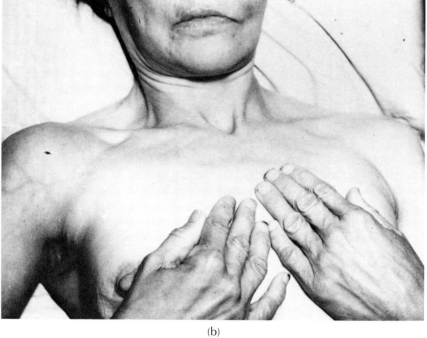

(b)

Fig. 11-7 Advanced pellagra (a) showing dermatitis outling the exposed area of the neck as well as the lesions of the back of the hands. The same patient (b) after nicotinamide therapy. (Courtesy The Upjohn Company, Kalamazoo, Michigan.)

228

Riboflavin Consumption and Deficiency in the United States

Ten-State Nutrition Survey The mean riboflavin intake for infants and young children, adolescents, pregnant and lactating women, and persons 60 years and older were much higher than the standard used for evaluating the intake of the vitamin (0.55 mg riboflavin per 1000 kcal [4184 kJ]) (6). However, riboflavin status, measured by urinary levels, was less satisfactory than it was for the vitamin thiamin. A high prevalence of "deficient" and "low" values was found among individuals 17 years of age and under. The percentage of "deficient" and "low" riboflavin urine values was higher for the black population. In general, riboflavin status was poor among blacks and young people of all ethnic groups (5).

First Health and Nutrition Examination Survey, United States (HANES) Only the clinical signs attributed to a human riboflavin deficiency have been reported (1); values for the dietary intake and urinary excretion levels of the vitamin will be presented in the final report of HANES (2). Clinical signs related to a riboflavin deficiency were found more often among blacks than whites in the below-poverty group. For example, the high values were 5.3 percent, cheilosis (Negro males, 18–44 years); 6.8 percent, nasolabile seborrhea (white males, 12–17 years); and 2.7 percent, angular scars of the lips (Negroes, 6–11 years).

Niacin

Pellagra, a disease produced by a deficiency of niacin, has existed for centuries. It was once of *endemic* proportions in the United States South, but Africa is the only continent in which pellagra is now a public health problem (18). Pellagra affects the skin, the gastrointestinal tract, and the nervous system. Because of its specific lesions, pellagra has often been referred to as the disease of the "three d's" (*dermatitis*, diarrhea, and *dementia*). Its characteristic dermatitis, which is aggravated by sunlight and heat, is bilaterally symmetrical and appears on the hands, feet, face, forearms, and elsewhere (Fig. 11.7). The skin becomes red and the lesions itch and burn. When the mucous membranes of the gastrointestinal tract are affected, the early symptoms include *glossitis*, anorexia, and abdominal pains. As the disorder becomes more severe, there is also diarrhea. Insomnia, irritability, fear, depression, and forgetfulness are the first obvious neurological changes, but later on there may be dementia and paralysis. If the disease is not treated, it may prove fatal.

Goldberger and his coworkers (8) were the first to induce and cure pellagra in healthy men by dietary means. In 1937, a compound called nicotinamide was isolated from a liver concentrate, and the first successful treatment of human pellagra with either nicotinic acid or nicotinamide was reported.

In order to avoid confusion with the word "nicotine," the name of the vitamin, "nicotinic acid," was changed to "niacin" soon after its discovery. Cowgill at Yale coined the word "niacin" from the letters of the three words: *ni*cotinic, *ac*id, and vitam*in*.

Properties of Compounds with Niacin Activity

The two compounds that exhibit niacin activity are nicotinic acid (niacin) and nicotinamide (niacinamide) (Fig. 11.8). The two forms are equal in niacin acitivity. Nicotinic acid appears as colorless needlelike crystals that have a very bitter taste, whereas nicotinamide is a crystalline powder. Both are soluble in water and are not destroyed by acids, bases, light, air, or heat.

229

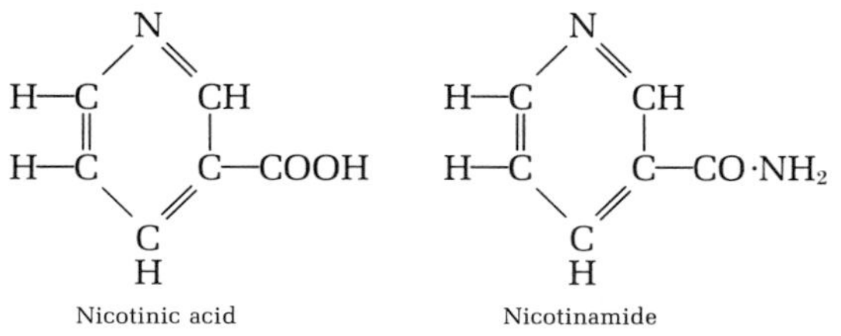

Fig. 11.8 The chemical formulas of nicotinic acid and nicotinamide.

Metabolism of Niacin

Niacin is absorbed from the intestinal tract, but little is stored in the body. The excess is excreted in the urine in the form of *metabolites* of niacin, principally N-methylnicotinamide and N-methyl pyridone (in about equal quantities). With a low niacin intake, there is a low level of metabolite excretion.

Niacin is found in the tissues largely as part of the coenzymes NAD and NADP. A deficiency of niacin decreases the level of the coenzymes in the liver and muscles but not in the blood.

The clinical signs used to assess a human niacin deficiency involve the appearance of the tongue—a scarlet-colored, beefylike tongue, fissures (slits) on the tongue, swelling of the tongue, and changes in the papillae (small nipple-shaped elevations) of the tongue (1).

The measurement of the niacin metabolite, N^1-methylnicotinamide, in the urine is the only practical biochemical method for nutrition surveys, but data from this assay has proven to be less than satisfactory (20).

Functions of Niacin

The principal role of niacin is as a constituent of two important coenzymes in the body: nicotinamide-adenine dinucleotide (NAD) and nicotinamide-adenine dinucleotide phosphate (NADP).

These coenzymes work with a group of enzymes known as the dehydrogenases, which help remove hydrogen from certain compounds and transfer it to other compounds in a series of complex reactions. Some of these more than 50 enzymes are required for reactions of the tricarboxylic acid cycle and others for fat synthesis and tissue respiration.

There has been interest in niacin in coronary heart disease research; CHOL levels have been reduced by 15 to 20 percent with niacin therapy (17).

The Tryptophan-Niacin Relationship It was demonstrated in 1945 that one of the essential amino acids, tryptophan, can be converted into niacin in the bodies of both animals and humans (16). The conversion ratio of tryptophan to niacin in adult men (14, 15) and adult women (12) was found to be about 60 to 1, that is, 60 mg of dietary tryptophan is equivalent to 1 mg of niacin. Studies with both pregnant and nonpregnant women (23) indicate that the conversion of tryptophan to niacin is more efficient in pregnant women.

Effects of a Niacin Deficiency

The first report of experimentally induced pellagra in human beings by dietary means was made by Goldberger and Wheeler in 1915 (8). They used a diet made up of the same foods eaten by *pellagrins*. After niacin was identified as the antipellagra factor in 1937, numerous researchers tried unsuccessfully to produce experimental pellagra by depriving their subjects of niacin. Finally, in 1952 (after the tryptophan-niacin relationship was understood), Goldsmith and her associates (9) at Tulane University succeeded in producing pellagra by using a corn diet that was low in both niacin and tryptophan. The subjects of Goldsmith's study developed pellagra after 50 days on this diet; then they were cured with tryptophan, which further demonstrated the importance of this amino acid in niacin metabolism. Before this study, it had been assumed that the intake of B-complex vitamins (other than niacin) would improve the multiple lesions of pellagra. However, although the diet in this study included those vitamins, the typical lesions of pellagra still appeared. Thus it is clear that pellagra is caused by a deficiency of one specific factor—niacin—and nothing else.

It is interesting to note that pellagra is rarely reported in Central America where corn is a staple food; the reason is that the niacin present in the corn in the bound form (niacytin) is released when the food is treated with lime (a common step in the preparation of corn for consumption in this region) (10, 18).

Recommended Dietary Allowances for Niacin

The RDA for niacin (as in the case of thiamin) is based on recommended energy intakes (19). The daily niacin recommendation for men and women 19 to 22 years of age is 20 mg and 14 mg, respectively, or 6.7 mg of niacin per 1000 kcal (4184 kJ) (Table 11.2).

The term "niacin equivalent" is no longer used in the RDA, but it is recognized that, on the average, 1 mg of niacin is derived from each 60 mg of dietary tryptophan (19).

Niacin in College Meals   Niacin (preformed) in meals served at 50 American colleges averaged 19.66 mg per person per day with a range of 12.39 to 27.74 mg (22). When the calculated tryptophan content of the meals was added to the analyzed preformed niacin content, the RDA for niacin was met at all the colleges.

Food Sources of Niacin

Although niacin occurs in both plant and animal products, the best sources are liver, kidney, brewer's yeast, and tunafish; muscle meats, poultry, peanuts, and peanut butter are also excellent sources. Milk, although low in actual niacin content, is a good antipellagra food because of its high tryptophan content. Fruits and vegetables vary in their niacin content. Cereals as a group tend to be low in niacin, but whole-grain and enriched products contain more than refined cereals (Table 11.5).

It has been reported that ground coffee contains about 10 mg of niacin per 100 g (11, 21) and instant powdered coffee about 30.6 mg per 100 g. Apparently, the niacin level depends upon the degree of roasting: a light roast provides about 1 mg of niacin per cup, and a dark roast provides 2.4 to 3.4 mg niacin per cup (11). In certain areas of the world where the diet of the people is low in niacin and tryptophan, their high consumption of coffee may explain their low incidence of pellagra.

Niacin Losses during Cooking and Processing
Niacin is the most stable of the B-complex vitamins because it is not affected by exposure to light, air, or high temperatures. However, because niacin is water soluble foods may lose some of this nutrient when boiled; using a small amount of cooking water will minimize this loss.

Total Niacin Values of Various Foods

It is more realistic to express food values in total niacin values; food tables give niacin values in terms of preformed vitamin (Table 11.5). To illustrate the contribution of tryptophan, the total niacin value of some foods has been calculated (Table 11.6). The niacin value of 1 cup of milk is listed as 0.2 mg. This portion of milk contains about 120 mg tryptophan. Using the conversion factor, 60 mg of tryptophan equals 1 mg of niacin, 1 cup of milk contributes 2.0 mg of niacin from its tryptophan. One cup of milk contains 2.2 mg of total niacin, not 0.2 mg.

Table 11.5 Niacin Content of Various Foods as Served

Food	Per 100 g of food, Niacin, mg	Per average serving		
		Size of serving		Niacin, mg
		g		
Brewer's yeast	37.5	8	1 tbsp	3.0
Coffee (instant, freeze-dried)	33.3	.9	1 tsp	0.3
Liver (beef, fried)	16.5	85	3 oz	14.0
Peanut butter	15.0	16	1 tbsp	2.4
Tuna (canned, drained solids)	11.9	85	3 oz	10.1
Bran flakes, 40 percent	11.7	18	½ c	2.1
Heart (beef, braised)	7.7	85	3 oz	6.5
Chicken leg (fried)	7.1	38	1.3 oz	2.7
Ground beef (broiled)	5.4	82	2.9 oz patty	4.4
Almonds (chopped)	3.5	65	½ c	2.3
Bread (white, enriched)	3.2	28	1 sl	.9
Bread (whole wheat)	2.9	28	1 sl	.8
Peas, green (frozen, cooked)	1.8	80	½ c	1.4
Potatoes (baked)	1.7	156	1 med	2.7
Cornmeal (degermed, enriched, cooked)	.5	120	½ c	.6
Orange juice (frozen, reconstituted)	.4	124	½ c	.5
Milk (whole)	.1	244	1 c	.2
Butter	tr	14	1 tbsp	tr
Egg	tr	50	1 lg	tr
Sugar (white)	0	12	1 tbsp	0

From *Nutritive Value of Foods*, Home and Garden Bull. No. 72, revised. Washington, D.C.: U.S. Dept. Agr., 1977.

Niacin in the United States' Food Supply

In 1976, the niacin available per person per day was 25.3 mg (4) as compared with 17.1 in 1935–1939 (7), just before the enrichment of cereals began. The 1974 enrichment standard has increased the niacin content of white flour products (50 percent for flours and 25 to 50 percent for breads and rolls) (3). The niacin values in Tables 11.4, 11.5, and A-3 include these increases.

In the 1976 food supply 45.2 percent of the niacin came from meat, poultry, and fish; 27.4 percent from cereals; 9.8 percent from vegetables, fruits, and legumes; 1.4 percent from dairy products; 0.2 percent from eggs; and 16.0 percent from all other foods, including coffee and chocolate (4).

Niacin Consumption and Deficiency in the United States

Ten-State Nutrition Survey Because the niacin available from protein (tryptophan) elevates the total niacin value of the diet, no special data were presented on dietary niacin in this survey (6) and no biochemical measurements were made (5).

Table 11.6 Approximate Total Niacin Value of Various Foods

Food	Measure[a] Serving	g (A)	Tryptophan content mg/100g (B)	Niacin from tryptophan[d] mg/serving (C)	Niacin content[a] mg/serving (D)	Total niacin mg/serving (C + D)
Beans, green	1 c	135	33[c]	.7	.5	1.2
Bread (white, enriched)	1 sl	24	91[b]	.4	.8	1.2
Brewer's yeast	1 tbsp	8	429[c]	.6	3.0	3.6
Carrots	1	72	8[c]	.1	.4	0.5
Cheese (Cheddar)	1 oz	28	341[b]	1.6	trace	1.6
Chicken	1/2 broiler	176	205[c]	6.0	15.5	21.5
Corn (canned)	1 c	210	12[b]	.4	2.3	2.7
Egg	1 lg	50	184[c]	1.5	trace	1.5
Ground beef	2.9 oz	82	198[c]	2.7	4.4	7.1
Lettuce	1/4 head	135	10[c]	.2	.4	.6
Milk (whole)	1 c	244	50[c]	2.0	.2	2.2
Orange juice	1 c	249	6[c]	.3	.9	1.2
Peanut butter	1 tbsp	16	305[c]	.8	2.4	3.2
Peas, green	1 c	160	66[c]	1.8	2.7	4.5
Potato (white)	1 med	156	33[c]	.9	2.7	3.6
Salmon (pink, canned)	3 oz	85	200[b]	2.8	6.8	9.6
Tomato	1 med	135	9[c]	.2	.9	1.1

[a] From *Nutritive Value of Foods*, Home and Garden Bull. No. 72, revised. Washington, D.C.: U.S. Dept. Agr., 1977.

[b] From *Amino Content of Foods*, Home Econ. Res. Rept. No. 4. Washington, D.C.: U.S. Dept. Agr., 1957.

[c] From *Amino Acid Content of Foods and Biological Data on Proteins*, FAO Nutritional Studies No. 24. Rome: Food and Agr. Organ., 1970.

[d] Calculation: $(A \times B)/ 100 \div 60$.

First Health and Nutrition Examination Survey (HANES) The measurement of clinical signs of niacin deficiency showed a marked prevalence of "high" and "moderate" risk signs among the groups surveyed in HANES. Negroes had a higher incidence of these signs than did whites (for example, fissures of the tongue, 7.6 percent in Negro men and 2.2 percent in white men). Most of the signs were found in older age groups; this might indicate a chronic niacin deficiency (1).

Dietary intake of niacin will be presented in the final HANES report; biochemical measurements of niacin were not made (2).

Summary

Thiamin, unstable to heat and alkali, functions as the coenzyme thiamin diphosphate in several enzyme systems involved in the metabolism of carbohydrates. The vitamin also appears to be involved in the function of peripheral nerves. A severe deficiency of thiamin results in beriberi, a disease characterized by polyneuritis, either edema or emaciation, and disturbances of the heart. Mild deficiencies of thiamin (loss of appetite, malaise, and general weakness of the legs) are common in countries prone to beriberi (southeastern Asia). The RDA for 19-to-22-year-old men and women is 1.5 mg and 1.1 mg thiamin, respectively. Pork products, legumes, and whole-grain and enriched cereals are the best sources of the vitamin in the American diet. The thiamin content of the United States' food supply in 1976 was 2.06 mg per capita per day.

Riboflavin, unstable to light and alkali, functions as part of the coenzymes flavin mono-nucleotide (FMN) and flavin adenine dinucleotide (FAD) that are involved in the oxidation of carbohydrates, fats, and proteins. A deficiency of this vitamin does not cause a serious disease; sore lips, inflammation of the tongue, cracks at the corner of the mouth, facial dermatitis, and scrotal dermatitis are lesions found in ariboflavinosis. College men and women, 19 to 22 years of age, are recommended 1.8 mg and 1.4 mg riboflavin per day, respectively. Milk, cheese, eggs, veal, beef, leafy green vegetables, and whole-grain and enriched cereal products are good riboflavin sources. The 1976 riboflavin content of the United States' food supply was 2.47 mg per capita per day.

Niacin, the most stable of the B-complex vitamins, serves as a part of the coenzymes nicotinamide adenine dinucleotide (NAD) and nicotinamide adenine dinucleotide phosphate (NADP), which are required for reactions of the tricarboxylic acid cycle and for fat synthesis and tissue respiration. The essential amino acid tryptophan is converted to niacin in the body; the conversion factor is 60 to 1 (60 mg tryptophan is equivalent to 1 mg niacin). Pellagra, once endemic in the United States South, is characterized by dermatitis, diarrhea, and dementia. The RDA for college men and women, 19 to 22 years, is 20 mg and 14 mg, respectively. Liver, kidney, brewer's yeast, tunafish, muscle meats, poultry, peanuts, and peanut butter are excellent sources of niacin. The niacin available per capita per day in the United States' food supply in 1976 was 25.3 mg.

Is it possible to ingest too much thiamin, riboflavin, or niacin? Only large doses of niacin, sometimes given to individuals with a mental ill-ness, are known to be toxic (13). Large doses of niacin may produce flushing, itching, liver damage, elevated blood glucose, elevated blood enzymes, and/or peptic ulcer.

Glossary

anorexia: loss or lack of appetite for food.

ariboflavinosis: a deficiency of riboflavin.

beriberi: a deficiency disease caused by an insufficient intake of thiamin and characterized by polyneuritis, edema (in some cases), emaciation, and cardiac disturbances (enlargement of the heart and an unusually rapid heart beat).

coenzyme: an organic molecule that is required for the activation of an apoenzyme to an enzyme; the vitamin coenzymes are thiamin, riboflavin, niacin, pyridoxine, folacin, and pantothenic acid.

dementia: a psychosis (mental disorder) characterized by serious mental impairment and deterioration.

dermatitis: an inflammation of the skin.

edema: an abnormal accumulation of fluid in the intercellular spaces of the body.

electrocardiogram (ECG and EKG): a tracing representing the heart's electrical action that is made by amplifying the minutely small electrical impulses normally generated by the heart.

emaciation: excessive leanness; a wasted condition of the body.

endemic: see page 60.

glossitis: an inflammation of the tongue.

malaise: a feeling of illness or depression.

metabolite: see page 197

neuritis: inflammation of the peripheral nerves (which link the brain and spinal cord with the muscles, skin, organs, and other parts of the body).

nicotinamide-adenine dinucleotide (NAD): one of the coenzyme forms of niacin that participates in oxidation-reduction reactions in the cells.

nicotinamide-adenine dinucleotide phosphate (NADP): another coenzyme form of niacin that is involved in the oxidation-reduction reactions in the cells.

pellagrins: individuals suffering from pellagra.

polyneuritis: an inflammation encompassing many peripheral nerves.

transketolase: an enzyme that uses thiamin diphosphate as a coenzyme; it is involved in the synthesis of the five-carbon sugar ribose and NADP from carbohydrates.

Study Questions and Activities

1. Identify the following: glossitis, dermatitis, coenzyme, beriberi, nicotinic acid, cheilosis, niacytin, and total niacin value of a food.
2. Describe the physical and chemical properties of thiamin, riboflavin, and niacin.
3. Describe the symptoms of a mild form of beriberi.
4. How may thiamin, riboflavin, and niacin be lost or inactivated in preparing a food?
5. What is the relationship between the amino acid tryptophan and the vitamin niacin?
6. What are good food sources of thiamin, riboflavin, and niacin?

References

Thiamin

1. Abraham, S., F. W. Lowenstein, and D. E. O'Connell (1975). *Anthropometric and Clinical Findings:* Preliminary Findings of the First Health and Nutrition Examination Survey, United States, 1971–1972, DHEW Publ. No. (HRA) 75-1229. Rockville, Md.: U.S. Dept. Health, Educ., and Welfare.
2. Abraham, S., F. W. Lowenstein, and C. L. Johnson (1974). *Dietary Intake and Biochemical Findings:* Preliminary Findings of the First Health and Nutrition Examination Survey, United States, 1971–1972, DHEW Publ. No. (HRA) 74-1219-1. Rockville, Md.: U.S. Dept. Health, Educ., and Welfare.
3. Adams, C. F. (1975). *Nutritive Value of American Foods in Common Units.* Agr. Handbook No. 456. Washington, D.C.: U.S. Dept. Agr., pp. 273–279.
4. Agricultural Statistics (1977). Washington, D.C.: U.S. Dept. Agr., pp. 561–564.
5. Barchi, R. L. (1976). Thiamine triphosphatases in the brain. In *Thiamine,* edited by C. J. Gubler, M. Fujiwara, and P. M. Dreyfus. New York: John Wiley and Sons, Inc., p. 195.
6. *Biochemical,* Ten-State Nutrition Survey, 1968–1970 (1972). DHEW Publ. No. (HSM) 72-8132. Atlanta, Ga.: Center for Disease Control, U.S. Dept. Health, Educ., and Welfare.
7. Bradford, R. B. (1974). Biochemical detection of thiamin deficiency in infants and children in Thailand. *Am. J. Clin. Nutrition,* **27:** 1399.
8. *Dietary,* Ten-State Nutrition Survey, 1968–1970 (1972). DHEW Publ. No. (HSM) 72-8133. Atlanta, Ga.: Center for Disease Control, U.S. Dept. Health, Educ., and Welfare.
9. Friend, B. (1967). Nutrients in the United States food supply: A review of trends, 1909–1913 to 1965. *Am. J. Clin. Nutrition,* **20:** 907.
10. Henderson, F. W. (1960). Beriberi heart disease in the elderly patient. *Geriatrics,* **15:** 398.
11. Horwitt, M. K., E. Liebert, O. Kresler, and P. Wittman (1948). *Investigations of Human Requirements for B-Complex Vitamins.* Natl. Acad. Sci.-Natl. Research Council Bull. No. 116, Washington, D.C.: Natl. Research Council.
12. Jolliffe, N., R. Goodhart, J. Gennis, and J. K. Cline (1939). The experimental production of vitamin B_1 deficiency in normal subjects. The dependence of urinary excretion of thiamine on the dietary intake of B_1. *Am. J. Med. Sci.,* **198:** 198.
13. Keys, A., A. Henschel, H. L. Taylor, O. Mickelsen, and J. Brozek (1945). Experimental studies on man with restricted intake of B vitamins. *Am. J. Physiol.,* **144:** 5.
14. Passmore, R., B. M. Nicol, M. N. Rao, G. H. Beaton, and E. M. Demayer (1974). *Handbook on Human Nutritional Requirements.* Geneva: World Health Organ., p. 36.
15. *Recommended Dietary Allowances, Eighth Edition* (1974). Natl. Acad. Sci.-Natl. Research Council. Washington, D.C.: Natl. Research Council.
16. Reed, L. J. (1976). Regulation of mammalian pyruvate dehydrogenase complex by phosphorylation. In *Thiamine,* edited by C. J. Gubler, M. Fujiwara, and P. M. Dreyfus. New York: John Wiley and Sons, Inc., p. 19.

17. Sauberlich, H. E., J. H. Skala, and R. P. Dowdy (1974). *Laboratory Tests for the Assessment of Nutritional Status.* Cleveland, Ohio: CRC Press, p. 22.
18. von Muralt, A. (1962). The role of thiamine in neurophysiology. *Ann. New York Acad. Sci.,* **98:** 499.
19. Walker, M. A. and L. Page (1975). Nutritive content of college meals. Proximate composition and vitamins. *J. Am. Dietet. Assoc.,* **66:** 146.
20. Williams, R. R., H. L. Mason, B. F. Smith, and R. M. Wilder (1942). Induced thiamine (vitamin B₁) deficiency and the thiamine requirement of man. *Arch. Int. Med.,* **69:** 721.

Riboflavin

1. Abraham, S., F. W. Lowenstein, and D. E. O'Connell (1975). *Anthropometric and Clinical Findings:* Preliminary Findings of the First Health and Nutrition Examination Survey, United States, 1971–1972, DHEW Publ. No. (HRA) 75-1229. Rockville, Md.: U.S. Dept. Health, Educ., and Welfare.
2. Abraham, S., F. W. Lowenstein, and C. L. Johnson (1974). *Dietary Intake and Biochemical Findings:* Preliminary Findings of the First Health and Nutrition Examination Survey, United States, 1971–1972, DHEW Publ. No. (HRA) 74-1219-1. Rockville, Md.: U.S. Dept. Health, Educ., and Welfare.
3. Adams, C. F. (1975). *Nutritive Value of American Foods in Common Units.* Agr. Handbook No. 456. Washington, D.C.: U.S. Dept. Agr., pp. 273–279.
4. Agricultural Statistics (1977). Washington, D.C.: U.S. Dept. Agr., pp. 561–564.
5. *Biochemical,* Ten-State Nutrition Survey, 1968–1970 (1972). DHEW Publ. No. (HSM) 72-8132. Atlanta, Ga.: Center for Disease Control, U.S. Dept. Health, Educ., and Welfare.
6. *Dietary,* Ten-State Nutrition Survey, 1968–1970 (1972). DHEW Publ. No. (HSM) 72-8133. Atlanta, Ga.: Center for Disease Control, U.S. Dept. Health, Educ., and Welfare.
7. Friend, B. (1967). Nutrients in the United States food supply: A review of trends, 1909–1913 to 1965. *Am. J. Clin. Nutrition,* **20:** 907.

8. Goldsmith, G. A. (1975). Riboflavin deficiency. In *Riboflavin,* edited by R. S. Rivlin. New York: Plenum Press, p. 221.
9. Hills, O. W., E. Liebert, D. L. Steinberg, and M. K. Horwitt (1951). Clinical aspects of dietary depletion of riboflavin. *Arch. Int. Med.,* **87:** 682.
10. Horwitt, M. K. (1972). Riboflavin. V. Occurrence in food. In *The Vitamins,* edited by W. H. Sebrell, Jr. and R. S. Harris, 2nd ed., vol. 2. New York: Academic Press, p. 46.
11. Jusko, W. J. and G. Levy (1975). Absorption, protein binding, and elimination of riboflavin. In *Riboflavin,* edited by R. S. Rivlin. New York: Plenum Press, p. 99.
12. Passmore, R., B. M. Nicol, M. N. Rao, G. H. Beaton, and E. M. Demayer (1974). *Handbook on Human Nutritional Requirements.* Geneva: World Health Organ., p. 43.
13. *Recommended Dietary Allowances, Eighth Edition* (1974). Natl. Acad. Sci.-Natl. Research Council. Washington, D.C.: Natl. Research Council.
14. Sauberlich, H. E., J. H. Skala, and R. P. Dowdy (1974). *Laboratory Tests for the Assessment of Nutritional Status.* Cleveland, Ohio: CRC Press, p. 30.
15. Sebrell, W. H., Jr. and R. E. Butler (1938). Riboflavin deficiency in man: A preliminary note. *Public Health Rept.* (U.S.), **53:** 2282.
16. Singh, R. P., D. R. Heldman, and J. R. Kirk (1975). Kinetic analysis of light-induced riboflavin loss in whole milk. *J. Food Sci.,* **40:** 164.
17. Tucker, R. G., O. Mickelsen, and A. Keys (1960). The influence of sleep, work, diuresis, heat, acute starvation, thiamine intake, and bed rest on human riboflavin excretion. *J. Nutrition,* **72:** 251.
18. Walker, M. A. and L. Page (1975). Nutritive content of college meals. Approximate composition and vitamins. *J. Am. Dietet. Assoc.,* **66:** 146.
19. West, D. W. and E. C. Owen (1969). Metabolites of riboflavine in man. *Brit. J. Nutrition,* **23:** 889.

Niacin

1. Abraham, S., F. W. Lowenstein, and D. E. O'Connell (1975). *Anthropometric and Clinical Findings:* Preliminary Findings of the First Health

and Nutrition Examination Survey, United States, 1971–1972, DHEW Publ. No. (HRA) 75-1229. Rockville, Md.: U.S. Dept. Health, Educ., and Welfare.

2. Abraham, S., F. W. Lowenstein, and C. L. Johnson (1974). *Dietary Intake and Biochemical Findings: Preliminary Findings of the First Health and Nutrition Examination Survey, United States, 1971–1972, DHEW Publ. No. (HRA) 74-1219-1.* Rockville, Md.: U.S. Dept. Health, Educ., and Welfare.

3. Adams, C. F. (1975). *Nutritive Value of American Foods in Common Units.* Agr. Handbook No. 456. Washington, D.C.: U.S. Dept. Agr., pp. 273–279.

4. Agricultural Statistics (1977). Washington, D.C.: U.S. Dept. Agr., pp. 561–564.

5. *Biochemical,* Ten-State Nutrition Survey, 1968–1970 (1972). DHEW Publ. No. (HSM) 72-8132. Atlanta, Ga.: Center for Disease Control, U.S. Dept. Health, Educ., and Welfare.

6. *Dietary,* Ten-State Nutrition Survey, 1968–1970 (1972). DHEW Publ. No. (HSM) 72-8133. Atlanta, Ga.: Center for Disease Control, U.S. Dept. Health, Educ., and Welfare.

7. Friend, B. (1967). Nutrients in the United States food supply: A review of trends, 1909–1913 to 1965. *Am. J. Clin. Nutrition,* **20:** 907.

8. Goldberger, J. and G. A. Wheeler (1915). Experimental pellagra in the human subject brought about by a restricted diet. *Public Health Rept.* (U.S.), **30:** 3336.

9. Goldsmith, G. A., H. P. Sarett, U. D. Register, and J. Gibbens (1952). Studies of niacin requirement in man. I. Experimental pellagra in subjects on corn diets low in niacin and tryptophan. *J. Clin. Invest.,* **31:** 533.

10. Goldsmith, G. A., J. Gibbens, W. G. Unglaub, and O. N. Miller (1956). Studies of niacin requirement in man. III. Comparative effects of diets containing lime-treated and untreated corn in the production of experimental pellagra. *Am. J. Clin. Nutrition,* **4:** 151.

11. Goldsmith, G. A., O. N. Miller, W. G. Unglaub, and K. Kercheval (1959). Human studies of biologic availability of niacin in coffee. *Proc. Soc. Exp. Biol. Med.,* **102:** 579.

12. Goldsmith, G. A., O. N. Miller, and W. G. Unglaub (1961). Efficiency of tryptophan as a niacin precursor in man. *J. Nutrition,* **73:** 172.

13. Hathcock, J. N. (1976). Nutrition: toxicology and pharmacology. *Nutrition Rev.,* **34:** 65.

14. Horwitt, M. K. (1955). Niacin-tryptophan relationships in the development of pellagra. *Am. J. Clin. Nutrition,* **3:** 244.

15. Horwitt, M. K., C. C. Harvey, W. S. Rothwell, J. L. Cutler, and D. Haffron (1956). Tryptophan-niacin relationships in man. Studies with diets deficient in riboflavin and niacin together with observations on the excretion of nitrogen and niacin metabolites. *J. Nutrition,* **60:** Suppl. 1, 32.

16. Krehl, W. A., L. J. Teply, P. S. Sarma, and C. A. Elvehjem (1945). Growth-retarding effect of corn in nicotinic acid-low rations and its counteraction by tryptophane. *Science,* **101:** 489.

17. Kritchetsky, D. (1971). Final words. In *Metabolic Effects of Nicotinic Acids and Its Derivatives,* edited by K. F. Gey and L. A. Carlson. Bern, Switzerland: Hans Huber Publishers, p. 1149.

18. Passmore, R., B. M. Nicol, M. N. Rao, G. H. Beaton, and E. M. Demayer (1974). *Handbook on Human Nutritional Requirements.* Geneva: World Health Organ., p. 40.

19. *Recommended Dietary Allowances, Eighth Edition* (1974). Natl. Acad. Sci.-Natl. Research Council. Washington, D.C.: Natl. Research Council.

20. Sauberlich, H. E., J. H. Skala, and R. P. Dowdy (1974). *Laboratory Tests for the Assessment of Nutritional Status.* Cleveland, Ohio: CRC Press, p. 13.

21. Teply, L. J. and R. F. Prier (1957). Nutritional evaluation of coffee, including niacin bioassay. *J. Agr. Food Chem.,* **5:** 375.

22. Walker, M. A. and L. Page (1975). Nutritive content of college meals. Proximate composition and vitamins. *J. Am. Dietet. Assoc.,* **88:** 146.

23. Wertz, A. W., M. E. Lojkin, B. S. Bouchard, and M. B. Derby (1958). Tryptophan-niacin relationship in pregnancy. *J. Nutrition,* **64:** 339.

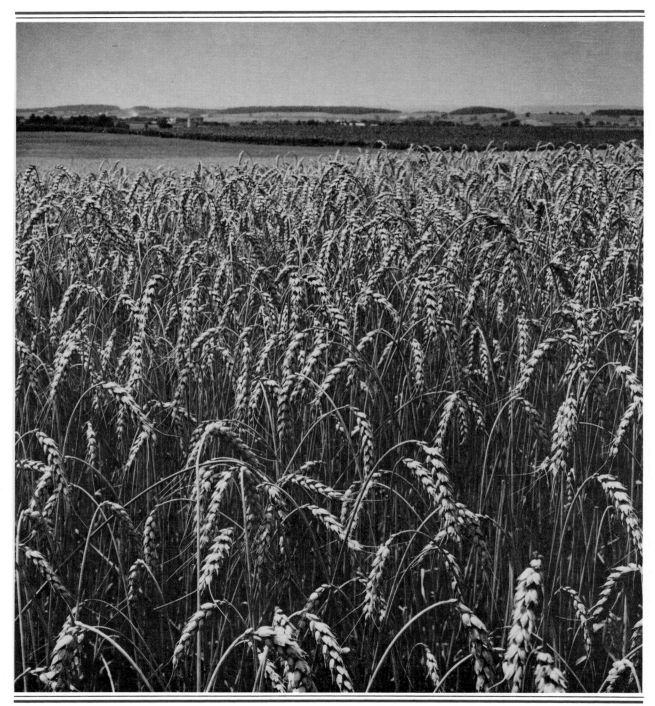

Wheat, with its generous supply of the B vitamins, has been a staple food since early times.

Chapter 12

The B-Complex Vitamins II

Abbreviations

acetyl CoA: acetyl coenzyme A
ACP: acyl carrier protein
ATP: adenosine triphosphate
CHOL: cholesterol
CO_2: carbon dioxide
CoA: coenzyme A
HANES: Health and Nutrition Examination
   Survey, United States

IF: intrinsic factor
PA: pernicious anemia
PGA: pteroylmonoglutamic acid
RBC: red blood cells
RDA: Recommended Dietary Allowance
TAC: tricarboxylic acid cycle
WBC: white blood cell

Vitamin B-6

Vitamin B-6 comprises three closely related chemical compounds with potential vitamin B-6 activity: pyridoxine, pyridoxal, and pyridoxamine (12). The pyridoxal and pyridoxamine forms occur primarily in animal products, whereas pyridoxine is found largely in vegetable products. The chemical formulas of pyridoxine, pyridoxal phosphate, and pyridoxamine phosphate are presented in Fig. 12.1, and the crystalline structure of pyridoxine is depicted in Fig. 12.2.

Metabolism of Vitamin B-6

Vitamin B-6 is readily absorbed by the intestinal mucosa and enters the body by the portal vein. The vitamin is present in most animal tissues, with a high concentration in the liver. Vitamin B-6 is excreted by way of the kidney. Measurement of the vitamin in the urine is the assay method used for nutrition surveys (39).

Functions of Vitamin B-6

Vitamin B-6 functions in the form of its coenzymes, usually as pyridoxal phosphate and some-

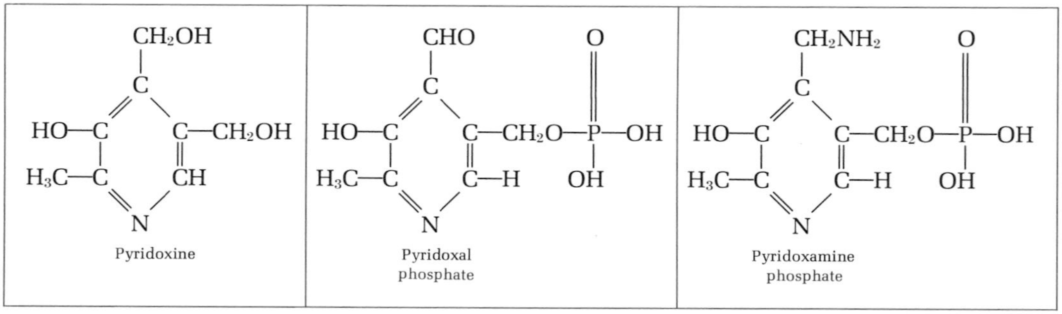

Fig. 12.1 Chemical formulas of pyridoxine, pyridoxal phosphate, and pyridoxamine phosphate.

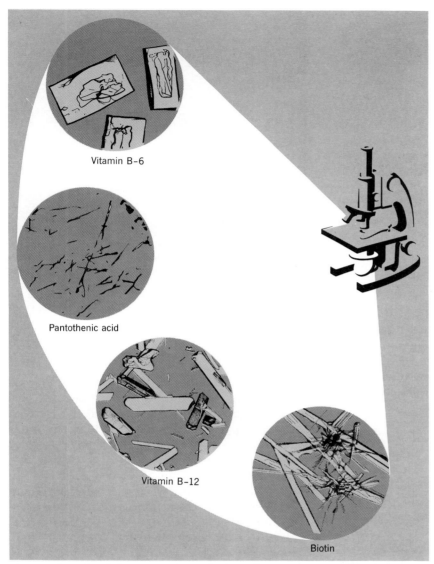

Fig. 12.2 Crystals of vitamin B-6, pantothenic acid, vitamin B-12, and biotin. (Courtesy Merck, Sharpe and Dohme Research Laboratories, Rahway, New Jersey.)

times as pyridoxamine phosphate (17) (Fig. 12.1). Riboflavin is needed for the conversion of pyridoxal to pyridoxal phospahte (44). More than 50 pyridoxal phosphate-dependent enzymes have been identified.

Vitamin B-6-containing enzymes are necessary in the metabolism of amino acids and protein (13). Pyridoxal phosphate aids the removal of CO_2 from the carboxyl groups (—COOH) of tyrosine, arginine, glutamic acid, and other amino acids

241

(decarboxylation). The coenzyme functions in the transfer of amino groups ($-NH_2$) from one compound to another (transamination) and in the transfer of sulfur from the amino acid methionine to form the amino acid cysteine (transulfuration). The conversion of the amino acid tryptophan to niacin requires the coenzyme. The transport of amino acids into the cells, important chemical reactions in the nervous system and brain, and the formation of a precursor of heme (a constituent of hemoglobin) also are dependent on pyridoxal phosphate.

The vitamin B-6 coenzyme functions in carbohydrate metabolism as part of an enzyme (phosphorylase) needed in the breakdown of glycogen to glucose.

Effects of a Vitamin B-6 Deficiency

Deprivation studies have shown that infants and adults need vitamin B-6. The symptoms of vitamin B-6 deficiency include anemia, skin lesions, convulsive seizures, and reduced antibody production. However, a deficiency seldom occurs naturally because the vitamin is found in so many foods.

The effects of vitamin B-6 deprivation in adults were first demonstrated by Vilter and coworkers (45), who used a low vitamin B-6 diet and one of the *antagonists* of the vitamin—desoxypyridoxine. After 2 or 3 weeks, all except one of the subjects had developed a greasy scaliness on their skin near their nose, mouth, and eyes (Fig. 12.3). These lesions were not improved by an intake of thiamin, riboflavin, or niacin, but they did disappear several days after vitamin B-6 was administered.

Symptoms of nervous irritability and convulsive seizures in about 300 infants less than six months of age were reported in the United States in the early 1950s (13). It was found that all of these babies had been fed the same commercially canned, liquid-milk formula. At 4 weeks of age one of these babies appeared to be irritable and

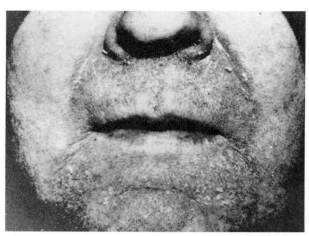

Fig. 12.3 Dermatitis in man due to a pyridoxine deficiency induced by the antivitamin desoxypyridoxine. The skin is red and rough in the nasolabial folds and on the chin, and the greasy scales are clearly visible. (Courtesy R. W. Vilter et al. (1953). The effect of vitamin B-6 deficiency induced by desoxypyridoxine in human beings. *J. Lab. Clin. Med.* 42: 335.)

showed a stiffening of the body, and at 2½ months of age went into convulsive seizures. The baby was given an intramuscular injection of 100 mg of pyridoxine hydrochloride; 3 minutes later, the convulsions stopped and the child began to react normally. It is now known that these seizures were caused by a lack of vitamin B-6 in the canned milk formula; the vitamin had been destroyed by heat during the canning process. Since that experience, processed milk formulas are now analyzed to make sure that they contain a sufficient amount of vitamin B-6. The effects of vitamin B-6 deprivation appear to be more dramatic in infants than in adults (13, 40).

Vitamin B-6 Inborn Errors of Metabolism These inherited disorders (once called vitamin B-6 dependency syndromes) occur in a very small number of people and require very large supplements of vitamin B-6 daily to reverse the symptoms of convulsions or anemia (15, 28).

Table 12.1 Recommended Dietary Allowances for Vitamin B-6, Folacin, and Vitamin B-12

	Age (years)	Vitamin B-6		Folacin		Vitamin B-12	
		mg	mg/1000 kcal[a]	μg	μg/1000 kcal[a]	μg	μg/1000 kcal[a]
Infants	0.0–0.5	.3	—	50	—	.3	—
	0.5–1.0	.4	—	50	—	.3	—
Children	1–3	.6	.5	100	77	1.0	.8
	4–6	.9	.5	200	111	1.5	.8
	7–10	1.2	.5	300	125	2.0	.8
Males	11–14	1.6	.6	400	143	3.0	1.1
	15–18	2.0	.7	400	133	3.0	1.0
	19–22	2.0	.7	400	133	3.0	1.0
	23–50	2.0	.7	400	148	3.0	1.1
	51+	2.0	.8	400	167	3.0	1.3
Females	11–14	1.6	.7	400	167	3.0	1.3
	15–18	2.0	1.0	400	191	3.0	1.4
	19–22	2.0	1.0	400	191	3.0	1.4
	23–50	2.0	1.0	400	200	3.0	1.5
	51+	2.0	.8	400	222	3.0	1.7
Pregnant		2.5	—	800	—	4.0	—
Lactating		2.5	—	600	—	4.0	—

[a] Calculated.

From *Recommended Dietary Allowances, Eighth Edition.* Natl. Acad. Sci.–Natl. Research Council. Washington, D.C.: Natl. Research Council, 1974.

Recommended Dietary Allowances for Vitamin B-6

The RDA for vitamin B-6 is 2.0 mg per day for everyone 19 years of age and over (35) (Table 12.1). Because vitamin B-6 is needed for protein metabolism, this amount allows for a daily protein intake of 100 g or more. The RDA per 1000 kcal (4184 kJ) for men and women, 19 to 22 years, is 0.7 and 1.0 mg vitamin B-6, respectively (Table 12.1).

Vitamin B-6 College Meals The vitamin B-6 content of meals served in 50 American colleges averaged 1.43 mg per person per day, with a range of 0.65 to 2.91 mg (47). More than 80 percent of the values were below the daily RDA of 2.0 mg, and about one-fourth of the colleges served meals with only 50 percent of the needed vitamin B-6.

Food Sources of Vitamin B-6

Vitamin B-6 is widely distributed among plant and animal foods, but the best sources are muscle meats, liver, vegetables, and whole-grain cereals. The vitamin B-6 content of various foods is given in Table 12.2 (32).

The amount of vitamin B-6 available in the 1976 American food supply was about 2.31 mg per capita per day (2). Over one-half of it came

243

Table 12.2 Vitamin B-6, Folacin, Vitamin B-12, Pantothenic acid, and Biotin Content of 100-Gram Portions of Various Foods

Food	Vit. B-6,[a] mg	Folacin,[b] μg	Vit. B-12,[a] μg	Pantothenic acid,[a] mg	Biotin,[c] μg
Apple	0.030	2.0	0	0.105	0.9
Apricots, canned	0.054	4.0	0	0.092	—
Banana	0.510	27.0	0	0.260	4.4
Beans, lima	—	—	0	0.470	—
Beans, snap, green	0.080	6.0	0	0.190	—
Beef, round	0.435	3.0	1.8	0.620	2.6
Bread					
white	0.040	17.0	tr	0.430	1.1
whole wheat	0.180	—	0	0.760	1.9
Broccoli	0.195	—	0	1.170	—
Carrots	0.150	3.0	0	0.280	2.5
Cheese (Cheddar)	0.080	6.0	1.0	0.500	3.6
Chicken					
dark	0.325	7.0	0.4	1.000	10.0
white	0.683	7.0	0.5	0.800	11.3
Egg	0.110	30.0	2.0	1.600	22.5
Ham	0.400	3.0	0.6	0.675	5.0
Liver, beef	0.840	—	80.0	7.700	96.0
Milk, whole	0.040	8.5	0.4	0.340	4.7
Orange	0.060	45.0	0	0.250	1.9
Peas, green	0.160	8.0	0	0.750	9.4
Pineapple, canned	—	2.0	0	0.140	—
Spinach	0.280	29.0	0	0.300	6.9
Tunafish, canned	0.425	—	2.2	0.320	3.0

[a] M. L. Orr (1969). *Pantothenic Acid, Vitamin B-6, and Vitamin B-12 in Foods*. Home Econ. Res. Rept. No. 36. Washington, D.C.: U.S. Dept. Agr., Agr. Res. Service.
[b] A. D. F. Hurdle, D. Barton, and I. H. Searles (1968). A method for measuring folate in food and its application to a hospital diet. *Am. J. Clin. Nutrition.* **21:** 1202. Used by permission.
[c] M. G. Hardinge and J. Crooks (1961). Lesser known vitamins in foods. *J. Am. Dietet. Assoc.,* **38:** 240.

from animal foods (meat, poultry, and fish, 46.2 percent; eggs, 1.8 percent; and dairy products, 10.3 percent) and the remainder from vegetables, fruits, cereals, and nuts.

Folacin (Folic Acid)

In 1931, Dr. Lucy Willis and her colleagues described a *macrocytic* anemia in pregnant women in India, which improved when they were given

a concentrated yeast preparation. Later it was shown that the factor in yeast was a group of chemically related vitamins with folic acid activity (folic acid pteroylmonoglutamic acid [PGA] and related compounds called polyglutamates), which have been given the generic name folacin (12). The biological active form of folacin is a reduction product called tetrahydrofolic acid.

Long before folacin was either isolated or synthesized, its deficiency symptoms had been described in humans, animals, and microorganisms, and it had been called by various names — vitamin M, factor U, vitamin B_c, and *Lactobacillus casei* factor. The research related to folacin has been described as the most complicated chapter in the story of the B-complex vitamins (48).

Metabolism of Folacin

Folacin occurs in food in two forms — free folates and bound folates (polyglutamates). The free folates, about 25 percent of the food intake, are thought to be absorbed readily by the intestinal tract. The bound folates (which must be digested before absorption) are changed to PGA by an enzyme found in the mucosa of the small intestine. As the PGA passes through the intestinal wall, it undergoes chemical change and enters the portal circulation as 5-methyltetrahydrofolate (16, 38). The vitamin is excreted by way of the kidney.

The measurement of folacin levels in both blood serum and red blood cells (RBC) is the procedure used to evaluate folacin nutriture in human beings (39).

Functions of Folacin

The coenzyme forms of folacin (17, 20) function in conjunction with enzymes in the transfer of single carbon units, which are important in the metabolism of many body compounds. Examples of such transfers include the formation of the essential amino acid methionine from its preform (homocystine) and the formation of the three-carbon amino acid serine from the two-carbon amino acid glycine.

The coenzymes of folacin working with other enzymes also take part in the synthesis of choline (see p. 252), in the formation of the amino acid tyrosine from the essential amino acid phenylalanine, and in the synthesis of the *purines* and *pyrimidines* which form part of the nucleoproteins that are found in the nuclei of all cells and are essential to living matter.

Effects of a Folacin Deficiency

Characteristic symptoms of a human folacin deficiency include macrocytic anemia (in which the red cells are larger than normal), *megaloblastic* anemia (in which there are large immature red cells [with nuclei]), inflammation of the tongue (glossitis), and disturbances of the intestinal tract (diarrhea) (19). The deficiency may be caused by inadequate dietary intake, impaired absorption or utilization, or an unusual need (caused by increased losses or requirements) by the body's tissues (20).

The classic megaloblastic anemia of folacin deficiency includes fewer white blood cells (WBC) than normal (leukopenia) and fewer blood platelets than normal (thrombocytopenia). The peripheral blood contains large elliptical RBCs and WBCs with misshapen nuclei. As the deficiency becomes worse, some of the normal RBCs (normoblasts) are replaced by large, abnormal RBCs (megaloblasts). Many of these cells fail to mature and are destroyed within the bone marrow itself; those that do enter the blood stream are short-lived. It should be noted that the anemia due to a folacin deficiency is very similar to that caused by a vitamin B-12 deficiency (20). The two can only be distinguished by measuring the serum folate level; in a folacin deficiency, it is lower than normal, and in a vitamin B-12 deficiency, it is either normal or high.

The Relationship of Folacin to Other Nutrients and Alcohol It is now believed that the factor(s) responsible for the symptom of megaloblastic anemia may be a defect in metabolism which affects the formation and/or activity of the folacin coenzymes (20, 46). When vitamin B-12 is deficient, for example, folacin cannot be recycled back to its coenzyme form, and a secondary folacin deficiency occurs (21). A severe deficiency of vitamin C (scurvy) causes the oxidation and inactivation of the biological form of folacin, and the megaloblastic anemia of scurvy

245

results (42). (Large doses of vitamin C, 500 mg or greater, have been reported by some researchers to destroy [by a reducing action] appreciable amounts of vitamin B-12 in the diet and may indirectly interfere with the formation of the folacin coenzymes [21]; others dispute this [29].) A defect in the body's use of folacin also may occur when the intake of dietary iron is insufficient (46, 48). Alcohol (ethanol) interferes with the normal absorption and metabolism of folacin (4, 37); this is of nutritional significance because of the prevalence of chronic alcoholism throughout the world.

Because this vitamin deficiency may result either from a shortage of folacin itself or from a related substance that interferes with the normal function of the folacin coenzymes, folacin deficiencies are thought to be a major health problem in this country (37) and throughout the world (36).

Prevalence of Folacin Deficiency Anemias

Surveys to determine the prevalence of folacin deficiency anemias were undertaken by the WHO Expert Group of Nutritional Anaemias in the 1960s (30), but it was found that there was insufficient information available to evaluate the relative importance of this vitamin deficiency (31). It has been suggested, however, that a high global prevalence of folacin deficiency does occur among pregnant women (9). The fortification of maize, rice, and bread with folacin among population groups in South Africa has been shown to be an effective measure to prevent the development of megaloblastic anemia in pregnancy (10, 11).

Folacin Therapy in Macrocytic Anemias Folacin is effective in relieving the symptoms of those who have tropical and nontropical sprue, nutritional macrocytic anemia, macrocytic anemia of pellagra, megaloblastic anemia of pregnancy, and megaloblastic anemia of infancy (9, 41). In pernicious anemia, folacin therapy normalizes the blood symptoms, but the neurologic symptoms remain unchanged; vitamin B-12, not folacin, should be used to treat this disorder (20). Microcytic anemia (when the majority of the RBC are smaller than normal) does not respond to folacin therapy.

Use of Folacin Antagonists in Leukemia The most potent folacin antagonist or antivitamin, aminopterin, has been used in the treatment of leukemia, a disease in which there is a marked increase in the production of leucocytes (white blood cells). This folacin antagonist may bring about a temporary relief (remission) but not a cure for leukemia.

Recommended Dietary Allowances for Folacin

The RDA for folacin is 400 μg per day for all persons 11 years and older (35) (Table 12.1). The folacin RDA per 1000 kcal (4184 kJ) for men and women, 19 to 22 years of age, is 133 and 191 μg, respectively (Table 12.1).

Folacin in College Meals The folacin content of meals offered at 50 American colleges averaged 338 μg per person per day with a range of 217 to 505 μg (47). About three-fourths (74 percent) of the meals failed to meet the RDA for the nutrient.

Food Sources of Folacin

Folacin is widely distributed in plants, especially in the green parts — hence the name folacin. Rich food sources include liver and leaf lettuce; other leafy green vegetables and legumes are also good sources.

The folacin in food can be classified into two main groups — free folate and total folate. The

246

amount of total folate available in the human food intake has not been established, but studies from Canada suggest that it may be in the range of 200 μg per day (24). Table 12.2 presents only the free folate values; some food values for free and total folates are now available (33).

Folacin Consumption and Deficiency in the United States

Neither the Ten-State Nutrition Survey nor HANES collected dietary data on folacin intake.

Serum and RBC folacin data from the Ten-State Nutrition Survey suggested that folacin intakes were generally acceptable among the population surveyed (8). Folacin data from HANES will be presented in the final report (1).

Vitamin B-12

After Minot and Murphy found in 1926 that pernicious anemia (PA) could be controlled by the ingestion of whole liver, many laboratories sought to discover what factor in liver was responsible. But it was not until 1948 that scientists finally isolated the substance that, in very small amounts, relieves this form of anemia; it was named vitamin B-12.

The compounds with vitamin B-12 activity are cyanocobalamin (vitamin B-12), hydroxocobalamin (vitamin B-12a, vitamin B-12b), and nitritocobalamin (vitamin B-12c) (12). Cyanocobalamin is a red crystalline compound (Fig. 12.2) whose complex formula ($C_{63}H_{88}N_{14}O_{14}PCo$) contains two minerals—cobalt and phosphorus.

Metabolism of Vitamin B-12

Vitamin B-12 is probably the only vitamin that requires a specific gastrointestinal tract secretion for its absorption. This substance, called the *intrinsic factor* (IF) by Castle (who first recognized its existence), is a mucoprotein secreted by the stomach. IF combines with vitamin B-12 and transports it across the intestinal wall. The formation of this combination (B-12-IF) is only the first step in the absorption of vitamin B-12. In the small intestine B-12-IF forms a complex with calcium and then enters the intestinal cells. Within the cells, vitamin B-12 is released from the B-12-IF and combines with the cell protein for transport across the cell wall. The serum protein that carries the vitamin to the blood-forming tissues is known as transcobalamin II; B-12 binding glycoprotein transports it to the liver (14, 21). Whenever vitamin B-12 is not needed for immediate use is stored in the liver. The vitamin is excreted by way of the kidneys and in bile.

The most useful measurement for the detection of a vitamin B-12 deficiency is the serum vitamin B-12 level (39). A low vitamin B-12 level indicates PA.

Functions of Vitamin B-12

The existence of a vitamin B-12 coenzyme was first reported by Barker in 1958 (5). It is now known that there are two vitamin B-12 coenzymes active in human beings—coenzyme B-12 (adenoslycobalamin) and methyl B-12 (methylcobalamin) (21, 26). The former serves as an intermediate hydrogen carrier and the latter as a methyl group carrier in the body cells (3, 34).

Vitamin B-12 appears to be needed for the metabolism of nucleic acid and the vitamin folacin. Without vitamin B-12, reduced folacin coenzymes apparently cannot be formed or function effectively to assist in the production of normal RBCs in the bone marrow (20).

Causes of a Vitamin B-12 Deficiency

Vitamin B-12 deficiency may be caused by a variety of intestinal disorders leading to defective absorption of the nutrient. It can result from *ideal resection*, competitive parasites (fish tapeworm), increased nutritional requirements (pregnancy), severe malnutrition, or a deficiency of IF

247

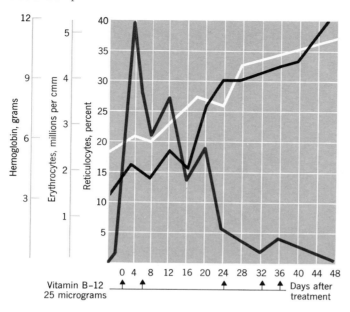

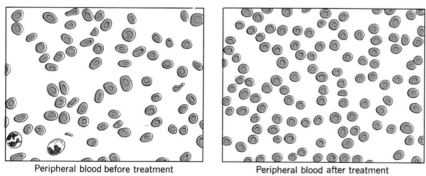

Peripheral blood before treatment Peripheral blood after treatment

Fig. 12.4 Patient with pernicious anemia in relapse; typical hematologic response to treatment with vitamin B-12. (Courtesy Merck, Sharpe and Dohme Research Laboratories, Rahway, New Jersey.)

(PA) (7). The two general symptoms of a B-12 deficiency are megaloblastic anemia and a variety of neurological disorders.

Vitamin B-12 and Pernicious Anemia

PA is a chronic disease that tends to afflict persons in their 50s and 60s. It is of genetic origin (that is, a dominant gene is responsible for an abnormality of the gastric mucosa, resulting in failure of the mucosa to secrete the IF). PA is characterized by abnormally large red blood cells (macrocytes), glossitis, and neurological disturbances such as stiffness of the limbs, irritability, drowsiness, and depression. When liver was used to treat the disease, Castle postulated

248

that a substance in the food (extrinsic factor) combined with a substance in the gastric juice (IF) to form the antipernicious-anemia factor. Vitamin B-12 is now recognized as the extrinsic factor. It has been found that minute doses of vitamin B-12 (10 to 15 μg per day) given by injection (intramuscularly) can relieve the disorder, and 100 μg given every month can prevent the recurrence of PA symptoms (21, 27) (Fig. 12.4). Intramuscular administration of vitamin B-12 is effective in PA because it bypasses the stomach and the need for absorption; it is not affected by the failure of the intestinal mucosa to secrete the IF, which is essential for the absorption of vitamin B-12.

Recommended Dietary Allowances for Vitamin B-12

The RDA for vitamin B-12 is 3 μg per day for all persons 11 years and over (35) (Table 12.1). The vitamin B-12 RDA per 1000 kcal (4184 kJ) for men and women, 19 to 22 years, is 1.0 and 1.4 μg per day, respectively.

Vitamin B-12 in College Meals Although the average vitamin B-12 content of meals served at 50 American colleges was 6.28 μg per person per day (range between 2.00 and 15.58 μg), nearly two-fifths (38 percent) of the colleges offered meals with vitamin B-12 levels below the 3.0 μg of the RDA (47).

Food Sources of Vitamin B-12

Animal protein foods are the chief dietary sources of vitamin B-12; cereal grains, vegetables, fruits, and legumes have virtually none at all. A 100-g serving of liver provides about 27 times the RDA for vitamin B-12 (32) (see Table 12.2).

Vegans (those who consume no animal products at all) eat a diet that may be seriously deficient in vitamin B-12. Lacto-ovo-vegetarians (those who consume no flesh foods) obtain some vitamin B-12 from eggs and milk products.

It is the practice of some vegans to supplement their diet with vitamin B-12. Brewer's yeast is a source of the vitamin that might be considered by vegans.

The amount of vitamin B-12 in the United States' food supply in 1976 was about 9.6 μg per person per day (2). It came from the following sources: meat, poultry, and fish (70.2 percent); eggs (8.1 percent); dairy products (20.1 percent); and flour and cereal products, because of the fortification of some cereals (1.5 percent).

Pantothenic Acid

About 1940, pantothenic acid received widespread attention as a possible remedy for gray hair. Since it had been observed that the black fur of a rat would turn gray when the animal was deprived of the vitamin, studies were undertaken to see if pantothenic acid could help human beings. No consistent benefits were observed, however.

Metabolism of Pantothenic Acid

Pantothenic acid, like other B vitamins, is readily absorbed through the mucosa of the small intestine and enters the portal circulation. Most of the pantothenic acid is used in the biosynthesis of coenzyme A (CoA) but a significant amount found in the cells is bound to protein in a compound known as acyl carrier protein (ACP).

Pantothenic acid is present in all living tissue, with high concentrations in the liver and kidney. (Large amounts of CoA are found in the liver, with lesser amounts in the adrenal glands.) The vitamin is excreted from the body by way of the kidneys.

Methods for measuring the status of the vitamin are limited because of a lack of interest in human pantothenic acid requirements (39); however, urinary excretion levels of pantothenic acid have been used in human studies.

Functions of Pantothenic Acid

Pantothenic acid (Fig. 12.2) functions in the body as part of two coenzymes—CoA and ACP (17, 51). CoA plays a vital role in the series of chemical reactions that break down carbohydrates and fats to release energy; it also is vital in the synthesis of cholesterol (CHOL), fatty acids, and other compounds (see Fig. 2.6). The oxidation of pyruvate to acetyl CoA is necessary for carbohydrate to enter the tricarboxylic acid cycle (TAC). (CoA has been described as the "gateway" to the TAC.) The oxidation of fatty acids requires CoA (two carbon fragments are liberated at a time from the carbon chain; these fragments are acetyl CoA) (see Fig. 5.3). The other coenzyme form of pantothenic acid, ACP, is required by the cells in the biosynthesis of fatty acids (CoA is involved in their breakdown).

Effects of a Pantothenic Acid Deficiency

In a study of experimental pantothenic acid deficiency in six young men, all were placed on a low pantothenic acid intake. (A natural pantothenic acid deficiency in man occurs rarely.) Two of the subjects were given an antagonist of the vitamin, omega-methyl pantothenate; two were given a supplement of pantothenic acid to serve as a control; and two merely had the deficient diet. In a few weeks the two taking the antagonist became irritable and restless, alternated between periods of insomnia and sleepiness, became fatigued after mild exercise, and developed gastrointestinal symptoms and a staggering gait. A few weeks later the men on the deficient diet alone also manifested the same symptoms (23).

A pantothenic acid deficiency in both animals and human beings curtails the production of antibodies (22). Subjects deficient in either pantothenic acid or pyridoxine appeared to form antibodies sluggishly, but men deficient in both failed completely to form antibodies in response to injections of typhoid and tetanus antigens, even though they had previously been immunized with these antigens in military service.

Suggested Allowance for Pantothenic Acid

A daily pantothenic acid intake of 5 to 10 mg has been suggested by the Food and Nutrition Board for children and adults, even though the daily need for this vitamin has not yet been determined (35).

Food Sources of Pantothenic Acid

Because this vitamin is found in all plant and animal tissues, its name (which was coined from the Greek and means "from everywhere") is quite appropriate. The best sources of this nutrient are liver, kidney, yeast, egg yolk, and fresh vegetables. As with the other B-complex vitamins, whole-grain breads and cereals contain appreciably more pantothenic acid than do refined cereal products. Milk is also a good source (0.8 mg of pantothenic acid per cup). For the pantothenic acid content of various foods, see Table 12.2 (32).

Biotin

The development of a deficiency syndrome in animals fed a diet containing uncooked egg white led to the discovery of biotin. Now it is known that the deficiency (called egg-white injury) occurs when the biotin in food combines with a factor in uncooked egg white (called avidin). When egg whites are cooked, avidin (a protein-carbohydrate complex) is inactivated. In the early studies, liver and yeast offered protection against egg-white injury because they both contained sufficiently large amounts of biotin

250

to completely saturate the avidin and leave a surplus of biotin available to meet the needs of experimental animals.

Metabolism of Biotin

Biotin is absorbed from the gastrointestinal tract by way of the intestinal cells and enters the portal circulation. (Avidin, the antagonist found in raw egg white, binds biotin and prevents its absorption from the intestinal tract.) A large part of the daily human biotin need comes from that supplied by intestinal bacteria; it has been found that three to six times more biotin is excreted in the urine than is ingested (35). Biotin is excreted by way of the kidneys and in the feces.

Measurements of biotin levels in the blood and urinary excretion levels of biotin both provide evidence of biotin status in human beings.

Functions of Biotin

Biotin (Fig. 12.2) is needed for certain intermediary reactions in the metabolism of carbohydrates, fats, and proteins. The vitamin forms part of the coenzymes that are necessary in reactions that add CO_2 to other compounds (49, 50). One biotin-containing coenzyme helps to lengthen the carbon chain in fatty acid synthesis; another has a role in the breakdown of the amino acid leucine; and yet another (that contains four molecules of biotin), known as pyruvic carboxylase, catalyzes the addition of CO_2 to pyruvic acid to form oxaloacetate in the presence of ATP. The formation of oxaloacetate is important because it is the starting point of the TAC, in which the potential energy of nutrients (ATP) is released for use by the body.

Almost 30 years ago, Professor H. A. Krebs stated that the biotin enzymes participated either directly or indirectly in the TAC (25). Professor Krebs himself called the cycle the tricarboxylic acid cycle, but it is also known as the Krebs cycle to honor the man who contributed to our understanding of it.

Effects of a Biotin Deficiency

A biotin deficiency has been experimentally induced by feeding male subjects a diet that was low in biotin and included a substantial amount of raw egg white (30 percent of the total energy value) (43). By the end of the first month, all the subjects had developed a fine scaliness on their skin. During the ninth and tenth week, the men experienced mild depression, extreme weariness, sleepiness, muscular pains, and highly sensitive skin. Later on they also developed *anorexia* and nausea. Because these symptoms disappeared so quickly after biotin was restored to their diets, it was concluded that this vitamin is essential for man.

A case history has been reported of biotin deficiency in a 62-year-old woman who added six raw eggs and two quarts of skim milk daily to her regular diet. This diet was recommended to her to provide a high intake of essential amino acids as part of the treatment for *liver cirrhosis* (6). After 18 months on this regime, the woman experienced loss of appetite, vomiting, glossitis, pallor, depression, lassitude, substernal pain, and scaly dermatitis (Fig. 12.5). However, after

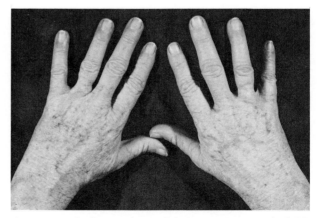

Fig.12.5 Hands showing biotin deficiency (From Baugh, C. M., J. H. Malone, and C. E. Butterworth Jr. (1968). Human biotin deficiency *Am. J. Clin. Nutrition* 21: 173-182. Used by permission.)

251

2 to 5 days of biotin therapy, all of her symptoms improved.

Suggested Allowance for Biotin

The Food and Nutrition Board has not yet established a biotin allowance because it is not known exactly how much biotin is synthesized by microorganisms in the intestinal tract (35). Because biotin is found in most foods and is also produced in the intestinal tract, a deficiency is seldom found.

Food Sources of Biotin

Biotin is found in foods of both plant and animal origin. The richest sources are kidney and liver; good sources include chicken, eggs, milk, most fresh vegetables, and some fruits. Meat, wheat products, and corn products are poor sources (Table 12.2). The raw egg presents an interesting situation; avidin is found in the white of the egg and biotin in the yolk. Quantitative determinations show an excess of avidin over biotin in the whole raw egg.

Two Related Compounds: Choline and Myo-Inositol

Possibly choline and myo-inositol should not be included with the other B-complex vitamins because both factors are found in the body in large amounts and neither has been shown to be missing in human deficiency symptoms. Choline can be synthesized in the body when enough methionine is available; myo-inositol may be a component of body tissues rather than a specific nutrient because it is required by animals and microorganisms in amounts far larger than any of the eight B-complex vitamins. In any event, choline and myo-inositol are included here because they are related to the B-complex group and because they are found in food.

Choline

This compound, first isolated from bile in 1849, functions in protein and fat metabolism and is a source of labile methyl (CH_3) groups, which play a role in the synthesis of vital protein substances such as epinephrine (adrenalin), a hormone of the adrenal gland. Choline is also a constituent of phospholipids and serves as a precursor of a related compound—acetylcholine—which is required for the transmission of nerve impulses.

It is estimated that an ordinary American diet contains 400 to 900 mg of choline per day, including its natural precursor, betaine (35). Rich sources of choline include brains, liver, kidney, eggs, yeast, and wheat germ; cheese, milk, beef, and vegetables contain lesser amounts.

Myo-Inositol

Even though many organisms (fungi, yeasts, and others) require myo-inositol as a growth factor, very little is known about its functions. One role of myo-inositol appears to be as a precursor for the phosphoinositides, which are found in various body tissues, but especially the brain. Good food sources of myo-inositol include heart, liver, brains, wheat germ, yeast, and whole-grain cereals.

Summary

The coenzyme of vitamin B-6, pyridoxal phosphate, functions in the metabolism of amino acids and proteins. Deficiency symptoms (produced by a B-6 antagonist) in human beings are skin lesions of the face, which are relieved with vitamin B-6; if B-6 is deficient in the diets of infants, convulsive seizures may occur. The RDA for B-6 is 2.0 mg per day for everyone 19 years of age and over. The best food sources of B-6 are muscle meats, liver, vegetables, and whole-grain cereals.

Folacin functions as a coenzyme in the metabolism of certain amino acids and in the synthesis

252

of choline, purines, and pyrimidines. A deficiency results in a megaloblastic anemia, inflammation of the tongue, and diarrhea. Factors other than folacin (for example, deficiency of vitamins B-12 and C, alcoholism) may indirectly cause the megaloblastic anemia by interfering with the metabolism of the folacin coenzymes. The RDA for folacin is 400 μg per day for all persons 11 years of age and over. Folacin is found in liver, leaf lettuce, leafy green vegetables, and legumes.

Vitamin B-12 functions as coenzymes in the metabolism of nucleic acid and folacin. For its absorption B-12 requires the intrinsic factor (IF), which is secreted by stomach cells. When IF is lacking, B-12 is not absorbed and pernicious anemia (PA) occurs. PA is characterized by a megaloblastic anemia and neurological symptoms. PA can be relieved by small muscular injections of B-12 (10 to 15 μg per day); 100 μg B-12 every month prevents the recurrence of PA. The RDA for B-12 is 3 μg per day for all persons 11 years and older. Animal proteins are the chief food source of B-12.

Pantothenic acid functions as part of the important factor coenzyme A (CoA). Acetyl CoA has been described as the "gateway" to the tricarboxylic acid cycle and is involved in reactions necessary to release energy from carbohydrates and fats and in the synthesis of other compounds. A deficiency of the vitamin (produced by a pantothenic acid antagonist) results in irritability, drowsiness, fatigue, staggering gait, and gastrointestinal disturbances in men. There is no RDA for pantothenic acid, and it is found in liver, kidney, yeast, egg yolk, and fresh vegetables.

Biotin, through its coenzymes, is needed for reactions in the metabolism of carbohydrates, fats, and proteins. Using a diet low in biotin and high in uncooked egg whites, men developed symptoms of depression, weariness, sleepiness, muscular pain, and skin lesions. There is no RDA for biotin; kidney and liver are rich sources of biotin, and chicken, eggs, milk, and most fresh vegetables are good sources.

Choline and myo-inositol are two compounds included with the B vitamins. Choline, a source of methyl groups, synthesizes body compounds including acetylcholine, which is required for the transmission of nerve impulses. Little is known of the function of myo-inositol. Both factors are found in yeast, wheat germ, liver, and kidney.

Are any of the other B vitamins toxic if ingested in large amounts? At this time (1978), it is known that only a high folacin intake is dangerous, but not toxic (18). Folacin intakes greater than 1 mg (1000 μg) per day may prevent the diagnosis of pernicious anemia by relieving the megaloblastic anemia of a vitamin B-12 deficiency but not the neurologic effects of it.

Glossary

anorexia: see page 234.

antagonist: a substance that exerts a nullifying or opposing effect to another substance.

antivitamin: a substance that interferes with the metabolism or synthesis of a vitamin.

fortification: see page 197.

ileal resection: removal of part of the ileum section of the small intestine where the vitamin B-12 intrinsic factor complex is absorbed.

intrinsic factor (IF): an enzyme secreted by the mucosal cells of the stomach which is required for the absorption of vitamin B-12 through the intestinal wall; a lack of the factor results in pernicious anemia.

liver cirrhosis: a progressive destruction of the liver cells and an abnormal increase of connective tissue.

macrocyte: the largest type of red blood cell.

megaloblast: a large, nucleated, immature type of cell; it is found in the blood in cases of pernicious anemia, vitamin B-12 deficiency, and folacin deficiency.

pernicious anemia: caused by a lack of the intrinsic factor (IF) necessary for the absorption of vitamin B-12; characterized by megaloblastic anemia and neurological symptoms.

purines: the parent substance of the purine bases; adenine and guanine are the major purine bases of nucleic acids; other important purines are uric acid and xanthine.

pyrimidine: the parent substance of several nitrogenous compounds found in nucleic acids—uracil, thymine, and cytosine.

sprue: a chronic disease caused by the imperfect absorption of nutrients (especially fat) from the small intestine; it is characterized by diarrhea, subnormal body weight, and sensations of fatigue.

Study Questions and Activities

1. Identify the following: coenzyme A, megaloblastic anemia, intrinsic factor, pyridoxal phosphate, methylcobalamin, avidin, and choline.
2. What are the functions of vitamin B-6, folacin, vitamin B-12, pantothenic acid, and biotin?
3. Describe the effects of the following vitamin deficiencies in human beings: vitamin B-6, folacin, vitamin B-12, and biotin.
4. Describe a treatment for pernicious anemia, and explain why it is effective.
5. Name several important food sources of vitamin B-6, vitamin B-12, folacin, pantothenic acid, and biotin.
6. What are the Recommended Dietary Allowances of vitamin B-6, folacin, and vitamin B-12 for college-age men and women?
7. Which B-complex vitamin must a vegan make a special effort to obtain? In what ways can he obtain an adequate amount of that vitamin?
8. What factors may interfere with either the production or activity of the folacin coenzymes and cause a megaloblastic anemia?

References

1. Abraham, S., F. W. Lowenstein, and C. L. Johnson (1974). *Dietary Intake and Biochemical Findings:* Preliminary Findings of the First Health and Nutrition Examination Survey, United States, 1971– 1972, DHEW Publ. No. (HRA) 74-1219-1. Rockville, Md.: U.S. Dept. Health, Educ., and Welfare.
2. *Agricultural Statistics* (1977). Washington, D.C.: U.S. Dept. Agr., pp. 561–564.
3. Babior, B. M. (1975). Cobamides as cofactors: Adenosylcobamide-dependent reactions. In *Cobalamin Biochemistry and Pathophysiology,* edited by B. M. Babior. New York: John Wiley and Sons, Inc., p. 287.
4. Baker, H., O. Frank, R. K. Zetterman, K. S. Rajan, W. ten Hove, and C. M. Leevy (1975). Inability of chronic alcoholics with liver disease to use food as a source of folates. *Am. J. Clin. Nutrition,* **28:** 1377.
5. Barker, H. A. (1958). A coenzyme containing pseudovitamin B_{12}. *Proc. Natl. Acad. Sci.,* **44:** 1093.
6. Baugh, C. M., J. M. Malone, and C. E. Butterworth, Jr. (1968). Human biotin deficiency: A case history of biotin deficiency induced by raw egg consumption in a cirrhotic patient. *Am. J. Clin. Nutrition,* **21:** 173.
7. Beck, W. S. (1975). Metabolic features of cobalamin deficiency in man. In *Cobalamin Biochemistry and Pathophysiology,* edited by B. M. Babior. New York: John Wiley and Sons, Inc., p. 405.
8. *Biochemical,* Ten-State Nutrition Survey, 1968– 1970 (1972). DHEW Publ. No. (HSM) 72-8132. Atlanta, Ga.: Center for Disease Control, U.S. Dept. Health, Educ., and Welfare.
9. Colman, N., E. A. Barker, M. Barker, R. Green, and J. Metz (1975). Prevention of folate deficiency by food fortification. IV. Identification of target group in addition to pregnant women in an adult rural population. *Am. J. Clin. Nutrition,* **28:** 471.
10. Colman, N., R. Green, and J. Metz (1975). Prevention of folate deficiency by food fortification. II. Absorption of folic acid from fortified staple foods. *Am. J. Clin. Nutrition,* **28:** 459.
11. Colman, N., J. V. Larsen, M. Barker, E. A. Barker, R. Green, and J. Metz (1975). Effect in pregnant subjects of varying amounts of added folic acid. *Am. J. Clin. Nutrition,* **28:** 465.
12. Committee on Nomenclature, American Institute

254

of Nutrition (1974). Tentative rules for generic descriptors and trivial names for vitamins and related compounds. *J. Nutrition,* **104:** 144.

13. Coursin, D. B. (1964). Vitamin B$_6$ metabolism in infants and children. *Vitamins and Hormones,* **22:** 755.

14. Ellenbogen, L. (1975). Absorption and transport of cobalamin: Intrinsic factor and the transcobalamins. In *Cobalamin Biochemistry and Pathophysiology,* edited by B. M. Babior. New York: John Wiley and Sons, Inc., p. 287.

15. Gershoff, S. M. (1976). Vitamin B-6. In *Nutrition Reviews' Present Knowledge in Nutrition.* 4th ed. New York: The Nutrition Foundation, Inc., p. 149.

16. Halsted, C. H., A. Reisenauer, and G. S. Gotterer (1977). Process of digestion and absorption of pterolypolyglutamate. In *Folic Acid Biochemistry and Physiology in Relation to the Human Nutrition Requirement.* Washington, D.C.: Natl. Acad. Sci., p. 136.

17. Harper, H. A. (1975). *Review of Physiological Chemistry.* 15th ed. Los Altos, Calif.: Lange Medical Publications, pp. 104–125.

18. Hathcock, J. N. (1976). Nutrition: toxicology and pharmacology. *Nutrition Rev.,* **34:** 65.

19. Herbert, F. (1976). Vitamin B-12. In *Nutrition Reviews' Present Knowledge in Nutrition.* 4th ed. New York: The Nutrition Foundation, Inc., p. 191.

20. Herbert, V. (1968). Folic acid deficiency in man. *Vitamins and Hormones,* **26:** 525.

21. Herbert, V. (1973). The five possible causes of all nutrient deficiency: Illustrated by deficiencies of vitamin B-12 and folic acid. *Am. J. Clin. Nutrition,* **26:** 77.

22. Hodges, R. E., W. B. Bean, M. A. Ohlson, and R. E. Bleiler (1962). Factors affecting human antibody response. V. Combined deficiencies of pantothenic acid and pyridoxine. *Am. J. Clin. Nutrition,* **11:** 187.

23. Hodges, R. E., M. A. Ohlson, and W. B. Bean (1958). Pantothenic acid deficiency in man. *J. Clin. Invest.,* **37:** 1642.

24. Hoppner, K., B. Lampi, and D. C. Smith (1977). Data on folacin activity in foods: Availability, applications, and limitations. In *Folic Acid Biochemistry and Physiology in Relation to the Human Nutrition Requirement.* Washington, D.C.: Natl. Acad. Sci., p. 69.

25. Krebs, H. A. (1949). The tricarboxylic acid cycle. *Harvey Lecture Series,* **44:** 165.

26. Linnell, J. C. (1975). The fate of cobalamins *in vivo.* In *Cobalamin Biochemistry and Pathophysiology,* edited by B. M. Babior. New York: John Wiley and Sons, Inc., p. 287.

27. McCurdy, P. R. (1975). "B-12 shots" flip side. *J. Am. Med. Assoc.,* **231:** 289.

28. Mudd, S. (1971). Pyridoxine-responsive genetic disease. *Federation Proc.,* **30:** 970.

29. Newmark, H. L., J. Scheiner, M. Marcus, and M. Prabhudesai (1976). Stability of vitamin B-12 in the presence of ascorbic acid, *Am. J. Clin. Nutrition,* **29:** 645.

30. *Nutritional Anaemias* (1968). WHO Tech. Rept. Series 405. Geneva: World Health Organ., pp. 21–23, 37.

31. *Nutritional Anaemias* (1972). WHO Tech. Rept. Series 503. Geneva: World Health Organ. pp. 1–27.

32. Orr, M. L. (1969). *Pantothenic Acid, Vitamin B$_6$, and Vitamin B$_{12}$ in Foods.* Home Econ. Res. Rept. 36. Washington, D.C.: U.S. Dept. Agr.

33. Perloff, B. P. and R. R. Butrum (1977). Folacin in selected foods. *J. Am. Dietet. Assoc.,* **70:** 161.

34. Poston, J. M. and T. C. Stadtman (1975). Cobamides as cofactors: Methylcobamides and the synthesis of methionine, methane, and acetate. In *Cobalamin Biochemistry and Pathophysiology,* edited by B. M. Babior. New York: John Wiley and Sons, Inc., p. 111.

35. *Recommended Dietary Allowances, Eighth Edition* (1974). Natl. Acad. Sci.-Natl. Research Council. Washington, D.C.: Natl. Research Council.

36. *Requirements of Ascorbic Acid, Vitamin D, Vitamin B$_{12}$, Folate, and Iron* (1970). WHO Tech. Rept. Series 452. Geneva: World Health Organ, p. 43.

37. Rosenberg, I. H. (1975). Folate absorption and malabsorption. *New Engl. J. Med.,* **293:** 1303.

38. Rosenberg, I. H. (1977). Role of intestinal con-

jugase in the control of the absorption of poly-glutamyl folates. In *Folic Acid Biochemistry and Physiology in Relation to the Human Nutrition Requirement*. Washington, D.C.: Natl. Acad. Sci., p. 136.

39. Sauberlich, H. E., J. H. Skala, and R. P. Dowdy (1974). *Laboratory Tests for the Assessment of Nutritional Status*. Cleveland, Ohio: CRC Press, p. 60.

40. Snyderman, S. E., L. E. Holt, Jr., R. Carretero, and K. Jacobs (1953). Pyridoxine deficiency in the human infant. *Am. J. Clin. Nutrition*, **1**: 200.

41. Spies, T. D. (1962). The pteroylglutamites and vitamin B_{12} in nutrition. In *Clinical Nutrition*, edited by N. Joliffe. New York: Harper and Row, p. 635.

42. Stokes, P. L., V. Melikian, R. L. Leeming, H. Portman-Graham, J. A. Blair, and W. T. Cooke (1975). Folate metabolism in scurvy. *Am. J. Clin. Nutrition*, **28**: 126.

43. Sydenstricker, V. P., S. A. Singal, A. P. Briggs, N. M. deVaughn, and H. Isbell (1942). Observations on the "egg-white injury" in man. *J. Am. Med. Assoc.*, **118**: 1199.

44. The interrelationship between riboflavin and pyridoxine (1977). *Nutrition Rev.*, **35**: 237.

45. Vilter, R. W., J. F. Mueller, H. S. Glazer, T. Harrold, J. Abraham, C. Thompson, and V. R. Hawkins (1953). The effect of vitamin B_6 deficiency induced by desoxypyridoxine in human beings. *J. Lab. Clin. Med.*, **42**: 335.

46. Vilter, R. W., J. J. Will, T. Wright, and D. Rullman (1963). Interrelationships of vitamin B_{12}, folic acid, and ascorbic acid in the megaloblastic anemias. *Am. J. Clin. Nutrition*, **12**: 130.

47. Walker, M. A. and L. Page (1975). Nutritive value of college meals. Proximate composition and vitamins. *J. Am. Dietet. Assoc.*, **66**: 146.

48. Wagner, A. F. and K. Folkers (1964). *Vitamins and Coenzymes*. New York: John Wiley and Sons, Inc. (interscience), p. 123.

49. Wood, H. G. (1976). The reactive group of biotin in catalyses by biotin enzymes. *Trends in Biochem. Sci.*, **1**: 4.

50. Wood, H. G., G. K. Zwolinski, and M. D. Lane (1977). Transcarboxylase: Role of biotin, metals, and subunits in the reaction and its quaternary structure. *CRC Critical Rev. in Biochem.*, **4**: 47.

51. Wright, L. D. (1975). Pantothenic acid. In *Nutrition Reviews' Present Knowledge in Nutrition*. 4th ed. New York: The Nutrition Foundation, Inc., p. 226.

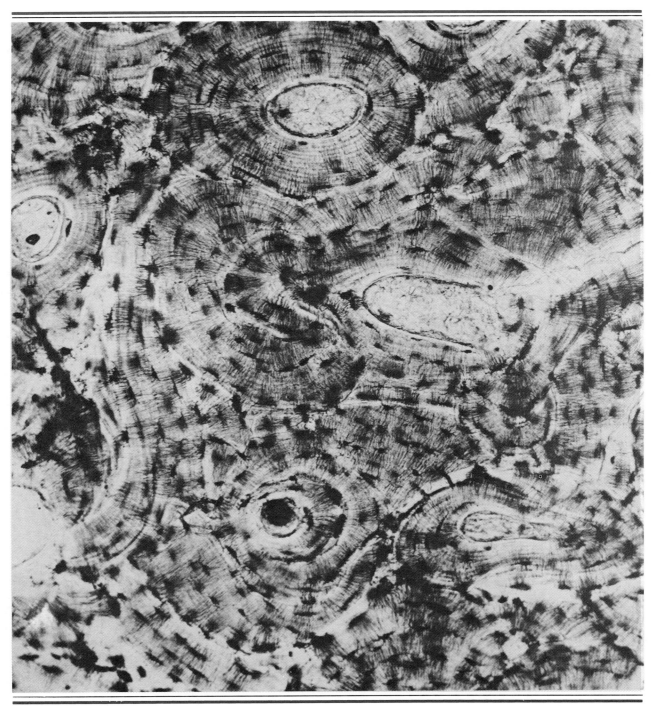

Bones (as shown in this cross section) are one of the body's main uses of calcium and phosphorus. These minerals, which provide strength for the bones, are deposited into a matrix, which is composed of a ground substance and collagen fibers.

Abbreviations

ATP: adenosine triphosphate
Ca: calcium
Ca:P: calcium to phosphorus
DNA: deoxyribonucleic acid
HANES: Health and Nutrition Examination
  Survey, United States

Mg: magnesium
meq or mEq: milliequivalent
P: phosphorus
PTH: parathyroid hormone
RDA: Recommended Dietary Allowances
S: sulfur

Introduction to Minerals

Minerals Required by the Human

The organic compounds—carbohydrates, lipids, and proteins—are composed mainly of carbon, oxygen, hydrogen, and nitrogen. Together with water, these organic compounds comprise about 96 percent of the total body weight; the rest is made up of mineral elements.

The mineral elements are also referred to as inorganic or ash constituents. On combustion of a substance such as coal or wood, for example, the organic matter burns while the inorganic does not; hence the term "ash constituents." In the body the mineral components of food remain after the organic compounds of which they were a part have been oxidized.

The adult body content of some minerals is shown in Table 13.1. Such data are difficult to obtain; those in Table 13.1 are the most recent available. The values are the means of the chemical analyses done between 1951 and 1956 on five adults (36).

At this time it is known that the human requires 14 different mineral elements for good health and growth. Certain ones—calcium, phosphorus, sodium, chlorine, potassium, magnesium, and sulfur—are found in the body in appreciable amounts (0.05 percent or more) and are therefore called macrominerals; the others—iron,

iodine, manganese, copper, zinc, cobalt, and fluorine—appear only in very small amounts or traces and are thus called trace elements or microminerals. There are indications that three other

Table 13.1 Composition of Adults

	Subjects
Sex	4 men, 1 woman
Age (average in years)	44
Weight (average in kg)	61

Composition per kilogram of fat-free body tissue mean values	
Water (g)	720
Total N (g)	34
Sodium (meq)	80[a]
Potassium (meq)	69
Chlorine (meq)	50
Calcium (g)	22.4
Phosphorus (g)	12.0
Magnesium (g)	0.47
Iron (mg)	74
Copper (mg)	1.7
Zinc (mg)	28
Cobalt (mg)	0.021

[a] Mean of two subjects only.
From E. M. Widdowson and J. W. T. Dickerson. *Chemical composition of the body.* In *Mineral Metabolism, An Advanced Treatise*, vol. 2, *The Elements.* Part A, edited by C. L. Comar and F. Bronner. New York: Academic Press, 1964, p. 9.

Table 13.2 Mineral Elements Associated with Enzymes, Either as Components or Cofactors

Mineral	Enzyme	Reaction
Copper	Tyrosinase	Reduction of molecular oxygen
	Ascorbic acid oxidase	Respiratory oxidation
Iron	Peroxidase	Breakdown of peroxides
	Cytochrome oxidase	Reduction of molecular oxygen
	Catalase	Release of molecular oxygen from hydrogen peroxide
Magnesium	Hexokinase	Conversion of glucose to glucose-6-phosphate in carbohydrate metabolism
	Cocarboxylase	Conversion of pyruvate to coenzyme A in carbohydrate metabolism
Manganese	Arginase	Conversion of amino acid arginine to urea
Potassium	Fructokinase	Conversion of fructose to fructose-1-phosphate in carbohydrate metabolism
Zinc	Alcohol dehydrogenase	Conversion of ethyl alcohol to acetylaldehyde in carbohydrate metabolism
	Carbonic anhydrase	Removal of carbon dioxide from carbonic acid to form water in gastric mucosa during digestion
	Carboxypeptidase	Peptide (COOH group) converted to amino acid and peptide in protein digestion

From P. L. Altman and D. S. Dittmer, eds. *Metabolism.* Bethesda, Md.: Fed. Am. Soc. Expt. Biol., 1968, pp. 284, 285, 318, 319, 424, 425.

elements—selenium, molybdenum, and chromium—may also be important in the nutrition of the human. Traces of aluminum, boron, and vanadium have been found in animal tissues, but there is as yet no conclusive evidence that any of them has a specific biological function.

General Functions of Minerals

Body Building Functions Minerals serve as structural constituents in the hard tissues of the body, the bones and teeth, giving rigidity to these structures. And they are components of soft tissues—muscle protein contains sulfur and nervous tissue contains phosphorus. Some compounds essential to the functioning of the body contain minerals; iodine is present in thyroxine, zinc in insulin, cobalt in vitamin B-12, sulfur in thiamin, and iron in hemoglobin. And there are many others.

Body Regulating Functions *Maintenance of Acid-Base Balance.* Minerals contribute to the maintenance of approximate neutrality in the blood and body tissues by helping to protect against either the accumulation of too much acid or too much base (alkali). The normal reaction of the body is near neutral, slightly on the basic side. The chief base-forming elements are: sodium, potassium, calcium, and magnesium. The acid-forming elements are chlorine, phosphorus, and sulfur. For further discussion, see chapt. 15.)

261

Maintenance of Water Balance. The water in the body is in two compartments: inside the cells—intracellular *fluid*—and outside the cells—extracellular fluid. A *semipermeable* membrane separates the compartments. Water in the body contains *electrolytes* (minerals) in solution. The movement of fluid between the cells and the surrounding aqueous medium is related to the concentration of minerals in the solution. Sodium, potassium, chloride, and *bicarbonate ions* play a major role in the movement of fluid in the body. (For further discussion, see chapt. 15.)

Essential for the Functioning of Some Enzymes
Some enzymes contain a metal as an integral part of the molecule; these enzymes are called metalloenzyme. If the metal is removed (this can only be accomplished in the laboratory), the enzyme loses its capacity to function. For another and larger group of enzymes, the metals are *cofactors* which serve only to *activate* the enzyme and are not bound to it. Different metals may function to activate the same enzyme. The enzyme and the activating metal are called metal-enzyme complexes (16, 17). In Table 13.2 metal ions that serve as constituents of enzymes or as cofactors are listed with the appropriate enzymes.

Transmission of Nerve Impulses Sodium, potassium, and calcium each have specific functions in the transmission of nerve impulses. When a stimulus is applied to a nerve, the membrane, which is electrically charged, becomes more permeable; sodium, which is in greater concentration outside the cell, enters it and potassium passes out of the cell. Investigations have demonstrated that transmission of the impulse results chiefly from the movement of sodium ions into the nerve fiber during the early rising part of the impulse, and there is a movement outward of potassium ions later during the fall of the *action potential.* It is hypothesized that calcium contributes to the increased permeability of the membrane and thus to sodium conductance of the impulse in this way: sodium ions

(*monovalent* ions) enter the membrane displacing the divalent calcium ions from their binding sites, increasing the permeability of the membrane (27).

Calcium (Ca)

The body contains more calcium than any other mineral. Approximately 2 percent (0.9 to 1.4 kg) of the body weight of an adult is calcium, about 99 percent of which is in the bones and teeth. A newborn infant's skeleton is only partly mineralized; the calcium content is around 0.8 percent of the total body weight. Using values for the calcium content of the body at birth and at adulthood and the rate of growth during childhood, values for calcium content of the body at different ages were calculated to be as follows (11):

Age (yr)	Weight (kg)	Ca content (g)
1	10.6	100
5	19.1	219
10	33.3	396
15	55.0	806
20	67.0	1078

Metabolism of Calcium

Absorption The extent of calcium absorption varies widely among individuals; the greatest absorption occurs in childhood when the need is large. Infants fed human milk were found to absorb 50 to 70 percent of the calcium ingested, but adults absorb only 10 to 40 percent of the calcium in a mixed diet. As the amount in the diet increases, the percent of the intake absorbed tends to decrease. Because calcium salts are more soluble in an acid medium, most calcium absorption takes place in the upper part of the small intestine where the contents are slightly acid following gastric digestion. The process of absorption is chiefly by active transport, with some taking place by passive diffusion.

Dietary Factors that Improve Absorption *Vitamin D.* Certain nutrients in the diet have been found to improve the absorption of calcium. Vitamin D is one of these. The mode of action of vitamin D_3 (cholecalciferol) is now clear; it is discussed on page 183.

Lactose. Lactose in the diet favors the absorption of calcium in adults (15) and in infants (14). Intestinal absorption of calcium was less when lactose-free milk was fed than when milk with lactose was fed. The precise way in which lactose increases the absorption of calcium is not yet clear.

Dietary Factors that Interfere with Absorption Fewer calcium ions can be absorbed when insoluble calcium salts are formed in the intestine. Two food constituents that produce insoluble salts are oxalic acid and phytic acid.

Oxalic acid and calcium combine to form the insoluble calcium oxalate. Oxalic acid is found in beet greens, chard, rhubarb, spinach, and some cocoa. Although the calcium in these foods exists as the insoluble oxalate and therefore cannot be absorbed, they should not be ignored; the leafy green vegetables are high in vitamin A activity and iron.

Researchers wondered whether the free oxalic acid in these foods would combine with calcium from other foods consumed at the same time, thus making that calcium insoluble. In a study of children five to eight years of age who had enough dietary calcium (1.3 g daily for the older children; 0.8 g for the younger ones), it was found that the absorption of calcium was not lowered by a daily serving of spinach (4). At the same level of calcium intake, balance studies with and without a serving of spinach and with and without an amount of oxalic acid equivalent to that in spinach (0.7 g) showed little difference in calcium retention.

Phytic acid is found in the bran of whole wheat. It combines with calcium to form insoluble calcium phytate, which cannot be absorbed. It is not a problem in whole wheat bread because the action of the enzyme phytase during the leavening and baking processes changes the phytic acid phosphorus to orthophosphate, which forms a soluble salt with calcium (9).

Fiber is being found to be responsible for preventing the absorption of minerals. In a balance study, when two adults were changed from a diet low in fiber content, with white bread at each meal, to one of high fiber content, with wholemeal (wheat) bread at each meal, negative calcium (and magnesium, zinc, and phosphorus) balances developed. The increased loss of each element was by way of the feces. This loss correlated closely with increased fecal dry matter weight, which in turn was directly proportional to fecal fiber excretion (26).

Blood Calcium Calcium absorbed from the intestine is transported by the blood to all parts of the body. The normal blood calcium level of 9 to 11 mg/100 ml is remarkably constant and maintained so by the action of the *parathyroid hormone* (PTH), vitamin D, and *calcitonin* (a hormone secreted by the thyroid gland). If the blood level falls, PTH provides more calcium by stimulating its release from storage in the bone, decreasing calcium excretion from the kidney, and, with the cooperative action of vitamin D, increasing its absorption. Calcitonin inhibits calcium release from bone and thereby lowers the blood calcium when it is higher than normal.

Storage Bone serves as a labile storage place for calcium. The *trabeculae* of *spongy (cancellous) bone* is the place of storage. The trabeculae are fine interlacing partitions enclosing cavities that contain marrow. At the exterior of the spongy bone is the *compact bone* (Fig. 13.1). The labile stores are utilized when calcium is needed by the tissues or the blood. Teeth do not store labile calcium; consequently the calcium contained in them cannot be released.

263

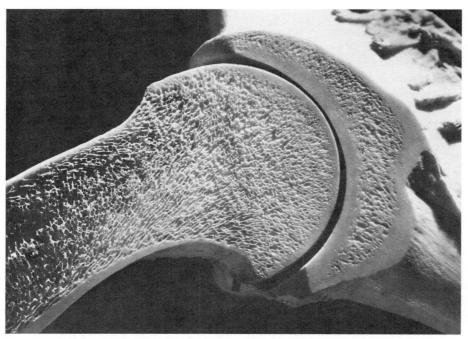

Fig. 13.1 Photograph of a section of the humerus at the shoulder joint. The figure illustrates the appearance and distribution of spongy and compact bone. (A. Feininger Life Magazine © Time, Inc.)

Excretion: Urinary The urinary excretion of calcium is fairly constant within individuals but varies widely from person to person. Calcium intake exerts a variable influence on the excretion. Bed rest markedly increases the urinary loss of calcium as does sitting quietly, but standing quietly does not. It appears that weight-bearing on the long bones is important in conserving body calcium (34).

The level of dietary protein has a notable influence on urinary calcium; increasing the protein consumed from 47 to 142 g daily on a constant calcium intake (500 mg or 800 mg or 1400 mg daily) caused the amount of urinary calcium to approximately double, in a study with young men (13). In another series of investigations with adults, when the protein intake was around 560 g daily, the urinary calcium excretion was 800 percent more than when they were consuming a protein-free diet irrespective of the calcium intake (from 100 to 2300 mg daily) (20).

Excretion: Fecal Fecal calcium is made up of unabsorbed food calcium and unabsorbed *endogenous* calcium. Endogenous calcium is that amount excreted on a calcium-free diet.

Excretion: Sweat Calcium may be lost in significant amounts in sweat under conditions of elevated temperatures, amounting to as much as 30 percent of the total excretion. Urinary calcium is not decreased in compensation for that lost in sweat (11).

Functions of Calcium

Calcium has two important functions: to help build bones and teeth and to regulate certain

264

body processes. Obviously the need for calcium is greatest during childhood (the years of growth), but the need continues into adulthood as well. Once bone is formed, new bone continues to be built and old bone to be destroyed simultaneously. Calcium circulating in the blood and tissues is required for transmission of nerve impulses, muscle contraction, blood clotting, regulation of cell membrane permeability, and other functions.

Building Bones and Teeth Calcium, as well as other mineral elements, gives rigidity and permanence to the bones and teeth. Bones, therefore, can support the body and serve as the "lever whereby muscular contraction results in closely coordinated movements ranging from locomotion to fine hand movements, thus providing man and other vertebrates their great mobility and dexterity" (22). Bone forms protective cavities for the heart and lungs as well as the brain. Although bone can withstand almost as much weight as cast iron before breaking, it is itself light in weight.

Bone is a highly specialized type of connective tissue; it is formed through two separate processes: matrix formation and mineral deposition. Three cellular components of bone are associated with specific functions: osteoblasts with bone formation, osteocytes with bone resorption, and osteoclasts with bone resorption.

The osteoblasts form collagen — a protein substance that is arranged in bundles of long fibers. The collagen fibers are the organic matrix in which minerals are deposited. The chief minerals in bone are calcium and phosphorus, with small amounts of sodium, magnesium, and fluorine. Bone minerals exist in the form of extremely small crystals and comprise 60 to 70 percent of the weight of dry bone.

Studies with radioactive calcium have shown that bone is continually being formed and broken down; it is estimated that about 20 percent of adult bone calcium is resorbed and replaced each year.

Teeth are composed of three highly calcified

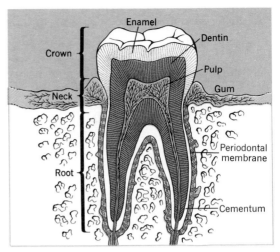

Fig. 13.2 Longitudinal section of a molar tooth in its alveolus.

tissues: *enamel,* the outermost covering; *dentin,* the portion beneath the enamel and surrounding the tooth pulp; and *cementum,* the calcified portion covering the root of the tooth. In the center of the tooth, enclosed in these calcified tissues, is the pulp — the soft connective tissue that contains the blood vessels, lymphatics, and nerves. The pulp extends into the *periodontal membrane* (Fig. 13.2).

Enamel, the hardest tissue in the body, is approximately 97 percent mineral (5). The major minerals — calcium, phosphorus, magnesium, and carbonate — are embedded in an enamel protein matrix. Dentin, which forms the largest portion of the tooth, lies beneath the enamel and surrounds the pulp. Its composition is similar to bone, approximately 60 percent mineral (5). Dentin is formed and nourished by the odontoblasts; they continue to form secondary dentin throughout the life of the tooth. When a carious lesion is developing, the formation of secondary dentin proceeds at an accelerated pace. The odontoblasts are located around the periphery of the pulp and are in contact with the inner surface of the dentin (29). The calcium salts of phosphate and carbonate (of which dentin is largely

265

composed) are embedded in a network of protein (collagen) fibers. The chemical composition of cementum is assumed to be similar to bone and dentin, but little is known about it (23).

There are three significant differences between the calcified tissues of teeth and the other body tissues (29). First, enamel and dentin contain no microscopically detectable capillary or lymphatic vessels to act as transport for nutrients. There may be some diffusion from the saliva to the enamel and from the blood, by way of the odontoblastic layer of the pulp, to the dentin. Second, enamel cannot repair areas that have been improperly formed or inadequately calcified during formation, nor can teeth repair themselves from destruction caused by tooth decay or mechanical injury. By contrast, the long bones are able to heal diseased or fractured areas. Thus it is especially important that the teeth have an optimal amount of protein and minerals during their developmental period and that measures be taken to prevent partial destruction afterward. Last, the calcified tissues of the teeth undergo a partial change of environment during their life history. Before eruption the teeth have systemic contact through normal vascular (blood) and neural (nerve) pathways. However, when the teeth emerge into the oral cavity, the blood supply to the enamel is severed, and the enamel comes in contact with saliva, microorganisms, food debris, and other substances present in the mouth.

Body Regulating Function *Transmission of Nerve Impulses.* When a nerve impulse arrives at the junction of a nerve and muscle (neuromuscular junction), the chemical compound *acetylcholine* is released. It is believed that calcium promotes the release of acetylcholine. Acetylcholine bridges the gap between the nerve and the muscle fibers, making it possible for the nerve impulse to pass to the muscle (3).

Muscle Contraction and Relaxation. Muscle contraction is a complicated process requiring muscle proteins, enzymes, and minerals. Precisely what happens when muscles contract and what chemical changes take place are still being studied. Only a few of the key points will be presented here.

Actin, myosin, and *troponin* are the proteins in the skeletal muscle that are most directly involved in muscle contraction and mechanical work. The stimulus that produces muscle contraction is an electrical impulse delivered by the motor nerve to the muscle cell. It travels along the membrane of the muscle fiber. The electrical activity increases the permeability of the membranes of the *sarcoplasmic reticulum* to calcium ions. The ions pour into the cytoplasm, activating the troponin-inhibited contractile mechanism. Troponin inhibits muscle contraction by blocking the interaction of the proteins actin and myosin, unless it is combined with calcium.

After contraction, calcium is quickly removed and returned to the storage sacs in the sarcoplasmic reticulum, and the muscle relaxes (7, 32). Potassium, sodium, and magnesium are also essential components in the muscle contraction-relaxation processes (3).

Blood Clot Formation Calcium is one of the essential factors in the clotting of blood. Freshly drawn blood coagulates rapidly. However, if blood is drawn into a tube containing oxalic acid, no clot is formed because the calcium in the blood combines with the oxalic acid to form an insoluble salt, thus making the calcium unavailable for functioning in the coagulation process.

The process of blood clotting is complex and as yet incompletely understood. There seems to be agreement among most research workers in the field on the following three steps (8):

1. A substance called *prothrombin activator* is formed in response to the rupture of a blood vessel.

2. The prothrombin activator *catalyzes* the conversion of prothrombin to *thrombin.*

3. The thrombin acts as an enzyme to convert *fibrinogen* into fibrin threads that enmesh *red blood cells* and plasma to form the clot itself.

266

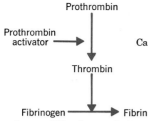
Fig. 13.3 Simple scheme of blood coagulation.

The least well-established of the three steps is the mechanism by which the prothrombin activator is formed. In Fig. 13.3 the changes from prothrombin (a protein normally present in the blood) to fibrin (the blood clot) are shown. Calcium plays a role in the conversion of prothrombin to thrombin.

Regulation of Cell Membrane Properties Cell membranes are composed of lipid protein complexes, which are freely permeable to lipid-soluble substances. The membrane is believed to have many minute pores that pass from one side of the membrane to the other. It is through these pores that lipid-insoluble substances of very small size, such as water, are believed to pass into and out of the cell. The pore permeability varies under different conditions. Excess calcium in the extracellular fluid causes a decrease in membrane permeability; a decrease in calcium concentration causes increased membrane permeability (8, 19).

Regulation of Strontium Absorption Strontium-90, a *radioactive isotope* of strontium, occurs in the fallout from nuclear explosions. Strontium and calcium are similar in metabolic behavior and distribution in the body. More than 95 percent of both minerals is deposited in the bones and teeth. The body preferentially absorbs calcium and preferentially excretes strontium by

way of the kidney (6, 35). This discrimination helps safeguard the body against the accumulation of radioactive strontium. A metabolism study done in 1973 of adults showed that calcium does not reduce significantly the absorption of strontium-90 (31); these findings are contrary to the accepted metabolic relationship between calcium and strontium.

Absorption of Vitamin B-12 The presence of calcium is necessary for vitamin B-12 absorption from the intestine (for discussion see p. 247).

Calcium to Phosphorus Ratio

Bone loss is observed in adult experimental animals (mice, rats, dogs) when they are fed an excess of dietary phosphorus or an insufficiency of dietary calcium. Bone resorption occurs when the calcium to phosphorus (Ca:P) ratio is less than 2:1 (twice as much calcium as phosphorus in the ration) whether the calcium intake is high or low. Even though it is recognized that such findings cannot be applied directly to the human, concern is expressed that the customary adult diet, higher in phosphorus than calcium content, may be conducive to bone loss common in the aging. The Ca:P ratio of the food supply available for consumption has been 1:1.7 during this decade (the 1970s) and has been near that for a long time: 1:1.6 in 1935–1939 and 1:1.9 in 1909–1913 (21). The Committee on Dietary Allowances (25) noted that the usual recommendation for Ca:P ratio lies between 1:2.1 and 1:1.2.

A reassuring finding from a study with adults whose calcium intakes ranged from 200 to 2000 mg daily and phosphorus 800 mg and 2000 mg daily, was that increasing the phosphorus intake from 800 mg to 2000 mg daily with the calcium intake remaining constant did not diminish the absorption of calcium nor alter the calcium balances (30). In an earlier study (24), similar results were obtained. The calcium balances in young adults fed three levels of calcium (344,

267

944, and 1544 mg daily) and three levels of phosphorus (766, 1066, and 1366 mg daily) with Ca:P ratios varying from 2:1 to 1:1.4 were not changed by an increase in phosphorus intake at all dietary levels of calcium. These studies show that the Ca:P ratio in human adults, at least within the limits observed, is not of importance in the calcium balance.

Calcium Deficiency

Irwin and Kienholz (12) completed a thorough review of the literature on calcium needs of man in 1973 and concluded that it was difficult to find clear-cut symptoms of calcium deficiency. In the first Health and Nutrition Examination Survey (HANES) carried out in 1971–1972, the clinical test used to assess calcium status and detect deficiency was Chvostek's sign (contraction of the perioral muscles [around the mouth] on tapping the malar [cheek bone] process) (2). Contraction of the perioral muscles indicates a hyperirritability of the neuromuscular system due to calcium deficiency or calcium-phosphorus imbalance. Persons 12 to 17 years of age in the income group below the poverty level had the highest prevalence of positive Chvostek's sign (Negroes, 18.9 percent, and whites, 14.8 percent) among all age-sex and income groups. Women aged 18 to 44 years at both income levels also showed a high incidence of positive Chvostek's sign (Negroes, 15.1 percent, and whites, 13.0 percent). For all other groups the prevalence was considerably less.

As another part of HANES the dietary intake of calcium was determined and the findings evaluated by established standards of calcium intake expressed in mg per day (1). The HANES standards for dietary intake are presented in Appendix Table A-27. The diets of women age 18 years and older in both the above and below poverty levels failed to meet the standard for calcium intake. All other age-sex-race and income groups met the standards. The prevalence of Chvostek's sign and low dietary calcium were not always found in the same groups. In women, 18 to 44 years, however, both the clinical and dietary assessment indicated an inadequacy in calcium nutrition.

Bone Disorders   It is generally believed that the bone disorder osteomalacia may occur when there has been a low calcium intake; it sometimes afflicts women after repeated pregnancies or a long period of lactation. Osteomalacia is characterized by a deficiency of minerals in the bone matrix, which produces a softening of the bones. However, the primary cause of this disorder appears to be a vitamin D deficiency, which prevents the efficient use of available calcium.

Another disorder, osteoporosis, is characterized by a generalized decrease in total bone mass (18) and tends to occur in older persons. The condition occurs in 25 percent of white women and 6 percent of white men older than 60 years (28). There is evidence that osteoporosis is sometimes associated with a prolonged negative calcium balance, which may be due to a low calcium intake, malabsorption, or high urinary output. Since there may be other causes as well, calcium therapy is not always beneficial (12, 22). (See chapt. 21 for more information on osteoporosis).

Excessive Calcium Intake

Any useful effects of exceeding the RDA for calcium have not been observed, nor have any ill effects. High calcium intake appears not to be a causal factor in abnormal conditions such as high blood calcium in infancy, accretions of calcium in soft tissues, and kidney stones; however, low intake is a part of the therapy for those conditions (10).

Recommended Dietary Allowances for Calcium

The need for calcium is usually estimated by the calcium balance method; this procedure is similar to that which is used for nitrogen balance (see

Table 13.3 Recommended Dietary Allowances for Calcium

	Age, years	RDA mg	RDA mg/1000 kcal
Infants	0.0–0.5	360	—
	0.5–1.0	540	—
Children	1–3	800	615
	4–6	800	444
	7–10	800	333
Male	11–14	1200	428
	15–18	1200	400
	19–22	800	267
	23–50	800	296
	51+	800	333
Female	11–14	1200	500
	15–18	1200	571
	19–22	800	381
	23–50	800	400
	51+	800	444
Pregnant		1200	—
Lactating		1200	—

From *Recommended Dietary Allowances, Eighth Edition* (1974). Washington, D.C.: Natl. Acad. Sciences.

p. 92). For adults of all ages the Recommended Dietary Allowance for calcium is 800 mg (0.8 g) daily (25). The calcium needs for age and sex groups expressed as RDA and RDA per 1000 kcal are given in Table 13.3. The effect of protein intake on calcium balance was taken into consideration in establishing this recommendation. As protein intake increases, a greater amount of calcium is excreted in the urine. To maintain calcium equilibrium, adults who consume about the RDA for protein only need 500 mg of calcium per day. However, since most people in the United States eat more than the RDA for protein, a higher allowance for calcium was established (25).

Food Sources of Calcium

Milk and milk products are the best and most dependable sources of calcium. Without milk or milk products, it is difficult for the diet alone to provide the Recommended Dietary Allowance for calcium, but including them in reasonable amounts will probably assure an adequate intake. For older adolescents three cups of milk (or their equivalent), together with other foods, are usually enough to meet the daily allowance. For adults two cups of milk are enough. (For a discussion of filled milk and imitation milk, see chapt. 16.)

The calcium content of a variety of foods is given in Table 13.4. Green leafy vegetables—kale, mustard greens, and others (excluding members of the goosefoot family, such as spinach and chard, which contain oxalic acid)—rank next to dairy products as good sources of calcium. Broccoli is a good source; citrus fruits, soybeans, and other legumes are fair sources; meats, nuts, and grains are relatively poor sources (but the use of milk in bread and other baked goods will improve their calcium content).

Calcium in the United States' Food Supply

The amount of calcium in the food supply of the United States has increased during this century. The food supply contained about 816 mg of calcium per person per day in 1909–1913, 950 mg in 1967, and 940 mg in 1977 (21).

Sources of calcium in the American diet in 1977 were as follows: dairy products, 74.6 percent; vegetables, 7.4 percent; meat, fish, and poultry, 4.0 percent; flour and cereal products, 3.4 percent; dry beans, peas, and soya products, 2.9 percent; fruits, 2.2 percent; eggs, 2.2 percent; sugars and other sweeteners, 2.2 percent; and miscellaneous foods, 0.8 percent (21).

Meals served to students were collected for seven consecutive days at 50 colleges (in 31 states) and analyzed for various nutrients. The calcium content of the meals averaged 1216 mg per person per day with a range of 899 to 1531 mg (33). All colleges served meals with calcium content above the recommended allowance for young adults (Table 13.3).

269

Table 13.4 Calcium Content of Various Foods as Served

Food	Per 100 g of food — Calcium, mg	Per average serving — Size of serving, g	Per average serving — Calcium, mg
Cheese (Cheddar)	729	1 oz 28	204
Molasses, light	165	1 tbsp 20	33
Mustard greens, cooked	138	½ c 70	97
Ice cream	133	½ c 66	88
Kale (frozen), cooked	120	½ c 65	78
Milk, whole	119	1 c 244	291
Cream, light	93	1 tbsp 15	14
Broccoli, stalks, cooked	87	½ c 78	68
Bread (white, enriched)	86	1 sl 28	24
Bread (whole wheat)	86	1 sl 28	24
Cheese (cottage, creamed)	61	¼ c 56	34
Egg (medium)	56	1 50	28
Peanut butter	51	2 tbsp 32	18
Green beans, cooked	51	½ c 62	32
Orange	41	1 med 131	54
Peas, green, canned	26	½ c 85	22
Lima beans (frozen), cooked	20	½ c 85	17
Oatmeal, cooked	9	½ c 120	11
Potato, baked	9	1 med 156	14

From *Nutritive Value of Foods*, Home and Garden Bull. No. 72. Washington, D.C.: U.S. Dept. Agr., 1977.

Phosphorus (P)

Phosphorus, together with organic materials, forms structural units in every body cell and functions in almost every aspect of metabolism. Inorganic phosphorus and calcium comprise most of the mineral content of the bones and teeth. Phosphorus constitutes about 1 percent of the body weight and ranks after calcium as an abundant mineral element in the body. Because phosphorus is widely distributed in foods, the body's need is easily supplied. Phosphorus deficiency in man does not occur under normal circumstances. It is usually accorded less space than calcium, chiefly because phosphorus is easily supplied in the diet.

Metabolism of Phosphorus

In food, phosphorus is found in a variety of organic and inorganic compounds. Enzymatic action in the digestive tract frees the inorganic phosphorus from its organic combinations. It is absorbed from the small intestine (mainly in the upper part of the duodenum, because it is less alkaline), chiefly as inorganic phosphorus. Approximately 70 percent of the amount ingested is absorbed. Excretion takes place mainly through the kidneys; the amount excreted depends upon how much has been absorbed from the intestinal tract. Excretion is controlled by the parathyroid gland, which seems to be the main regulator of phosphorus homeostasis.

Functions of Phosphorus

Bone and Tooth Formation Calcification (mineralization) of the skeleton cannot take place unless enough phosphorus is available. Phosphorus combines with calcium to form a relatively insoluble compound that makes the bones and teeth strong and rigid. The phosphorus content of bone is about one-half that of calcium. Approximately 85 percent of the phosphorus in the body is in the mineralized bones and teeth. Phosphorus, like calcium, is needed for maintenance of the skeletal structure.

Constituent of Essential Body Compounds Phosphorus is found in nucleic acids in the nuclei of cells. It is a constituent of phospholipids found in cell membranes and also in the blood plasma and portions of the nervous system. The important compounds DNA and RNA contain phosphorus. By the process of *phosphorylation*, phosphorus-containing compounds are produced; sugars are phosphorylated, facilitating the absorption of glucose from the intestine and its passage through the cell membranes of the body; and vitamins such as pyridoxal that take part in enzyme systems must first be phosphorylated.

Storage and Release of Energy Organic phosphorus compounds play a role in the oxidative breakdown of carbohydrates, proteins, and fats and in the capture and transfer of chemical energy released during this process. One phosphorus-containing compound, adenosine triphosphate (ATP), serves as a link between processes that release and those that require energy. It is one of a group of compounds that contain "energy-rich" or "high-energy" phosphate bonds. In living cells there is a simultaneous breakdown of organic compounds with the release of energy and a synthesis of others that require energy. The energy-rich compounds play an essential part in bringing together the production of energy from foodstuffs and the utilization of that energy by the cell for its many functions (see p. 17).

Recommended Dietary Allowances for Phosphorus

It is recommended that an adult consume 800 mg of phosphorus daily, the same as for calcium (25). The phosphorus needs for age and sex groups expressed as RDA and RDA per 1000 kcal are given in Table 13.5.

Food Sources of Phosphorus

High-protein foods such as meat, poultry, fish, and eggs are excellent sources of phosphorus. Cereal grains (especially wheat germ and whole grains) provide a very good source. The high

Table 13.5 Recommended Dietary Allowances for Phosphorus

	Age, years	RDA mg	RDA mg/1000 kcal
Infants	0.0–0.5	240	—
	0.5–1.0	400	—
Children	1–3	800	615
	4–6	800	444
	7–10	800	333
Males	11–14	1200	428
	15–18	1200	400
	19–22	800	267
	23–50	800	296
	51+	800	333
Females	11–14	1200	500
	15–18	1200	571
	19–22	800	381
	23–50	800	400
	51+	800	444
Pregnant		1200	—
Lactating		1200	—

From *Recommended Dietary Allowances, Eighth Edition* (1974). Washington, D.C.: Natl. Acad. Sciences.

271

phosphorus content of whole-grain products, however, may be misleading because of the large amount of phytin phosphorus, which is not readily utilized by the body. Dried beans and peas contain appreciable amounts of phosphorus, and milk and dairy products are excellent sources. Vegetables and fruits as a whole, however, are rather low in phosphorus (see Table 13.6). A diet that has enough protein and calcium can be assumed to contain sufficient phosphorus. Data from the U.S. Department of Agriculture for 1977 show that generous amounts of phosphorus are available in the food supply for the American consumer—about 1.57 g per person per day (21), an amount that has been almost constant for two decades. Sources of phosphorus in the diet are: dairy products, 35.0 percent; meat, fish, and poultry, 28.5 percent; flour and cereal products, 12.2 percent; vegetables, 9.1 percent; dry beans, peas, nuts, and soya products, 6.1 percent; fruits, 1.8 percent; and other foods, 2.3 percent (21).

Meals served to students were collected for seven consecutive days at 50 colleges (in 31 states) and analyzed for various nutrients. The phosphorus content of the meals averaged 1725 mg per person per day with a range of 1153 to 2348 mg. All colleges served meals with a phosphorus content above the recommended allowance for young adults (Table 13.5) (33).

Table 13.6 Phosphorus Content of Various Foods as Served

Food	Per 100 g of food Phosphorus, mg	Per average serving Size of serving, g	Per average serving Phosphorus, mg
Liver, calf, fried[a]	537	3 oz	85	456
Cheese (Cheddar)	518	1 oz	28	145
Shredded wheat	388	1 biscuit	25	97
Bread (whole wheat)	254	1 sl	28	71
Haddock, fried	247	3 oz	85	210
Beef, round, lean, braised	268	3 oz	68	182
Egg, fried, medium	174	1	46	80
Ice cream, regular	102	½ c	66	67
Bread (white, enriched)	96	1 sl	28	27
Milk, whole	93	1 c	244	228
Baked beans, with pork and tomato	92	½ c	128	118
Corn, cooked, kernels	73	½ c	82	60
Oatmeal, cooked	57	½ c	120	68
Broccoli, frozen, cooked	56	⅔ c	123	69
Green beans, cooked	37	½ c	62	23
Orange (without peel)	20	1 med	131	26
Grapefruit (with peel)	8	½ med	241	19

[a] *Nutritive Value of American Foods*, Agr. Handbook No. 456. Washington, D.C.: U.S. Dept. Agr., 1975.
From *Nutritive Value of Foods*, Home and Garden Bull. No. 72. Washington, D.C.: U.S. Dept. Agr., 1977.

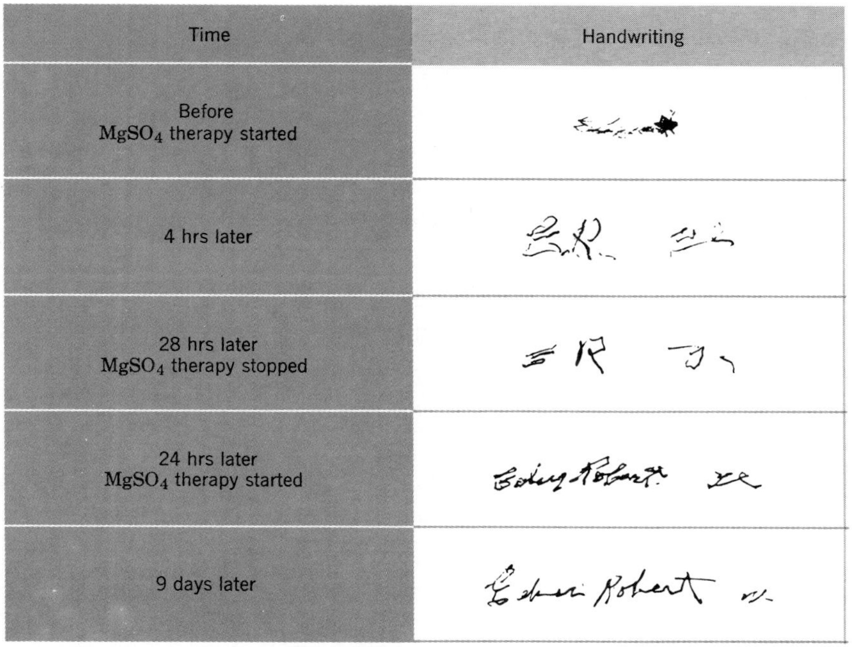

Time	Handwriting
Before MgSO$_4$ therapy started	
4 hrs later	
28 hrs later MgSO$_4$ therapy stopped	
24 hrs later MgSO$_4$ therapy started	
9 days later	

Fig. 13.4 Samples of handwriting obtained from a patient with low serum magnesium levels at various times as indicated. Part of the name has been obliterated. (Courtesy Flink, E. B., et al (1954). Magnesium deficiency after prolonged parenteral fluid administration and after chronic alcoholism complicated by delirium tremens, *J. Lab. Clin. Med.* 43: 169.)

Magnesium (Mg)

The adult human body contains about 20 to 25 g of magnesium; about one-half of it is concentrated in the bones and the remainder is in the soft tissues (primarily the muscles and liver) and extracellular fluids (10). The magnesium in the bones is not readily available to the body cells.

Metabolism of Magnesium

Absorption and Excretion Magnesium is absorbed in the small intestine. Because the salts of magnesium are sparingly soluble, only about one-third of the amount ingested is absorbed (8). It is the relative insolubility of magnesium sulfate that makes it a laxative when taken in large amounts; it brings about an increase in osmotic pressure, which draws water into the intestine.

Magnesium and calcium are absorbed from the intestinal tract by a common pathway; a low intake of either one will increase the absorption of the other. Unlike calcium, however, magnesium is not excreted from the bloodstream into the intestine; the magnesium in the feces has merely not been absorbed. Most of the excretion of magnesium is by way of the feces.

Blood Magnesium The blood magnesium level remains fairly constant over a wide range of intakes because of the intestinal and renal conservation when the intake is low and the increased renal excretion when the intake is high (2). Unlike for calcium, there are no hormones to regulate the serum level of magnesium.

273

Functions of Magnesium

Magnesium is mainly an activator of certain peptidases, certain enzymes in carbohydrate metabolism (see Table 13.2), and enzymes that split and transfer phosphate groups (among them the phosphatases and the enzymes that are involved in ATP reactions). Because ATP is necessary for many reactions in the body, magnesium plays an important, but indirect, role in the body's anabolic and catabolic processes. It also is involved in protein synthesis through its roles in binding messenger RNA to ribosomes and in the synthesis and degradation of DNA (9). Magnesium is important in neuromuscular transmission; at some points it functions cooperatively with calcium, at others antagonistically (13).

Magnesium Deficiency

A study of magnesium deficiency induced by a limited dietary intake in normal adult volunteers gave an opportunity to observe deficiency symptoms uncomplicated by disease conditions. Symptoms have been observed in the human but in conjunction with abnormal states — chronic alcoholism with malnutrition, acute or chronic renal disease (involving dysfunction of the tubules), childhood malnutrition disorders of the parathyroid gland, prolonged *parenteral fluid administration,* and other conditions (9, 13). In experimental magnesium deficiency there was observed: a drop in magnesium blood level, and also in urinary and fecal excretions; a drop in calcium blood level, despite an adequate intake, normal absorption, and a drop in urinary excretion. Most (six of the seven subjects) developed low blood potassium. Neurological signs occurred in five of the seven, as did anorexia, nausea, and apathy. Spontaneous generalized muscle spasms and tremors were observed; personality changes developed. Normality was restored with the reinstitution of a magnesium-containing diet (Fig. 13.4). Shils (11, 12), whose study it was, concluded that magnesium is es-

sential for the normal metabolism of potassium and calcium and for the mobilization of calcium from bone, and that the signs and symptoms observed are associated with complex electrolyte changes that take place in magnesium deficiency.

Recommended Dietary Allowances and Food Sources of Magnesium

The RDA for men is 350 mg per day and for women 300 mg per day. These recommendations were based upon magnesium balance studies (1, 3, 5, 6, 7). The magnesium needs for age and sex groups expressed as RDA and RDA per 1000 kcal are given in Table 13.7.

Some excellent sources of magnesium are green leafy vegetables, nuts, soybeans, and snails (6); meat also is a good source. The magnesium content

Table 13.7 Recommended Dietary Allowances for Magnesium

	Age, years	RDA mg	RDA mg/1000 kcal
Infants	0.0–0.5	60	—
	0.5–1.0	70	—
Children	1–3	150	115
	4–6	200	111
	7–10	250	104
Males	11–14	350	125
	15–18	400	133
	19–22	350	117
	23–50	350	130
	51+	350	146
Females	11–14	300	125
	15–18	300	143
	19–22	300	143
	23–50	300	150
	51+	300	167
Pregnant		450	—
Lactating		450	—

From *Recommended Dietary Allowances, Eighth Edition* (1974). Washington, D.C.: Natl. Acad. Science.

Table 13.8 Magnesium Content of Various Foods

Food	Magnesium, mg/100 g	Food	Magnesium, mg/100 g
Apple, raw,	0.035	Orange juice, frozen,	
Baked beans	0.2	reconstituted	8.2
Beef, uncooked, ground	<0.02	Potato, fresh, uncooked	14.0
Bread (white, enriched)	0.25	Peanut butter	172.0
Cheese (American)	<0.4	Sugar, brown	62.0
Eggs, whole	<0.02	white	<1.0
Flour, bleached, enriched	0.4	Tomato, fresh	4.3
Ice cream (vanilla)	<0.01	Tunafish, canned	
Milk, whole	<0.01	(without salt)	23.0

From A. Gormican, Inorganic elements in foods used in hospital menus. (Copyright ©, The American Dietetic Association. Reprinted by permission from *J. Am. Dietet. Assoc.*, **56**: 397, 1970.)

of a variety of foods is presented in Table 13.8. The ordinary American diet has been estimated to contain about 120 mg of magnesium per 1000 kcal of food (4). Meals served to students at 50 colleges were found to contain less magnesium than the recommended allowance. The average amount in the meals was 251 mg per person per day (14).

Sulfur (S)

Sulfur is found in every cell of the body. It is present in the sulfur-containing amino acids (methionine, cystine, and cysteine); in the vitamins thiamin and biotin; and in body compounds including coenzyme A and insulin.

Daily Need for and Food Sources of Sulfur

Because symptoms of a dietary deficiency have never been observed in human beings, man's need for sulfur, if there is one, is not known. Sulfur is an integral part of protein nutrition; if there is a requirement for this mineral, it is probably related to that of protein.

Sulfur is found in generous amounts in wheat germ, lentils, cheese, lean beef, kidney beans, peanuts, and clams. The major source of sulfur in the diet appears to be the amino acid cysteine.

Summary

The mineral elements, also referred to as inorganic or ash constituents, comprise about 4 percent of the total body weight. There are 14 different mineral elements known to be essential for the human.

Calcium, one of the essential minerals, is present in the body in a greater amount than any other mineral. It has two important functions: one, the building of bones and teeth, and the other, body regulating functions, including a role in the transmission of nerve impulses, muscle contraction and relaxation, blood clot formation, regulation of the permeability of cell membranes, and absorption of vitamin B-12. The absorption of calcium is more efficient when the need is greater; vitamin D and lactose improve absorption. Oxalic acid, phytic acid, and fiber present in foods may interfere with absorption. Blood calcium is main-

275

tained at the normal level by two hormones— the parathyroid hormone, which stimulates the release of calcium from its storage place in the bone, and calcitonin, which inhibits the release of calcium from bone. The urinary excretion of calcium is fairly constant within an individual but varies widely among individuals. The level of dietary protein has a notable effect on urinary calcium excretion; increasing the protein intake increases the calcium excretion.

The HANES results on the prevalence of calcium deficiency using the Chvostek's sign as the criterion showed persons 12 to 17 years of age, in the below-poverty group, to have the highest incidence of positive Chvostek's sign of all groups. Women aged 18 to 44 years of both income levels followed next. For all other groups the prevalence was rather limited. The diets of women 18 years and older in both income groups failed to meet the intake used as standard in this survey (600 mg daily). All other age-sex groups met the respective standards established.

The RDA for calcium is 800 mg daily for all adults. Good food sources of calcium are dairy products and green leafy vegetables.

Phosphorus constitutes about 1 percent of the body weight and ranks after calcium as an abundant mineral in the body; approximately 85 percent is in the bones and teeth. Phosphorus is a component in many of the essential body compounds, including nucleic acid in the nuclei of cells, phospholipids in cell membranes, blood plasma, and parts of the nervous system, in DNA and RNA, and many more compounds. Phosphorus functions in the maintenance of acid-base balance and plays a role in the oxidative breakdown of carbohydrates, proteins, and fats and in the capture and transfer of chemical energy released in this process.

The RDA for phosphorus is the same as for calcium (800 mg daily). Phosphorus is distributed widely in foods; it is found in meats, dairy products, cereals, and legumes.

The amount of magnesium in the adult human body is about 20 to 25 g; about one-half of the magnesium is in the bones, the remainder is in the soft tissues and extracellular fluid. Magnesium functions chiefly as an activator of certain enzymes (the peptidases and enzymes that split and transfer phosphate groups).

Sulfur is found in every cell in the body. The sulfur-containing amino acids, the vitamins thiamin and biotin, insulin, and coenzyme A are all important sulfur-containing compounds. Sulfur deficiency has never been observed in the human.

Glossary

acetylcholine: a chemical compound normally present in many parts of the body; essential to the conveying of nerve impulses.

actin: a major protein in voluntary muscle.

action potential: the electrical energy of a stimulated membrane, produced by the flow of ions across the membrane with the change in its permeability on stimulation.

activate: to render a substance, such as an inactive compound, capable of exerting its proper effect.

biocarbonate ion: the prefix "bi" indicates the presence of hydrogen; the bicarbonate ion is ($^-HCO_3$).

blood cells: also known as corpuscles; include red blood cells (erythrocytes) and white blood cells (leukocytes).

bone, cancellous (or spongy): a porous type of bone located at the end of the long bones, surrounded by compact bone.

bone, compact: a dense type of bone; forms the outer layer of the long bones (bones of the arms, legs, and clavicele) surrounding the marrow in the shaft and the spongy bone at the end of the bone.

calcitonin: hormone formed by the thyroid gland that lowers the blood calcium levels; elevated plasma calcium stimulates its secretion.

catalyze: to accelerate the rate of a chemical reaction through the action of an element or compound (a catalyst) that remains unchanged during the reaction or is regenerated to its original form at the end of the reaction.

cementum: calcified tissue covering the root of a tooth.

cofactor: a nonprotein component that may be required by an enzyme for its activity.

dentin: the chief substance of the tooth, which surrounds the tooth pulp and is covered by enamel on the exposed part of the tooth (crown) and by cementum on the roots.

electrolyte: compound that, when dissolved in water, separates into charged ions capable of conducting an electric current. For example, NaCl dissociates into the ions Na^+ and Cl^-.

enamel: the calcified tissue covering the crown of a tooth.

endogenous: produced within the organism.

fibrinogen: a protein in blood that through the action of the enzyme thrombin is converted to fibrin (the insoluble protein essential to the clotting of blood).

fluid: liquid.

monovalent: having a valence (the power of an atom to combine with another atom) of one. The valence of the hydrogen atom is one. Sodium (Na^+) has a valence of one; it combines with chloride (Cl^-) to form sodium chloride (NaCl).

myosin: one of the two main proteins of muscle; involved with actin in the contraction of muscle fibers.

parathyroid hormone: see page 96.

parenteral fluid administration: see page 96.

periodontal membrane: provides the connection between the root of the tooth and its socket in the bone.

phosphorylation: see page 19.

prothrombin activator: a complex substance that splits prothrombin (present in blood) to form thrombin, an essential step in the clotting process. When tissue is injured it releases two factors (tissue factor and tissue phospholipids) that initiate the formation of prothrombin activator; or within the circulatory system, injury to the blood can initiate the formation of the prothrombin factor.

radioactive isotope: see page 11.

sarcoplasmic reticulum: a network of smooth-surfaced tubules surrounding the myofibrils (small, contractile, threadlike structures within the cytoplasm of a muscle fiber) of a muscle, such as a skeletal or a cardiac muscle.

semipermeable membrane: a membrane that allows the passage of only certain solids but is freely permeable to water.

thrombin: an enzyme that catalyzes the conversion of fibrinogen to fibrin.

trabeculae: calcified portion of spongy bone.

troponin: one of the minor proteins in muscle; myosin and actin make up about 80 percent of the proteins involved in the contraction process.

Study Questions and Activities

1. Identify the main locations of calcium in the body and relate location to function.
2. Identify the factors that increase and decrease calcium absorption.
3. Define or explain the following: bone trabeculae, osteoporosis, calcium oxalate, phytic acid, labile calcium.
4. What factors affect one's requirement for calcium?
5. Plan a menu for an individual for two days that will provide 800 mg of calcium each day.
6. Discuss some of the functions of phosphorus in the body.
7. Did you consume the recommended amount of calcium and phosphorus yesterday?
8. What would you say to an adult who told you: "I don't drink milk because I associate it with infancy and childhood"?
9. Name three good food sources of magnesium.

References

Introduction to Minerals, Calcium, and Phosphorus

1. Abraham, S., M. D. Carroll, C. M. Dresser, and C. L. Johnson (1977). *Dietary Intake Findings, United States, 1971–1974*. Washington, D.C.: U.S. Dept. Health, Educ. and Welfare; Natl. Center for Health Statistics.

2. Abraham, S., F. W. Lowenstein, and D. E. O'Connell (1975). *Anthropometric and Clinical Findings*. First Health and Nutrition Examination Survey, United States, 1971–72. Rockville, Md.: U.S. Dept. Health, Educ. and Welfare, Natl. Center for Health Statistics.

3. Banks, P., W. Bartley, and L. M. Birt (1976). *The Biochemistry of the Tissues*. 2nd ed. New York: John Wiley and Sons, p. 340.

4. Bonner, P., F. C. Hummel, M. F. Bates, J. Horton, H. A. Hunscher, and I. G. Macy (1938). The influence of a daily serving of spinach or its equivalent in oxalic acid upon the mineral utilization of children. *J. Pediatrics*, **12:** 188.

5. Brudevald, F. (1962). Chemical composition of the teeth in relation to caries. In *Chemistry and Prevention of Dental Caries*, edited by R. F. Sognnaes. Springfield, Ill.: Charles C Thomas, p. 12.

6. Comar, C. L. and J. C. Thompson, Jr. (1973). Radioactivity in foods. In *Modern Nutrition in Health and Disease*, 5th ed., edited by R. S. Goodhart and M. E. Shils. Philadelphia: Lea and Febiger, p. 442.

7. Endo, M. (1977). Calcium release from the sarcoplasmic reticulum. *Physiol. Rev.*, **57:** 71.

8. Guyton, A. C. (1976). *A Textbook of Physiology*. 5th ed. Philadelphia: W. B. Saunders Co., p. 101.

9. Harrison, H. E. (1976). Phosphorus. In *Present Knowledge in Nutrition*, 4th ed., edited by D. M. Hegsted, Chm., and Editorial Committee. Washington, D.C.: The Nutrition Foundation, Inc.

10. Hegsted, D. M. (1973). Calcium and phosphorus. In *Modern Nutrition in Health and Disease*, 5th ed., edited by R. S. Goodhart and M. E. Shils. Philadelphia: Lea and Febiger, p. 268.

11. Irving, J. T. (1973). *Calcium and Phosphorus Metabolism*. New York: Academic Press, p. 34.

12. Irwin, M. I. and E. W. Kienholz (1973). A conspectus of research on calcium requirements of man. *J. Nutrition*, **103:** 1019.

13. Johnson, N. E., E. N. Alcantra, and H. M. Linksweiler (1970). Effect of level of protein intake on urinary and fecal calcium and calcium retention of young adult males. *J. Nutrition*, **100:** 1425.

14. Kobayashi, A., S. Kawai, Y. Ohbe, and Y. Nagashima (1975). Effects of dietary lactose and a lactase preparation on the intestinal absorption of calcium and magnesium in normal infants. *Am. J. Clin. Nutrition*, **28:** 681.

15. Kocian, J., I. Skala, and K. Bakos (1973). Calcium absorption from milk and lactose-free milk in healthy subjects and patients with lactose intolerance. *Digestion*, **9:** 317.

16. Lehninger, A. L. (1975). *Biochemistry*. 2nd ed. New York: Worth Publishers, p. 185.

17. Li, T.-K. and B. L. Vallee (1973). The biochemical and nutritional role of trace elements. In *Modern Nutrition in Health and Disease*, 5th ed., edited by R. S. Goodhart and M. E. Shils. Philadelphia: Lea and Febiger, p. 375.

18. Linkswiler, H. M. (1976). Calcium. In *Present Knowledge in Nutrition*, 4th ed., edited by D. M. Hegsted, Chm., and Editorial Committee. Washington, D.C.: The Nutrition Foundation, Inc., p. 232.

19. Manery, J. F. (1969). Calcium and membranes. In *Mineral Metabolism, vol. 3, Calcium Physiology*, edited by C. L. Comar and F. Bronner. New York: Academic Press, p. 405.

20. Margen, S., J.-Y. Chu, N. A. Kaufmann, and D. H. Calloway (1974). Studies in calcium metabolism. I. The calciuretic effect of dietary protein. *Am. J. Clin. Nutrition*, **27:** 584.

21. Marston, R. and B. Friend (1978). Nutrient content of the national food supply. *National Food Situation*, NFR 1, January, p. 13.

22. McLean, F. C. and M. R. Urist (1968). *Bone*. 3rd ed. Chicago: Univ. of Chicago Press, p. 245.

23. Nizel, A. E. (1972). *Nutrition in Preventive Dentistry: Science and Practice*. Philadelphia: W. B. Saunders, p. 8.

24. Patton, M. B., E. D. Wilson, J. M. Leichsenring, L. M. Norris, and C. M. Dienhart (1953). The relation of calcium-to-phosphorus ratio to the utilization of those minerals by 18 young college women. *J. Nutrition*, **50:** 373.

25. *Recommended Dietary Allowances, Eighth Edition* (1974). Washington, D.C.: National Research Council.

26. Reinhold, J. G., B. Faradji, P. Abadi, and F. Ismail-

Beigi (1976). Decreased absorption of calcium, magnesium, zinc, and phosphorus by humans due to increased fiber and phosphorus consumption as wheat bread. *J. Nutrition,* **106**: 493.

27. Schwartz, I. L. and G. J. Siegel (1973). Excitation, conduction, and transmission of the nerve impulse. In *Best and Taylor's Physiological Basis of Medical Practice,* 9th ed., edited by J. R. Brobeck. Baltimore: Williams & Wilkins Co., pp. 1–49.

28. Shapiro, J. R., W. T. Moore, H. Jorgensen, J. Reid, E. E. Epps, and D. Whedon (1975). Osteoporosis. *Arch. Int. Med.,* **135**: 563.

29. Shaw, J. H. and E. A. Sweeney (1973). Nutrition in relation to dental medicine. In *Modern Nutrition in Health and Disease,* 5th ed., edited by R. S. Goodhart and M. E. Shils. Philadelphia: Lea and Febiger, p. 733.

30. Spencer, H., L. Kramer, and C. Norris (1975). Calcium absorption and balance during high phosphorus intake in man. *Federation Proc.,* **34**: 888.

31. Spencer, H., L. Kramer, J. Samachson, E. P. Hardy, Jr., and J. Rivera (1973). Strontium-90 calcium interrelationships in man. *Health Physics,* **24**: 525.

32. Szent-Gyorgi, A. G. (1975). Calcium regulation of muscle contraction. *Biophysical J.,* **15**: 707.

33. Walker, M. A., and L. Page (1977). Nutritive content of college meals. *J. Am. Dietet. Assoc.,* **70**: 260.

34. Walser, M. (1969). Renal excretion of alkaline earths. In *Mineral Metabolism, vol. 3, Calcium Physiology,* edited by C. L. Comar and F. Bronner. New York: Academic Press, p. 235.

35. Wasserman, R. H., E. M. Romney, M. W. Skovgstad, and R. Siever (1977). *Strontium.* In *Geochemistry and the Environment, Vol. II. The Relation of Other Selected Trace Elements to Health and Disease.* Washington, D.C.: National Academy Sciences, p. 73.

36. Widdowson, E. M., and J. W. T. Dickerson (1964). Chemical composition of the body. In *Mineral Metabolism, vol. 2, The Elements, Part A,* edited by C. L. Comar and F. Bronner. New York: Academic Press, p. 9.

Magnesium and Sulfur

1. Hathaway, M. L. (1962). *Magnesium in Human Nutrition.* Home Econ. Res. Rept. No. 19. Washington, D.C.: U.S. Dept. Agr.

2. Heaton, F. W. (1969). The kidney and magnesium homeostasis. *Ann. N.Y. Acad. Sci.,* **162**: 775.

3. Leverton, R. M., J. M. Leichsenring, H. Linkswiler, and F. Meyer (1961). Magnesium requirement of young women receiving controlled intakes. *J. Nutrition,* **74**: 33.

4. Manalo, R., R. E. Flora, and J. E. Jones (1967). A simple method for estimating dietary magnesium. *Am. J. Clin. Nutrition,* **20**: 627.

5. McKey, B. V., F. M. LaFont, G. L. Borchers, D. A. Navarrete, and J. O. Holmes (1962). Magnesium studies in adult men. *Federation Proc.,* **21**: 310.

6. Nelson, G. Y. and M. R. Gram (1961). Magnesium content of accessory foods. *J. Am. Dietet. Assoc.,* **38**: 437.

7. *Recommended Dietary Allowances, Eighth Edition* (1974). Washington, D.C.: National Research Council.

8. Seelig, M. S. (1964). The requirements of magnesium by the normal adult. Summary and analysis of the published data. *Am. J. Clin. Nutrition,* **14**: 342.

9. Shils, M. E. (1976). Magnesium. In *Present Knowledge in Nutrition,* 4th ed., edited by D. M. Hegsted, Chm., and Editorial Committee. Washington, D.C.: The Nutrition Foundation, Inc., p. 247.

10. Shils, M. E. (1973). Magnesium. In *Modern Nutrition in Health and Disease,* 5th ed., edited by R. S. Goodhart and M. E. Shils. Philadelphia: Lea and Febiger, p. 287.

11. Shils, M. E. (1969). Experimental human magnesium depletion. *Medicine* (Baltimore), **48**: 61.

12. Shils, M. E. (1964). Experimental human magnesium depletion. I. Clinical observations and blood chemistry alterations. *Am. J. Clin. Nutrition,* **15**: 133.

13. Wacker, W. E. C. and A. F. Parisi (1968). Magnesium metabolism. *New Engl. J. Med.,* **278**: 712.

14. Walker, M. A. and L. Page (1977). Nutritive content of college meals. *J. Am. Dietet. Assoc.,* **70**: 260.

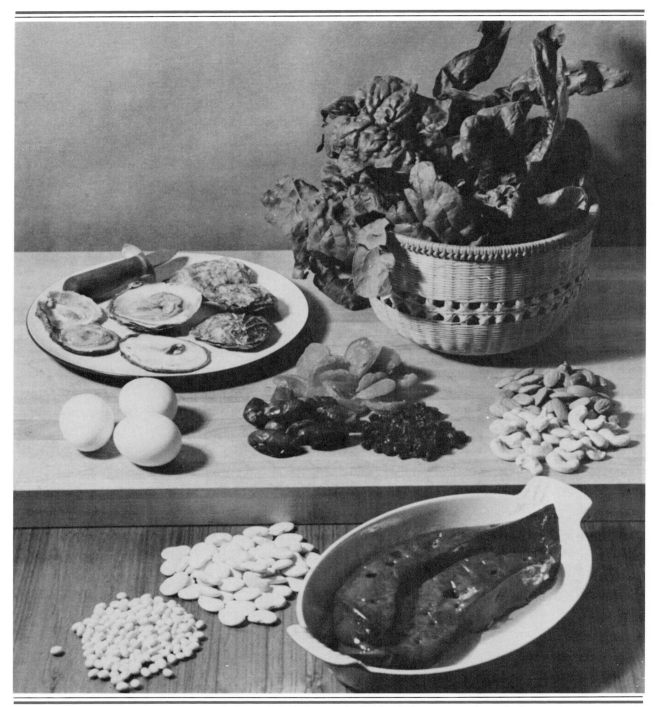

Iron, which is supplied in high quantity by all of these foods (oysters, spinach, eggs, dried apricots, dates, raisins, almonds, cashews, lima beans, navy beans, and liver), is required to form hemoglobin, which enables the blood to transport oxygen throughout the body.

Chapter 14

The Microminerals

Abbreviations

Acetyl CoA: acetyl coenzyme A
ATP: adenosine triphosphate
CHOL: cholesterol
DIT: diiodotyrosine
DMF: decayed, missing, filled
DNA: deoxyribonucleic acid
GT: glucose tolerance
GTF: glucose tolerance factor
HANES: Health and Nutrition Examination
   Survey, United States

MIT: monoiodotyrosine
NAF: sodium fluoride
PBI: protein-bound iodine
RBC: red blood cells
RDA: Recommended Dietary Allowances
RNA: ribonucleic acid
T_4: tetraiodothyronine
T_3: triiodothyronine
TSH: thyroid-stimulating hormone
ppm: parts per million

Iron

The iron content of the body is relatively small: for women it is about 25 mg per kg of body weight, and for men about 35 mg per kg. Men tend to have greater iron stores than women.

Metabolism of Iron

The iron used in the body comes from three sources: that salvaged from the breakdown of hemoglobin, that released from stores in the body, and that absorbed from the gastrointestinal tract. Of these three sources, the destruction (hemolysis) of red cells normally contributes the largest amount. In a normal man about 20 to 25 mg of iron per day comes from that source, whereas only about 1 mg comes directly from food.

Absorption Conditions influencing the absorption of iron are many; they may be classified roughly as physiological factors and factors affecting the availability of iron in food eaten (6). The amount of iron in the body is regulated by the amount absorbed. In the case of most nutrients, excesses can be excreted; with iron, excretion is limited—control rests in absorption (32).

Physiological Factors. Under normal conditions in adults, absorption and excretion are in equilibrium, amounting to about 0.5 to 2.0 mg of iron daily. Most of the absorption takes place in the duodenum and upper small intestines (13). The body conserves its iron, reusing it rather than excreting it.

There has been much speculation as to the role of the intestinal mucosa in controlling absorption of iron. The movement of iron across the intestinal mucosa begins with its entrance into the outer border *(brush border)* of the cells, an energy-dependent process. Part of the iron then attaches to a *plasma* protein (*transferrin,* which has a specific property of binding iron) and is transported into the blood. The remaining iron, retained in the mucosal cells, is returned to the lumen of the intestine with the cells as they are sloughed off (28).

Two major factors enter into the control of iron absorption: the status of body stores of iron and the rate of red cell formation *(erythropoiesis).* Decreased stores are associated with increased iron absorption and vice versa. Women have a lower store of iron than do men and a higher rate of absorption (Table 14.1). During pregnancy and in anemias (due to a deficiency of iron), conditions in which the need for iron is greater, the absorp-

282

Table 14.1 Iron Absorption and Bodily Distribution in Healthy Young Adult
Men and Women

Component	Men, 70 kg	Women, 58 kg
Dietary iron, mg/day		
RDA	10	18
Actual intake	16	11
Absorbed iron	0.9 (6 percent)	1.3 (12 percent)
Body iron, mg/person		
Total	3,450	2,450
Hemoglobin	2,100	1,750
Tissue	350	300
Storage	1,000	400
Serum ferritin	0.3	0.1

From H. N. Munro, Iron absorption and nutrition. Reprinted from *Federation Proc.*, **36:** 2015 (1977).

tion is greater than in nonpregnant women and in persons of normal iron status.

When the formation of red cells increases, the absorption of iron increases. When one ascends to a higher altitude with the accompanying increase in red cell formation, absorption increases. Blood loss through *hemorrhage* or a blood donation increases erythropoiesis and absorption (26). The mechanism whereby the mucosal cell responds to the status of iron stores and rate of erythropoiesis to divide the iron between that to be absorbed into the blood and that to remain in the cell to be returned to the intestine has not been discovered.

Factors Affecting Iron Availability. Iron is absorbed in two forms: *heme* and *nonheme* iron (4, 13, 26). Heme iron (found in meat, fish, and poultry) is highly available and not affected by the composition of the diet; nonheme iron (found in cereals and vegetables) is much less *available*, and its absorption is greatly influenced by dietary composition (13). Because it enters the mucosal cell as an intact *porphyrin* complex, heme iron is protected from the influence of dietary components.

The absorption of heme and nonheme iron can be measured quantitatively by using separate extrinsic *radioiron tags* (4). In studies with young men (using the radioiron tag method) whose daily iron intake from diets typical for them was 17.4 mg (1 mg of which was heme iron and the remainder nonheme iron), the absorption of heme iron averaged 37 percent and of nonheme iron, 5.3 percent (4). In another investigation, the absorption of heme and nonheme iron from a meal of various foods (containing a total of 4.5 mg iron, 1.5 mg of which was heme iron) was 27 percent and 6 percent, respectively (24). The poor absorption of nonheme iron is obvious in these results.

The major source of iron for the greater share of the population is nonheme iron. Means of enhancing its absorption is actually a necessity for combating iron deficiency *anemia*. Meats (beef, veal, pork, fish, and poultry) improve the absorption of nonheme iron; dairy products (eggs, milk, and cheese) do not. To illustrate, when dairy products were substituted for beef in a meal of lean beef, corn meal, potatoes, bread, margarine, peaches, and ice milk, absorption decreased by 60 to 80 percent (8). Where beef, lamb, pork, liver, fish, or chicken was substituted for *ovalbumin* in a semisynthetic meal of dextrimaltose (as carbohydrate), corn oil (as fat), and ovalbumin

283

(as protein), iron absorption increased two to four times.

Vitamin C increases the absorption of nonheme iron by reducing the ferric form (Fe^{+++}), which occurs commonly in foods, to the more soluble and better absorbed ferrous form (Fe^{++}). Two studies are cited to show the effect of vitamin C on absorption: in one, 60 mg of vitamin C was added to a rice diet and absorption of iron more than tripled; in another, 150 g papaya (66 mg vitamin C) was added to maize with an increase in iron absorption of more than five times (26). To determine the effect of different amounts of vitamin C on iron absorption, a range of intakes varying from 25 to 1000 mg daily was given to male adults consuming a semisynthetic diet. At the 25 mg level, the absorption was 1.65 times greater than with no supplement, and at the other extreme, at the 1000 mg level, the absorption was 9.57 times greater. An important observation is that for vitamin C to influence iron absorption it must be fed simultaneously with the meal (9).

Two foods that interfere with iron absorption are bran and tea. The addition of bran to rolls made from ferrous sulfate-enriched flour reduced significantly iron absorption in a study of young men: with the addition of 1.7 percent bran, absorption was reduced about 20 percent; with the addition of 10 percent bran, absorption was reduced about 50 percent (3). The two components of bran that are implicated in interfering with iron absorption are fiber (9 to 12 percent) and *phytate* (around 4 percent). There are *in vitro* studies on the mineral binding capacity of fiber (35) and balance studies with animals on the influence of fiber and of phytate on absorption (31, 35, 37). However, few studies have been done with humans, and the laboratory and animal findings cannot be extrapolated to the human. Preliminary studies indicate that about one-half the iron in whole wheat is monoferric phytate, a soluble compound of high availability (evaluated in animal studies) (31), which would tend to indicate that phytate is not the interfering factor in bran. Further support for fiber being suspect of

causing the interference comes from preliminary findings from balance studies in which two young men consumed with their food 10 g cellulose (100 percent fiber) daily for 14 days in the form of filter paper dispersed in applesauce; a significant decrease in the absorption of iron occurred (35). Further studies with the human are needed before a definitive explanation can be made for the interference of bran with iron absorption.

Drinking tannin-containing beverages, such as tea, with meals that consist largely of vegetable foods causes a decrease in iron absorption. Tea inhibits the absorption of nonheme iron to a notable extent, as was seen when tea was taken with iron salts, or with bread, or a rice meal (11).

There are other factors that affect iron absorption but which are not sufficiently well-defined for the human to be included in this discussion.

In conclusion, it must be said that knowledge of the iron content of a diet may be a relatively poor indicator of nutritional "adequacy" or "inadequacy." The availability of the iron in the food combination in which it is consumed is equally important.

Transport Approximately 3 to 4 mg of iron circulates in the blood plasma, accounting for 0.2 percent of the total iron in the blood. Iron is transported in the blood by the iron-binding protein transferrin. Transferrin delivers iron to the bone marrow for incorporation in new hemoglobin molecules, to other tissues requiring iron, and to the storage depots. The level of transferrin is quite constant from day to day; its level increases with iron depletion.

Storage A good index of iron stores in healthy persons is the concentration of *ferritin* in the blood. The range for adults is between 12 and 300 μg/L; in patients with iron deficiency anemia, the concentration is 12 μg/L; and in patients with iron overload, it may be as high as 10,000 μg/L (22). During pregnancy blood ferritin falls to an iron-deficient level at 30 weeks and remains

284

there until term unless supplemental iron is given. A quantitative estimate has been made that 1 μg/L of blood ferritin is equivalent to 8 mg storage iron (41). The storage reserve in men is about 0.5 to 1.5 g and in women about 0.3 to 1.0 g; in iron-deficiency anemia, there is no storage iron (Fig. 14.1). Iron is stored chiefly in the liver, spleen, and bone marrow (Fig. 14.2). When the ferritin storage capacity is fully utilized, iron accumulates as *hemosiderin*. By weight the iron content of hemosiderin is around 25 to 30 percent and may be as much as 37 percent; the iron content of ferritin is around 23 percent (12). Both ferritin and hemosiderin can be mobilized when the need for iron arises.

Excretion Once iron enters the bloodstream, it tends to be used and reused. Only about 0.3 to 0.5 mg of iron is excreted daily in the feces, which comes from blood loss into the intestine and desquamated intestinal mucosal cells. In addition

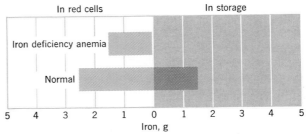

Fig. 14.1 **Relative distribution of iron between RBCs and storage in normal and iron-deficient persons. (From Wallerstein, R. O., 1977. Marrow iron. J. Am. Med. Assoc., 238: 1661. Copyright © 1977, American Medical Association.**

there is in the feces the unabsorbed food iron. Less than 0.1 mg of iron is ordinarily excreted in the urine per day (5).

The only way in which significant amounts of iron leave the body after absorption into the bloodstream is through loss of blood due to blood

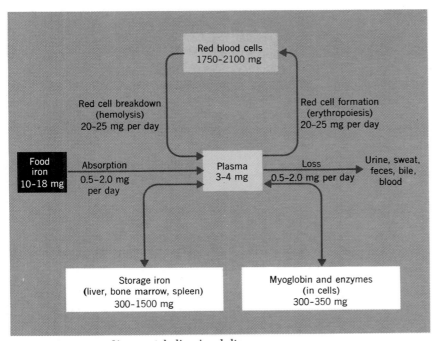

Fig. 14.2 Summary of iron metabolism in adults.

donations, abnormal hemorrhage resulting from accidents or illness, and menstruation. A donation of 500 ml of iron four times per year is enough to raise the daily iron requirement of the male donor from less than 1 mg to between 3 and 4 mg. Menstruation can produce a large loss of iron. Hallberg and co-workers reported that the mean menstrual loss of iron amounts to about 0.5 mg per day (18, 20). However, about 5 percent of the women in the Hallberg study lost more than 1.4 mg per day. These aspects of iron metabolism are summarized graphically in Fig. 14.2.

Functions of Iron in the Body

In the Red Cells of the Blood Most of the iron in the blood is located in the *red cells* (erythrocytes); it is found there in hemoglobin, a compound made up of an iron-containing pigment (heme) and a protein (globin). The location of iron in the body is shown in Table 14.1. There are four atoms of iron in a molecule of hemoglobin (Fig. 14.3). Even though iron constitutes less than

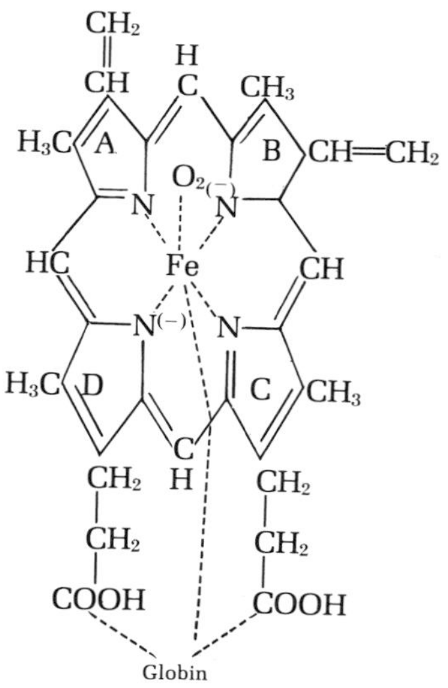

Fig. 14.3 Heme with molecule of globin. Hemoglobin is formed of four heme molecules and the protein globin.

1 percent of the hemoglobin molecule, it is the essential component. Erythrocyte formation (erythropoiesis) takes place in the bone marrow. In the early stage of development, the erythrocytes are large, contain a nucleus, and have little or no hemoglobin. The mature erythrocyte has no nucleus and is essentially hemoglobin. Because the red cell cannot produce the materials necessary for its continued existence, its life is terminated after about 120 days. Since the body contains approximately 20,000 billion erythrocytes, this life span suggests that they are destroyed (and produced) at the rate of 115 million per minute (36). Destroyed red cells are removed from the circulation, chiefly by the spleen, and the iron salvaged for reuse.

In the lungs hemoglobin combines loosely with oxygen to form oxyhemoglobin; this compound carries oxygen to the tissues and releases it there. The high oxygen pressure in the lungs facilitates the combination of atmospheric oxygen and hemoglobin. In the tissues, where the oxygen pressure is low, oxygen is readily released. Oxyhemoglobin from which oxygen has been released is called reduced hemoglobin. Reduced hemoglobin then returns to the lungs (by way of the veins) to secure oxygen in the form of oxyhemoglobin, and the cycle is repeated (Fig. 14.4).

Carbon dioxide diffuses from the tissues to the *capillaries* (as carbon dioxide molecules), where 10 percent of it is carried by hemoglobin. The major portion, however, is changed to the *bicarbonate ion*. In the lungs, hemoglobin releases the carbon dioxide and picks up oxygen.

In Muscle Tissue Iron is found in the muscle cells in two combinations—as myoglobin and as a constituent of certain enzymes. Myoglobin is similar to hemoglobin in structure and function; it also is made up of an iron-containing pigment and a protein. Myoglobin has only one atom of iron per molecule. Myoglobin accepts oxygen from hemoglobin; it can store oxygen temporarily in the muscle for use primarily in aerobic metabolism with the formation of ATP, which can be used for muscle contraction and also for any other energy demands—synthesis of protein, glucose, fatty acids, or other compounds.

In All Cells The cytochromes are heme-containing proteins that function in oxidation-reduction reactions in the mitochondria of the cell. They are needed in the final steps of biological oxidation when water is formed and useful energy trapped in the form of ATP (see Fig. 2.6).

Assessment of Iron Status

Iron deficiency can be assessed by methods which indicate not only that a deficiency exists but the severity of the condition (14). First, the stored iron is used where there is an iron deficiency; then, with the depletion of iron stores, blood ferritin decreases, iron absorption increases, and blood transferrin level *(iron-binding capacity)* increases. As the deficiency continues, the iron level in the blood falls, and there is impairment in the erythropoietic process due to lack of iron. A few months more of continued lack of sufficient iron results in iron deficiency anemia characterized by smaller than normal erythrocytes (micro-cytes) that contain less hemoglobin than normal *(hypochromic)*; the condition is microcytic hypochromic anemia. Measures used for the diagnosis of iron deficiency include the determination of serum iron and percent saturation of blood transferrin (13); *hematocrit* and hemoglobin determinations are diagnostic of iron deficiency anemia. Acceptable values and those that are low (indicate anemia) are presented in Table 14.2. In iron deficiency the percent saturation of transferrin is low—there is insufficient iron for transferrin to bind; the hematocrit is low (percent of blood that is cells) because the erythrocytes are smaller than normal; the hemoglobin level is low because there is insufficient iron for its formation. Other anemias are explained in the glossary at the end of this chapter.

Iron Deficiency

For the 32,669 individuals whose hemoglobin levels were determined in the Ten-State Nutrition Survey, 1968–1970, a high prevalence of low values (adult males, less than 14 g/100 ml; adult females, less than 12 g/100 ml) was found. These preliminary findings showed a tendency for lower hemoglobin levels to be associated with lower dietary iron intakes. The sample was

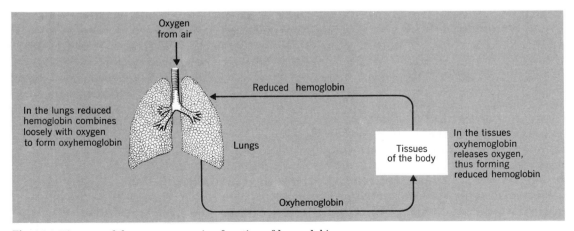

Fig. 14.4 Diagram of the oxygen-carrying function of hemoglobin.

Table 14.2 Guidelines for Interpretation of Blood Data Diagnostic of Iron Deficiency Anemia

	Acceptable		Low	
	Men	Women	Men	Women
Transferrin saturation, percent	20–29	15–29	< 20	< 15
Hematocrit, percent	44–52	38–48	< 44	< 38
Blood hemoglobin, g/100 ml	14–16.5	12–14.5	< 14	< 12

From S. Abraham, F. W. Lowenstein, and C. L. Johnson (1974). Preliminary Findings of the First Health and Nutrition Examination Survey, United States, 1971–1972: *Dietary Intake and Biochemical Findings*. DHEW Publ. No. (HRA) 74-1219-1. Rockville, Md.: U.S. Dept. Health, Education, and Welfare, Health Resources Adm., Natl. Center for Health Statistics, p. 182.

representative of low-income families of the area studied, but not of the moderate- and high-income families (21, 38).

Further assessment of iron deficiency in the United States was obtained as a part of the first Health and Nutrition Examination Survey (HANES) of the nutritional status of the civilian, noninstitutionalized population between the ages of 1 and 74 years. The preliminary findings were based on the examinations of 10,126 individuals (1). Used as indicators of iron deficiency in the HANES were serum iron and total iron-binding capacity (transferrin saturation) measurements. As indicators of anemia (due to iron deficiency), hemoglobin and hematocrit determinations and red cell counts were made.

The complete guidelines used are presented in Appendix Table A-25.

The HANES data gave evidence of iron deficiency among children and adolescents of ages 1 through 17 years based on a relatively high percentage of low transferrin saturations. For the adults 18 years and over the percentages of low hemoglobin and low hematocrit values (indicating anemia) were relatively high, more so for women than men and particularly so for Negroes 60 years and over. (Fig. 14.5 shows the distribution of hemoglobin values.) The percentages of low serum iron and percent transferrin saturation (indicating iron deficiency) were not high in adults. It would

appear that the cause of the low hemoglobin and hematocrit values (indicators of iron deficiency anemia) was not really lack of iron. (No information is available on the possible role of folate and vitamin B-12 deficiency to explain the high percentage of low hemoglobin and hematocrit values. (See pp. 245 and 247 for the role of folate and vitamin B-12 in anemias.)

Racial differences were observed in *serum* iron, transferrin saturation, hemoglobin, and hematocrit values, with Negroes usually having the lower ones. Lower income groups usually had lower values.

Food consumption was part of the HANES study. Iron was one of the nutrients for which the intake was calculated; the other nutrients were calcium and vitamins A and C. The age groups whose mean intakes met the standard least well at both income levels were women 18–44 years of age (mean intakes were 41 to 51 percent below the standard); children 1–5 years (mean intakes were 31 to 40 percent below the standard); and adolescents 12–17 years (mean intakes were 23 to 33 percent below the standard) (1). The dietary intake standards are shown in Appendix Table A-27.

The iron intake data and the biochemical findings concur that in children and adolescents, 1–17 years, a low iron intake may have been responsible for the anemia observed. Adults,

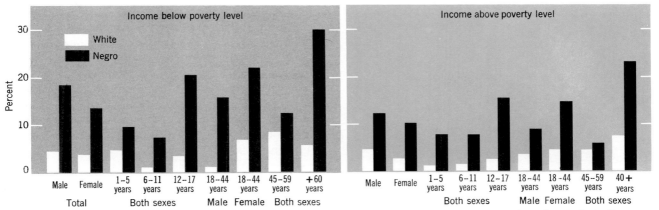

Fig. 14.5 Percent of persons with low hemoglobin values by age, sex, and race for income levels, United States, 1971–1972 (HANES Preliminary). (From Preliminary Findings of the First Health and Nutrition Examination Survey, United States, 1971–1972: Dietary Intake and Biochemical Findings. DHEW Publ. No. (HRA) 74-1219-1. Rockville, Md.: Health Res. Adm., Natl. Center for Health Statistics, U.S. Dept., Health, Educ., and Welfare, 1974 p. 12.)

18 years and beyond, with low intakes of iron (especially women) did not have low serum iron or low percent of transferrin saturation, indicating that iron deficiency was not the prime cause of the anemia and that other factors must have been involved.

In tropical areas, parasite infestation is a major cause of iron deficiency anemia. In hookworm infestation, the worm *Necator americanus* attaches to the tips of the intestinal villi in the small intestine and draws blood from the submucosal blood vessels, causing microcytic hypochromic anemia (42).

Blood donors experience a lowering of their hemoglobin level when they give blood. The decrease may average 2.3 g per 100 ml of blood when about 500 ml is donated, as found in a study of 200 persons at the University of Iowa (15). This group's mean hemoglobin level before donation was 12.8 g. The length of time required for the hemoglobin to return to its usual level after such a donation may vary from 2 weeks to 4 months, depending upon the amount of iron stored; the average time required by the Iowa group was 50 days. Women tend to require longer than men. After giving blood, the taking of medicinal iron and adhering to a high iron diet will help restore the hemoglobin level.

Iron Deficiency and Work Capacity A reduction in the hemoglobin concentration decreases the oxygen-carrying capacity of the blood, which reduces oxygen delivery to tissues in exercise (7). The level of hemoglobin influences work performance. In a study of 65 women with hemoglobin levels ranging from 6.1 to 15.9 g per 100 ml, the work time that they could endure on a standardized treadmill was 10.4 min versus 18.0 min for the lowest hemoglobin group and the highest, respectively (17) (Fig. 14.6). In another study, hemoglobin and hematocrit concentrations of sugarcane cutters showed a direct relationship to their scores on the Harvard step test (stepping up 20 in. on a platform and stepping back down at timed intervals). When these agricultural workers received iron supplementation of 100 mg/day for 6 months, their hemoglobin

289

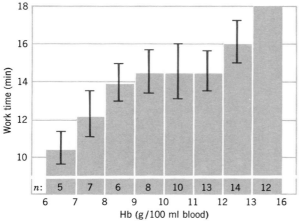

Fig. 14.6 Maximum treadmill work time in different Hb groups. The bar represents mean work time; the line (I) represents standard error of the mean (From Gardner, G. W., V. R. Edgerton, B. Senewiratne, R. J. Barnard, and Y. Ohira, (1977). Physical work capacity and metabolic stress in subjects with iron deficiency anemia. Am. J. Clin. Nutrition, 30: 910.)

concentration and step test score increased in parallel fashion; a control group given placebos showed no change in either hemoglobin or exercise performance (7, 39).

Iron Overload

An excessive body load of iron can be caused by a greater than normal absorption of iron from the intestine, by parenteral injection, or by a combination of the two. There are disorders in which an excessive amount of iron is absorbed; one of these is *idiopathic hemochromatosis*, a genetic disorder. Excessive intake, also, results in excessive absorption; the normal controls over absorption are ineffective. In the case of the Bantu of South Africa whose diets contain an excessive amount of iron, which is derived from the iron cooking pots used by them and from drums used in the preparation of the fermented beverage, kafir beer. In adult males the intake may exceed 100 mg of iron daily. An abnormally large amount of iron

is deposited in the liver (siderosis). When the concentration of iron in the liver becomes too great, a redistribution takes place with hemosiderin being deposited in many organs, particularly the pancreas and heart muscle (myocardium) (30). An excessive deposit of iron in the liver causes dysfunction. Prolonged administration of iron to persons who do not need it causes iron overload and symptoms indistinguishable from hemochromatosis (13).

Recommended Dietary Allowances for Iron

Iron need is estimated by measuring the loss from the body and determining the amount of dietary iron needed to replace the loss (6). The total excretion of iron is about 1.0 mg per day. An additional 0.5 mg is assumed to be needed by women each day to compensate for menstrual losses. Since the amount of iron absorbed from food is believed to be about 10 percent, 10 mg daily is recommended for all adult men and for women 51 years of age and over; 18 mg is recommended for females 11 to 50 years of age (34). The higher allowance for women of child-bearing age would permit the accumulation of iron to satisfy the demands of pregnancy. The iron needs for age and sex groups expressed as RDA and RDA in mg per 1000 kcal are given in Table 14.3.

Meals served to students in 50 colleges had an average iron content of 16.0 mg per person per day with a range of 6.8 to 26.0 mg. For each 1000 kcal of the college meals, the average value for iron was 6.0 mg, which exceeds the recommendation for men 19 to 22 years of age but fails to meet the recommendation for women of that age (see Table 14.3) (40).

Food Sources of Iron

Liver is an excellent source of iron. Other meats, egg yolks, legumes, and dark green leafy vegetables also contain noteworthy amounts. Fruits and other vegetables have lesser amounts. Certain dried fruits (raisins, prunes, and apricots) contain fairly large quantities, as do enriched and whole-grain cereals (Table 14.4).

The availability of iron for absorption varies among foods. Iron in meat, fish, and poultry (heme iron) is much better absorbed than that from vegetable sources (nonheme iron) (see p. 283). Most of the iron comes from nonheme sources in the United States' food supply and to an even greater extent in developing countries. The provision of an adequate iron intake entails concern for both quantity and availability.

Iron in the United States' Food Supply

The amount of iron in the United States food supply has been increasing since 1935–1939, partly because of the enrichment of cereal grains in 1941 (this enrichment may have increased the amount of iron in the food supply by about one-fifth) and the increased use of meat and poultry (16). The amount of iron available per capita for daily consumption in 1977 was 18.6 mg (29).

The percentage of iron contributed by groups of foods in the United States in 1977 was as follows: beef, pork, poultry, and fish, 30.9; flour and cereal products, 27.9; vegetables, 14.7; sugars and sweeteners, 6.8; dry beans, peas, nuts, and soya flour, 6.3; eggs, 4.7; fruits, 4.1; dairy products, 2.5; and miscellaneous foods, 2.2 (29).

Iron Fortification

Proposals to increase the level of iron fortification of cereal products generated opposition and controversy (8). Women and young children might have profited by additional iron, whereas most male adults need no additional iron and some of them might have suffered risk of iron overload (19). It is settled for now, however. There appeared in the Federal Register, November 18, 1977, an order withdrawing the amendment to increase the level of iron fortification of enriched flour and bread products and restoring the former provisions for these products (see chap. 17).

Table 14.3 Recommended Dietary Allowances for Iron

	Age, years	RDA mg	RDA mg/1000 kcal
Infants	0.0–0.5	10	—
	0.5–1.0	15	—
Children	1–3	15	11.5
	4–6	10	5.6
	7–10	10	4.2
Male	11–14	18	6.4
	15–18	18	6.0
	19–22	10	3.3
	23–50	10	3.7
	51+	10	4.2
Female	11–14	18	7.5
	15–18	18	8.6
	19–22	18	8.6
	23–50	18	9.0
	51+	10	5.6
Pregnant		18+[a]	—
Lactating		18	—

[a] This increased requirement cannot be met by ordinary diets; therefore, the use of supplemental iron is recommended. From *Recommended Dietary Allowances, Eighth Edition* (1974). Washington, D.C.: Natl. Acad. Sciences.

Research has been done (2, 10, 23, 25, 27, 33) on the question of iron fortification. The iron salt to be used, the food to be fortified (iron is poorly available in cereals), and the combination with another nutrient for fortification (vitamin C enhances the absorption of iron) are questions that will no doubt continue to be studied.

Iodine

The total amount of iodine in an adult's body is about 9 to 10 mg (7), and about 8 mg of it is in the thyroid; about 1.2 mg is in the blood and extrathyroidal tissues. The thyroid gland, located at the base of the neck and weighing about 20 to 25 g, consists of two lobes, one on either side of

Table 14.4 Iron Content of Various Foods as Served

	Per 100 g of food	Per average serving	
Good	Iron, mg	Size of serving	g	Iron, mg
Liver, pork, fried[a]	29.6	2 oz	55	16.3
Molasses, blackstrap	16.0	1 tbsp	20	3.2
Liver				
calf, fried[a]	14.5	2 oz	55	8.0
beef, fried	8.8	2 oz	55	4.8
chicken, cooked[a]	8.4	2 oz	57	4.8
Molasses, light	4.5	1 tbsp	20	0.9
Raisins, seedless	3.6	1 pkg (1½ tbsp)	14	0.5
Beef, lean, ground, broiled	3.5	3 oz	85	3.0
Bread				
whole wheat	3.2	1 sl	25	0.8
white, enriched	2.5	1 sl	28	0.7
Spinach, cooked	2.2	½ c	90	2.0
Egg, hard-cooked	2.0	1 med	50	1.0
Peanut butter	1.9	1 tbsp	16	0.3
Peas, green, canned	1.9	½ c	85	1.6
Chicken, breast, fried	1.6	2.7 oz	79	1.3
Tomato juice	0.9	½ c	122	1.1
Rice, white, enriched, cooked	0.9	½ c	102	0.9
Salmon, pink, canned	0.8	3 oz	85	0.7
Broccoli, stalks, cooked	0.8	½ c	78	0.6
Potato, baked, peeled	0.7	1 med	156	1.1
Cheese (Cheddar)	0.7	1 oz	28	0.2
Carrots, cooked	0.6	½ c	78	0.5
Cabbage, raw, shredded	0.4	1 c	70	0.3
Orange	0.4	1 med	131	0.5
Milk, whole	tr	8 oz	244	0.1

[a] *Nutritive Value of American Foods*, Agr. Handbook No. 456. Washington, D.C.: U.S. Dept. Agr., 1975.
From *Nutritive Value of Foods*, Home and Garden Bull. No. 72. Washington, D.C.: U.S. Dept. Agr., 1977.

the trachea, connected by an isthmus across the front of the trachea. It is in the thyroid gland that the thyroid hormones thyroxine (tetraiodothyronine, T_4), containing four atoms of iodine, and triiodothyroxine (T_3), containing three atoms of iodine, are formed (8).

Metabolism of Iodine

Absorption Most iodine is absorbed from the small intestine, but some of it enters the bloodstream directly from the stomach. Iodine is absorbed rapidly: using a Geiger counter, radio-active iodine has been detected in the hand within 3 to 6 minutes after it had been ingested by mouth (13). Absorption is virtually 100 percent.

Utilization After absorption most of the iodine goes to the thyroid gland and the kidneys. Under normal conditions the thyroid cells remove about 25 percent of the absorbed iodine from the plasma and concentrate it to a level 20 or even 50 times higher than that of the plasma. The iodine is rapidly incorporated into the thyroglobulin mole-cule, a large glycoprotein comprising 70 to 80 percent of the protein of the gland. Iodinated thyroglobulin has four iodine-containing com-pounds, all derivatives of the amino acid tyrosine: monoiodotyrosine (MIT), diiodotyrosine (DIT), thyroxine (tetraiodothyronine, T_4), and triiodo-thyronine (T_3) (see Fig. 14.7). MIT and DIT are not active as hormones (9); T_4 and T_3 are. They are released intact from thyroglobulin and enter the blood, where the ratio of the concentration of thyroxine to T_3 is around 50:1 (6). The thyroid

hormones are bound to protein carriers in the blood and taken to the target cells of their action. T_4 can be converted to T_3 by a process of *mono-deiodination* in the liver, kidney, and other tis-sues, normally accounting for about two-thirds of the T_3 available in the body (2, 25).

The most important regulator of the action of the thyroid gland is the thyroid-stimulating hor-mone (TSH) of the anterior pituitary gland. A fall in the output of thyroid hormones causes an in-crease in TSH secretion and stimulation of the thyroid gland; an increase in the level of the thyroid hormones in the blood causes a decrease in TSH secretion and a lessening of the stimula-tion of the thyroid gland (3).

The portion of the absorbed iodine entering the kidneys may be partially reabsorbed into the plasma; the remainder is excreted (8).

Storage Thyroglobulin, the storage form of iodine, is deposited in the colloid portion of the gland (Fig. 14.8). The thyroid gland of a nor-mal adult has in the stored thyroglobulin suf-

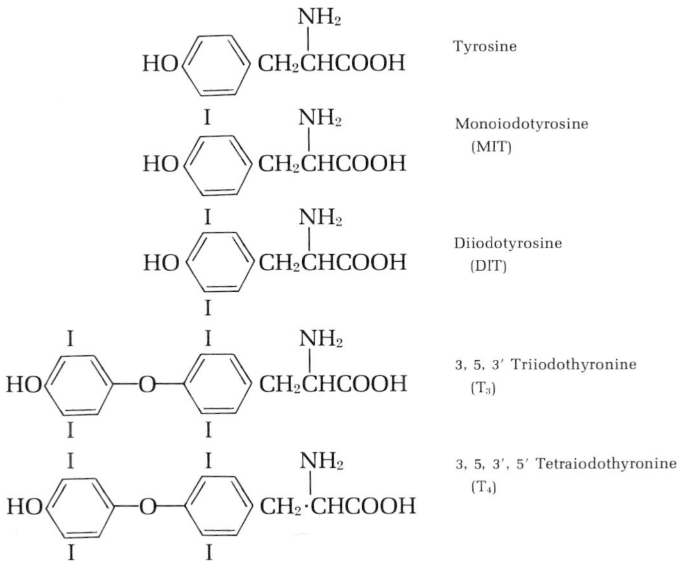

Fig. 14.7 Structure of tyrosine and its important iodinated derivatives.

293

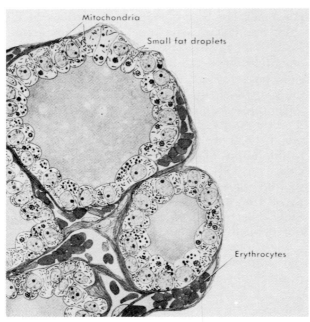

Mitochondria

Small fat droplets

Erythrocytes

Fig. 14.8 Section through several follicles of human thyroid. Aniline-acid fuchsin. (Courtesy W. B. Saunders Company, from Bloom W. and D. W. Fawcett, A TEXTBOOK OF HISTOLOGY, 10th edition, 1975. Photo by R. R. Bensley.)

ficient thyroxine to maintain the body in the normal state for two months (8, 24).

The body conserves its iodine supply. Iodine from deiodinated MIT and DIT is returned to the iodine pool where it is available for reincorporation into thyroglobulin.

Excretion The chief pathway of excretion is through the kidneys; lesser amounts are excreted through the intestine and in perspiration. Most iodine in the feces is in the unchanged thyroid hormones. During lactation iodine is secreted into the milk.

Function of Iodine in the Body

It is believed that iodine's only function in the body is as an essential component of the thyroid hormones.

In the body cells, the hormones increase the rate of oxidation, raising the basal metabolic rate (8). The hormones cause the mitochondria in most cells to enlarge in size and number, increasing the permeability of the mitochondrial membrane, and thereby facilitating the entry and exit of substances involved in respiratory activity and energy transfer (*in vitro* studies). Other actions include stimulation of protein synthesis and an inhibiting (uncoupling) action on *oxidative phosphorylation* (causing less ATP to be formed and more heat to be produced, which explains why the hyperthyroid person becomes thin).

Assessment of Iodine Status

The most useful method for assessment of iodine status is measurement of the free thyroxine concentration in the blood. Formerly, the protein-bound iodine (PBI)-level in the blood was the most commonly used method; however, by this method, all iodinated proteins are measured and not the thyroid hormones specifically. Because of its lack of specificity, the PBI method is being replaced by the direct determination of free T_4 in the blood. Most of T_4 exists in the blood in a bound form (99.97 percent), with the remainder (0.03 percent) present as free thyroxine. It is generally considered that the level of free T_4 determines the metabolic status of an individual; the level is abnormally high in hyperthyroid patients and low in those with hypothyroidism (3).

Radioactive iodine makes it possible to trace the utilization of iodine in the body. A common technique for assessing thyroid function is measuring the amount of radioiodine taken up by the thyroid gland 24 hours after a specified dose has been given. Normally, the thyroid will take up between 10 and 40 percent of the radioiodine in 24 hours. In hypothyroid patients the uptake is usually less than 20 percent (3, 23).

A dietary insufficiency of iodine is accompanied by a less than normal excretion of iodine in the urine. Excretions of less than 50 μg/g

294

creatinine are considered to be indicative of a deficiency (23).

Effects of Iodine Deficiency

Insufficient iodine produces endemic goiter, which is a worldwide problem (10). The highest incidence has been in the Alps, the Pyrenees, the Himalayas, the Thames Valley (England), certain regions of New Zealand, several countries of South America, and the Great Lakes and Pacific Northwest regions of the United States. The preventive use of iodine has lowered the incidence. The goiter areas of the world (where preventive measures are essential) are shown in Fig. 14.9. In 1972, the incidence of goiter and cretinism in the areas considered to be the most seriously affected, the Himalayas, was reassessed. In a village (Wapaa) 10,000 ft (3050 meters) above sea level, the incidence of visible goiter among the population was 70 percent and of palpable goiter, 90 percent (16). Here, preventive treatment had not been used.

Women and girls tend to develop endemic goiter more often than men and boys do. The greatest vulnerability to limited iodine intake occurs during adolescence, when girls are especially inclined to develop enlarged thyroid glands.

Without sufficient iodine, the level of thyroid hormones in the blood is low (hypothyroidism), with proportionately more T_3 and less T_4. When the level of thyroid hormones is low, the pituitary gland secretes more TSH. TSH causes the thyroid gland to enlarge by increasing both the number and the size of its epithelial cells in an effort to maintain normal secretion of the hormones. An enlarged thyroid gland with low hormone secretion is called simple, or nontoxic, goiter. If there are numerous cases in a given geographical area, simple goiter is called "endemic goiter." A woman with endemic goiter is shown in Fig. 14.10.

Cretinism (congenital hypothyroidism) results from an insufficiency of iodine in the intrauterine and early postnatal life. Its manifestations differ from varying degrees of mental debility only to

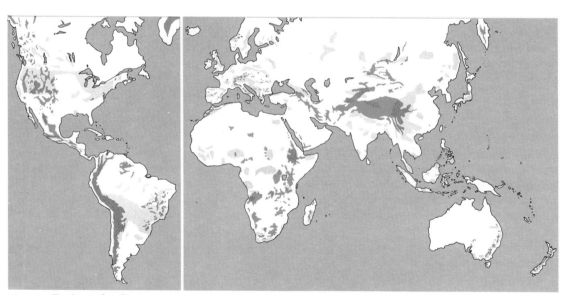

Fig. 14.9 Regions of endemic goiter in 1960. (From "Endemic Goiter" by R. B. Gillie. Copyright © 1971 by Scientific American, Inc. All rights reserved.)

295

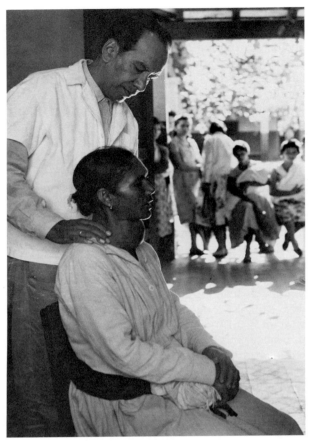

Fig. **14.10** Woman with endemic goiter being examined at a Health Center in Paraguay. (W.H.O.)

is probable that the thyroid gland had never functioned properly. If treatment is started as soon as the condition is detected, many of its symptoms can be reversed. However, the longer the condition persists, the more permanent its effects will be. Cretinism tends to be found in the endemic goiter areas of the world where adequate preventive measures have not been instituted or effectively applied (10, 16).

Adults in whom the thyroid gland has been destroyed surgically or by radioactive iodine develop myxedema, a state resembling cretinism but coming on in adult life. Occasionally, myxe-

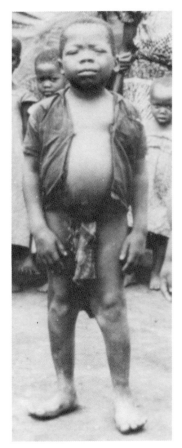

Fig. **14.11** A cretin. (F.A.O.)

the clearcut symptoms, mental and physical, of cretinism (28). The maternal thyroid, it appears, takes precedence over the placenta and developing fetus for whatever iodine is available. The growth rate of cretins is retarded; their facial features appear coarse and swollen; their abdomens protrude and are enlarged; their skin appears thick, dry, and pasty, and is often deeply wrinkled; their tongues are enlarged; and their lips are thick and usually remain parted (Fig. 14.11). Although cretinism is usually not recognizable until three or four months after birth, it

296

dema follows chronic *thyroiditis,* and sometimes the cause is unknown. This condition is characterized by thick and puffy skin and subcutaneous tissues, particularly of the face and extremities, and the face tends to be expressionless. The individual is lethargic and inactive; his body temperature and pulse rate are lowered; he usually gains weight; and all of his bodily and mental processes become retarded.

Iodine is essential for normal reproduction in both human beings and animals. For centuries it has been observed that women often develop a goiter during pregnancy, indicating a greater need for thyroxine. Animals in low-iodine areas sometimes manifest sterility or give birth to deformed offspring. Pigs have been born without hair; sheep, swine, horses, and cattle have developed enlarged thyroid glands during pregnancy; and the mortality rates have been high among the young.

Iodine Consumption and Goiter Incidence

The use of iodized salt is believed to be the major factor in the decline of endemic (simple) goiter in the United States. Iodized salt first appeared in this country in 1924; it was put on sale in Michigan, accompanied by a well-planned educational program. At that time, a survey of four Michigan counties showed that 38.6 percent of the school children had simple goiter. A resurvey of the same counties in 1951 showed that the incidence was only 1.4 percent (14). The amount of iodine added to salt in the United States is 0.5 to 1.0 part in 10,000 in the form of potassium iodide (11). Benefits of iodized salt in several goitrous areas of the world have been documented by the Joint FAO/WHO Expert Committee on Nutrition (17). In spite of the use of iodized salt in the United States, some goiters have persisted. It has been assumed that the goiters were due to a continuing iodine deficiency. However, findings from the Ten-State Nutrition Survey, 1968–

1970, indicated that very few of the almost 40,000 persons examined were iodine deficient (urinary iodine excretions were high, indicating an adequate iodine intake). The sample was representative of low-income families of the areas studied. The over-all prevalence of goiter was 3.1 percent, with the highest occurrence among adolescents and adults (15, 30).

The preliminary data obtained on 10,126 persons in the Health and Nutrition Examination (HANES), 1971–1972, showed an incidence of 10 percent or less of moderate thyroid enlargement and less than 5 percent of markedly enlarged glands. Interpretation of the findings must await the results on urinary iodine excretion to establish if the goiter was associated with a deficient or possibly an excessive iodine intake (1).

To examine further the relationship between the incidence of goiter and iodine status, Trowbridge and co-workers (31) made a study of 7785 children, 10 to 15 years of age, in the states of Michigan, Kentucky, Texas, and Georgia. The average prevalence of goiter was 6.8 percent. The 520 children with goiter had a higher urinary iodine excretion than their nongoitrous controls (matched for race, age, sex, height, and weight). Food consumption information was obtained from 754 of the children. Some foods from each area studied were analyzed; those high in iodine content were bread (made using iodine-containing dough conditioners), milk, and iodized salt (4). Iodine deficiency was not the cause of the goiters found in these children. One explanation proposed by the investigators (19, 30) for the goiters is that there may have been a deficiency of iodine at an earlier time; such goiters do not recede even though the iodine intake later becomes adequate.

In Canada, the National Nutrition Survey (1970–1972) revealed moderate enlargement of the thyroid in the general population, which could not be attributed to iodine deficiency. The data for urinary iodine excretion indicated adequate or even high intakes in some individuals (20, 22).

297

Table 14.5 Average Iodine Intake for Young
Adult United States Males

Reference period	Iodine intake, μg per day	Energy intake, kcal
1960	100–150	—
Prior to 1970	454	2400
Fiscal year 1974	600[a]	2800
	1050[b]	2800
Fiscal year 1975	538[a]	2800

[a] Without iodized salt.
[b] Upper limit with iodized salt.
From J. M. Talbot, K. D. Fisher, and C. J. Carr (1976). *A Review of the Effects of Dietary Iodine on Certain Thyroid Disorders.* Bethesda, Md.: Fed. Am. Soc. Exptl. Biol., p. 12.

Information on the iodine consumption of young adult males (15 to 20 years of age) obtained from the 1975 Food and Drug Administration Survey showed an estimated daily average intake of 538 μg (2800 kcal diet) and 750 μg (3900 kcal diet) (5). The increase in iodine intake in 1975 over that of young men in 1960 was about five times (4, 8) (Table 14.5). Corresponding increases can be assumed for females and others of the population as well (27).

In seeking a cause for the rise in intake of iodine, the sales of iodized salt were examined. In 1969–1970, 55 percent of the packaged salt for home use was iodized; in 1974–1975, 58 percent was iodized (27). The increase was small and could not account for the large increase in dietary iodine. Another source of iodine in some localities is the water supply; iodine is sometimes used as a disinfectant in drinking water. Iodine-supplemented rations for animals increase the iodine consumption of humans; kelp meal fed to hens increases the iodine content of eggs. Iodine compounds used as sanitizers in dairies are found to increase the amount of iodine in milk (6). When iodate dough conditioners are used, bread is high in iodine content. Since 1974, the use of iodate

dough conditioners has been decreasing (27). Some vitamin-mineral supplements contain iodine (12).

Moderate increases in iodine intake, that is, up to around ten times the recommended allowance, lead to no problems. The gland for a time takes up more iodine than it releases with the formation of thyroglobulin; within a few weeks the gland returns to taking up a normal amount even though the high intake continues (34). Some individuals appear to be able to adapt to excessive intakes of iodine with continuing normal synthesis of the thyroid hormones. Some are unable to adapt. Goiters developed in persons drinking water in which 1 mg iodine was added per liter as an antispetic against the intestinal parasite *Endamoeba histolytica* (29). The goiter that accompanies high iodine intake is designated "iodide goiter." This type of goiter occurs in about 10 percent of the population of the coastal regions of Hokkaido, the northern island of Japan, where the diet is permanently high in iodine content due to the consumption of the iodine-rich seaweed, kelp (26, 32).

Dietary Goitrogens

These chemical compounds inhibit the synthesis of hormones by the thyroid gland. Enlargement of the thyroid gland has been produced in experimental animals that were fed turnips and cabbage, even though their diet contained suficient iodine. Endemic goiter in the United States has not been linked to the consumption of any particular food (24). However, endemic goiter has been found among children in Australia and Tasmania who drank the milk of cows that had been fed a certain type of kale (marrowstem).

Goitrin, an antithyroid compound, is found in plants in the precursor form—progoitrin—which is changed to goitrin by enzymatic action. Progoitrin has been identified in the seeds of most of the mustard family and in the edible portions of cabbage, kale, rape, rutabagas, and white

298

turnips. Progoitrin is heat-labile and inactivated by cooking (3).

Recommended Dietary Allowances for Iodine

The daily iodine requirement for prevention of goiter in adults is 50 to 75 μg or approximately 1 μg/kg body weight. The RDA provides a safety margin above the prevention level: for men, 19 to 22 years of age, the RDA is 140 μg; for those 23 to 50 years, 130 μg; and for those 51 years and over, 110 μg. For women from 19 to 50 years, the RDA is 100 μg and for those 51 years and over, 80 μg (21). The iodine needs for age and sex groups expressed as RDA and μg per 1000 kcal are given in Table 14.6.

Table 14.6 Iodine Needs Expressed as RDAs and Nutrient Densities

	Age, years	RDA	
		μg	μg/1000 kcal
Infants	0.0–0.5	35	—
	0.5–1.0	45	—
Children	1–3	60	46
	4–6	80	44
	7–10	110	46
Male	11–14	130	46
	15–18	150	50
	19–22	140	47
	23–50	130	48
	51+	110	46
Females	11–14	115	48
	15–18	115	55
	19–22	100	48
	23–50	100	50
	51+	80	44
Pregnant		125	—
Lactating		150	—

From *Recommended Dietary Allowances, Eighth Edition* (1974). Washington, D.C.: Natl. Acad. Sciences.

Food Sources of Iodine

The amount of iodine in most foods is exceedingly small and can only be determined by sensitive chemical methods. The content varies widely among foods and even for the same food under different soil and fertilizer conditions. Seafood and seaweed are the best sources of iodine. Saltwater fish have much more iodine than do freshwater fish. Fish (such as cod) that feed on marine algae and other organisms that contain iodine have a relatively high iodine content.

The amount of iodine in land plants depends mainly upon the amount in the soil where they were grown. The leaves and flowers of plants appear to have a higher concentration than do the roots. However, most vegetables, cereal grains, and legumes have little iodine. Bread may be a notable source of iodine (35–95 μg/25 g slice) when iodate is used as a dough conditioner (18). The amount in dairy products and eggs varies according to the amount of iodine in the food consumed by the animals. In Table 14.7 mean values for iodine content of food groups is given (33). Iodized salt is the most dependable source of iodine in the diet.

Table 14.7 Iodine Content of Composites of Food Categories

Food category	Number of samples	Iodine (g/kg, wet wt.)	
		Mean ± S.E.	Median
Sea foods	7	660 ± 180	540
Vegetables	13	320 ± 100	280
Meat products	12	260 ± 70	175
Eggs	11	260 ± 80	145
Dairy products	18	130 ± 10	139
Bread and cereals	18	100 ± 20	105
Fruits	18	40 ± 20	18

From R. L. Vought and W. T. London (1964). Dietary sources of iodine. *Am. J. Clin. Nutrition,* **14:** 186. (American Society of Clinical Nutrition, reprinted by permission.)

Manganese

Manganese is found in all animal tissues thus far examined but especially in the liver, skin, bones, and muscles. There is a total of about 12 to 20 mg in a 70-kg man.

Metabolism of Manganese

Manganese is not easily absorbed. In the blood it is transported bound to a protein. The chief pathway of excretion of manganese is by way of the feces; it enters the feces as a constituent of bile.

Functions of Manganese

Manganese is an activator of enzymes (*cofactor*) in numerous reactions but a constituent of an enzyme (*metalloenzyme*) in only a few (12, 22). The synthesis of CHOL from acetyl CoA requires manganese as a cofactor as do certain enzymatic reactions in which ATP participates as a phosphate donor. The manganese cofactor is also involved in fatty acid metabolism and protein synthesis (Table 13.2). The metalloenzyme pyruvate carboxylase, which contains both manganese and the vitamin biotin, catalyzes the conversion of pyruvate to oxaloacetate in carbohydrate metabolism.

Effects of a Manganese Deficiency and Toxicity in Human Beings

At present (1978), the effects of a manganese deficiency in human beings have not been demonstrated. Although manganese poisoning is not common, it was recognized as early as 1837 among men who worked at loading manganese-rich ores. In a study of manganese poisoning of 150 Moroccan miners, the symptoms were as follows: a peculiar, masklike expression on the face; involuntary laughing; a low voice with blurred speech; walking with a spastic gait; and tremors of the hands (20) (Fig. 14.12).

Daily Need for and Food Sources of Manganese

A daily requirement for manganese has not yet been determined. Several human balance studies have been made that indicate a need: young women retained about 1.54 mg daily (14), young men retained about 3.34 mg daily (11), and preadolescent girls retained from 0.15 to 0.24 mg on intakes ranging from 2.13 to 2.43 mg (4). A dietary intake of 2.5 to 7 mg per day appears to meet the human need for manganese (19).

Manganese in College Meals The manganese content of meals served at 50 American colleges

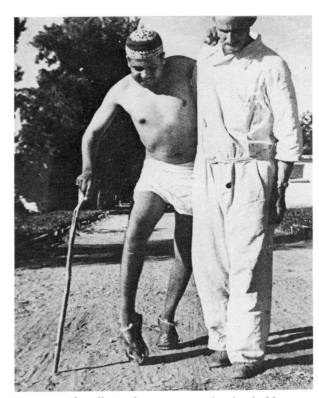

Fig. 14.12 The effects of manganese poisoning in Morrocan miners. The patient cannot walk without help. (From collection of J. Rodier, courtesy the author and Brit. J. Ind. Med., 12, 1955, 21.)

300

Table 14.8 Manganese, Copper, Zinc, and Chromium in Various Foods

Food	mg per 100/g			
	Manganese	Copper	Zinc	Chromium
Apple, raw	0.035	0.014	0.012	<0.015[a]
Baked beans	0.2	0.170	1.7	<0.060
Beef, uncooked, ground	<0.02	0.061	3.4	<0.030
Bread (white, enriched)	0.25	0.110	0.75	<0.060
Cheese (American)	<0.4	0.110	4.1	0.170
Eggs, whole	<0.02	0.053	1.8	0.052
Flour, bleached, enriched	0.4	0.130	0.93	<0.060
Ice cream (vanilla)	<0.01	0.005	0.53	<0.015
Milk, whole	<0.01	0.005	0.43	<0.015
Orange juice, frozen, reconstituted	<0.008	0.0075	0.015	0.012
Potato, fresh, uncooked	0.042	0.052	0.2	<0.03
Peanut butter	1.9	0.61	2.9	<0.06
Sugar				
brown	<0.04	<0.02	0.029	<0.06
white	<0.04	<0.02	<0.02	<0.06
Tomato, fresh	<0.02	<0.01	0.046	<0.03
Tunafish, canned (without salt)	<0.02	0.011	0.44	<0.03

[a] <0.015 indicates that the chromium content of 100 g of apple is less than 0.015 mg.
From Gormican, A. (1970). Inorganic elements in foods used in hospital menus. *J. Am. Dietet. Assoc.*, **56:** 397.

averaged 3.35 mg per person per day with a range of 2.37 to 5.05 mg (24). All the colleges but two had meals within the range of 2.5 to 7 mg per day.

Food Sources of Manganese In analyzing 128 foods for manganese, it was found that the best sources were dry tea, instant powdered coffee, cocoa powder, bran flakes, shredded wheat, oatmeal, walnuts, peanut butter, canned pineapple, and whole wheat bread (6) (see Table 14.8).

Copper

The importance of copper in nutrition was first demonstrated by Hart and others at the University of Wisconsin in a series of studies that began in 1925. When rats and rabbits were given a milk diet, they developed an anemia that was not alleviated by iron supplements; they improved only when they were given the copper-containing ash of certain foods.

There is a total of about 100 to 150 mg of copper in most human adults; the highest concentrations are found in the liver, kidneys, hair, and brain.

Metabolism of Copper

Copper is absorbed from the small intestine into the bloodstream where most of it becomes bound to a protein called ceruplasmin. This protein functions in the body's utilization of iron. The pathway of excretion of copper is by way of the bile into the feces.

301

Functions of Copper

Copper is present in a number of respiratory enzymes. For example, it acts as a cofactor for the enzyme tyrosinase, which is needed in one of the series of reactions to oxidize the amino acid tyrosine to the pigment melanin (the dark pigment of the skin and hair) (Table 13.2). Ascorbic acid oxidase, another copper-containing enzyme, aids in the conversion of the reduced form of vitamin C to its oxidized form (dehydroascorbic acid). The copper-containing enzymes, the amine oxidases, are necessary to *collagen* and *elastin* synthesis.

Copper is essential for the development of young red blood cells. When there is a copper deficiency, the number of red cells is reduced. As observed in experimental animals (13), a copper deficiency causes iron not to be released at the normal rate from its storage sites but to be removed from the blood to help form the red cell precursors in the bone marrow. If enough copper is given to restore the red blood cell level to normal, the iron level is also quickly raised.

From the standpoint of human health, copper is necessary for normal blood formation (hemopoiesis), maintenance of vascular and skeletal structures (blood vessels, tendons, and bones), and the structure and functioning of the central nervous system (15).

Effects of a Copper Deficiency

The human infant is born with enough copper and iron in his liver to last until he begins to consume foods other than milk; milk is low in both minerals. If the infant is malnourished, however, two types of copper-related deficiencies may occur (7, 23). The first, occurring early in life, involves an untreated iron deficiency with insufficient copper; both iron and copper are needed to relieve the symptoms of anemia, *hypoproteinemia*, and low serum iron and copper levels. The second, a copper deficiency in the presence of adequate iron, results in anemia, *neutropenia*, low serum copper levels, and "scurvylike" bone changes; all symptoms are relieved by copper therapy alone.

Except in isolated cases of feeding intravenous formulas low in copper (22), adults do not tend to develop a copper deficiency even during long periods of malnutrition. This fact was substantiated by observing 38 Americans who had been held captive in World War II; they had received an inadequate food intake for about 3¹/₃ years (2).

Daily Need for and Food Sources of Copper

As of 1978, no copper requirement had been established for man (19). Human balance studies seem to indicate that an ordinary diet completely satisfies man's need for this nutrient.

It has been noted that adults maintain a copper balance on an intake of 2 mg per day. Preadolescent girls retained from 0.48 to 0.77 mg of copper on daily intakes that ranged between 1.55 and 1.70 mg (4, 18), indicating that their diet was providing them with enough of this mineral.

Copper in College Meals The copper content of meals served at 50 American colleges averaged 3.37 mg per person per day, with a range of 1.74 to 12.51 mg (24). Only four colleges had meals slightly below the 2.0 mg level, the other 46 college meals contained 2.0 mg copper or more.

Food Sources of Copper The copper content of various foods is presented in Table 14.8. The richest dietary sources are cocoa powder, dry tea, beef and pork liver, pecans, walnuts, bran flakes, and peanut butter (6).

Zinc

Small amounts of zinc are found in both plants and animals. The human body contains a total of about 2 g of zinc, mainly in the hair, bones, eyes, and sex glands and secretions.

Zinc deficiency among human beings has been recognized for more than a decade in countries where the diet consists mainly of cereal grains (Iran and Egypt). There is evidence that marginal states of zinc nutrition do exist in the United States (19).

Metabolism of Zinc

Only a small percentage of ingested zinc appears to be absorbed from the intestinal tract, and the absorption mechanism is unknown (9). Zinc is excreted from the body by way of the feces.

Functions of Zinc

Zinc is a component of numerous metalloenzymes (Table 13.2). At this time, about 70 zinc-containing metalloenzymes have been identified (22). One of them, DNA polymerase, is involved in DNA and RNA metabolism. Another, pancreatic carboxypeptidase, is needed in the digestion of protein. As a cofactor, zinc increases the activity of a number of other enzymes as well.

Effects of a Zinc Deficiency

The symptoms of a zinc deficiency in adolescent boys are retarded growth, retarded sexual development, rough skin, poor appetite, and mental lethargy; impaired sense of taste, poor healing of wounds, and susceptibility to infection also may occur (Fig. 14.13) (17). It was once thought that the human zinc deficiency syndrome was limited only to males. However, two Iranian females (19 and 20 years old), with the same clinical symptoms as males, have responded to treatment with large doses of zinc salts (21).

Hair zinc levels of less than 70 parts per million (ppm), impaired sense of taste, poor appetite, and suboptimal growth were observed among apparently healthy children in Denver (10). The symptoms of this marginal zinc deficiency were relieved with an increased intake of zinc.

That a secondary zinc-deficient state may occur

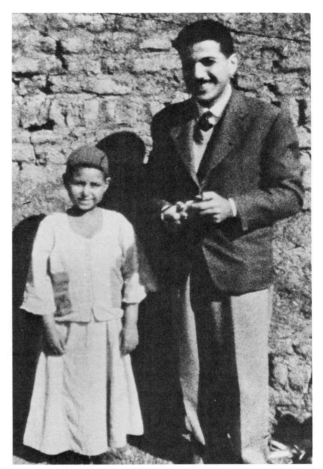

Fig. 14.13 Zinc deficiency dwarfism seen in a sixteen-year-old Egyptian boy. The man at the right is of normal height. (Courtesy Harold H. Sandstead, M.D. Reproduced with permission of *Nutrition Today* Magazine, Annapolis, Maryland, © March, 1968.)

in other diseases is seen in *sickle cell anemia* (1). Some of the manifestations of the disease in adults are improved with zinc therapy.

Recommended Dietary Allowances for and Food Sources of Zinc

The RDA for zinc is 15 mg for all those 11 years of age and older (19). The RDA per 1000 kcal

303

Table 14.9 Recommended Dietary Allowances for Zinc

	Age, years	Zinc	
		mg	mg/1000 kcal[a]
Infants	0.0–0.5	3	—
	0.5–1.0	5	—
Children	1–3	10	7.7
	4–6	10	5.6
	7–10	10	4.2
Males	11–14	15	5.4
	15–18	15	5.0
	19–22	15	5.0
	23–50	15	5.6
	51+	15	6.3
Females	11–14	15	6.3
	15–18	15	7.1
	19–22	15	7.1
	23–50	15	7.5
	51+	15	8.3
Pregnant		20	—
Lactating		25	—

[a] Calculated.

From *Recommended Dietary Allowances, Eighth Edition.* Washington, D.C.: Natl. Acad. Sciences, 1974.

(4184 kJ) for college men and women, 19 to 22 years, is 5.0 and 7.1 mg, respectively (Table 14.9).

Zinc in College Meals The average zinc intake of the meals offered at the 50 American colleges was 11.03 mg per person per day, with a range of 6.36 to 16.11 mg (24). Only 4 colleges served meals whose average zinc content met the 15 mg allowance of the RDA.

Food Sources of Zinc There is evidence that zinc in plant protein is less available to human beings than that in animal protein due to the presence of phytates (16). Nutrition research workers presently believe that diets containing the recommended amounts of animal protein will satisfy the need for zinc, but those limited to vegetable protein may not. (The meals served at the 50

American colleges were high in protein, but no breakdown was made of the sources of animal and vegetable proteins [24].) Zinc is found in most ordinary foods (Table 14.8). The richest dietary sources are meat, poultry, seafood, eggs, cheese, milk, peanut butter, and whole-grain cereal products (5, 6, 8).

Cobalt

Cobalt has been found to be essential for human beings and animals (23).

Function of Cobalt

The only function of cobalt in humans and animals appears to be as a constituent of the vitamin B-12 molecule. The pathway of cobalt from the soil to vitamin B-12 in the ingested food of human beings and nonruminant animals is sometimes called the cobalt cycle. Plants obtain cobalt from the soil. Ruminant animals (for example, cattle, sheep, goats) eat the plants, and the bacteria in their rumina use the cobalt to manufacture vitamin B-12. These animals absorb the vitamin, which is distributed throughout their body tissues. Human beings and nonruminant animals ingest the meat and milk of these animals and thereby obtain vitamin B-12.

Effects of a Cobalt Deficiency and Toxicity in Human Beings

Nothing is known about the effects of a cobalt deficiency in human beings. If humans ingest cobalt in large amounts, the number of red blood cells increases; this condition is called polycythemia. Experimental polycythemia has been produced by giving people 150 mg of cobalt salts per day (3). After 7 to 22 days, the subjects showed a 16 to 21 percent increase in the number of red cells. Polycythemia is a natural condition in all those who live at very high altitudes; the additional red blood cells compensate for the lower percentage of oxygen in the air at such elevations.

Daily Need for and Food Sources of Cobalt

The Food and Nutrition Board has not established Recommended Dietary Allowances for cobalt (19). Studies with preadolescent girls, however, indicate that about 7.7 μg of cobalt is needed for balance; therefore Engel and co-workers suggested a daily allowance of 15 μg for this age group (4). Little information is available on the cobalt content of foods.

Molybdenum

The importance of molybdenum in animal nutrition was established only in 1953. The effects of insufficient molybdenum have not been observed in man.

Functions of Molybdenum

The importance of molybdenum in the nutrition of human beings has not been established. Molybdenum is an essential nutrient for the rat, dog, lamb, turkey poult, and chick in order to form and maintain the flavin enzyme xanthine oxidase (flavin coenzymes contain riboflavin). Found in liver and milk, xanthine oxidase catalyzes the oxidation of hypoxanthine to xanthine (breakdown products of nucleic acid metabolism) and the latter to uric acid.

Daily Need for and Food Sources of Molybdenum

It is not known how much molybdenum man may require but the estimated intake in the United States of 45–500 μg per day probably meets this need (19). Molybdenum is widely distributed in many foods; good sources include legumes, cereal grains, certain dark-green vegetables, liver, and kidney.

Fluorine

Fluorine is now considered to be an essential nutrient because it is incorporated in the structure of teeth and is necessary for maximal resistance to dental caries (40). A fluoride (salt of fluorine) level of 1 part per million (ppm) in drinking water seems to be a safe, economical, and efficient way to reduce the incidence of dental caries. The Food and Nutrition Board now recommends the fluoridation of public water supplies in the United States in areas of low fluoride concentrations. The Canadian Council on Nutrition (10) also recommended fluoridation of Canadian public water supplies and suggested the use of a fluoride supplement for caries prophylaxis where there are no communal water supplies or where they are not fluoridated. Water fluoridation also has been undertaken in Brazil, Chile, Colombia, Czechoslovakia, Finland, Ireland, Japan, the Netherlands, New Zealand, Puerto Rico, Switzerland, the United Kingdom, and the U.S.S.R. (13).

Metabolism of Fluorine

Balance studies indicate what proportion of a fluoride dosage is retained by the body. Most of the absorption takes place in the intestine. At daily intakes of 4 to 5 mg, the subjects excreted almost all of the fluoride ingested (33). When the subjects were given 12 to 25 mg of fluoride per day, more than one-half of the ingested amount was retained, but the body stores were slowly depleted after the intake level was returned to normal (29).

Fluorides and Bone Structure

Evidence exists that fluoride may help prevent the bone destruction that is associated with aging.

305

X-rays were used to study the effect of fluoride ingestion on the bone structure of men and women over 45 years of age from high-fluoride (4.0 to 5.9 ppm) and low-fluoride (0.15 to 0.3 ppm) areas in North Dakota (5). Those from the low-fluoride areas tended to have a lower *bone density* and a greater incidence of *osteoporosis*. In Watford, England (which has fluoridated water), there was less osteoporosis among women than in Leigh (which does not have fluoridation) (2).

The use of large doses (around 20 to 70 mg daily) of sodium fluoride to treat osteoporosis and other bone disorders helped to improve the calcium balance without producing evident toxic effects (6, 41). The Mayo Clinic reported that after 7 to 25 months of fluoride feeding, osteoporotic patients appeared to simulate new bone formation (25). Without calcium and vitamin D, however, the new bone was largely uncalcified; but with calcium and vitamin D, the new bone tissue appeared to be relatively normal. (For a discussion of osteoporosis, see chapt. 21.)

The Effects of Various Fluoride Levels on Human Tissue

The effect of minimal amounts of fluoride on the skeletal tissues of man has been studied both *radiologically* and *histologically* in individuals who have consumed water containing fluorides throughout their lives (52). It has been reported that fluorosis, the skeletal index of excessive exposure to fluorides, has never been observed in persons who drank water containing less than 4 ppm of fluoride. Furthermore, none of the characteristic lesions of fluorosis have been found in histological sections of rib bones from deceased persons who had always lived in an area where the drinking water contained 1.9 ppm of fluoride.

One of the unexpected but interesting findings from the North Dakota study mentioned above was the degree of calcification of the subjects, abdominal aorta. There was significantly less calcification of this artery among those who were living in the high-fluoride areas than among those in the low-fluoride areas. This was particularly true for the men in the study (5).

Like iodine, which belongs in the same chemical group, fluorine is excreted by way of the kidneys.

Food Sources of Fluoride

Fluoride is found in plant, fish, and animal foods. Seafood contains from 5 to 15 ppm of fluoride and dry tea as much as 75 to 100 ppm.

Diets, exclusive of drinking water, vary in fluoride content; 0.3 mg in low-fluoride areas and 3.1 mg in high-fluoride ones (40). Hospital diets, very constant in fluoride content (1.6 to 1.9 mg per day over a six-year period), contained about one-half the amount of fluoride when the drinking water was temporarily not fluoridated (39). Foods absorb the mineral when they are cooked.

Fluoride and Dental Caries

The relationship between fluoride and tooth physiology was recognized as a public health problem in this country and elsewhere when it was found in the 1930s that the tooth enamel of persons in certain communities became mottled. Teeth exposed to excessive fluoride in the drinking water became dull and chalky in appearance; some showed signs of pitting and corrosion; and in severe cases they became stained a color ranging from yellow to black. By analyzing the fluoride content of the water supplies in a number of communities, investigators concluded that mottling could be prevented by either avoiding water with excessive amounts of the mineral or removing the excess amounts by chemical means. From these same studies (24) it was found that children who ingested water containing natural fluorides in amounts of 1 part per million (ppm) not only had no mottling, but exhibited a low incidence of dental caries (Fig. 14.14).

Since then, important findings about fluorides and dental health have been made (1). If fluorides are continuously consumed from early child-

306

hood, maximum protection will be given to the deciduous and permanent teeth. The easiest way to supply fluoride to an entire community is to fluoridate the drinking water. The desirable level of fluoride has been set at 1.0 to 1.2 ppm in the temperate zone and somewhat less in warmer regions.

Controlled Fluoridation Studies

Before controlled studies of water fluoridation were undertaken, all that was known about the role of fluoride in dental health was based on the experience of individuals who were born and continued to live in a natural fluoride area.

The study of fluoridation can be divided into phases. The first phase includes all of the early work as well as the announcement of the relationship between mild dental fluorosis and a low rate of dental decay in children. The second phase, or period of controlled experimentation, began in 1945 with the initiation of the famous fluoridation studies (Newburgh–Kingston, New York, and Grand Rapids–Muskegon, Michigan). Since that time other communities, both here and abroad, have undertaken similar fluoridation studies, but only the Newburgh–Kingston study will be described here.

The Newburgh–Kingston Study A 10-year experiment began in May, 1945, in these two New York communities located 30 miles apart on the Hudson River. The inhabitants of both towns were of similar racial and economic backgrounds, and the populations were about equal in number (30,000). The water supply of Newburgh was treated with sodium fluoride (1.0 to 1.2 ppm), whereas that of Kingston was not. Annual dental examinations and periodic medical evaluations were made of selected children from these two communities.

At the end of 10 years, medical officers reported that there was no significant difference in the height, weight, selected laboratory tests, or X-ray studies of the children of Newburgh and Kings-

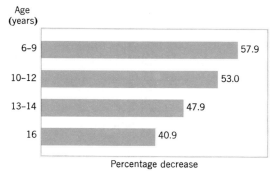

Fig. 14.14 Percentage reduction in DMF (decayed, missing, filled) teeth of children from 6 to 16 years after 10 years of fluoridation in Newburgh, New York. (Adapted from *Fluorides and Human Health* [1970]. *Geneva:* World Health Organ., p. 298.)

ton (45). However, the dental team reported that clinical and X-ray dental examinations showed that the DMF (decayed, missing, and filled teeth) count of the permanent teeth was lower among the children from Newburgh than among those from Kingston (4).

Other Observations

In a study of 138,000 recruits at the Great Lakes Naval Training Center (1970 to 1974), 12 percent of whom were from cities with fluoridated water supplies and 11 percent from cities without fluoridation, the cities with fluoridated water accounted for approximately ten times as many caries-free recruits as the cities without it (26).

Other Methods of Fluoride Administration

It is not always possible to fluoridate water supplies. Approximately 67 million persons are consuming fluoride-deficient public water and an additional 47 million whose water supply is other than a public facility, such as occurs in most rural areas (30). Other methods have been used — the ingestion of sodium fluoride tablets, local application of fluoride solutions to the

307

tooth enamel (topical application), toothpastes that contain fluoride, and rinsing the mouth with a fluoride solution. A sodium fluoride tablet that contains 1 mg of fluoride was given each day to 221 children for periods of up to 15 years (44). The rates of DMF corresponded to those found among children who drank water of 1 ppm of fluoride for comparable periods of time (1). The topical application of fluoride involves swabbing the teeth with a fluoride solution at prescribed intervals of time. It is reported that the incidence of dental caries was reduced by 40 percent the following year when a 2 percent solution of sodium fluoride was used on the teeth of a large number of children (27). Researchers at the Dental School at Indiana University (22) found that greater protection was provided by topically applied stannous chlorofluoride than by sodium fluoride (1).

Kyes and his co-workers (28) conducted clinical trials on various fluoridated toothpastes but found that they were not all successful in combating tooth decay. It is difficult to produce a satisfactory stannous fluoride toothpaste because, with storage, there is a decrease in the available fluoride and stannous ions; also, saliva reacts with the fluoridated toothpaste, thereby reducing the fluoride available to the teeth (43).

Rinsing the mouth with a sodium fluoride (NaF) solution was found to reduce notably the incidence of new carious surfaces in school children. A 16 percent reduction in DMF surfaces was observed in first-grade children and a 14 percent reduction in fifth-grade children who rinsed with a 0.2 percent NaF solution once a week for two school years (19). Fluoride mouth-rinsing is suggested as a caries prevention plan satisfactory for use as a school program (30).

Effect of Fluorides on Dental Caries in Adults

There is a lower reduction in dental decay when the ingestion of fluorides is begun after childhood. Muhler (36) reported that a year after a single topical application of 10 percent stannous fluoride, 200 university students showed a 24 percent reduction in the increment of DMF teeth. (The reduction for children is 40 to 60 percent; see p. 307).

In Aurora, Illinois, a study was made of the incidence of dental caries among 1000 persons between the ages of 18 and 59 who had consumed 1.2 ppm of naturally fluoridated water almost continuously during their lifetime (12). It was found that they had between 40 and 50 percent fewer caries than a similar group in Rockford, Illinois, who had ingested fluoride-free water most of their lives. The actual differences in DMF values between the two groups, however, decreased with age (1). For those 20 to 24 years of age, the difference was 48.2 percent, but only 31.5 percent for those aged 55 to 59. This difference may be due to the fact that the uptake of fluoride by enamel appears to cease at about 30 years of age (24).

The Action of Fluoride on the Teeth

Two theories, one involving systemic action, the other, oral environment, have been advanced to explain the mode of action of fluoride in reducing dental decay (24). One theory is that the mineral reduces the solubility of the enamel in acid by being incorporated into it. A laboratory demonstration has shown that when enamel is exposed to a fluoride solution (as little as 1.0 ppm), it becomes less soluble in acid. The other suggests that fluoride inhibits the bacterial enzymes that produce the acid that attacks the enamel. It is possible that fluoride works in several ways simultaneously.

Chromium

In the 1950s, it was found that chromium plays a role in the glucose tolerance (GT) of human beings (34, 48). GT is the time required for the blood sugar to return to normal after a fasting individual ingests only sugar. The length of time is normally 2½ hours; if a person has an impaired GT, it is longer.

Metabolism of Chromium

Only a small part of the chromium ingested in the food is absorbed by human beings. It has been observed that insulin-requiring diabetics absorb two to four times more chromium in the 24 hours after intake than do normal subjects (11). (More research is needed, however, to learn whether or not chromium nutrition is related to diabetes.) Two forms of chromium appear to circulate in the blood plasma, and the chief pathway of excretion is in the urine.

Functions of Chromium

It now appears that chromium is part of a complex called the glucose tolerance factor (GTF) (11, 17, 35). Although the exact chemical structure of GTF is unknown, it may have two molecules of nicotinic acid per atom of chromium and several amino acid residues. (Nicotinic acid is the vitamin niacin.) The richest known source of GTF is brewer's yeast. At this time (1978), it is postulated that GTF is necessary to work with the hormone insulin for the disposal of ingested carbohydrate in the body (11).

Chromium in Human Nutrition

Evidence is accumulating that human chromium deficiencies do exist (11, 17, 35). Malnourished Jordanian and Nigerian infants with impaired GT responded in some cases to chromium therapy (18). In the case of diabetes only some of the subjects responded with improved GT after chromium treatment (14, 46). There is some evidence of altered GT with aging, and chromium has improved the GT of some older and middle-aged adults (31). The GT of a patient receiving long-term parenteral nutrition also improved with chromium feeding (23).

What can cause a chromium deficiency? If it is assumed that chromium is essential for carbohydrate metabolism, then there ought to be enough in carbohydrate foods. High-carbohydrate foods, such as wheat and sugar, do contain chromium (whole wheat flour, 53 μg chromium per 100 kcal [418 kJ]; raw sugar, 6.0–8.8 μg chromium per 100 kcal [418 kJ]). However, if these two foods are refined or processed, chromium is lost (white flour, 6.6 μg chromium per 100 kcal [418 kJ]; refined sugar, 0.3–2.5 μg chromium per 100 kcal [418 kJ]). Following processing and refining, whole wheat flour and raw sugar lose as much as 87 percent and 72 to 95 percent, respectively, of their original chromium (21, 46).

Daily Need for and Food Sources of Chromium

As of 1978, no requirement has been established for chromium (40).

Chromium in College Meals The average daily chromium content of meals served in 50 colleges in the United States was 0.077 mg per person, with a range of 0.033 to 0.125 mg (51). These data compare well with the 0.06 mg estimated to be in the average diet.

Food Sources of Chromium Chromium values for various foods are listed in Table 14.8. The best dietary sources appear to be brewer's yeast, American cheese, dry beans, peanut butter, meat, and whole grains (15).

Selenium

Both selenium toxicity (from an excessive intake) and deficiency (from an inadequate intake) have been observed in livestock; some evidence of toxicity but not of deficiency has been observed in human beings (49).

In the Great Plains region of the United States

309

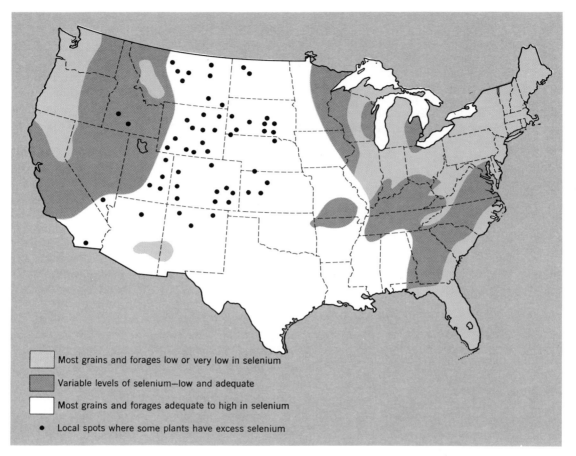

Fig. 14.15 Selenium in crops in relation to animal needs. (From *Science for Better Living*, U.S. Yearbook of Agriculture [Washington, D.C.: U.S. Dept. Agr., 1968], p. 366.)

in the 1930s, grazing animals suffered from "alkali disease" ("blind staggers"), characterized by a stiffness and lameness, loss of hair, deformed hooves, blindness, and often death. This condition was due to an excess of selenium; because the soil had a high selenium content, so did the grasses that the animals consumed.

Metabolism of Selenium

Ingested selenium is absorbed from the intestine into the blood, where it is taken up by a protein and transported in this form. Selenium is found in the highest concentrations in the liver, kidney, heart, and spleen. The main pathway of excretion is by way of the kidneys.

Functions of Selenium

Selenium functions as a constituent of the enzyme glutathione peroxidase, which detoxifies products of oxidized fats and is found in the RBC (42). It is also credited as a protective agent against mercury poisoning in animals (7).

Selenium Toxicity in Human Beings

Evidence of toxicity in human beings differs from symptoms that occur in animals. Studies of Oregon school children suggest that the incidence of dental caries and gingivitis (inflammation of the gums) was significantly higher among children in high selenium (seleniferous) than in low selenium (nonseleniferous) areas (16, 50). But more research is needed before this relationship can be definitely established.

Other signs of human selenium toxicity reported include loss of hair, brittleness of fingernails, garlic odor of the breath, fatigue, and irritability (3).

Selenium in Human Nutrition

Reduced blood selenium values have been reported in children suffering from protein-calorie malnutrition (7, 8). However, further studies are needed in order to understand the significance of this observation and to know whether or not selenium is an essential element for man.

Because of the uneven distribution of selenium in the soils of the United States (Fig. 14.15), there has been an association made of increased incidence of certain human disease with low levels of the mineral in the soil and promotion of supplementary selenium for various human diseases (such as cancer, heart disease, and arthritis). The 1977 Statement of the Food and Nutrition Board (3) concludes that "There is no evidence at this time to suggest that the food supply in the United States contains either too little or too much selenium. There is reason, however, to suspect that indiscriminate selenium supplementation of the diet is potentially hazardous...."

Food Sources of Selenium

The amount of selenium in food varies widely from one region to another (Fig. 14.15). For example, the selenium content of eggs and milk produced in two different sections of Oregon was found to differ tenfold. Meat, eggs, milk, seafood, and whole-grain cereals are good sources of selenium (15).

Other Trace Elements

Deficiencies of nickel, tin, vanadium, and silicon have been produced in experimental animals under conditions meant to eliminate metallic contamination from the environment (37, 38, 47). It appears that nickel is involved in liver metabolism, tin in the growth rate, vanadium in bone development and reproductive performance, and silicon in bone calcification. At this time (1978), there is no evidence that these elements are related to human nutrition (40).

Summary

Iron as a component of hemoglobin in RBCs carries oxygen from the lungs to the tissues and releases it there. Some of the carbon dioxide produced in the tissues (10 percent) is carried by hemoglobin to the lungs where it is released. Iron also is a component of the cytochromes that function in oxidation-reduction reactions in the mitochondria of the cell. The amount of iron in the body is regulated by the amount absorbed; with most nutrients excesses can be excreted, with iron it is difficult. Absorption of iron is more efficient when the need is greater, as during pregnancy and in iron deficiency anemia. The absorption of iron from meat, fish, and poultry (heme iron) is much greater than the absorption from cereals and vegetables (nonheme iron). Taking vitamin C with a meal of nonheme iron improves the absorption; bran and tea are foods that interfere with iron absorption because of the fiber and tannin content, respectively. The RDA for all adult men and for women 51 years and over is 10 mg; for females 11 to 50 years of age, the RDA is 18 mg. The following foods contribute a good quantity of iron to the diet: liver, meats, egg yolk, legumes, leafy green vegetables, and enriched and whole-grain cereals; availability varies with the source. Data from the first HANES showed evidence of iron deficiency in children and adolescents (1 through 17 years of age) but not in adults.

Iodine is an essential component of the hormones of the thyroid gland. In the body cells, the hormones increase the rate of oxidation, stimulate protein synthesis, and have an inhibiting action on oxidative phosphorylation (causing less ATP to be formed and more heat to be produced). The RDA for men 19 to 22 years of age is 140 μg; for those 23 to 50 years, 130 μg; and for those 51 years and over, 110 μg. For women 19 to 50 years the RDA is 100 μg and for those 51 years and over, 80 μg. The amount of iodine in plant sources depends upon the amount in the soil where they were grown; the amount in dairy products and eggs varies according to the amount consumed by the animals. Seafood is high in iodine content. Iodized salt is the most reliable source. Insufficient iodine causes endemic goiter; the decline in its incidence in the United States is attributed to the use of iodized salt, which began in 1924. Women and girls tend to develop endemic goiter more often than do men and boys. Results from the Ten-State Nutrition Survey showed an incidence of thyroid enlargement of 3.1 percent, whereas very few persons had an inadequate intake of iodine based on the level of urinary iodine excretion. The investigators are puzzled and are seeking an explanation for the thyroid enlargement observed.

Manganese, found in the enzyme pyruvic carboxylase, for example, functions in carbohydrate, lipid, and protein metabolism. Only the toxic effects of manganese in human beings have been observed; there is no RDA for it. Dry tea, peanut butter, and whole-grain cereals are good manganese foods.

Copper is present in several enzymes involved in normal blood formation, in maintaining vascular and skeletal structures, and in the structure and functioning of the nervous system. Anemia, neutropenia, low serum copper levels, and changes in the bone are the symptoms in the human infant that respond only to copper therapy. Adults are not prone to copper deficiency; there is no RDA for copper. Dry tea, beef and pork liver, and peanut butter are good sources of food copper.

There are about 70 enzymes that contain zinc; one of them, DNA polymerase, is needed in DNA and RNA metabolism. Retarded growth, retarded sexual development, and poor appetite are among the symptoms of a zinc deficiency in males and females. The signs of a marginal zinc deficiency include poor appetite, suboptimal growth, and impaired sense of taste. The RDA for zinc is 15 mg daily for all those 11 years and older. Meat, eggs, milk, and whole-grained cereals are some of the rich zinc foods.

Cobalt's only function is as a constituent of the vitamin B-12 molecule. There is no RDA for cobalt, and little is known about cobalt in foods.

Molybdenum is a part of the enzyme xanthine oxidase, and it is widely distributed in many foods. There is no RDA for the element.

Fluorine, added to drinking water at a level of 1 ppm, gives maximal resistance to dental caries in human beings. It also helps to prevent bone destruction associated with human aging. Fluorine is found in plant, fish, and animal foods.

Chromium appears to be involved in carbohydrate metabolism as part of the enzyme called the GTF. Whether or not chromium is related to human diabetes remains to be proven. Cheese, dry beans, and brewer's yeast are some of the best sources of the element. There is no RDA for chromium.

Only the human toxic effects of selenium are known. Selenium is a constituent of the enzyme glutathione peroxidase. At this time, there is neither an RDA nor a need for selenium supplementation in the United States. Meats, milk, seafood, and whole-grain cereals are good food sources of the element.

Deficiencies of nickel, tin, vanadium, and silicon have been produced in experimental animals, but there is no evidence that these elements are related to human nutrition.

Glossary

anemia: reduction in number of erythrocytes per cu mm, the quantity of hemoglobin, or the volume of packed red cells per 100 ml of blood.

 iron deficiency: microcytic (red cells, small in size), hypochromic (hemoglobin level low) caused by deficiency of iron in the diet, blood loss, inadequate absorption.

 pernicious: low red cell count; macrocytic (larger than normal) red cells; caused by a lack of intrinsic factor in gastric juice and consequently failure to absorb vitamin B-12. See page 248 for discussion.

 folic acid deficiency: failure of the synthesis and maturation of the red blood cells, with formation of megaloblasts (large immature red cells). See page 246 for discussion.

availability: in nutrition, free to be absorbed from the intestine into the blood.

bicarbonate ion: see p. 276.

bone density: the mineral compactness of bone.

brush border: minute cylindrical processes (microvilli) on the surface of a cell, greatly increasing the surface area; found in the intestinal epithelium.

carbon dioxide: a colorless, odorless gas, CO_2, resulting from the oxidation of carbon; formed in the tissues and eliminated by the lungs.

capillary: a minute blood vessel between the arterioles (minute arteries) and venules (small veins); the interchange of material between the blood and the tissues takes place through the capillary walls.

cofactor: see p. 277.

collagen: see p. 28.

elastin: a major connective tissue protein of elastic structures (i.e., large blood vessels); a yellow, elastic, fibrous mucoprotein.

erythropoiesis: the production of erythrocytes.

extrinsic radioiron tags: radioactive iron added to food, making it possible to identify the iron in the body.

ferritin: see p. 119.

hematocrit: percentage of whole blood volume that is erythrocytes.

heme: see p. 119.

hemochromatosis: a disorder of iron metabolism characterized by excess deposition of iron in the tissues, especially in the liver and pancreas, and by bronze pigmentation of the skin. Occurs in conditions of iron overload.

hemorrhage: escape of blood from the vessels; bleeding.

hemosiderin: an insoluble form of storage iron.

histology: microscopic anatomy; deals with minute structure, composition, and function of tissues.

hypochromic: pertains to a condition in which there is an abnormal decrease in the hemoglobin content of the erythrocytes.

hypoproteinemia: abnormally small amounts of total protein in the circulating blood plasma.

idiopathic: a condition of spontaneous origin; of unknown causation.

iron-binding capacity: the relative saturation of the iron-binding protein transferrin—the amount of the transferrin bound to iron in relation to the amount remaining free to combine with iron.

metalloenzyme: an enzyme containing a metal (ion) as an integral part of its active structure; examples are cytochromes (iron, copper), carbonic anhydrase (zinc).

monodeiodination: removal of one atom of iodine from a compound.

neutropenia: the presence of abnormally small numbers of mature white blood cells in the granulocytic series (neutrophils).

nonheme: iron that is not a part of the hemoglobin molecule; a designation for iron in foods of plant origin.

osteoporosis: a reduction in the normal quantity of bone.

ovalbumin: an albumin found in egg whites.

oxidative phosphorylation: see p. 19.

phytate: a salt of phytic acid (a phosphorus compound occurring in outer layers of cereal grains); the calcium

313

of the insoluble calcium phytate is unabsorbable from the intestine.

plasma: fluid portion of the blood in which the corpuscles (erythrocytes [red cells], leukocytes [white cells], and platelets) are suspended.

porphyrin: a compound present in hemoglobin; a tetrapyrrole ring structure.

radiologically: studied by the examination of X-rays.

red blood cells: also called erythrocytes or red corpuscles; when mature they consist chiefly of hemoglobin and a supporting framework.

seleniferous: areas in which the soil is high in the mineral selenium.

serum (blood): the clear, straw-colored fluid that remains after blood has clotted; the liquid portion of plasma without fibrinogen.

sickle cell anemia: a genetic disorder characterized by the presence of crescent-shaped red blood cells, excessive hemolysis, and active blood formation (hemopoiesis); symptoms are leg ulcers, arthritic manifestations, pain, and abnormal hemoglobin (85 percent is sickle cell hemoglobin and the remainder fetal hemoglobin).

thyroiditis: inflammation of the thyroid gland.

transferrin: blood protein that binds and transports iron.

veins: a vessel through which blood passes on the way to the heart, carrying blood that has given up most of its oxygen.

Study Questions and Activities

1. What are the main locations of iron in the body, and how do they relate to the functions of iron?

2. What foods or dietary nutrients affect iron absorption favorably? Unfavorably?

3. Define or explain the following: hemoglobin, ferritin, hypochromic anemia, simple goiter, cretinism, endemic goiter, and T_3 and T_4.

4. Discuss the absorption, use, and excretion of iron by the body.

5. Plan meals for two days that will provide approximately 18 mg of iron each day.

6. What evidence is there that the iodization of salt is a good public health practice?

7. Question three families to learn if they use iodized salt. Interview two grocers to find out about the comparative sale of iodized versus plain salt.

8. Identify the following: polycythemia, xanthine oxidase, glucose tolerance, manganese poisoning symptoms.

9. What are the signs of copper deficiency and zinc deficiency in human beings?

10. What are three good food sources of copper? Zinc?

11. How do copper, cobalt, and manganese function in the body?

12. Describe some of the findings that have linked fluorine with the maintenance of bone structure in man.

13. Does the community in which you are living or attending college have fluoridated water?

14. Discuss some of the latest findings about the role of chromium and selenium in human nutrition.

References

Iron

1. Abraham, S., F. W. Lowenstein, and C. L. Johnson (1974). *Preliminary Findings of the First Health and Nutrition Examination Survey, United States, 1971–1972: Dietary Intake and Biochemical Findings.* DHEW Publ. No. (HRA) 74-1219-1. Rockville, Md.: Health Resources Adm., Natl. Center for Health Statistics, U.S. Dept. Health, Educ., and Welfare, pp. 10 and 14.

2. Amine, E. K., and D. M. Hegsted (1974). Biological assessment of available iron in food products. *J. Agr. Food Chem.,* **22:** 470.

3. Björn-Rasmussen, E. (1974). Iron absorption from wheat bread; influence of various amounts of bran. *Nutrition and Metab.,* **16:** 101.

4. Björn-Rasmussen, E., L. H. Allberg, B. Isaksson, and B. Avidsson (1974). Food iron absorption in man. Applications of the two-pool extrinsic tag method to measure heme and nonheme iron ab-

sorption from the whole diet. *J. Clin. Invest.,* **53:** 247.

5. Bothwell, T. H. (1970). Total iron loss and relative importance of different sources. In *Iron Deficiency,* edited by L. Hallberg, H.-G. Harwerth, and A. Vannotti. New York: Academic Press, p. 151.

6. Bowering, J., A. M. Sanchez, and M. I. Irwin (1976). A conspectus of research on iron requirements of man. *J. Nutrition,* **106:** 985.

7. *Control of Nutritional Anemia with Special Reference to Iron Deficiency* (1975). Tech. Rept. Series 580. Geneva: World Health Organ., p. 6.

8. Cook, J. D. (1977). Absorption of food iron. *Federation Proc.,* **36:** 2028.

9. Cook, J. D. and E. R. Monsen (1977). Vitamin C, the common cold, and iron absorption. *Am. J. Clin. Nutrition,* **30:** 235.

10. Disler, P. B., S. R. Lynch, R. W. Charlton, T. H. Bothwell, R. B. Walker, and F. Mayet (1975). Studies on the fortification of cane sugar with iron and ascorbic acid. *Brit. J. Nutrition,* **34:** 141.

11. Disler, P. B., S. R. Lynch, R. W. Charlton, J. D. Torrance, T. H. Bothwell, R. B. Walker, and F. Mayet (1975). The effect of tea on iron absorption. *Gut,* **16:** 193.

12. Fairbanks, V. F., J. L. Fahey, and E. Beutler (1971). *Clinical Disorders of Iron Metabolism.* 2nd ed. New York: Grune and Stratton, p. 52.

13. Finch, C. A. (1976). Iron metabolism. In *Present Knowledge in Nutrition,* edited by D. M. Hegsted, Chm., and Editorial Committee. Washington, D.C.: The Nutrition Foundation, Inc., p. 280.

14. Finch, D. A. (1970). Diagnostic value of different methods to detect iron deficiency. In *Iron Deficiency,* edited by L. Hallberg, H.-G. Harwerth, and A. Vannotti. New York: Academic Press, p. 409.

15. Fowler, W. M. and A. P. Barer (1942). Rate of hemoglobin regeneration in blood donors. *J. Am. Med. Assoc.,* **118:** 421.

16. Friend, B. (1967). Nutrients in the United States food supply: A review of trends, 1909–1913 to 1965. *Am. J. Clin. Nutrition,* **20:** 907.

17. Gardner, G. W., R. Edgerton, B. Senewiratne, R. J. Barnard, and Y. Ohira (1977). Physical work capacity and metabolic stress in subjects with iron deficiency anemia. *Am. J. Clin. Nutrition,* **30:** 910.

18. Hallberg, L., A. Hogdhal, L. Nilsson, and G. Rybo (1966). Menstrual blood loss: A population study. Variation at different ages and attempts to define normality. *Acta Obstet. Gynecol. Scand.,* **45:** 320.

19. Hegsted, D. M. (1976). Food fortification. In *Nutrition in the Community,* edited by D. S. McLaren. New York: John Wiley and Sons, p. 203.

20. Heinrich, H. C. (1970). Intestinal absorption in man—methods of measurement, dose relationship, diagnostic and therapeutic applications. In *Iron Deficiency,* edited by L. Hallberg, H.-G. Harwerth, and A. Vannotti. New York: Academic Press, p. 253.

21. *Highlights, Ten-State Nutrition Survey, 1968–1970* (1972). DHEW Publ. No. (HSM) 72-8134. Atlanta, Ga.: Center for Disease Control, U.S. Dept. Health, Educ., and Welfare.

22. Jacobs, A. (1977). Serum ferritin and iron stores. *Federation Proc.,* **36:** 2024.

23. Layrisse, M. and C. Martinez-Torres (1977). Fe(III)–EDTA complex as iron fortification. *Am. J. Clin. Nutrition,* **30:** 1166.

24. Layrisse, M. and C. Martinez-Torres (1972). Model for measuring dietary absorption of heme iron—Test with a complete meal. *Am. J. Clin. Nutrition,* **25:** 401.

25. Layrisse, M., C. Martinez-Torres, J. D. Cook, D. Walker, and C. A. Finch (1973). Iron fortification of food: Its measurement by the extrinsic tag method. *Blood,* **41:** 333.

26. Layrisse, M., C. Martinez-Torres, and M. Gonzalez (1974). Measurement of the total daily dietary iron absorption by the extrinsic tag model. *Am. J. Clin. Nutrition,* **27:** 152.

27. Layrisse, L., C. Martinez-Torres, M. Renzi, F. Velez, and M. Gonzalez (1976). Sugar as a vehicle for iron fortification. *Am. J. Clin. Nutrition,* **29:** 8.

28. Linder, M. C. and H. N. Munro (1977). The mech-

anism of iron absorption and its regulation. *Federation Proc.*, **36**: 2017.

29. Marston, R. and B. Friend (1976). Nutrition review. NSF 158. *National Food Situation*. ERS, U.S. Dept. Agr., November, p. 25.

30. Moore, C. V. (1973). Iron. In *Modern Nutrition in Health and Disease*, 5th ed., edited by R. S. Goodhart and M. E. Shils. Philadelphia: Lea and Febiger, p. 803.

31. Morris, E. R. and R. Ellis (1976). Phytate as carrier for iron — A breakthrough in iron fortification of foods? In *Proc. Ninth National Conference on Wheat Utilization Research*. ARS-NC-40. Peoria, Ill.: Agr. Res. Service, U.S. Dept. Agr., p. 163.

32. Munro, H. N. (1977). Iron absorption and nutrition. *Federation Proc.*, **36**: 2015.

33. Pennell, M. D., M. I. Davies, J. Rasper, and I. Motzok (1976). Biological availability of iron supplements for rats, chicks and humans. *J. Nutrition*, **106**: 265.

34. *Recommended Dietary Allowances, Eighth Edition* (1974). Washington, D.C.: National Academy Sciences, p. 92.

35. Reinhold, J. G., F. Ismail-Beigi, and B. Faradji (1975). Fibre vs. phytate as determinant of the availability of calcium, zinc and iron of breadstuffs. *Nutrition Reports Int.*, **12**: 75.

36. Rogers, T. A. (1961). *Elementary Physiology*. New York: John Wiley and Sons.

37. Stiles, L. W. (1976). Effect of fiber on the availability of minerals. In *The Role of Fiber in the Diet*, edited by D. L. Downing. Special Report No. 21. Ithaca, N.Y.: New York State Cooperative Extension.

38. *Ten-State Nutrition Survey in the United States, 1968–1970* (1971). Atlanta, Ga.: Center for Disease Control, U.S. Dept. Health, Educ., and Welfare.

39. Viteri, F. E. and B. Torien (1974). Anaemia and physical work capacity. *Clin. Haematol.*, **3**: 609.

40. Walker, M. A. and L. Page (1977). Nutritive content of college meals. *J. Am. Dietet. Assoc.*, **70**: 260.

41. Walters, G. O., F. Miller, and M. Worwood (1973).
Serum ferritin concentration and iron stores in normal subjects. *J. Clin. Path.*, **26**: 770.

42. Zamcheck, N. and S. A. Broitman (1973). Nutrition in diseases of the intestine. In *Modern Nutrition in Health and Disease*, 5th ed., edited by R. S. Goodhart and M. E. Shils. Philadelphia: Lea and Febiger, p. 803.

Iodine

1. Abraham, S., F. W. Lowenstein, and D. E. O'Connell (1975). *Anthropometric and Clinical Findings. First Health and Nutrition Examination Survey, United States, 1971–1972*. DHEW Publ. No. (HRA) 75-1229. Rockville, Md.: Public Health Service, U.S. Dept. Health, Educ., and Welfare, p. 22.

2. Brown, J., I. J. Chopra, J. S. Cornell, J. M. Hershman, D. H. Solomon, R. P. Uller, and A. J. Van Herle (1974). Thyroid physiology in health and disease. *Ann. Intern. Med.*, **81**: 68.

3. Cavalieri, R. R. (1973). Iodine. In *Modern Nutrition in Health and Disease*, 5th ed., edited by R. S. Goodhart and M. E. Shils. Philadelphia: Lea and Febiger, p. 362.

4. *Compliance Program Evaluation: FY'74 Selected Minerals in Foods Survey* (1975). Bureau of Foods program circular 7320.08C. Washington, D.C.: Food and Drug Adm., U.S. Dept. Health, Educ., and Welfare.

5. *Compliance Program Evaluation: FY'75 Selected Minerals in Foods Survey* (1976). To be published as Bureau of Foods program circular 7320.08 (adult data), and 7320.33 (infants and toddlers data). Washington, D.C.: U.S. Dept. Health, Educ., and Welfare.

6. Conrad, L. M., III and R. W. Hemken (1975). Milk iodine as influenced by iodophor teat dip. *J. Dairy Science*, **58**: 752.

7. DeGroot, L. J. (1966). Kinetic analysis of iodine metabolism. *J. Clin. Endocrinol.*, **26**: 149.

8. DeGroot, L. J. and J. B. Stanbury (1975). *The Thyroid and Its Diseases*. 4th ed. New York: John Wiley and Sons.

9. Dunn, J. T. (1974). Thyroglobulin and other factors in the utilization of iodine by the thyroid. In *Endemic Goiter and Cretinism: Continuing Threats to World Health*, edited by J. T. Dunn and G. A. Medeiros-Neto. Scientific Publ. No. 292. Washington, D.C.: Pan Amer. Health Organ., p. 17.

10. Dunn, J. T. and G. A. Medeiros-Neto, eds. (1974). *Endemic Goiter and Cretinism: Continuing Threats to World Health*, Scientific Publ. No. 292. Washington, D.C.: Pan Amer. Health Organ., p. 17.

11. Endemic Goiter (1960). In *Legislation on Iodine Prophylaxis*. Geneva: World Health Organ., p. 14.

12. Fisher, K. D. and C. J. Carr (1974). *Iodine in Foods: Chemical Methodology and Sources of Iodine in the Human Diet*. Bethesda, Md.: Life Sciences Research Office, Fed. Am. Soc. Exptl. Biol.

13. Hamilton, J. G. (1948). The rates of absorption of the radioactive isotopes of sodium, potassium, chlorine, bromine, and iodine in normal human subjects. *Am. J. Physiol.*, **124**: 667.

14. Hamwi, J. G., A. W. Van Fossen, R. E. Whetstone, and I. Williams (1955). Endemic goiter in Ohio school children. *Am. J. Public Health*, **45**: 1344.

15. *Highlights, Ten-State Nutrition Survey, 1968–1970* (1972). DHEW Publ. No. (HSM) 72-8134. Atlanta, Ga.: Center for Disease Control, U.S. Dept. Health, Educ., and Welfare.

16. Ibbertson, H. K., P. D. Gluckman, M. S. Croxson, and L. J. W. Strang (1974). Goiter and cretinism in the Himalayas: A reassessment. In *Endemic Goiter and Cretinism: Continuing Threats to World Health*, edited by J. T. Dunn and G. A. Medeiros-Neto. Scientific Publ. No. 292. Washington, D.C.: Pan Amer. Health Organ., p. 129.

17. Joint FAO/WHO Expert Committee on Nutrition (1967). *Seventh Report*, FAO Nutrition Meeting Rept. Series No. 42. Rome: Food and Agr. Organ., p. 35.

18. Kidd, P. S., F. L. Trowbridge, J. B. Goldsby, and M. Z. Nichaman (1974). Sources of dietary iodine. *J. Am. Dietet. Assoc.*, **65**: 420.

19. Matovinovic, J., M. A. Child, M. Z. Nichaman, and F. L. Trowbridge (1974). Iodine and endemic goiter. In *Endemic Goiter and Cretinism: Continuing Threats to World Health*, edited by J. T. Dunn and G. A. Medeiros-Neto. Scientific Publ. No. 292. Washington, D.C.: Pan Amer. Health Organ., p. 17.

20. Murray, T. K. (1977). Prevalence of goiter in Canada. *Am. J. Clin. Nutrition*, **30**: 1573.

21. *Recommended Dietary Allowances, Eighth Edition* (1974). Washington, D.C.: National Academy Sciences, p. 96.

22. Sabry, Z. I. (1973). *Nutrition Canada, National Survey*. Ottawa: Information Canada, p. 114.

23. Sauberlich, H. E., J. H. Skala, and R. P. Dowdy (1974). *Laboratory Tests for the Assessment of Nutritional Status*. Cleveland, Ohio: CRC Press, p. 124.

24. Stanbury, J. B. (1970). Importance of goitrogens, with particular reference to the United States. In *Iodine Nutriture in the United States*. Washington, D.C.: National Academy Sciences, p. 40.

25. Sterling, K., M. A. Brenner, and E. S. Newman (1970). Conversion of thyroxine to triiodothyronine in normal human subjects. *Science*, **169**: 1099.

26. Suzuki, H., T. Higuchi, K. Sawa, S. Ohtaki, and Y. Horiuchi (1965). "Endemic coast goiter" in Hokkaido, Japan. *Acta Endocrinol.*, **50**: 161.

27. Talbot, J. M., K. D. Fisher, and C. J. Carr (1976). *A Review of the Effects of Dietary Iodine on Certain Thyroid Disorders*. Bethesda, Md.: Life Sciences Research Office, Fed. Am. Soc. Exptl. Biol.

28. Thilly, C. H., F. Delange, M. Camus, H. Berquist, and A. M. Ermans (1974). Fetal hypothyroidism in endemic goiter: The probable pathogenic mechanism of endemic cretinism. In *Endemic Goiter and Cretinism: Continuing Threats to World Health*. Washington, D.C.: Pan Amer. Health Organ., p. 121.

29. Thomas, W. C., Jr., A. P. Black, G. Freund, and R. N. Kinman (1969). Iodine disinfection of water. *Arch. Environ. Health*, **19**: 124.

30. Trowbridge, F. L., K. A. Hand, and M. Z. Nichaman (1975). Findings relating to goiter and iodine in the Ten-State Nutrition Survey. *Am. J. Clin. Nutrition*, **28**: 712.

31. Trowbridge, F. L., J. Matovinovic, G. D. McLaren, and M. Z. Nichaman (1975). Iodine and goiter in children. *Pediatrics*, **56:** 82.

32. Underwood, E. J. (1973). Trace elements. In *Toxicants Occurring Naturally in Foods*. 2nd ed. Washington, D.C.: National Academy Science, p. 74.

33. Vought, R. L. and W. T. London (1964). Dietary sources of iodine. *Am. J. Clin. Nutrition*, **14:** 186.

34. Wolff, J. (1969). Iodide goiter and the pharmacologic effects of excess iodide. *Am. J. Med.*, **47:** 101.

Manganese, Copper, Zinc, Cobalt, Molybdenum

1. Brewer, G. J., A. S. Prasad, F. J. Oelshlegel, Jr., E. B. Schoomaker, J. Ortega, and D. Oberleas (1976). Zinc and sickle cell anemia. In *Trace Elements in Human Health and Disease, Volume I, Zinc and Copper*, edited by A. S. Prasad and D. Oberleas. New York: Academic Press, p. 283.

2. Cartwright, G. E. and M. M. Wintrobe (1946). Hematologic survey of repatriated American military personnel. *J. Lab. Clin. Med.*, **31:** 886.

3. Davis, J. E. and J. P. Fields (1955). Cobalt polycythemia in humans. *Federation Proc.*, **14:** 331.

4. Engel, R. W., N. O. Price, and R. F. Miller (1967). Copper, manganese, cobalt, and molybdenum balance in preadolescent girls. *J. Nutrition*, **92:** 197.

5. Freeland, J. H. and R. J. Cousins (1976). Zinc content of selected foods. *J. Am. Dietet. Assoc.*, **68:** 526.

6. Gormican, A. (1970). Inorganic elements in foods used in hospital menus. *J. Am. Dietet. Assoc.*, **56:** 397.

7. Graham, G. G. and A. Cordano (1976). Copper deficiency in human subjects. In *Trace Elements in Human Health and Disease, Volume I, Zinc and Copper*, edited by A. S. Prasad and D. Oberleas. New York: Academic Press, p. 391.

8. Haeflein, K. A. and A. I. Rasmussen (1977). Zinc content of selected foods. *J. Am. Dietet. Assoc.*, **70:** 610.

9. Halsted, J. A., J. C. Smith, Jr., and M. J. Irwin (1974). A conspectus of research on zinc requirements in man. *J. Nutrition*, **104:** 345.

10. Hambidge, K. M., C. Hambidge, M. Jacobs, and J. D. Baum (1972). Low levels of zinc in hair, anorexia, poor growth, and hypogeusia in children. *Pediatrics Res.*, **6:** 868.

11. Lang, V. M., B. B. North, and L. M. Morse (1965). Manganese metabolism in college men consuming vegetarian diets. *J. Nutrition*, **85:** 132.

12. Leach, R. M., Jr. (1976). Metabolism and function of manganese. In *Trace Elements in Human Health and Disease, Volume II, Essential and Toxic Elements*, edited by A. S. Prasad and D. Oberleas. New York: Academic Press, p. 235.

13. Lee, G. R., D. M. Williams, and G. E. Cartwright (1976). Role of copper in iron metabolism and heme biosynthesis. In *Trace Elements in Human Health and Disease, Volume I, Zinc and Copper*, edited by A. S. Prasad and D. Oberleas. New York: Academic Press, p. 373.

14. North, B. B., J. M. Leichsenring, and L. M. Norris (1960). Manganese metabolism in college women. *J. Nutrition*, **72:** 217.

15. O'Dell, B. L. (1976). Biochemistry and physiology of copper in vertebrates. In *Trace Elements in Human Health and Disease, Volume I, Zinc and Copper*, edited by A. S. Prasad and D. Oberleas. New York: Academic Press, p. 291.

16. O'Dell, B. L., C. E. Burpo, and J. E. Savage (1972). Evaluation of zinc availability in foodstuffs of plant and animal origin. *J. Nutrition*, **102:** 653.

17. Prasad, A. S. (1976). Deficiency of zinc in man and its toxicity. In *Trace Elements in Human Health and Disease, Volume I, Zinc and Copper*, edited by A. S. Prasad and D. Oberleas. New York: Academic Press, p. 1.

18. Price, N. O., G. E. Bunce, and R. W. Engel (1970). Copper, manganese, and zinc balance in preadolescent girls. *Am. J. Clin. Nutrition*, **23:** 258.

19. *Recommended Dietary Allowances, Eighth Edition* (1974). Natl. Acad. Sci.-Natl. Research Council. Washington, D.C.: Natl. Research Council.

20. Rodier, J. (1955). Manganese poisoning in Moroccan miners. *Brit. J. Ind. Med.*, **12:** 21.

21. Ronaghy, H. A. and J. A. Halsted (1975). Zinc deficiency occurring in females. Report of two cases. *Am. J. Clin. Nutrition*, **28**: 831.

22. Ulmer, D. D. (1977). Trace elements. *New Engl. J. Med.*, **297**: 318.

23. Underwood, E. J. (1977). *Trace Elements in Human and Animal Nutrition*. 4th ed. New York: Academic Press.

24. Walker, M. A. and L. Page (1977). Nutritive content of college meals. III. Mineral elements. *J. Am. Dietet. Assoc.*, **70**: 260.

Fluorine, Chromium, Selenium, Other Trace Elements

1. Adler, P. (1970). Fluorides and dental health. In *Fluorides and Human Health*. Geneva: World Health Organ., p. 323.

2. Ansell, B. M. and J. S. Lawrence (1966). Fluoridation and the rheumatic disease. A comparison of rheumatism in Watford and Leigh. *Ann. Rheum. Dis.*, **25**: 67.

3. Are selenium supplements needed (by the general public)? Statement of the Food and Nutrition Board, Division of Biological Sciences, Assembly of Life Sciences, National Research Council (1977). *J. Am. Dietet. Assoc.*, **70**: 249.

4. Ast, D. B., D. J. Smith, B. Wachs, and K. T. Cantwell (1956). Newburgh–Kingston caries–fluorine study. XIV. Combined clinical and roentgenographic dental findings after ten years of fluoride experience. *J. Am. Dental Assoc.*, **52**: 314.

5. Bernstein, D. S., N. Sadowsky, D. M. Hegsted, C. D. Guri, and F. J. Stare (1966). Prevalence of osteoporosis in high- and low-fluoride areas in North Dakota. *J. Am. Med. Assoc.*, **198**: 499.

6. Bernstein, D. S. and P. Cohen (1967). Use of sodium fluoride in the treatment of osteoporosis. *J. Clin. Endocrinol. Metab.*, **27**: 197.

7. Burk, R. F. (1976). Selenium in man. In *Trace Elements in Human Health and Disease, Volume II, Essential and Toxic Elements*, edited by A. S. Prasad and D. Oberleas. New York: Academic Press, p. 105.

8. Burk, R. F., Jr., W. N. Pearson, R. P. Wood, II, and F. Viteri (1967). Blood-selenium levels and *in vitro* red blood cell uptake of ^{75}Se in kwashiorkor. *Am. J. Clin. Nutrition*, **20**: 723.

9. Carlos, J. P., A. M. Gittelsohn, and W. Haddon, Jr. (1962). Caries in deciduous teeth in relation to maternal ingestion of fluoride. *Public Health Rept.* (U.S.), **77**: 658.

10. Dietary standard for Canada (1964). *Can Bull. Nutrition*, **4**: No. 1.

11. Doisy, R. J., D. H. P. Streeten, J. M. Freiber, and A. J. Schneider (1976). Chromium metabolism in man. In *Trace Elements in Human Health and Disease, Volume II, Essential and Toxic Elements*, edited by A. S. Prasad and D. Oberleas. New York: Academic Press, p. 79.

12. Englander, H. R. and D. A. Wallace (1962). Effect of naturally fluoridated water on dental caries in adults: Aurora–Rockford, Illinois, Study III. *Public Health Rept.* (U.S.), **77**: 887.

13. Fluoridation and dental health (1969). *WHO Chronicle*, **23**: 505.

14. Glinsman, W. H. and W. Mertz (1966). Effect of trivalent chromium on glucose tolerance. *Metab. Clin. Exp.*, **15**: 510.

15. Gormican, A. (1970). Inorganic elements in foods used in hospital menus. *J. Am. Dietet. Assoc.*, **56**: 397.

16. Hadjimarkos, D. M. (1965). Effect of selenium on dental caries. *Arch. Environ. Health*, **10**: 893.

17. Hambidge, K. M. (1974). Chromium nutrition in man. *Am. J. Clin. Nutrition*, **27**: 525.

18. Hopkins, L. L. Jr., O. Ransome-Kuti, and A. S. Majaj (1968). Improvement of impaired carbohydrate metabolism by chromium (III) in malnourished infants. *Am. J. Clin. Nutrition*, **21**: 203.

19. Horowitz, H. S., W. F. Creighton, and B. J. McClendon (1971). The effect on human dental caries of weekly oral rinsing with a sodium fluoride mouthwash. A final report. *Arch. Oral Biol.*, **16**: 609.

20. Horowitz, H. S. and S. B. Heifetz (1967). Effects of prenatal exposure to fluoridation on dental caries. *Public Health Rept.* (U.S.), **82**: 297.

319

21. Howard, A. N. and I. M. Baird, eds. (1973). *Nutritional Deficiencies in Modern Society*. London: Newman Books, Ltd., pp. 67–70.

22. Howell, C. L. and J. C. Muhler (1954). Effect of topically applied stannous chlorofluoride on the dental caries experience in children. *Science*, **120**: 316.

23. Jeejeebhoy, K. N., R. C. Chu, R. B. Marliss, G. R. Greenberg, and A. Bruce-Robertson (1977). Chromium deficiency, glucose intolerance, and neuropathy reversed by chromium supplementation, in a patient receiving long-term parenteral nutrition. *Am. J. Clin. Nutrition*, **30**: 531.

24. Jenkins, G. N., P. Venkateswarlu, and I. Zipkin (1970). Physiological effects of small doses of fluoride. In *Fluorides and Human Health*. Geneva: World Health Organ., p. 203.

25. Jowsey, J., R. K. Schenk, and F. W. Reutter (1968). Some results of fluoride on bone tissue in osteoporosis. *J. Clin. Endocrinol. Metab.*, **28**: 869.

26. Keene, H. J., F. A. Catalanotto, and G. J. Mickel (1976). Prevalence of caries-free naval recruits from cities with fluoridated and nonfluoridated water supplies. *J. Dental Res.*, **55**: 704.

27. Knutson, J. W. and W. D. Armstrong (1943). The effect of topically applied sodium fluoride on dental caries experience. *Public Health Rept.* (U.S.), **58**: 1701.

28. Kyes, F. M., N. J. Overton, and T. W. McKean (1961). Clinical trial of caries inhibitory dentifrices. *J. Am. Dental Assoc.*, **63**: 189.

29. Largent, E. I. and F. F. Heyroth (1949). The absorption and excretion of fluorides. III. Further observations on metabolism of fluorides at high levels of intake. *J. Ind. Hyg. Toxicol.*, **31**: 134.

30. Leske, G. S. and L. W. Ripa (1977). Guidelines for establishing a fluoride mouth rinsing caries prevention program for school children. *Public Health Rept.* (U.S.), **92**: 240.

31. Levine, R. A., H. P. Streeten, and R. J. Doisy (1968). Effects of oral chromium supplementation on the glucose tolerance of elderly human subjects. *Metabolism*, **17**: 114.

32. McClure, F. J. (1970). *Water Fluoridation*. Bethesda, Md.: U.S. Dept. Health, Educ., and Welfare, National Institute of Dental Research, p. 158.

33. McClure, F. J., H. H. Mitchell, T. S. Hamilton, and C. A. Kinser (1945). Balances of fluorine ingested from various sources in food and water by five young men. *J. Ind. Hyg. Toxicol.*, **27**: 159.

34. Mertz, W. (1967). The role of chromium in mammalian nutrition. *Federation Proc.*, **26**: 186.

35. Mertz, W., E. W. Toepfer, E. E. Roginski, and M. M. Polansky (1974). Present knowledge of the role of chromium. *Federation Proc.*, **33** 2275.

36. Muhler, J. C. (1958). The effect of a single application of stannous fluoride on the incidence of dental caries in adults. *J. Dental Res.*, **37**: 415.

37. Nielsen, F. H. (1976). Newer trace elements and possible application in man. In *Trace Elements in Human Nutrition and Disease, Volume II, Essential and Toxic Elements*, edited by A. S. Prasad and D. Oberleas. New York: Academic Press, p. 379.

38. Nielsen, F. W., and D. A. Ollerich (1974). Nickel: A new essential trace element. *Federation Proc.*, **33**: 1767.

39. Osis, D., L. Kramer, E. Wistrowski, and H. Spencer (1974). Dietary fluoride intake in man. *J. Nutrition*, **104**: 1313.

40. *Recommended Dietary Allowances, Eighth Edition* (1974). Natl. Acad. Sci.-Natl. Research Council. Washington, D.C.: Natl. Research Council.

41. Rich, C., J. Ensinck, and P. Ivanovich (1964). The effect of sodium fluoride on calcium metabolism of subjects with metabolic bone diseases. *J. Clin. Invest.*, **43**: 545.

42. Rotruck, J. T., A. L. Pope, H. E. Ganther, A. B. Swanson, D. G. Hafeman, and W. G. Hoekstra (1973). Selenium: Biochemical role as a component of glutathione peroxide. *Science*, **179**: 588.

43. Rushton, M. A. (1963). Fluoridation. *Proc. Nutrition Soc.* (Cambridge), **22**: 79.

44. Schlesinger, E. R. (1965). Dietary fluorides and caries prevention. *Am. J. Public Health*, **55**: 1123.

45. Schlesinger, E. R., D. E. Overton, H. C. Chase, and K. T. Cantwell (1956). Newburgh–Kingston

caries–fluorine study. XIII. Pediatric findings after ten years. *J. Am. Dental Assoc.*, **52:** 296.

46. Schroeder, H. A. (1968). The role of chromium in mammalian nutrition. *Am. J. Clin. Nutrition*, **21:** 230.

47. Schwarz, K. (1974). Recent dietary trace element research, exemplified by tin, fluorine, and silicon. *Federation Proc.*, **33:** 1748.

48. Schwarz, K. and W. Mertz (1959). Chromium (III) and the glucose tolerance factor. *Arch. Biochem. Biophys.*, **85:** 292.

49. Scott, M. L. (1973). The selenium dilemma. *J. Nutrition*, **103:** 803.

50. Tank, G. and C. A. Storvick (1960). Effect of naturally occurring selenium and vanadium on dental caries. *J. Dental Res.*, **39:** 473.

51. Walker, M. A. and L. Page (1977). Nutritive content of college meals. III. Mineral elements. *J. Am. Dietet. Assoc.*, **70:** 260.

52. Weidman, S. M., J. A. Weatherell, and D. Jackson (1963). The effect of fluoride on bone. *Proc. Nutrition Soc.* (Cambridge), **22:** 105.

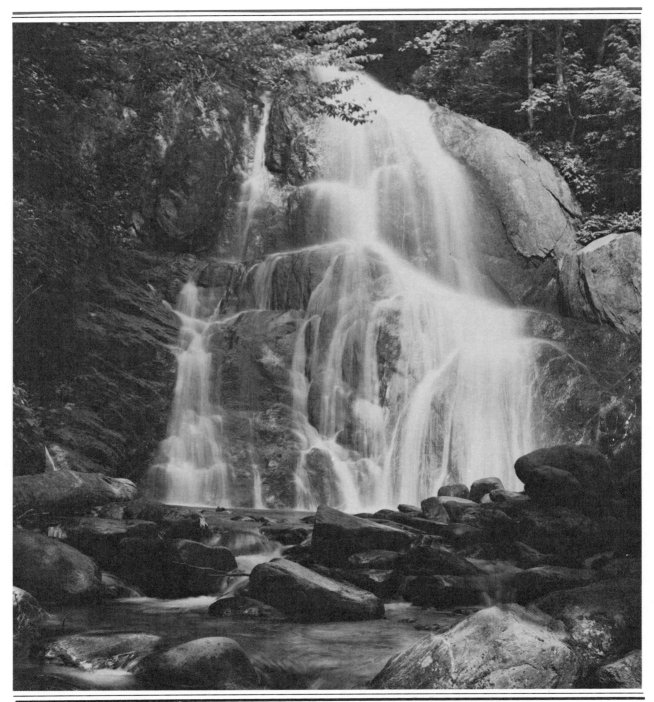

Pure drinking water is a natural resource sought by everyone.

Chapter 15

Water and Electrolytes

Abbreviations

ABS: alkyl benzene sulfonate
—NH₄: ammonium ion
CO₂: carbon dioxide
H₂CO₃: carbonic acid
Cl: chloride
DDT: dichlorodiphenyltrichloroethane

meq or mEq: milliequivalent
ml: milliliter
K: potassium
Na: sodium
STP: sodium tripolyphosphate
WHO: World Health Organization

Water

Water is required by the body, yet it is often overlooked in discussions of the various nutrients. Actually, it is possible to survive longer without food than without water. The survival time depends on the rate of water loss; one can live without food for more than a month but without water for only a few days.

Functions of Water

Water serves as a building material in each cell of the body. The tissues vary in their water content—fatty tissues, 20 percent; striated muscle, 75 percent; and blood plasma, 90 percent (Table 15.1).

As a solvent, water is used in digestion, where it aids in the mastication and softening of food, it supplies fluid for the digestive juices, and it facilitates the movement of material along the digestive tract. The nutrients, in a state of solution, are absorbed through the intestinal wall into the blood and are carried directly to the liver by way of the portal vein or into the lymph vessels, which enter the venous blood in the chest area. Within the cells, water is the medium in which intracellular chemical reactions take place. The blood, which is about 90 percent water, collects the waste products from the cells and carries them to the lungs, the kidneys, or skin for excretion.

Water also facilitates elimination by way of the intestine.

Water is the major constituent of all body fluids including digestive juices, blood, lymph, urine, and perspiration. It serves as a lubricant in the joints and between internal organs. It bathes the body cells, keeping them moist, permitting the passage of substances between the cells and blood vessels.

Water helps to regulate the body temperature. There is always some loss of heat by evaporation from the skin and the lungs. Even when the temperature is a comfortable 23° to 25°C (73.4° to 77°F), water loss is about 600 ml per day, and heat is dissipated at the rate of 12 to 18 kcal (56 to 75 kJ) per hour. This invisible loss of water via the skin and lungs is called insensible perspiration. (Because heat is continuously being produced in the body through metabolic processes, the constant loss of heat is offset and the body temperature remains unchanged.)

Sensible perspiration (sweating) varies according to the temperature of the environment and the amount of physical exertion; it could range from 0 to 2 liters or more per hour. Football players may lose 4.5 to 5 kg (10 to 11 lb) in body weight during a game (largely due to perspiration). The centers that regulate sweating are located in the *hypothalamus*. These centers respond to an elevation in blood temperature above normal, causing increased sweating, evaporation

324

(if the humidity is not too high), and a lowering of the body temperature.

Distribution of Body Water

The water in the body may be thought of as being in two compartments: inside the cells — *intracellular* fluid, and outside the cells — *extracellular* fluid. About 55 percent of the body water is intracellular (about 25 liters in a 70-kg man) and about 45 percent is extracellular (about 15 liters in a 70-kg man) (8). The extracellular compartment includes plasma, interstitial fluid and lymph, dense connective tissue and bone, and *transcellular water* (fluid of the salivary glands, pancreas, liver, mucous membranes of the respiratory and gastrointestinal tracts, cerebrospinal fluid, and ocular fluid) (Table 15.2).

Approximately 55 to 65 percent of the body weight of an adult man is water and of an adult woman, 45 to 55 percent. The difference between the sexes is related to the amount of body fat: adipose tissue contains less water than lean body mass (Table 15.1). The body fat in men 21 to 23 years of age of average build is around 12.4 percent and in women of the same age, 21.2 percent (2).

Table 15.1 Water Content of Various Tissues

Tissue	Water content, percent
Adipose tissue	20
Bone (marrow-free)	25–30
Connective tissue	60
Liver	70
Muscle (striated)	75
Kidney	80
Nervous tissue	
gray matter	85
white matter	70
Blood	
plasma	90
cells	65

Adapted from E. P. Cronkite (1973). Fluid distribution and exchange. In *Best and Taylor's Physiological Basis of Medical Practice*, 9th ed., edited by J. R. Brobeck. Baltimore: The Williams and Wilkins Co., p. 4–114.

Total body water as percentage of body weight is much higher for the young than for the adult; Fig. 15.1 shows the large portion of body weight that is extracellular fluid in premature and newborn infants and the much smaller portion in

Table 15.2 Body Water Distribution in an "Average" Normal Young Adult Male[a]

Compartment	Percent of body weight	Percent of total body water	Liters
Total extracellular	27	45	19
Plasma	4.5	7.5	3
Interstitial-lymph	12.0	20.0	8
Dense connective tissue and cartilage	4.5	7.5	3
Bone water	4.5	7.5	3
Transcellular	1.5	2.5	1
Total intracellular	33	55	23
Total body water	60	100	42

[a] All values rounded to nearest 0.5.
From I. S. Edelman and J. Leibman (1959). Anatomy of body water and electrolytes. *Am. J. Med.*, **27:** 256.

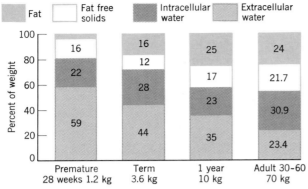

Fat | Fat free solids | Intracellular water | Extracellular water

Fig. 15.1 Comparison of water content as percent of total weight of premature and term infants, a child of 1 year, and a normal, adult 70-kg male. Total water decreases progressively as does extracellular water, whereas intracellular water increases with increase in body cell mass. (From Randall, H. T. [1973]. Water, electrolytes and acid-base balance in _Modern Nutrition in_ Health and Disease, 5th ed., edited by R. S. Goodhart and M. E. Shils. Philadelphia: Lea and Febiger, p. 329. Used with permission. Data taken from Widdowson (growth and composition of the fetus and newborn, in _Biology of Gestation, Vol. II, The Neonate,_ edited by N. S. Assali [New York: Academic Press, 1968] and Moore et al., _Body Cell Mass and its Supporting Environment: Body Composition in Health and Disease_ [Philadelphia: W. B. Saunders, 1963].)

adulthood. The high proportion of extracellular fluid (labile water) in infancy causes the young to be particularly ill-affected by conditions such as diarrhea that cause fluctuations in water balance. During growth, with the increase in body cell mass, the amount of intracellular water also increases.

Water Balance

An example of gross water balance for an adult in good health under conditions in which there is no sweating is presented in Table 15.3.

Carbohydrate | 275 g × 0.6 = 165 g of water of oxidation
Fat | 90 g × 1.1 = 99 g of water of oxidation
Protein | 75 g × 0.4 = 30 g of water of oxidation
Total | 94 g (1¼ cups)

Approximately 54 percent of the water intake comes from liquid, 37 percent from food, and 9 percent from metabolism. About 54 percent of the water is excreted through the urine, 43 percent through insensible loss (lungs and skin), and 4 percent through the feces.

Sources of Water for the Body _Liquids._ The largest fluid intake is from this source. The average person consumes a total of about 1 to 1½ liters of liquid (water, coffee, tea, soup, milk, fruit juice, and others) each day.

Solid Foods. The water content of foods varies widely, but most foods contain more than 70 percent. Figure 15.2 shows the percentage of water in various foods. An interesting comparison is that between green beans (a solid food), which is 92 percent water, and milk (a fluid food), which is 87 percent water. The similarity in the water content is hidden because of the difference in the carbohydrates of the two foods. In green beans some of the carbohydrate is cellulose, which is insoluble; the chief carbohydrate in milk is lactose, which is water soluble. The amount of water obtained from solid foods may vary from ½ to 1 liter per day, depending upon the foods eaten.

Metabolism of Energy Nutrients. Water is formed during the metabolism of carbohydrates, fats, and proteins. Water is continuously being supplied by this source because of the constant oxidation of food for energy. However, the amount of water formed by different foods varies: about 0.60 g of water is produced per g of carbohydrate, 1.07 g per g of fat, and 0.41 g per g of protein (1). An example of the water produced by the metabolism of a day's intake of food follows:

Table 15.3 Water Balance in an Adult Man (70 kg)

		Volume, ml
Water available	Liquid (water, coffee, milk, etc.)	1450
for use by body	Solid food	1000
	Oxidation	250
	Total	2700
Water output[a]	Urine	1450
	Insensible (lungs and skin)	1150
	Feces	100
	Total	2700

[a] In this example, it is assumed that there is no sweating.

Adapted from *Recommended Dietary Allowances. Seventh Edition* (1968). Washington, D.C.: Natl. Research Council, p. 66.

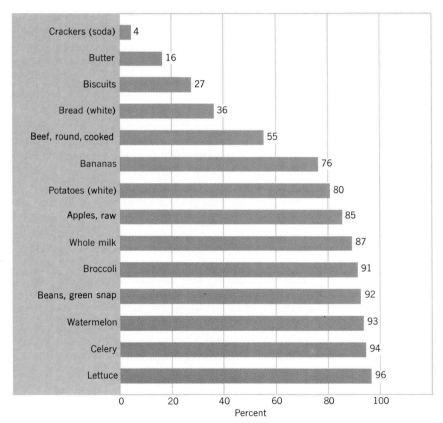

Fig. 15.2 Amount of water in 100 g of various foods. (From *Nutritive Value of American Foods,* Agr. Handbook No. 456. Washington, D.C.: U.S. Dept. Agr., 1975.)

Water Excretion   *Kidneys*. The largest amount of water normally lost from the body is through the kidneys, which excrete from 1 to 2 liters of urine each day. The urinary output varies according to the liquid intake, the type of food consumed, and the amount of water lost through the skin and lungs. Under normal conditions, the greater the amount of fluid ingested in drink and food, the greater the urinary excretion. However, when an individual is physically more active and the environmental temperature higher than usual, proportionately more water is lost through the skin and less by way of the kidney.

As the blood flows through the kidneys, its composition is modified according to the body's need for the various constituents it carries; in general when the body's need is greater, less of the constituent is excreted by the kidney. The kidney tubules function to maintain the composition of the blood within normal limits by selectively reabsorbing such vital substances as amino acids, plasma proteins, glucose, water, and electrolytes; and they excrete waste products of metabolism.

Skin. Water is lost from the skin through insensible perspiration and sweating. Less than 1 liter per day is lost by those who lead a sedentary life in a temperate climate; more than 10 liters per day may be lost by those who live in a hot desert climate. The amount of water lost through the skin depends upon physical activity, environmental and body temperature, humidity, and wind velocity.

Lungs. About 400 ml of water is lost (in the form of an insensible vapor) through the lungs each day. Breathing on a cold glass object results in condensation of moisture on it, giving visual evidence that the lungs are a pathway of water excretion.

Any condition that increases pulmonary ventilation will increase the water loss. If the inspired air is very dry, there will be a higher water loss. The cold, dry air of the mountains takes more moisture from the lungs than does the humid air at the seashore. At very high altitudes the losses are even greater because the low oxygen content of the air requires increased ventilation of the lungs. In Sir John Hunt's successful expedition to the top of Mt. Everest, each man had to drink 5 to 7 pints (2½ to 3½ liters) of water daily (4).

Intestinal Tract. Normally only a small amount of water (about 100 to 200 ml) is excreted through the feces. Most of the large volume of water that flows into the small intestine is reabsorbed. However, additional water may be lost due to diarrhea, vomiting, or an intestinal fistula.

Water Requirements

It has been suggested that, under ordinary circumstances, a reasonable water intake would be 1 ml of water per 1 kcal of food (9). Additional water is needed by those who consume high protein diets and those who live or travel in a hot environment.

Water Supply

Pollution   The matter of having enough pure water to drink in the years ahead is of serious concern. "Water is considered polluted when it is altered in composition or condition so that it becomes less suitable for any or all of the functions and purposes for which it would be suitable in its natural state" (6). Because of pollution, the quality of worldwide water supplies is declining. The chief pollutants are sewage and other liquid wastes from the domestic use of water, industrial wastes, and agricultural effluents.

Sewage and domestic waste water (that used for bathing, laundry, washing dishes, and so forth) increases with population growth. Pollution of the water supply by sewage may occur at the source itself or while it is being conveyed from the source to the consumer. Sewage invariably contains pathogenic bacteria, viruses, and intestinal *parasites*. In many developing countries, the pathogenic bacteria in the water supply

328

often cause infantile diarrhea, dysentery, and other *enteric* infections that are sometimes fatal. There is ample evidence that infectious hepatitis (caused by a presently unidentified virus) and amoebic dysentery (caused by the parasite *Entamoeba histolytica*) result from polluted water.

The contaminants found in sewage and waste water that definitely have a detrimental effect on water supplies include carbon, nitrogen, and phosphorus. Carbon compounds produced by sewage serve as the principal food for aquatic microorganisms; a proliferation of these microorganisms will consume the dissolved oxygen in a stream, thus producing stagnation with bad odors, discolored water, and decayed masses of vegetation. Phosphorus and nitrogen discharged into a receiving stream will encourage the growth of nuisance aquatic plants, such as bluegreen algae. For many years inorganic pollutants (such as nitrates and phosphates) were thought to be harmless. Nitrate fertilizers and animal wastes are the chief sources of nitrate pollution, and phosphate fertilizers and detergents, the chief sources of phosphate pollution (5).

In the 1950s, almost simultaneously in many places in the United States as well as in several European countries, huge banks of suds appeared in the rivers and creeks due to detergent contamination. The main ingredient in detergents (alkyl benzene sulfonate, ABS) could not be digested by bacteria in the water. In 1965, a biodegradable detergent (one that could be digested by bacteria and thus destroyed), a sodium tripolyphosphate (STP), was introduced in the United States (3).

Pesticides in the water supply come from two sources: industrial wastes (from manufacture of pesticides) and runoff from agricultural land. Among the organic pesticides that resist bacterial degradation, the most important are the chlorinated hydrocarbons—lindane, which is currently used and DDT (dichlorodiphenyltrichloroethane), aldrin, and dieldrin which may exist as residues in the soil even though no longer used. The U.S. Public Health Service has established limits for the use of these compounds. Because of their low solubility in water and their tendency to be absorbed by solid surfaces, only traces of these compounds are found in the water; much larger quantities are found in the mud and bottom sediment.

Pollution by radioactive wastes varies from place to place. Artificial radioactive substances discharged from nuclear power reactors and radioactive waste disposal are generally found in low concentrations in drinking water (10).

Available Supplies The demand for water increases as the standard of living rises. It is estimated that the average North American requires 6400 liters (approximately 1600 gallons) of water daily to sustain his life style. This amazing quantity embraces estimates for use in agriculture and industry, including steel, coal, and gasoline production required for supplying the goods that are a part of daily living (10). A small part of the total requirement for water is that for drinking and personal use, perhaps 45 to 50 gallons per person per day.

The reuse of waste water is believed to be an economical way to conserve and increase available water supplies. The total of all solids (or pollutants) represents less than 0.1 percent of the total weight of all water supplies. There are methods of desalting ocean water to provide new water supplies, but the cost is high. Rainmaking may be a possibility for providing water to dry areas (3). One approach (called water harvesting) is the collection and storage of water from land that has been treated to increase the runoff of rainfall and snowmelt (7).

For a discussion of the fluoridation of water supply, see page 305.

Electrolytes

Sodium, potassium, and chloride are appropriately discussed with water because of their unique relationships to body fluids. Sodium is the major *cation* (a positively charged ion) and chloride the major *anion* (a negatively charged ion) in extracellular fluid; potassium is the major cation in intracellular fluid.

Electrolytes: Sodium (Na)

The sodium content of the normal human adult is 80 mEq per kg (1.85 mg/kg) (Table 13.1). Sixty to 65 percent of the body's sodium is found in the blood plasma and in other fluids outside the cells; the remainder is found in the bones.

Functions of Sodium

Sodium is important in the maintenance of *isotonicity* in body fluids and control of the amount of body water; retention of sodium is accompanied by retention of water. It is also a part of the mechanism for the control of acid-base balance in the body (discussed on p. 337).

Sodium has a role in the transport of substances across cell membranes into the cell; for example, the absorption of glucose and of the amino acids is facilitated by the presence of sodium.

Metabolism of Sodium

Absorption and Excretion As much as 95 percent of the sodium ingested is absorbed. The chief pathway of excretion is by way of the kidneys; small amounts are excreted in the feces and some in insensible perspiration. The amount of sodium in sweat varies with the temperature of the environment and with the severity of physical exercise.

Excretion by way of the kidneys varies with the intake of sodium. When the intake of sodium is low, the kidneys conserve it by excreting less than normal; when the intake is moderate to high, the excretion is greater than normal. The kidneys

actually regulate, to a large extent, the sodium content of the body.

Loss of sodium in sweat is decreased in *acclimatized* individuals (9), and the loss is compensated for to some extent by a decreased urinary sodium excretion (5, 37). It takes about a week for men unaccustomed to heat to become fully acclimatized; this judgment was reached by noting the time required for men to do a job with the same ease and comfort in the heat as it was done at ordinary temperatures (30).

The practical question is whether or not additional salt should be taken when sweating is profuse. A WHO scientific group (16) indicated that "in many countries, the dietary intake of sodium chloride will support the production of a minimum of 5 liters of sweat per eight-hour shift in acclimatized men, without disruption of the salt balance. When occupations require higher rates of sweating, a supplementary intake of salt is recommended." To apply the WHO recommendation, information on the amount of sweat produced under varying temperature and intensity of labor conditions is needed. An early investigator (1947) made this information available, as depicted in Fig. 15.3, for climbing stairs, driving a car, and sitting reading at four different environmental temperatures—27°C (81°F), 32°C (90°F), 38°C (100°F), and 43°C (109°F). Activities equivalent in intensity to those shown in Fig. 15.3 can be found in Table 8.4, page 136.

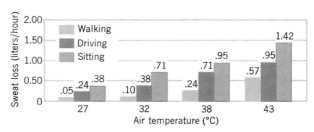

Fig. 15.3 Sweating rates for a clothed man in various activities and at various ambient temperatures. (From Adolph, E. F., et al. (1947). *Physiology of Man in the Desert*, New York: Interscience Publishers.)

Sodium Deficiency

Sodium deficiency due to inadequate consumption is rarely encountered in healthy individuals who have no abnormal losses (16, 19, 27). Depletion usually results from gastrointestinal losses (through vomiting or diarrhea); in such instances water also is lost. Profuse sweating may cause sodium and water depletion (see p. 336). If there is a disproportionately greater loss of sodium in relation to water, the sodium in the extracellular fluid becomes lower than normal, causing a marked decrease in osmotic pressure of this fluid. When this happens, water moves from the extracellular fluid into the cells, thereby raising the osmotic pressure of the extracellular fluid. The volume of the extracellular fluid, including blood, then falls, causing a drop in blood pressure. The lower than normal blood pressure enhances the output of renin (an enzyme liberated by the kidney when the blood pressure is low). Renin acts on a blood protein (angiotensin), which stimulates the production of the hormone aldosterone by the adrenal cortex. Aldosterone acts on the kidney to conserve sodium and water (22). Thus the volume of the extracellular fluid (including that of circulating blood) is restored.

Sodium Excess

When the sodium level in the body is above normal, the production of renin decreases, diminishing the formation of aldosterone and the absorption of sodium.

Acute toxicity with the development of edema has been found to occur in healthy adult men on an intake of 35 to 40 g of sodium chloride daily. Chronic sodium chloride toxicity occurs in many individuals at much lower intakes (21).

Sodium and Hypertension

An unequivocal statement cannot be made concerning salt intake as a cause of elevated blood pressure. In some persons hypertension is associated with high salt intake (11), for others it is not (15, 35). However, the blood pressure of hypertensive persons is reduced by a diet low in salt content (10, 13).

In a study of choice of liquid for drinking—distilled water or saline solution—among 10 hypertensive and 12 normal persons, the mean amount of sodium chloride ingested by the hypertensive was more than four times that consumed by those who were normal (34). Appetite for salt is an acquired taste (21).

Sodium-Restricted Diets

Since the 1950s, it has been the practice to restrict sodium in the diets of those suffering congestive heart disease, hypertension, kidney disease, cirrhosis of the liver, and toxemia of pregnancy. Dietitians and nutritionists have developed and refined the plans for sodium-restricted diets for use by those persons (8).

A sodium-restricted diet includes a minimum of foods from animal sources and prohibits the addition of any salt in preparation. Spices, herbs, and other condiments that are low in sodium can be used for flavor. To ensure the nutritional adequacy of such a diet, low-sodium milk is recommended for anyone required to consume less than 500 mg of sodium a day. The nutritive values of a quart of low-sodium and regular milk are as follows (17):

	Whole milk	
	Low-sodium	Regular
Energy (kcal)	675	675
Protein (g)	31.2	31.2
Carbohydrate (g)	46.0	46.0
Fat (g)	35.0	35.0
Sodium (mg)	< 50	550
Calcium (mg)	930	1150
Potassium (mg)	2300	1300
Thiamin (mg)	0.2	0.4
Riboflavin (mg)	0.8	1.7

Table 15.4 Sodium Content of Various Foods as Served

Food	Per 100 g of food, Sodium, mg	Per average serving Measure	Per average serving Weight, g	Per average serving Sodium, mg
Cracker, saltine	1118	1 packet, 4 crackers	11	123
Bacon	1020	2 med sl	15	153
Cheese, Cheddar	700	1 sl	24	168
Bread, white enriched	507	1 sl	28	142
Soup, tomato with equal volume of water	396	1 c	245	970
split pea with equal volume of water	384	1 c	245	941
Rice, white, cooked	374	1 c	205	767
Rice, white, precooked	273	1 c	165	450
Beans, green, snap, canned, solids	236	1 c	135	319
Peas, green, canned	236	1 c	249	588
Cake, yellow	227	1 pc	92	209
Coffee, instant, regular	125	1 tsp	0.8	1
Peas, frozen, cooked	115	1 c	160	184
Egg, medium, hard cooked	108	1 med	50	54
Pork, ham, baked	73	1 serving	85	637
Chicken, light-meat, roasted	64	1 c, chopped	140	90
Ice cream, regular	63	1 c	133	84
Beef, rump roast	57	1 serving	85	49
Milk, fluid, whole	50	1 c	244	122
Carrot, raw	42	1	81	34
Beans, green, snap, cooked	4	1 c	125	5
Peas, green, cooked	1	1 c	160	2
Banana, medium	0.6	1 med.	175	1

From: C. F. Adams, *Nutritive Value of American Foods*, Agr. Handbook No. 456. Washington, D.C.: U.S. Dept. Agr., 1975.

Low-sodium milk is prepared by an ion-exchange process; the sodium of the milk is replaced by an equivalent amount of potassium. The resulting product, however, contains only about 50 percent of the thiamin and riboflavin and 75 percent of the calcium of the original milk. Taste and flavor are only slightly affected. Low-sodium milk is available in powdered form at certain pharmacies and dairies.

Sodium in water used for beverages and food preparation must be summed with the calculated sodium in the daily food. Municipal and private water supplies should be checked frequently to determine the sodium level; water softeners in private homes should also be checked because they often add sodium to the water. Distilled water should be used if the water's sodium content is too high.

Daily Need for Sodium

The need for sodium chloride is based on water intake; 1 g of sodium chloride per liter of water is suggested. At normal temperatures the water requirement for adults is about 1 ml per kcal (4.18 kJ) daily. The energy RDA for men 19 to 22 years old is 3000 kcal (12.5 MJ) daily; the water need, 3 liters; and sodium chloride, 3 g daily. For women in the same age group (19 to 22 years) the energy RDA is 2100 kcal (8.8 MJ); the water need, 2.1 liters; and sodium chloride, 2.1 g daily. The actual consumption of salt by adults is much higher than that—from 2.3 to 6.9 g of sodium daily (6 to 18 g of sodium chloride daily) (27). For college students fed at 50 American colleges, the daily sodium intake was 5.1 ± 0.9 g (about 13 g sodium chloride) per person per day (36).

The increase in sodium requirement during pregnancy is estimated to be 4 mEq daily, which amounts to about 25 g sodium (64 g sodium chloride) total for the prenatal period (26).

Sources of Sodium

The principal sources of sodium in the diet include the salt used in food processing (ham, bacon, canned and frozen foods, crackers, and potato chips), in cooking at home, and additions at the table. Other sources of sodium include baked goods (baking powder contains sodium bicarbonate and sodium aluminum sulfate) and ready-to-eat foods (which often contain various sodium compounds—monosodium glutamate, sodium nitrite, sodium propionate, sodium citrate, sodium benzoate, etc.). The theoretical amount of sodium in table salt is 39 g per 100 g, or about 2.1 g per teaspoon (1). The sodium content of 100 g portions and of portions commonly served of various foods are listed in Table 15.4.

The sodium content of drinking water varies from area to area. The U.S. Public Health Service tested the sodium-ion content of about 2000 representative, nationwide community water supplies during 1963–1966 and found that 58 percent of the samples had less than 20 mg of sodium per liter (38).

Many common medications contain sodium compounds, such as alkalizers and antacids, headache remedies, sedatives, and cathartics (29). Also baking soda, often taken for indigestion, is a sodium compound.

Electrolytes: Potassium (K)

An adult's body contains about 69 mEq per kg (2.6 g per kg) (Table 13.1) of potassium. Potassium is concentrated primarily within the cells rather than in the extracellular fluids as is sodium, so that the body is better able to conserve it. The potassium content of an individual's body is considered to be sufficiently constant (in spite of some observed variation) that its measurement can be used as a means of determining lean body mass (that portion of body weight that is not adipose tissue) (25). Body fat contains a low concentration of potassium. Determinations of total body potassium in professional football players showed the amount to increase as the season progressed and to be higher than the amount in healthy young men taking only an average amount of exercise daily (7).

Functions of Potassium

Like sodium, potassium helps to maintain the normal osmotic pressure of body fluids and the acid-base balance of the body. Potassium contributes to the maintenance of the osmotic pressure

333

of the intracellular fluid; to a large extent it is bound to protein. It also functions to activate several enzyme reactions; one of them is pyruvate kinase (in the chemical reaction that produces pyruvic acid in carbohydrate metabolism, see p. 261). In muscle contraction and in the transmission of nerve impulses, potassium diffuses out of the cell into the extracellular fluid as sodium enters the cell; similarly, potassium re-enters the cell as sodium leaves it.

Metabolism of Potassium

Like sodium, potassium is well-absorbed — about 90 percent of the amount ingested is absorbed from the intestine. The pathway of excretion is by way of the kidneys.

Potassium Deficiency

Diet alone is not likely to produce a potassium deficiency. However, there may be a serious depletion in cases of cirrhosis of the liver, diarrhea, vomiting, *diabetic acidosis,* body burns (24), and severe protein-calorie malnutrition.

A person who has suffered serious burns may show a negative potassium balance because of large losses of the mineral from his body cells. It has been demonstrated that a potassium and nitrogen intake in the ratio of 6 to 1 (rather than the normal 4 to 1) is necessary to maintain equilibrium in burned patients (24).

The potassium deficiency that occurs in kwashiorkor has led researchers to believe that by treating this disorder initially with skim milk, the high potassium content of milk may be as important as protein in relieving the symptoms (14). Chemical analyses of the brain, liver, skeletal muscles, heart, and kidney tissues of children who died from protein-calorie malnutrition showed a depletion of potassium in all tissues (3), but the loss was greatest in the skeletal muscles.

Some medications cause an increase in urinary excretion of potassium and the necessity for its replacement. Adrenal steroids and some diuretics are among those drugs (6).

At the U.S. Medical Research and Nutrition Laboratory, it was found that fasting produced both a potassium deficiency and an abnormal tolerance of glucose. By taking potassium during a two-week fast period, six obese patients improved their glucose tolerance (4).

Clinical symptoms of potassium deficiency are muscular weakness and *lethargy.* Studies at the University of Glasgow, Scotland, indicated that muscular strength in elderly people, as measured by grip strength, decreased as the potassium intake fell below recommended levels (20).

Potassium Excess

Rarely is it possible to ingest enough potassium to cause an excess in the body. Potassium excess may occur as a result of renal disorders and failure to eliminate potassium normally. An excess causes abnormal heart muscle action (5). In conditions where there is an excess, the urinary excretion is increased; in an insufficiency, the excretion is lessened.

Daily Need for Potassium

The quantitative needs for potassium are not established. The usual diet of an adult is estimated to supply from 50 to 100 mEq daily as potassium or 3.7 to 7.4 g as potassium chloride (21). The average potassium content of meals served in 50 American colleges was 2.7 ± 0.4 g per person per day (36). For adults in good health the intake of potassium in the ordinary diet would appear to be adequate.

Sources of Potassium

Potassium is widely distributed in foods. Good sources are meat, fish, and poultry; fruits and vegetables are high in potassium content as are whole-grain cereals. Table 15.5 gives the potas-

Table 15.5 Potassium Content of Various Foods as Served

Food	Per 100 g of food, Potassium, mg	Per average serving		
		Size of serving		Potassium, mg
			g	
Cocoa, dry pwd.[a]	1518	1 tbsp	5.4	82
Liver, calf, fried[a]	453	1 sl	85	385
Beans, dry, navy, cooked	416	1 c	180	749
Chicken, light meat, roasted[a]	411	1 c chopped	140	575
Banana	370	1 med	119	440
Carrots	342	1	72	246
Celery	341	1 c chopped	120	409
Beef, relatively lean, roast	328	1 serv	85	279
Bacon	233	2 med sl	15	35
Milk, fluid, whole	152	1 c	244	370
Beans, snap, green, cooked	151	1 c	125	189
Peas, green, frozen, cooked	135	1 c	160	216
Egg, hard cooked	130	1 med	50	65
Crackers, saltine	118	1 packet 4 crackers	11	13
Apple	110	1 med	138	152
Bread, white, enriched	104	1 sl	28	29
Peas, green, canned	96	1 c	170	163
Beans, green, snap, canned	95	1 c	135	128
Soup, tomato, with equal volume of water	94	1 c	245	230
Cake, plain	79	1 pc	86	68

[a] *Nutritive Value of American Foods*, Agr. Handbook No. 456. Washington, D.C.: U.S. Dept. Agr., 1975.
From: *Nutritive Value of Foods*, Home and Garden Bull, No. 72. Washington, D.C. U.S. Dept. Agr., 1977.

sium content of some foods. Also see Appendix Table A-3 for a more extensive listing.

Electrolytes: Chloride (Cl)

Chloride, like sodium, is found largely in the extracellular compartment, the blood plasma and the fluids outside the cells; it is present also in gastric juice as a component of hydrochloric acid.

Functions of Chloride

As a major component of extracellular fluid, chloride helps in maintaining osmotic pressure in body fluids. Chloride also functions in the regulation of acid-base balance (see p. 337). Chloride and also phosphate, carbonate, sulfate groups, *organic acids*, and protein have an acid reaction. Passmore and Draper listed the distribution of certain mineral ions in a normal man, expressed

Water and Electrolytes

as mEq per liter of intracellular and extracellular fluid (23):

	Intracellular fluid	Extracellular fluid
Sodium (Na+)	10	145
Potassium (K+)	150	5
Calcium (Ca++)	2	2
Magnesium (Mg++)	15	2
	177	154
Chloride (Cl−)	10	100
Phosphate (PO$_4$−−−)	90	2
Carbonate (HCO$_3$−)	10	27
Sulfate (SO$_4$−−)	15	1
Organic acids	−	5
Protein	52	19
	177	154

Concerning the above values, the authors state that those for the extracellular fluid may be considered reliable; few analyses of intracellular fluid have been made, so these values "merely give some guidance as to the order of magnitude of the common ions in cells."

The chloride ion activates the starch-splitting enzyme of saliva, salivary amylase.

Metabolism of Chloride

Cells (parietal cells) of the stomach lining secrete hydrochloric acid into the stomach. The origin of the chloride ion for the hydrochloric acid secretion is the blood.

Chloride is readily absorbed from the intestine. The principal pathway of excretion is by way of the kidney. As with sodium and water and in contrast to potassium, aldosterone causes the kidney to conserve chloride. Chloride in excess is readily excreted by the kidney.

336

Daily Need and Sources of Chloride

The quantitative need for chloride has not been established. The chief source of chloride is from salt added to food.

Water and Electrolyte Balance

Effect of Physical Activity

Profuse sweating with resultant losses of water, sodium, and potassium are concerns for the well-being of athletes and their competency in physical performance. Losses are less for the acclimatized athlete than for the athlete who is not. It is recommended that before strenuous exercise in a hot climate the athlete should undergo a period of active acclimatization (39). A suggested procedure is to participate in moderate exercise in the heat for four to seven days or up to two weeks. With acclimatization, the individual undergoes several physiological adjustments that make for a better capacity to endure the stress of heat; the total blood volume increases, the flow of blood to the skin also increases, and the time required for blood to reach the skin is shortened (39).

Water replacement is of first concern. Symptoms of water deprivation appear very soon, as shown in Table 15.6. It is recommended that during rigorous exercise small, frequent drinks (2 to 3 oz [50 to 60 ml]) be taken instead of delaying and taking larger amounts less often. Darden (12) points out that an athelete soon recognizes the amount of fluid that is best for his body. In preparation for endurance events, large quantities of water may be taken the hour before the event; immediately prior .5 liter should cause no problems (39).

Under heavy sweat losses, controlled salt tablet intake may be advisable. Adding additional salt to food for salt replacement is used by some athletes; however, a taste for heavily salted food may develop and continue when the additional elec-

Table 15.6 Rate of Onset of Deficiency Syndromes in Working Men Exposed to Complete Deficiency

Nutrient	Time lapse before earliest deleterious effects appear	Earliest deficiency syndromes and end results
Water	A few hours	Easy fatigue, poor performance; eventual exhaustion from dehydration
Total kilocalories	2 or 3 days	Easy fatigue, poor performance
Sodium chloride	Several days	Easy fatigue, poor performance; eventually heat cramps

From C. F. Consolazio, R. E. Johnson, and L. J. Pecora. *Physiological Measurements of Metabolic Functions in Man.* New York: McGraw-Hill Book Co., © 1963, p. 345. Used with permission of McGraw-Hill Book Company.

trolyte is not needed. Salt tablets are taken with a liberal amount of water and should be taken only when the weight loss is over 5 to 6 lb (2.2 to 2.7 kg) (39). Potassium also is lost in sweat. Some success in the prevention of heat stress has been reported with the use of tablets containing potassium (33); another recommendation was that fruits, especially bananas, be included in the diet to increase the potassium intake (31).

In wrestling, most participants believe their chances for success are better at a body weight lower than their preseason weight. Studies of weight losses in high school and college wrestlers indicate that from 3 to 20 percent of the body weight (preseason) is lost before the weight is certified for the competition (32). Studies on the nature of the weight loss show that water, fats, and proteins are lost when not only food restriction but also fluid deprivation procedures are followed (18, 28). Concerned about the procedures used for achieving the desired weight by young competitors, the American College of Sports Medicine made a statement of their position, one point of which was that the daily energy requirement should be provided by a balanced diet and that it was "the responsibility of coaches, school officials, physicians, and parents to discourage wrestlers from securing less than their minimal needs without prior medical approval" (2).

Acid-Base Balance

Chemical Reaction of Body Fluids

Acid-base balance (also called hydrogen-ion balance) refers to the chemical reaction of body fluids. The blood and tissue fluids are weakly basic (pH 7.35 to 7.45) with two exceptions — gastric juice in the stomach (pH 1.77) and the fluid in the kidney tubules (urine has a mean pH of about 6.0, although the pH varies according to the body's acid-base equilibrium) (Fig. 15.4). The body cells cannot function if the pH varies too far from the narrow range of pH 7.35 to 7.45 (the extremes compatible with life are recognized to be pH 6.8 and pH 7.8). Effective mechanisms function in the body to control the pH and maintain it within the normal range. Since the processes that regulate acid-base equilibrium are complex, they will be presented here in a brief and simplified form.

Hydrogen-Ion Concentration

To understand the acid-base equilibrium mechanism, one must know something about hydrogen-ion (H^+) concentration. The acidic or basic reaction of a solution depends upon its concentration of hydrogen ions. The symbol pH was devised for

337

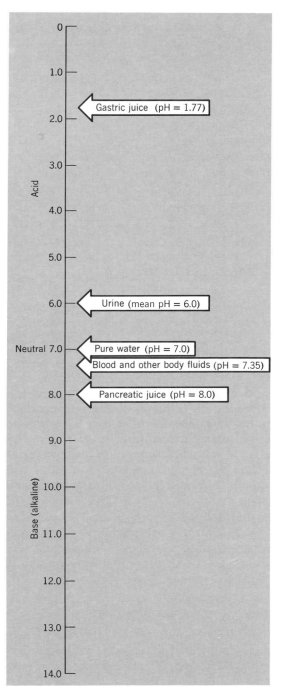

Fig. 15.4 The pH scale.

simplicity in expressing hydrogen-ion concentration (to avoid using large fractional numbers); it is the negative logarithm of the hydrogen-ion concentration. The pH scale ranges from 0 to 14.0, with the midpoint (7.0) neutral. The scale is acid from 0 to 7.0 and basic from 7.0 to 14.0. The lower the pH number, the greater the hydrogen-ion concentration (and thus the greater the acidity); the higher the pH number, the lower the hydrogen-ion concentration (and thus the greater the basicity).

Mechanisms for Controlling Acid-Base Balance

The principal mechanisms for controlling acid-base equilibrium are the *buffer systems* of the body and the excretory action of the lungs and the kidneys. The buffer systems are the principal mechanisms for short-term regulation of pH. Buffers are substances that can absorb large amounts of acids or bases without undergoing much change in hydrogen-ion concentration. Among the significant buffer systems of the body are those that combine a weak acid and its salts; for example, a sodium bicarbonate-carbonic acid buffer system is found in the extracellular fluids of the body (see p. 261). The phosphates in the body fluids are also important buffers, as are plasma proteins and the hemoglobin of the red cells (see p. 104).

A mechanism for minimizing changes in pH in the blood when the carbon dioxide tension and the concentration of the bicarbonate ion in the red blood cells increase is the diffusion of the bicarbonate ion from the red cells to the plasma and the movement of the chloride ion from the plasma to the red cells (removal from the plasma of a strong acid ion-Cl^- in exchange for a weak acid ion-HCO_3^- from the red cells). In the lungs, where the carbon dioxide tension and the bicarbonate concentration in the red cells decrease, the reverse movements take place, with the bicarbonate ion moving into the cell and the chloride ion shifting from it to the plasma. This process is known as the chloride shift.

The maintenance of a constant pH in the body ultimately depends upon the excretory action of the lungs and the kidneys. The lungs normally eliminate carbon dioxide (CO_2) from the body as rapidly as it is produced in the tissues. If the production becomes excessive, as in exhausting work or exercise, and the carbonic acid (H_2CO_3) content of the blood rises, the respiratory center in the brain is stimulated, increasing the breathing rate and the elimination of CO_2. If the hydrogen-ion concentration of the body fluids is lowered, the action of the respiratory center becomes depressed, lowering the breathing rate and the elimination of CO_2, and increasing the concentration of carbonic acid in the body fluids.

The kidneys excrete sulfuric, phosphoric, and hydrochloric acids (the end products of metabolism) in the form of salts. Sulfuric acid is produced by protein catabolism since most proteins are made up of some sulfur-containing amino acids. Phosphoric acid is also produced by protein catabolism. These acids may combine with sodium, potassium, magnesium, or calcium (but principally with sodium and potassium) to form salts.

An important mechanism for neutralizing acids is the production of ammonium ions ($-NH_4$) by the kidneys. The excretion of ammonium salts instead of sodium, potassium, magnesium, or calcium salts conserves these minerals within the body if the supply is limited. If the base is in excess (as may occur after prolonged vomiting), the kidneys excrete more sodium and potassium ions and fewer ammonium salts.

Acid-Forming and Base-Forming Foods

Because of the mechanisms for maintaining the body's acid-base balance within normal range, the acid-base reaction of the diet is of little practical importance. The following is a brief explanation of the meaning of acid-forming and base-forming foods. Foods classed as acid-forming have more phosphorus, sulfur, and chlorine than base-forming ions; those classed as base-forming have more sodium, potassium, calcium, and magnesium than acid-forming ions.

Acid-forming foods include meat, fish, poultry, eggs, cereals, and some nuts (peanuts and walnuts). Base-forming foods include vegetables, fruits, milk, and some nuts (almonds). After metabolism, the inorganic ions that remain from a usual mixed diet are base-forming. Sugar, butter, lard, oils, cornstarch, and tapioca contain no mineral elements and so are neither acid- nor base-forming.

Lemons, oranges, limes, and certain other fruits are acid to the taste; they are, however, base-forming foods. The acid taste is due to organic acids (such as citric and malic), which are oxidized completely to carbon dioxide and water, leaving the salts, which are predominantly basic in reaction. The organic acids in plums and prunes (benzoic acid) and in cranberries (quinic) are not metabolized in the body. Hence these fruits contribute to the acidity of body fluids.

Summary

Water is an essential nutrient without which the survival time is at best only a few days. Each cell of the body contains water; it serves as a solvent and as a lubricant, and it helps in the regulation of body temperature. The body contains more water than any other nutrient (55 to 65 percent in men, 45 to 55 percent in women). Body water comes from ingested liquids and solids and from water formed in the metabolism of carbohydrates, fats, and proteins. The major pathway of excretion is by way of the kidneys, with some loss through the skin and in exhalation. A suggested requirement under ordinary circumstances is 1 ml water per 1 kcal (4.8 kJ) of food.

Sodium, potassium, and chloride are the electrolytes important in the maintenance of isotonicity in body fluids and in the mechanisms of acid-base balance in the body. Sodium and chloride are present chiefly in the extracellular fluid

339

(compartment) and potassium in the intracellular fluid (compartment). The sodium content of the body is largely controlled by the kidneys through excreting less when the intake is low and more when the intake is high. The sodium lost in sweat by persons doing physical work in a hot atmosphere may need replacement by the introduction of extra salt. With acclimatization, the sodium content of sweat lessens. The need for sodium is based on water intake; the suggested amount is 1 g of sodium chloride (0.4 g sodium) per liter of water ingested. Principal sources of sodium in the diet are the salt in processed and home-cooked foods and the salt added at the table. Whether or not the level of salt intake is a possible cause of elevated blood pressure cannot be stated unequivocally; however, it is known that restriction in sodium intake reduces blood pressure in hypertensive individuals.

The potassium content of an individual's body is considered to be sufficiently constant for its measurement to be used as an index of lean body mass, the principal location of potassium in the body. In addition to functioning in the maintenance of normal osmotic pressure and acid-base balance, potassium is essential in the activation of certain enzyme reactions and in the processes of muscle contraction and transmission of nerve impulses. The quantitative need for potassium is not established. It is widely distributed in food so that dietary lack is not likely to be the cause of deficiency. There are conditions that increase the need for potassium, among them the taking of certain medications, including adrenal steroids and diuretics. Muscular weakness and lethargy are clinical symptoms of potassium deficiency.

The chloride ion, in addition to functioning in the maintenance of osmotic pressure and the regulation of acid-base balance, activates the starch-splitting enzyme salivary amylase and is a component of the hydrochloric acid secreted in the stomach. A quantitative need for chloride has not been established. Sodium chloride added to food is the chief source of it in the diet.

Large losses of water and electrolytes occur during severe physical activity in the heat. Water replacement is the first concern. When sweat losses are heavy, controlled salt intake may be advisable.

The reaction of blood and tissue fluids is weakly basic (pH 7.35 to 7.45) except for the stomach tissues that secrete hydrochloric acid, which are pH 1.77, and the fluid in the urinary tubules, which is around pH 6.0. The principal mechanisms for controlling the balance between acid and base in the body are the buffer systems and the excretory actions of the lungs and the kidneys.

Glossary

acclimatize: the process of becoming adjusted to a new environment.

aldosterone: an electrolyte regulating hormone secreted by the adrenal cortex.

angiotensin: a polypeptide present in blood which stimulates the secretion of aldosterone by the adrenal cortex.

anion: a negatively charged ion.

buffer system: buffers are substances that tend to stabilize the pH of a solution; a buffer is a mixture of either a weak acid and its salt or a weak base combined with an acid. An acid-base pair is made up of a proton donor and a proton acceptor. For example:

$$\frac{\text{bicarbonate}}{\text{carbonic acid}}, \frac{\text{HCO}_3^-}{\text{H}_2\text{CO}_3}, \frac{\text{proton (H}^+\text{) acceptor}}{\text{proton (H}^+\text{) donor}}$$

The pairs are called "buffer systems."

cation: a positively charged ion.

cirrhosis of the liver: progressive destruction of the liver cells and an abnormal increase of connective tissue.

diabetic acidosis: a relative decrease of alkali in body fluids in proportion to the content of acid.

electrolyte: any compound that, when dissolved in water, separates into charged particles (ions) capable of conducting an electric current, such as sodium chloride, which dissociates into Na^+ and Cl^-.

enteric: pertaining to the small intestine.

340

extracellular: outside of the cells.

hypertension: persistently high blood pressure.

hypothalamus: a portion of the brain lying at the base of the cerebrum (the main part of the brain occupying the upper part of the cranium).

intracellular: inside the cells.

isotonicity: the same osmotic pressure among fluids (solutions).

lethargy: a condition of drowsiness or indifference.

mEq or meq: milliequivalent; one mEq of an ion is equal to the atomic weight (mg) divided by the valence. For example, for sodium, it is $23/1 = 23$.

organic acid: contains one or more carboxyl groups (COOH); simple examples are formic acid (HCOOH) and oxalic acid $\begin{matrix}(COOH)\\|\\(COOH)\end{matrix}$

parasite, intestinal: an organism that lives in the intestine of man and animal, gaining its nourishment there.

proton: a particle of the nucleus of an atom that has a charge of plus one. A proton is a positive hydrogen ion (H^+).

renin: an enzyme produced by the kidney in response to diminished blood pressure; renin converts angiotensinogen present in the blood to angiotensin, which stimulates aldosterone secretion.

toxemia of pregnancy: a pathologic condition occurring in pregnant women, characterized by excessive vomiting (hyperemesis, gravidum), hypertension, albuminuria, and edema.

transcellular water: a term applied to the fluid of the salivary glands, the pancreas, liver, mucous membrane of the respiratory and gastrointestinal tracts, cerebrospinal fluid, and ocular fluids.

Study Questions and Activities

1. Explain the functions of water as a body-building material and in regulating body processes.
2. Define or explain the following: intracellular fluid, extracellular fluid, and water of oxidation.
3. Keep a record of your intake of all fluids for one day. Compare this record with an estimate of water from your food intake and your metabolism. Is your water consumption adequate?
4. How might one conserve body water?
5. Name three good food sources of sodium and of potassium.
6. What are the signs of potassium deficiency in human beings? What conditions are likely to produce this deficiency?
7. Do you believe that it is a good idea to use a large amount of salt in preparing food? If so, why? If not, why not?
8. Is it logical to discuss sodium, potassium, chloride, and water in the same chapter? If so, give your reasons; if not, explain why not.
9. Should individuals be careful about the acid-base reaction of the foods they eat? Justify your reply.

References

Water

1. Alper, C. (1968). Fluid and electrolyte balance. In *Modern Nutrition in Health and Disease*, 4th ed., edited by M. G. Wohl and R. S. Goodhart. Philadelphia: Lea and Febiger, p. 404.
2. Behnke, A. R. (1969). New concept of height-weight relationship. In *Obesity*, edited by N. L. Wilson. Philadelphia: F. A. Davis, Co., p. 27.
3. Behrman, A. S. (1968). *Water Is Everybody's Business*. Garden City, N.Y.: Doubleday.
4. Davidson, S., R. Passmore, J. F. Brock, and A. S. Truswell (1975). *Human Nutrition and Dietetics*. 6th ed. London: Churchill Livingstone, p. 96.
5. Grava, S. (1969). *Urban Planning Aspects of Water Pollution Control*. New York: Columbia Univ. Press.
6. *Health Hazards of The Human Environment* (1973). Geneva: World Health Organ. p. 47.
7. Myers, L. E. (1968). New-old water abracadabra reverses disappearing act. In *Science for Better Living: The Yearbook of Agriculture 1968*, edited by J. Hayes. Washington, D.C.: U.S. Dept. Agr., p. 135.

8. Randall, H. T. (1973). Water, electrolytes, and acid-base balance. In *Modern Nutrition in Health and Disease*, 5th ed., edited by R. S. Goodhart and M. E. Shils. Philadelphia: Lea and Febiger, p. 329.

9. *Recommended Dietary Allowances. Eighth Edition* (1974). Washington, D.C.: National Academy Sciences.

10. Thomas, G. W., S. E. Curl, and W. F. Bennett, Sr. (1976). *Food and Fiber for a Changing World. Third Century Challenge to American Agriculture.* Danville, Ill.: The Interstate Printers and Publishers, Inc., p. 77.

Electrolytes, Water and Electrolyte Balance, Acid-Base Balance

1. Adams, C. F. (1975). *Nutritive Value of American Foods in Common Units.* Agr. Handbook No. 456. Washington, D.C.: U.S. Dept. Agr., p. 142.

2. American College of Sports Medicine (1977). Position stand on weight loss in scholastic and collegiate wrestlers. Mimeographed statement. Madison, Wis.

3. Alleyne, G. A. O., D. Halliday, J. C. Waterlow, and B. L. Nichols (1969). Chemical composition of organs of children who died from malnutrition. *Brit. J. Nutrition.* 23 783.

4. Anderson, J. W., R. H. Herman, and K. L. Newcomer (1969). Improvement in glucose tolerance of fasting patients given oral potassium. *Am. J. Clin. Nutrition.* 22: 1589.

5. Ashworth, A. and A. D. B. Harrower (1967). Protein requirements in tropical countries: Nitrogen losses in sweat and their relation to nitrogen balance. *Brit. J. Nutrition.* 21: 833.

6. Beeson, P. B. and W. McDermott, eds. (1975). *Textbook of Medicine.* 14th ed. Philadelphia: W. B. Saunders, p. 1588.

7. Boddy, K., R. Hume, P. C. King, E. Weyers, and T. Rowan (1974). Total body plasma, and erythrocyte potassium and leucocyte ascorbic acid in "ultra-fit" subjects. *Clin. Sci. and Mal. Med.,* 46: 449.

8. Chicago Dietet. Assoc. Inc. and So. Suburban Dietet. Assoc. of Chicago, Inc. (1975). *Manual of Clinical Dietetics.* Downers Grove, Ill.: Johnson Printers, sec. VII, p. 1.

9. Consolazio, C. F., R. E. Johnson, and L. J. Pecora (1963). *Physiological Measurements of Metabolic Functions in Man.* New York: McGraw-Hill Book Co., p. 344.

10. Corcoran, A. C., R. D. Taylor, and I. H. Page (1951). Controlled observations on the effect of low sodium dietotherapy in essential hypertension. *Circulation.* 3: 1.

11. Dahl, L. K. (1961). Possible role of chronic excess salt consumption in the pathogenesis of essential hypertension. *Am. J. Cardiol.,* 8: 571.

12. Darden, E. (1976). *Nutrition and Physical Performance.* Pasadena, Calif.: The Athletic Press, pp. 122 and 159.

13. Dole, V. P., L. K. Dahl, G. C. Cotzias, D. D. Dziewiatkowski, and C. Harris (1951). Dietary treatment of hypertension. II. Sodium depletion as related to the therapeutic effect. *J. Clin. Invest.,* 30: 584.

14. Electrolyte metabolism in kwashiorkor (1957). *Nutrition Rev.,* 15: 101.

15. Gros, G., J. M. Weller, and S. W. Hoobler (1971). Relationship of sodium and potassium intake to blood pressure. *Am. J. Clin. Nutrition,* 24: 605.

16. *Health Factors Involved in Working Under Conditions of Heat Stress* (1969). WHO Tech. Report Series No. 142. Geneva: World Health Organ., p. 49.

17. Heap, B. (1968). Low-sodium milk — current status. *J. Am. Dietet. Assoc.,* 53: 43.

18. Herbert, W. G. and P. M. Rebisl (1972). Effects of dehydration upon physical work capacity of wrestlers under competitive conditions. *Res. Quart. Am. Assoc. for Health, Phys. Ed. and Recreation.* 43: 416.

19. Hunter, G. W., III, W. W. Frye, and J. C. Swartzwelder (1966). *A Manual of Tropical Medicine.* 4th ed. Philadelphia: W. B. Saunders Co., p. 638.

20. Low potassium may weaken grip in the aged (1969). *J. Am. Med. Assoc.,* 210: 25.

21. Meneely, G. R. and H. D. Battarbee (1976). Sodium and potassium. In *Present Knowledge in*

Nutrition, 4th ed., edited by D. M. Hegsted, Chm. and Editorial Committee. Washington, D.C.: The Nutrition Foundation, Inc., p. 259.

22. Mulrow, P. J. (1969). Aldosterone in hypertension and edema. In *Disease of Metabolism,* 6th ed., edited by P. K. Bondy and L. E. Rosenberg. Philadelphia: W. B. Saunders Co., p. 1092.

23. Passmore, R. and M. H. Draper (1964). The chemical anatomy of the human body. In *Biochemical Disorders in Human Disease,* 2nd ed., edited by R. H. S. Thompson and E. J. King. New York: Academic Press, p. 10.

24. Pearson, E., H. S. Soroff, G. K. Arney, and C. P. Artz (1961). An estimate of the potassium requirements for equilibrium in burned patients. *Surg., Gynecol., Obstet.,* **112:** 263.

25. Pierson, R. N., Jr., D. H. Y. Lin, and R. A. Phillips (1974). Total-body potassium in health: Effects of age, sex, height, and fat. *Am. J. Physiol.,* **226:** 206.

26. Pitkin, R. M., H. A. Kaminetsky, M. Newton, and J. A. Pritchard (1972). Maternal nutrition, a selective review of clinical topics. *J. Obstet. and Gynecol.,* **40:** 773.

27. *Recommended Dietary Allowances. Eighth Edition* (1974). Washington, D.C.: National Academy Sciences, p. 89.

28. Ribisl, P. and W. Herbert (1970). Effects of rapid weight reduction and subsequent dehydration upon the physical working capacity of wrestlers. *Res. Quart. Am. Assoc. Health, Phys. Ed. and Recreation,* **41:** 536.

29. Rivers, J. (1973). *Sources of Dietary Sodium.* Chicago: Water Facts Consortium.

30. Robinson, S., E. S. Turrell, H. S. Belding, and S. M. Horwath (1943). Rapid acclimatization to work in hot climates. *Am. J. Physiol.,* **140:** 168.

31. Rose, K. (1975). Warning for millions: Intense exercise can deplete potassium. *Physician and Sportsmed.,* **3:** 67.

32. Rowell, L. B. (1974). Human cardiovascular adjustments to exercise and thermal stress. *Physiol. Rev.,* **54:** 75.

33. Schamadan, J. L., W. R. Godfrey, and W. D. Snively, Jr. (1968). Evaluation of potassium-rich electrolyte solutions as oral prophylaxis for heat stress disease. *Indust. Med. Surg.,* **37:** 677.

34. Schechter, P. J., D. Horwitz, and R. I. Henkin (1973). Sodium chloride preference in essential hypertension. *J. Am. Med. Assoc.,* **225:** 1311.

35. Swaye, P. S., R. W. Gifford, Jr., and J. N. Berrettoni (1972). Dietary salt and essential hypertension. *Am. J. Cardiology,* **29:** 33.

36. Walker, M. A. and L. Page (1977). Nutritive content of college meals. III. Mineral elements. *J. Am. Dietet. Assoc.,* **70:** 260.

37. Wheeler, E. F., H. El-Neil, J. O. C. Wilson, and J. S. Weiner (1973). The effect of work level and dietary intake on water balance and the excretion of sodium, potassium, and iron in a hot climate. *Brit. J. Nutrition,* **30:** 127.

38. White, J. M., J. G. Wingo, L. M. Alligood, et al. (1967). Sodium ion in drinking water. *J. Am. Dietet. Assoc.,* **50:** 32.

39. Williams, M. H. (1976). *Nutritional Aspects of Human Physical and Athletic Performance.* Springfield, Ill.: Charles C Thomas, Publ.

3

Applied Nutrition

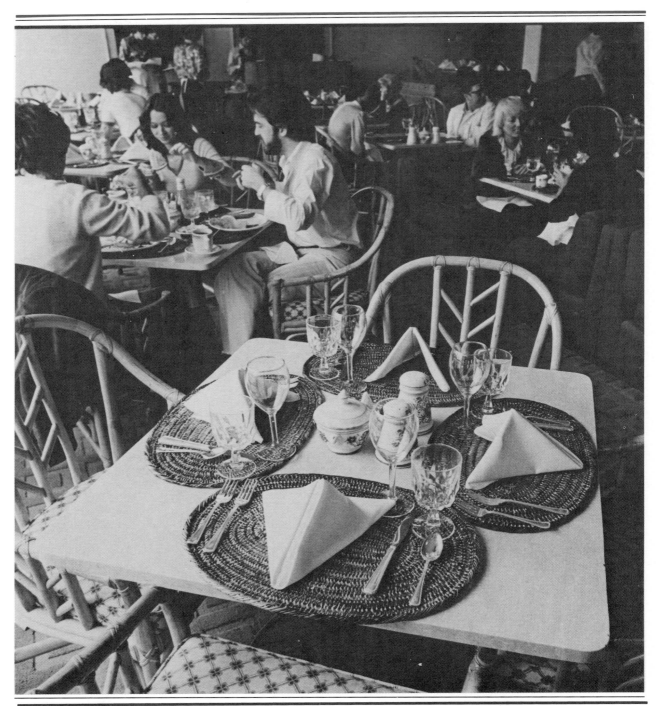

Pleasant surroundings and attractive table service make mealtime a special event.

Chapter 16

Selecting an Adequate Diet

Abbreviations

FDA: Food and Drug Administration
RDA: Recommended Dietary Allowances
USDA: United States Department of Agriculture

U.S.RDA: United States Recommended Daily Allowances

Introduction

An adequate diet is one that provides all of the essential nutrients in sufficient quantities for a given individual. Progress toward achieving this goal requires a plan so simple and so attractive that everyone, including the young as well as the old, can follow it. The Daily Food Guide provides such a practical and effective tool. It will be discussed in the pages that follow, along with other more precise procedures for planning an adequate food selection. The use of the Recommended Dietary Allowances (RDA), the Dietary Nutrient Guide, nutrition labeling as a guide, and indexes of the nutritive quality of foods are discussed.

Guides for Selecting an Adequate Diet

The Daily Food Guide

The Daily Food Guide is based on Four Food Groups, as shown in Fig. 16.1. The groups were chosen because of the specific nutrients contributed by each to the total diet. Foods on the basis of their composition have been assigned to the groups. The Guide is designed to direct the selection of foods and the quantities consumed to provide nutrients approximating the amounts specified by the RDA, forming the foundation of an adequate diet. To complete the energy needs (for the minimum number of servings recommended falls considerably short of providing enough energy) and also the RDA for some of the nutrients, additional food is needed, which may come from fats, sweets, and the Four Food Groups.

A day's menu comprised of the Four Food Groups is given in Table 16.1. These meals contain more than the minimum number of servings in three of the four food groups, as well as foods that are not included in any of the groups—sugars and fats. Eight nutrients and the energy value provided by the minimum recommended number of servings from the four groups, as well as the additional foods in the day's menu, are shown in Table 16.2. The percentage of the RDA provided by the minimum number of servings for these eight nutrients is presented graphically in Fig. 16.2. The RDA for all nutrients, with the exception of iron for young women, vitamin A, and thiamin for young men, and niacin and energy for both young men and young women were met completely or from 94 to 100 percent by the recommended minimum number of servings from each food group. With the additional foods all RDA were met except energy in the case of men and iron in the case of women (Table 16.2). Somewhat larger servings would readily solve the deficit for the men, but the solution of the iron deficit for women is more difficult. A concerted effort to select iron-rich foods can make it possible to attain the RDA; however, of notable importance is availability of the iron in the foods consumed and the effect of other foods eaten at the same time on the availability (see p. 283).

The four food groups and main nutrients contributed	Daily recommendations	Amount in one serving
Milk group: milk, cheese, ice cream, yogurt		
Calcium	children under 9 2–3 cups	one 8-oz (250 ml) cup
Riboflavin	children 9–12 3–4 cups	whole milk, skim milk, buttermilk,
Protein	adolescents 4 or more	powdered (reconstituted),
Phosphorus	adults 2 or more	evaporated (reconstituted)
	pregnant women 3 or more	Alternates for ½ cup whole milk:
	nursing mothers 4 or more	cheese, Cheddar-type, 1-in. cube
		creamed, cottage, ⅔ cup
		ice cream, 1 cup
		yogurt, 8 oz
Meat group[a]: beef, veal, pork, lamb, poultry, fish, eggs, with dry beans and peas, and peanut butter as alternates		
Protein	2 or more servings	2 to 3 oz (55 to 85 grams)
Phosphorus		lean cooked beef, veal, pork, lamb,
Iron		poultry, fish
B vitamins		1 egg
		⅔ cup cooked dry beans or peas
		2 tablespoons peanut butter
Vegetable–fruit group:		
Minerals	4 or more servings	½ cup vegetable or fruit
Vitamins	including:	1 medium vegetable or fruit
Cellulose	(a) one good source of	½ large vegetable or fruit
	vitamin C. Among the good	
	sources are: oranges,	
	lemons, grapefruit, cantaloupe,	
	strawberries, watermelon.	
	Broccoli, raw cabbage, kale,	
	mustard greens, potatoes,	
	spinach, tomatoes.	
	(b) one good source of	
	vitamin A value, at least	
	every other day. Good	
	sources of vitamin A	
	value are dark-green and	
	deep-yellow vegetables	
	such as broccoli, carrots,	
	chard, kale, pumpkin,	
	spinach, winter squash.	
Bread-cereals group: whole grain and enriched		
	4 or more servings	1 slice bread
		1 oz ready-to-eat cereal
		½ to ¾ cup cooked cereal, corn-meal, grits, macaroni, rice, noodles, or spaghetti

[a] Plans for adequate vegetarian diets are given on page 111.

Fig. 16.1 The four-food group plan. (Adapted from a daily food guide. *In Consumers All. The Yearbook of Agriculture.* Washington, D.C.: U.S. Dept. Agr., [1965], p. 394.)

Table 16.1 Menu Using the Daily Food Guide

Breakfast		Lunch		Dinner	
Orange juice	4 oz	Swedish meatballs	3 oz	Veal cutlet	3 oz
Egg, soft-cooked	1	Green beans	½ c	Potato, baked	1 med
Toast (whole wheat)	2 sl	Waldorf salad	¾ c	Broccoli	½ c
Butter	1 pat	Pan roll	1	Hard roll	1
Jelly	1 tbsp	Brownies	1	Butter	1 pat
Milk, whole	8 oz	Iced tea	8 oz	Lemon pie	1 sl
				Iced tea	8 oz
				Evening refreshment:	
				Milkshake	1½ c

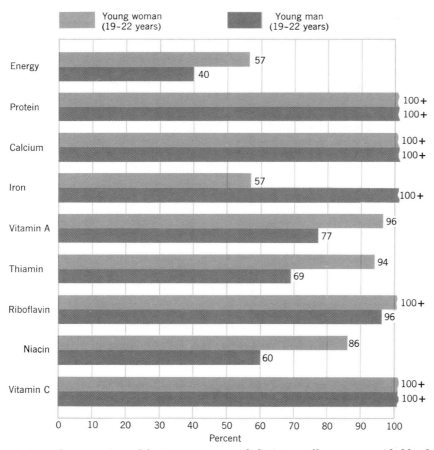

Fig. 16.2 The percentage of the 1974 Recommended Dietary Allowance provided by the minimum number of servings from the four groups for a 22 year-old man and woman based on the menu in Table 16.1.

Nutritive Value of Food Groups Each food individually as well as each group as a whole contributes important nutrients to the over-all diet. The four major groups will be discussed in turn.

Many of the food products to be discussed are regulated by standards of identity established by the Food and Drug Administration (FDA) (see p. 378 for more on FDA). The standard requires that the product contain certain ingredients in designated amounts. For example, for a product to be labeled "low fat milk" the composition must be as follows: fat, 0.5 percent to 2.0 percent; skim milk solids, 8.25 percent; vitamin A added, and the addition of vitamin D is optional. Proposals for a standard are published in the Federal Register. Opportunity is given for interested parties, manufacturers, consumers, and others to study the proposal and suggest changes. In case of controversy, public hearings are held. Food standards ensure uniformity and honesty in products.

Milk and Milk Products Milk has been described as nature's "most nearly perfect food." Most of the known essential nutrients are found in milk, but it is a much better source of some nutrients than others. Whole milk and whole milk products are excellent sources of calcium, protein, riboflavin, vitamin A, phosphorus, and thiamin; however, they are poor sources of iron and vitamin C. The nutritive value of milk and certain milk products is presented in Table 16.3. In order for adults to obtain enough calcium, nutritionists recommend that they consume 2 cups (or more) of fluid milk daily or an equivalent amount in the form of milk products, such as dried milk, evaporated milk, or cheese (Fig. 16.1).

Milk is available in several forms: fresh fluid, canned, and dried. Standards of identity are established for milk and cream products and cheeses and related products. The fresh fluid milk may be whole, containing all of its original fat (minimum of 3.25 percent), or skim (nonfat), containing no more than 0.5 percent of fat. Low-fat milk is the designation given to milk containing between 0.5 and 2.0 percent milk-fat. A concern about nonfat milk is that the vitamin A content is removed with the fat. However, most skim milk is fortified with 2000 IU of vitamin A and 400 IU of vitamin D per quart.

Each gram of whole milk contains about 1 mg of calcium, and 1 cup of milk supplies about one-third of the recommended calcium intake for a college-age man or woman. Milk also contains protein of high biological value; it complements the lower value protein of cereal products and legumes. If milk is served at each meal, either as a beverage or combined with other foods in prepared dishes, a good quality protein can be assured. An easy way to remember the approximate protein value of whole milk is that each ounce (about 30 g) contains about 1 g of protein; 1 quart of whole fluid milk supplies 32 g of protein.

Chocolate milk is whole milk to which chocolate syrup has been added; in chocolate-flavored milk, cocoa is used instead of chocolate. Chocolate drink is made with skim or lowfat milk, chocolate, and sweetener; in chocolate-flavored drink, cocoa is used instead of chocolate.

Cultured milks include buttermilk, yogurt, and acidophilus milk. Cultured buttermilk can be made by adding a lactic acid bacterial culture to whole milk, partially skimmed milk, or a reconstituted nonfat dry milk, but most of it is made from fresh fluid skim milk. Yogurt is made from whole, low fat, or nonfat milk, using a mixture of *Streptococcus thermophilus* and *Lactobacillus bulgaricus*. Acidophilus milk, used chiefly in modified diets, is prepared by adding *Lactobacillus acidophilus* to nonfat milk.

Canned milks include evaporated milk and sweetened condensed milk; the starting point of each is whole fluid milk. More than one-half of the water content of evaporated milk is removed and vitamin D is added. Heat sterilization of evaporated milk makes it possible to store unopened cans without refrigeration. Evaporated milk before reconstitution contains a minimum of 7.5 percent fat and 25.5 percent total milk solids.

351

Table 16.2 Nutrients and Energy Supplied by the Recommended Minimum Number of Servings in the Four-Group Plan, as Well as the Additional Foods from the Menu in Table 16.1

Food group	Food	Measure	Energy, kcal	Protein, g	Calcium, mg	Iron, mg	Vitamin A value, IU	Thiamin, mg	Ribo-flavin, mg	Niacin, mg	Vitamin C, mg
Milk	Milk	2 c	300	16	582	0.2	620	0.18	0.80	tr	4
	Total		300	16	582	0.2	620	0.18	0.80	tr	4
Meat	Egg	1	80	6	28	1.0	260	0.04	0.15	tr	0
	Ground beef	1 patty	185	23	10	3.0	20	0.08	0.20	5	0
	Total		265	29	38	4.0	280	0.12	0.35	5	0
Vegetable–fruit	Orange juice	½ c	60	1	13	0.1	270	0.12	0.02	tr	60
	Beans, green	½ c	15	1	32	0.4	340	0.05	0.06	tr	8
	Potato, baked	1 med	145	4	14	1.1	tr	0.15	0.07	3	31
	Broccoli, stalks	½ c	20	2	68	0.6	1940	0.07	0.16	1	70
	Total		240	8	127	2.2	2550	0.39	0.31	4	169
Bread–cereal	Bread (whole wheat)	2 sl	130	6	48	1.6	tr	0.18	0.06	1	tr
	Roll, pan	1	85	2	21	0.5	tr	0.11	0.07	1	tr
	Roll, hard	1	155	5	24	1.2	tr	0.20	0.12	2	tr
	Total		370	13	93	3.3	tr	0.49	0.25	4	tr
Total (recommended minimum number of servings)			1175	66	840	9.7	3450	1.18	1.71	13	173

Recommended Dietary Allowances

Women (19–22 years)		2100	46	800	18	4000	1.1	1.4	14	45
Men (19–22 years)		3000	54	800	10	5000	1.5	1.8	20	45
Additional foods										
Milk	½ c	75	4	146	0.1	155	0.04	0.20	tr	1
Egg	1	80	6	28	1.0	260	0.04	0.15	tr	0
Ice cream	½ c	135	3	88	0.1	270	0.03	0.16	tr	1
Veal cutlet	1	185	23	9	2.7	—	0.06	0.21	5	—
Apple	½	40	tr	5	0.2	60	0.02	0.02	tr	3
Celery	¼ c	5	tr	12	0.1	80	0.01	0.01	tr	3
Butter	1 tbsp	100	tr	3	tr	430	tr	tr	tr	0
Jelly	1 tbsp	50	tr	4	0.3	tr	tr	0.01	tr	1
Lemon pie	1 sector	305	4	17	1.0	200	0.09	0.12	1	4
Brownies	1	85	1	9	0.4	20	0.03	0.02	tr	tr
Mayonnaise	1 tbsp	65	tr	2	tr	30	tr	tr	tr	—
Total additional foods		1125	41	323	5.9	1505	0.32	0.09	6	12
Total for the day		2304	106	1163	15.6	4955	1.50	2.61	19	185

From *Nutritive Value of Foods*. Home and Garden Bull. No. 72 revised. Washington, D.C.: U.S. Dept. Agr., 1977.

353

Table 16.3 Nutritive Value of Milk and Certain Milk Products

Food	Measure	Energy, kcal	Protein, g	Calcium, mg	Iron, mg	Vitamin A value, IU	Thiamin, mg	Riboflavin, mg	Niacin, mg	Vitamin C mg
Milk, whole, 3.3 percent fat	1 c	150	8	291	0.1	310	0.09	0.40	tr	2
Milk, 2 percent fat[a]	1 c	120	8	297	0.1	500	0.10	0.40	tr	2
Milk, skim	1 c	85	8	302	0.1	500	0.09	0.37	tr	2
Milk, dry, nonfat	1 c	245	24	837	0.2	1610[b]	0.28	1.19	1	4
Yogurt, whole milk	1 c	140	8	274	0.1	280	0.07	0.32	tr	1
Evaporated milk	1 c	340	17	657	0.5	610[b]	0.12	0.80	1	5
Cheese										
Cheddar	1 cu. in.	70	4	124	0.1	180	tr	0.06	tr	0
cottage, creamed	1/2 c	118	14	68	0.2	185	0.02	0.18	tr	tr
Ice cream	1/2 c	135	2	88	0.1	270	0.02	0.17	tr	1

[a] 2 percent nonfat milk solids added.
[b] Applies to product with added vitamin A.
From *Nutritive Value of Foods*. Home and Garden Bull. No. 72 revised. Washington, D.C.: U.S. Dept. Agr., 1977.

More than one-half the water content of sweetened condensed milk is also removed; the standard for the minimum fat content is 8.5 percent and for total milk solids, 28.0 percent. The concentration of the added sugar (44 percent) is sufficiently high to act as a deterrent to bacterial growth, making heat treatment in the processing of this product unnecessary for safe storage without refrigeration.

Nonfat dry milk is a popular product. It is prepared by evaporating part of the water from pasteurized skim milk, followed by spraying it into a drying chamber to remove more water, so that the final product contains no more than 5 percent moisture. The fat content should not exceed $1\frac{1}{2}$ percent; vitamins A and D may be added to the product.

Cream is sold as light, coffee, or table cream, which has a fat content of 20.6 percent; light whipping or whipping cream, with a fat content of 31.3 percent; and heavy or heavy whipping cream, with 37.6 percent fat. Half-and-half consists of half milk and half light cream; the fat content is 11.7 percent. Sour cream is light cream which has been cultured under controlled conditions.

Filled milk, according to the Filled Milk Act (Public Law 513, 1923), is any milk to which a fat or oil other than butterfat has been added (3, 8). The fat used as a replacement for butterfat has been coconut oil, which has more than 90 percent of its fatty acids saturated, whereas butterfat has around 60 percent saturated. The Filled Milk Act prohibits the shipment of filled milk products across state lines.

Imitation milk is made to appear like milk but contains no complete milk ingredients. The protein used is often casein or soy proteins; the fat, a vegetable fat; and dextrose rather than lactose is used. Artificial color and flavor are used. Since there is no standard of identity for imitation milk, the ingredients and their quantities vary a lot (3, 8).

Another imitation product is coffee whiteners or lighteners, which substitute for cream in coffee. The product is generally composed of vegetable fat, a protein (casein), sweetener, emulsifiers, stabilizers, coloring, and flavoring.

Cheeses are produced by the action of rennet or lactic acid on milk. The casein coagulates and becomes semisolid, forming the cheese, and the whey separates out. On the market there are more than 400 varieties of cheese classified as hard, semisoft, soft, and process cheeses. Of the hard cheeses, the most extensively used are Cheddar (American cheese), Edam, Gouda, Swiss, and Parmesan; semisoft cheeses are Gorgonzola, Roquefort, blue, Muenster, and brick; soft cheeses include cottage, cream, Neufchâtel, Camembert, Brie, Limburger, and Liederkranz. Process cheese is a blend of cheeses to which water and an emulsifying agent (such as sodium citrate or disodium phosphate) are added, and pasteurized.

The nutritive value of cheese varies according to whether skim or whole milk is used, the moisture content of the final product, and the manufacturing process used. One ounce (about 28 g) of Cheddar-type cheese provides about the same nutritive value as a glass of milk. In the manufacture of cheese, some of the whey is discarded; this removes some of the water-soluble nutrients including lactose, the water-soluble vitamins, and minerals.

Meats, Fish, Poultry, Eggs, Legumes, and Nuts
Meat, fish, and poultry are somewhat similar in nutritive value, contributing significant amounts of protein, iron, and phosphorus, as well as some thiamin, riboflavin, and niacin. The protein in this group of foods, as in the milk group, is of high biological value. An 85 g (3 oz) serving of meat supplies approximately 20 to 25 g of protein, which is about one-half of the RDA for young adults.

There is a large amount of iron in organ meats, especially liver and kidney, and a smaller amount in muscle tissues. Meat is a poor source of calcium, but some fish products—chiefly shellfish and canned salmon (where some of the bone is edible)—are fair sources.

355

Table 16.4 Nutritive Value of Various Meats, Fish, Poultry, Egg, Legumes, and Nuts

Food	Measure	Energy, kcal	Protein, g	Calcium, mg	Iron, mg	Vitamin A value, IU	Thiamin, mg	Riboflavin, mg	Niacin, mg	Vitamin C, mg
Beef, round, braised	3 oz	220	24	10	3.0	20	0.07	0.19	5	—
Pork, lean and fat, loin, roasted	3 oz	310	21	9	2.7	0	0.78	0.22	5	—
Chicken, breast, boneless, fried	2.8 oz	160	26	9	1.3	70	0.04	0.17	12	—
Salmon, pink, canned	3 oz	120	17	167[a]	0.7	60	0.03	0.16	7	—
Egg, raw or cooked	1	80	6	28	1.0	260	0.04	0.15	tr	0
Beans, canned, pork and tomato sauce	½ c	155	8	69	2.3	165	0.10	0.04	1	3
Beans, red kidney, cooked	½ c	115	8	37	2.3	5	0.07	0.05	1	—
Peas, split, dry, cooked	½ c	115	8	11	1.7	40	0.15	0.09	1	—
Lentils, cooked	½ c	105	8	25	2.1	20	0.07	0.06	1	0
Liver, beef, fried	3 oz	195	22	9	7.5	45,390[b]	0.22	3.56	14	23
Peanut butter	2 tbsp	190	8	18	0.6	—	0.04	0.04	5	0
Peanuts, roasted, salted	½ c	420	19	54	1.5	—	0.23	0.10	12	0

[a] If the bones are discarded, this value will be greatly reduced.

* Value varies widely

From *Nutritive Value of Foods.* Home and Garden Bull. No. 72 revised. Washington, D.C.: U.S. Dept. Agr. 1977.

Pork muscle is high in thiamin, but other muscle meats contain only moderate amounts. Organ meats (liver, kidney, heart, and tongue) contain more riboflavin than do muscle meats. Liver, the storage place for vitamin A, is the only commonly eaten animal tissue that contains any appreciable amount of this vitamin.

Eggs are important for their protein, iron, phosphorus, vitamin A, and riboflavin content. Egg protein, which is found in both the yolk and the white, is of excellent biological value. One egg contains about 6 g of protein, approximately two-thirds the amount in one glass of milk. Phosphorus is distributed in both the yolk and the white, but iron and vitamin A are found only in the yolk.

In *Legumes in Human Nutrition*, Aykroyd (1) lists the 18 most common legumes, including kidney beans, soybeans, lentils, split peas, lima beans, cowpeas (black-eyed), and chick-peas (garbanzo). Although legume proteins have a somewhat lower biological value than do animal proteins, they are important in many areas of the world. One-half cup of cooked legumes supplies approximately 7 to 10 g of protein. Table 16.4 gives the nutritive value of various protein foods.

Although nuts contain protein in good quantity, they have a high fat content, which limits their consumption because of its high satiety value. The protein of the peanut (the only nut that has been studied to any extent) contains low amounts of lysine and threonine, with methionine the limiting amino acid. Even so, peanut butter should be recommended as a good source of protein in a mixed diet.

Vegetables and Fruits As a group, vegetables and fruits contribute minerals, vitamins (nearly all of the vitamin C and more than one-half of the vitamin A value in the Daily Food Guide plan), and cellulose to the diet. Not to be disregarded is their variety in color, flavor, and texture. For the sake of clarity, vegetables and fruits will be grouped together according to their principal nutrients.

In general, dark-green and deep-yellow vegetables and fruits have a high vitamin A value. Nutritionists recommend that adults eat one good source or two fair sources of vitamin A at least every other day. Leafy dark-green vegetables are also higher in calcium, iron, vitamin C, and the B vitamins than are other vegetables. Some green vegetables (spinach, chard, sorrel, and beet greens) contain oxalic acid, which combines with calcium to form an unabsorable salt (see p. 263); however, these vegetables provide generous amounts of iron, vitamin C, and vitamin A value.

Head lettuce, celery, cabbage, and other light-green vegetables are especially important for their cellulose content. The light-green vegetables are low in vitamin A value; thus it should be noted that the color green is not always associated with vitamin A value.

Citrus fruits and tomatoes are dependable sources of vitamin C, but tomato juice contains only about one-third as much as the citrus fruits. Other foods such as strawberries, cantaloupes, and green peppers are almost as rich in vitamin C as citrus fruits are, but because of their cost and seasonal nature, they do not fit into a regular diet as well as citrus fruits and tomatoes. Raw cabbage, broccoli, kale, and Brussels sprouts are also good sources of vitamin C.

Vegetables of the seed, root, and tuber classes (for example, lima beans, corn, green peas, and sweet and white potatoes) tend to be high in carbohydrate content because starch is stored in these areas of the plant; however, most vegetables and fruits are low in protein, fat, and energy value. Table 16.5 shows the nutritive value of various fruits and vegetables.

Bread and Cereal Products Cereals are seeds of the grass family—wheat, corn, rice, oats, buckwheat, rye, and barley. From these cereal grains, various flours (for example, wheat, corn, rice, buckwheat, oat, rye, and barley) are produced for making bread and other bakery goods, breakfast cereals, pasta, hominy, and so forth. Figure

Table 16.5 Nutritive Value of Various Fruits and Vegetables

Food	Measure	Energy, kcal	Protein, g	Calcium, mg	Iron, mg	Vitamin A value, IU	Thiamin, mg	Riboflavin, mg	Niacin, mg	Vitamin C, mg
Apple	1 med	80	tr	10	0.4	120	0.04	0.03	tr	6
Banana	1 med	100	1	10	0.8	230	0.06	0.07	1	12
Broccoli, cooked	½ c	20	2	68	0.6	1940	0.07	0.16	1	70
Cabbage, cooked	½ c	15	1	32	0.2	95	0.03	0.03	tr	24
Carrots, cooked	½ c	25	1	26	0.5	8140	0.04	0.04	tr	5
Green beans, cooked	½ c	15	1	32	0.4	340	0.05	0.06	tr	8
Kale, cooked	½ c	22	3	103	0.9	4565	0.06	0.10	1	51
Lettuce, iceberg	¼ hd	20	1	27	0.7	450	0.08	0.08	tr	8
Lima beans, cooked	½ c	105	7	32	2.4	200	0.08	0.04	1	11
Orange juice, frozen, reconstituted	½ c	60	1	13	0.1	270	0.12	0.02	tr	60
Peaches, canned	½ c	100	1	5	0.4	550	0.02	0.03	1	4
Potato (white), baked	1	145	4	14	1.1	tr	0.15	0.07	3	31
Tomato juice	½ c	23	1	9	1.1	970	0.06	0.04	1	20

From *Nutritive Value of Foods.* Home and Garden Bull. No. 72 revised. Washington, D.C.: U.S. Dept. Agr., 1977.

WHOLE WHEAT

Cross section of a grain of wheat showing the various nutrients in the different parts of the grain.

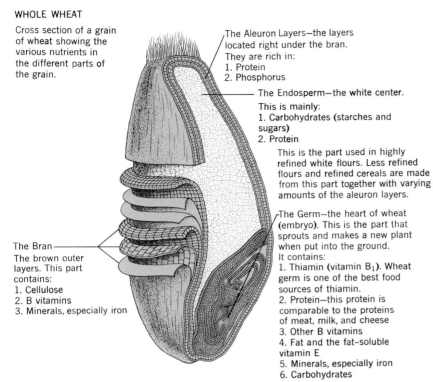

The Aleuron Layers—the layers located right under the bran. They are rich in:
1. Protein
2. Phosphorus

The Endosperm—the white center. This is mainly:
1. Carbohydrates (starches and sugars)
2. Protein

This is the part used in highly refined white flours. Less refined flours and refined cereals are made from this part together with varying amounts of the aleuron layers.

The Germ—the heart of wheat (embryo). This is the part that sprouts and makes a new plant when put into the ground. It contains:
1. Thiamin (vitamin B_1). Wheat germ is one of the best food sources of thiamin.
2. Protein—this protein is comparable to the proteins of meat, milk, and cheese
3. Other B vitamins
4. Fat and the fat-soluble vitamin E
5. Minerals, especially iron
6. Carbohydrates

The Bran
The brown outer layers. This part contains:
1. Cellulose
2. B vitamins
3. Minerals, especially iron

Fig. 16.3 The whole wheat kernel, its structure, composition, and nutritive value. (Courtesy the Ralston Purina Company.)

16.3 shows the parts of a kernel of wheat; other cereal grains are similar in structure. Whole wheat has the following percentage composition: carbohydrate, 72; protein, 12; moisture, 10; fat, 2; fiber, 2; and ash, 2.

In preparing cereal products for the market, it is common practice to remove parts of the grain. In the case of brown rice, only the outer husk is removed, whereas for white rice all of the outer coats are removed, leaving mainly the endosperm (center) portion. Whole wheat flour is made from the entire grain, except for the husk; white flour is made from just the endosperm. Most of the cellulose, minerals, and B vitamins are in the outer layers of the grain. The endosperm contains mostly carbohydrates and incomplete protein. The germ contains most of the fat of the grain and some of the thiamin. Because the fat tends to become rancid during storage and attracts insects, the germ is usually removed in milling.

Efforts are made to improve the nutritive value of the manufactured cereal products, making them equal to or exceeding the original whole grain in certain nutrients. (Of course, there are likely nutrient losses as yet unidentified that occur in the manufacturing process.) The products with added nutrients have designations that inform the consumer as to the type of nutritive improvement he is purchasing. Restored cereals are those that have the level of one or more nutrients contained in the original grain added back to the cereal product: restoration is a voluntary, unregulated process carried out at the discretion of the manufacturer. Enriched cereals have thiamin,

359

Table 16.6 Nutritive Value of Various Bread and Cereal Products as Served

Food	Measure	Energy, kcal	Protein, g	Calcium, mg	Iron, mg	Vitamin A value, IU	Thiamin, mg	Ribo-flavin, mg	Niacin, mg	Vitamin C, mg
Biscuit, enriched	1	105	2	34	0.4	tr	0.08	0.08	tr	tr
Bread										
white, enriched	1 sl	65	2	20	0.6	tr	0.10	0.06	1	tr
whole wheat	1 sl	65	3	24	0.8	tr	0.09	0.03	1	tr
Macaroni, cooked										
enriched	1 c	155	5	11	1.3	0	0.20	0.11	2	0
Muffin, enriched	1	120	3	42	0.6	40	0.09	0.12	1	tr
Oatmeal, cooked	1 c	130	5	22	1.4	0	0.19	0.05	tr	0
Rice (white, enriched)	1 c	225	4	21	1.8	0	0.23	0.02	2	0
Roll, pan, enriched	1	85	2	21	0.5	tr	0.11	0.07	1	tr

From *Nutritive Value of Foods*, Home and Garden Bull. No. 72 revised. Washington, D.C.: U.S. Dept. Agr., 1977.

riboflavin, niacin, and iron added at specified levels according to the federal standards of identity prescribed by the Food and Drug Administration. Calcium and vitamin D are optional ingredients, but if added they must be at the levels specified by the FDA. Any product labeled "enriched" must meet the FDA standard of identity. (See p. 379 for more on enrichment.) Fortified cereals are those to which nutrients are added that do not occur naturally in the grain or occur in relatively small amounts. Many breakfast cereals are fortified. The manufacturer decides which nutrients to add and at what levels. Nutrition labeling informs the consumer to what extent the product has been fortified. Whole wheat flour (graham flour, entire wheat flour) and whole wheat bread are regulated by FDA standards of identity. Whole wheat flour is prepared from cleaned whole wheat.

Cereal grains are easy to grow, easy to store, and will not readily spoil after the outer layers and germ have been removed. Cereals provide mainly energy, largely in the form of carbohydrates. Whole-grain or enriched cereal products also contribute thiamin, iron, riboflavin, niacin, cellulose, and some incomplete protein. However, when this protein is supplemented with milk, meat, or eggs, cereal proteins make a significant contribution to the diet; for further discussion on vegetable proteins, see p. 108. About 17 percent of the protein in an ordinary U.S. diet comes from bread and cereal products; for those on low-cost diets, the percentage is even higher. Table 16.6 presents the nutritive value of various bread and cereal products.

The RDA as a Guide

The RDA are goals to be aimed for in the selection of foods for the daily diet. When the nutrient content of self-chosen diets or planned ones is computed (using food composition tables), the inadequacies and surpluses can be identified. The task is a tedious, time-consuming one. First, several days' records of food consumption should be kept, with the amounts consumed estimated as accurately as possible. From the results of these computations, a pattern of foods for the meals of the day that would provide sufficient nutrients to approximate the Recommended Allowances could be arrived at.

Dietary Nutrient Guide

The Dietary Nutrient Guide is based on the use of a limited number of nutrients (index nutrients), the presence of which in daily diets predicts the presence of all essential nutrients (6). A shortened list of foods (mini-list) was devised for the purpose of evaluating the coexistence of nutrients in foods and for evaluating diets. The mini-list was evolved by having one food substitute for a number of foods similar in composition. For example, apples, raw, unpared, substitute in the mini-list for all apples (pared or unpared), raw pears, grapes, plums, watermelon, sweet cherries, honeydew melon, and casaba melon. The index nutrients are seven (vitamin B-6, magnesium, pantothenic acid, vitamin A, folacin, iron, and calcium). The author of the Guide (6) found that if a diet meets the recommended intakes for the seven index nutrients most likely all essential nutrients will be adequate in the diet.

Nutrition Labeling as a Guide

A variety of foods is needed in a day's diet to provide the recommended intake of essential nutrients. Since foods differ in the kinds and amounts of nutrients they contain, it is necessary to have an informed idea about the contribution to the diet of, at least, the common foods. Nutrition labeling helps to satisfy this need (7). Those foods in the marketplace that have nutrition information give on the label the percentage of the U.S. Recommended Daily Allowance (U.S. RDA) for protein, vitamin A, vitamin C, three of the B-vitamins (thiamin, riboflavin, and niacin), calcium, and iron furnished by a serving of the food as it comes in the container. (For an explanation

Table 16.7 Allowances for Food Energy and Percentages of the U.S. Recommended Daily Allowances Needed to Meet the Recommended Dietary Allowances for Children, Men, and Women of Different Ages

Age	Food energy[1]	Protein[2]	Vitamin A	Vitamin C	Thiamin	Ribo-flavin	Niacin[3]	Calcium	Iron
Years	_Calories_				_Percent of U.S. Recommended Daily Allowance_				
Child:									
1–3	1300	35	40	70	50	50	30	80	85
4–6	1800	50	50	70	60	65	35	80	60
7–10	2400	55	70	70	80	75	50	80	60
Male:									
11–14	2800	70	100	75	95	90	55	120	100
15–18	3000	85	100	75	100	110	55	120	100
19–22	3000	85	100	75	100	110	60	80	60
23–50	2700	90	100	75	95	95	45	80	60
51+	2400	90	100	75	80	90	35	80	60
Female:									
11–14	2400	70	80	75	80	80	45	120	100
15–18	2100	75	80	75	75	85	30	120	100
19–22	2100	75	80	75	75	85	35	80	100
23–50	2000	75	80	75	70	75	30	80	100
51+	1800	75	80	75	70	65	25	80	60
Pregnant	+300[4]	+50[4]	100	100	+20[4]	+20[4]	35	120	100+
Nursing	+500[4]	+35[4]	120	135	+20[4]	+30[4]	35	120	100

[1] Calorie needs differ depending on body composition and size, age, and activity of the person.

[2] U.S. RDA of 65 grams is used for this table. In labeling, a U.S. RDA of 45 grams is used for foods providing high-quality protein, such as milk, meat, and eggs.

[3] The percentage of the U.S. RDA shown for niacin will provide the RDA for niacin if the RDA for protein is met. Some niacin is derived in the body from tryptophan, an amino acid present in protein.

[4] To be added to the percentage for the girl or woman of the appropriate age.

Source: U.S. Recommended Daily Allowance, "Food Labeling," _Federal Register_, vol. 38, no. 49, part II, March 14, 1973. _Recommended Dietary Allowances, eighth edition_, 1974. National Academy Sciences, National Research Council.

From B. Peterkin, J. Nichols, and C. Cromwell (1975). _Nutrition Labeling, Tools for Its Use_. Washington, D.C.: U.S. Dept. Agr., p. 47.

of U.S. RDA, see p. 34). For most nutrients the U.S. RDA are higher than the RDA; therefore 100 percent of the U.S. RDA is not needed in most instances, but more than 100 percent is needed in some to meet the RDA (see Table 16.7). To use nutrition labeling as an aid in selecting an adequate diet, a record must be kept of the food intake for a day. For the amount of each food eaten for which there is nutrition labeling, record from the label the number of kilocalories and percentage of the U.S. RDA for each of the eight nutrients. For the remaining foods, the same information may be found in the bulletin _Nutrition Labeling, Tools for Its Use_ (7). The kilocalories and each of the nutrients are then totaled and compared with the percentages in Table 16.7. The diet should be checked each day for about a week to determine if persistent shortages of some nutrients occur.

Indexes of Nutritive Quality of Foods as Guides

Independent investigators are exploring ways of establishing an easy-to-use index to describe the nutritive quality of individual foods (2, 5, 9). In each plan the nutrient contribution of a food is related to its energy value. The expression of the nutrient values of a food in terms of each 1000 kilocalories provided by it is one proposal; the value is called Nutrient Density (2). Milk, for example, contains 1200 mg Ca per 1000 kcal, and tomato juice contains 378 mg Ca per 1000 kcal. The recommended intake of calcium for men 19 to 22 years of age expressed in Nutrient Density is 267 and for women of the same age, 381. To illustrate the method of computation of recommended nutrient intake daily in terms of Nutrient Density, the RDA for calcium (800 mg daily) and for energy (3000 kcal daily) for men 19 to 22 years are used: 800 divided by 3 is 267 mg per 1000 kcal.

Another plan is the Index of Nutritional Quality, which incorporates the factors of nutrient and energy needs. It is the ratio of the percentage of the recommended intake of the nutrient to the percentage of the energy requirement in a serving of the food (9). And still another proposal is the Nutrient-Calorie Benefit Ratio, which also incorporates the recommended intakes of the nutrients and of energy: The percentage contribution of the nutrient to the recommended intake divided by the percentage contribution of energy to the recommended intake. In this plan the computation is made for a unit portion of food (such as 100 g) (5).

These proposals for facilitating the selection of an adequate diet will surely be further developed and food tables based on them prepared. They will provide tools for the selection of food on the basis of nutritive quality that will be more concise than the Daily Food Guide. The Daily Food Guide remains, however, the one that helps ensure variety in the diet and is sufficiently simple for all to understand and follow.

Plans for Food Budgets

Ultimately, daily menus and a plan for purchasing food must be made by individuals, families, or institutions that prepare meals. The Consumer and Food Economics Research Division of the USDA has published materials that are useful in making plans for the purchase of foods. Weekly food recommendations for the nourishment of 20 age-sex groups using 11 categories of food at 4 cost levels—thrifty, low-cost, moderate-cost, and liberal-cost—are presented (4). The federal government helps needy families buy additional food through the Food Stamp Program and the Family Food Donation Program, both administered by the U.S. Department of Agriculture.

To plan a weekly food budget for a family of a certain size, one should total the quantities recommended for each member (Appendix Tables A-4, A-5, A-6, A-7). For example, the weekly amount of food suggested for a family consisting of a man and a woman who are both 33 years of age, a girl of 8, and a boy of 11 are summarized in Table 16.8. In developing food plans at different cost levels, the Department of Agriculture used the following criteria: (a) nutritional adequacy, (b) the relative cost of different food groups as sources of specified nutrients, and (c) the suitability of certain foods as related to meals commonly eaten in the United States. Obviously, meal planning must include knowledge of a family's food preferences, as well as the availability and prices of these foods.

For families on limited budgets, the thrifty and low-cost plans contain substantially more potatoes, legumes, and grain products. Lower-cost cuts of meat and certain organ meats usually provide as much (if not more) nutritive value as the higher-priced cuts. The moderate-cost and liberal-cost plans include more milk, eggs, meat, fruits, and vegetables. More expensive items, such as foods out of season, convenience foods, and fancy delicacies are included in the moderate-cost and liberal-cost plans.

363

Table 16.8 Quantity of Food Recommended for a Family of Four[a] for One Week[b]

Food group	Unit	Thrifty plan	Low-cost plan	Moderate cost plan	Liberal-cost plan
Milk, milk products	qt[c]	14.5	15.9	19.3	20.6
Meat, poultry, fish	lb[d]	8.3	12.4	15.8	18.9
Eggs	no.	13.8	14.8	15.3	15.4
Dry beans, peas, nuts	lb[e]	1.7	1.4	1.2	1.3
Dark-green, deep-yellow vegetables	lb	1.4	1.7	2.0	2.2
Citrus fruit, tomatoes	lb	6.3	8.4	10.3	12.4
Potatoes	lb	6.2	5.8	5.9	5.9
Other vegetables, fruit	lb	13.0	13.5	21.0	24.8
Cereal	lb	4.2	4.0	3.2	3.2
Flour	lb	3.0	2.3	2.0	2.1
Bread	lb	6.9	6.3	5.9	5.6
Other bakery products	lb	4.0	4.4	5.4	5.0
Fats, oils	lb	2.6	2.6	2.8	2.9
Sugar, sweets	lb	3.6	3.6	4.1	4.3

[a] The family: a man and woman both 33 years of age; a girl of 8; and a boy of 11.

[b] Amounts are for food as purchased or brought into the kitchen from garden or farm. Amounts allow for a discard of about one-fourth of the edible food as plate waste, spoilage, etc. For general use, round the total amount of food groups for the family to the nearest tenth or quarter of a pound. In addition to groups shown, most families use some other foods: coffee, tea, cocoa, soft drinks, punches, ades, leavening agents, and seasonings.

[c] Fluid milk and beverage made from dry or evaporated milk. Cheese and ice cream may replace some milk. Count as equivalent to a quart of fluid milk: natural or processed Cheddar-type cheese, 6 ounces; cottage cheese, 2½ pounds; ice cream or ice milk, 1½ quarts; unflavored yogurt, 4 cups.

[d] Bacon and salt pork should not exceed ⅓ pound for each 5 pounds of this group.

[e] Weight in terms of dry beans and peas, shelled nuts, and peanut butter. Count 1 pound of canned dry beans, such as pork and beans or kidney beans, as .33 pound.

From B. Peterkin, *Family Food Budgeting*. Home and Garden Bull. No. 94. Washington, D.C.: Agr. Res. Services, U.S. Dept. of Agr., 1976, pp. 4–7.

Resources in Nutrition Education

Knowledge of nutrition facilitates the selection of an adequate diet. It is good to acquaint children with some information about nutrition while they are still in the process of establishing their own food habits. It must be remembered that there is some good in the food practices of all present-day cultural groups that are in reasonably good health. People should be encouraged to maintain their food habits (if they are good) or to supplement their usual foods (if they are inadequate) in order to meet their nutritive needs. Nutrition education can be judged a success only if it is effective within an existing cultural pattern of foods, not if it attempts to replace the pattern (5, 7).

Who is the nutrition teacher? "He is anyone and everyone who imparts nutrition information and/or motivates the use of nutrition facts—authentic, misleading, and sometimes downright inaccurate. Every community has many teachers. Some are authoritative, some are unintentionally less than accurate, and some are deliberately misleading" (2).

364

The Society for Nutrition Education was established in 1968; its "overall goal is to promote nutritional well-being for all people—through education, communication and education-related research." The Society publishes the *Journal of Nutrition Education,* which is "designed for persons who are interpreters of nutritional sciences and motivators for the development of good nutritional practices." The Society for Nutrition Education and other sources of information about food and nutrition for the professional and lay person are as follows:

Agricultural and Home Economics Extension
    Service Departments
State Universities

County Agricultural Extension Offices

Foods and Nutrition Departments
Colleges and Universities

State Departments of Health

Agricultural Research Service
U.S. Department of Agriculture
Washington, D.C.
(Its publications are available from:
Superintendent of Documents
U.S. Government Printing Office
Washington, D.C. 20402

and

Office of Communication
U.S. Department of Agriculture
Washington, D.C. 20250

American Dietetic Association
430 North Michigan Avenue
Chicago, Illinois 60611

American Home Economics Association
2010 Massachusetts Avenue N.W.
Washington, D.C. 20036

Department of Foods and Nutrition
American Medical Association
535 North Dearborn Street
Chicago, Illinois 60610

Food and Nutrition Board
National Academy of Sciences–National
    Research Council
2101 Constitution Avenue
Washington, D.C. 20418

Food and Drug Administration
U.S. Department of Health, Education, and
    Welfare
Washington, D.C. 20204

Society for Nutrition Education
2140 Shattuck Avenue, Suite 1110
Berkeley, California 94704

Sources of International Publications:

Food and Agriculture Organization
UNIPUB
345 Park Avenue So.
New York, New York 10010

World Health Organization
WHO Publications Centre
49 Sheridan Avenue
Albany, New York 12210

League for International Food Education
1155 Sixteenth St. N.W.
Washington, D.C. 20036

Fallacies About Foods and Nutrition

A fallacy is a false or erroneous idea. When untrue or misleading health claims are made deliberately for a food, it is called food quackery. For example, an erroneous claim is sometimes made that grapefruit possesses special enzymatic properties that enable it to break down excess body fat. This claim may encourage obese persons to eat substantial quantities of grapefruit to the exclusion of other foods. Food fallacies originate because of lack of information, fear, misconceptions, superstitions, or a desire for financial gain by unscrupulous persons.

Fear of ill health or feelings of unrest and dis-

365

Table 16.9 Values for 100-Gram Portions of Honey, White Sugar, Brown Sugar[a]

Food	Energy, kcal	Protein, g	Carbo-hydrate, g	Cal-cium, mg	Iron, mg	Thiamin, mg	Ribo-flavin, mg	Niacin, mg	Vita-min C, mg
Honey, strained (approx. 5 tbsp)	304	0.3	82.3	5.0	0.5	tr	0.04	0.03	tr
Sugar									
white (½ c) (½ c)	385	0	99.5	0	0.1	0	0	0	0
brown (approx. ½ c packed)	373	0	96.4	86.0	3.4	0.01	0.03	0.2	0
Recommended Dietary Allowances[b]									
Men, 19–22 yrs	3000	54	—	800	10	1.5	1.8	20	45
Women, 19–22 yrs	2100	46		800	18	1.1	1.4	14	45

[a] From C. F. Adams, *Nutritive Value of American Foods.* Agr. Handbook No. 456. Washington, D.C.: U.S. Dept. Agr., 1975.
[b] From *Recommended Dietary Allowances, Eighth Edition.* Natl. Research Council Publication. Washington, D.C.: National Academy Sciences, 1974.

satisfaction may lead some persons to be susceptible to quackery. The nutritional value of a product may not really be the key issue, but the product may symbolize the search for a solution to more basic problems that are responsible for the sense of unrest (4). In a study done in New York State of 340 women who ranged in age from less than 30 to more than 60 years and were members of community organizations (such as PTAs, church groups, home demonstration units, and nutrition clubs), it was found that those who were most susceptible to food quackery tended to be older or from a lower income group (3).

Many people have a number of beliefs about food. Some of these beliefs can be considered folklore or "old wives' tales"; they are handed down — unquestioned — from one generation to the next. It may be wise to stop and consider food practices that differ from the ordinary, "run-of-the-mill" variety; certain uncommon beliefs about food sometimes have a grain of truth. Centuries ago, burned sponge was recommended for simple goiter; later on it was learned that sponge contains iodine, the element required to prevent goiter.

Some Misconceptions Related to Food Nutrients

Related to Protein in the Diet That *skim milk has little nutritive value.* Skim milk is whole milk with the butterfat removed. It remains a superior food, even though it is naturally low in fat and vitamin A content. However, most commercially available skim milk has been supplemented with vitamins A and D.

That *pasteurizing milk causes important losses in its nutritive value.* Pasteurization is necessary to destroy any harmful bacteria that might be present. There is some loss of vitamin C, but milk is not a good source of vitamin C in any event.

That *large amounts of gelatin dissolved in water and taken as a food supplement will strengthen the fingernails.* Fingernail formation is apparently affected by a number of factors, including one's overall nutritional status, the state of one's endocrine glands, one's general health, and the environment. Gelatin is a pure protein, but a protein of low quality. It possesses no particular fingernail-strengthening quality.

366

Table 16.10 Values for 100-Gram Portion of Peas

Peas	Food energy, kcal	Protein, g	Calcium, mg	Iron, mg	Vitamin A value, IU	Thiamin, mg	Ribo-flavin, mg	Niacin, mg	Vita-min C, mg
Green, immature, fresh, raw	84	6.3	26	1.9	641	.35	.14	2.9	27
Fresh, cooked	71	5.4	23	1.8	538	.28	.11	2.3	210
Canned	88	4.7	26	1.9	688	.09	.06	0.8	8
Frozen, cooked	68	5.1	19	1.9	600	.27	.09	1.7	13
Dry mature seeds (split without seedcoat), cooked	115	8.0	11	1.7	40	.15	.09	0.9	—

From C. F. Adams, *Nutritive Value of American Foods.* Agr. Handbook No. 456. Washington, D.C.: U.S. Dept. Agr., 1975.

Related to Carbohydrate in the Diet   That *honey is not fattening.* No particular food is either fattening or nonfattening. All energy consumed in excess of need is deposited as fat. A tablespoon of honey (21 g) is higher in energy value than a tablespoon of sugar (12 g) — 65 kcal and 45 kcal, respectively.

That *honey contributes a significant amount of minerals and vitamins to the diet.* Besides carbohydrate, honey contains some nutrients, but the amount is small in comparison with the day's total need (see Table 16.9).

That *brown sugar contributes significantly more nutrients to the diet than does white sugar.* Brown sugar does contain some nutrients that white sugar does not but in inconsequential amounts. Iron is present in a relatively greater concentration than the other nutrients; 100 g (½ cup packed) contains 3.4 mg iron (see Table 16.9).

That *sucrose (sugar) is poisonous.* Sugar is one of the purest foods on the market. It supplies only carbohydrate and energy. Sucrose is used in cow's milk formulas for infants (it has advantages over lactose in that it is universally available and less expensive). Sucrose is fairly widely distributed in unprocessed foods, such as apples, honey, green peas, and oranges (see Table 4.1, p. 48, and the original report for a more extensive list).

That *highly milled grains should never be used.* White flour is a perfectly wholesome food. However, when grains are milled, the outer coats of the grains are removed, causing the loss of a relatively large proportion of the higher quality protein, the minerals, the B vitamins, and all of the vitamin E that is found in the embryo. Therefore when buying flour and bread made from highly milled grains, it is best to buy enriched products.

Fallacies in General

That *all processed foods have no nutritive content.* The comparative composition of one cup of green, immature peas, fresh and cooked; canned; frozen, cooked; and mature dry, cooked is shown in Table 16.10. It is apparent from the values in Table 16.10 that processed peas contribute much to the diet.

That *water is fattening.* Water has no energy value; therefore although water may be held in the tissues, it cannot be converted to fat.

"Natural Foods," "Organic Foods," and "Health Foods"

No definitions or regulations have been established for natural, organic, or health foods. Natural food could be the designation for most of the food available to the consumer; it was grown in a garden or on a tree, or produced on a farm, or in a modern equivalent of a farm, with more confined quarters. Foods, almost without exception,

367

are organic; they are compounds containing carbon, hydrogen, and oxygen. Also nearly all edible foods provide needed nutrients and can be considered health foods. However, foods so designated have other connotations.

"Natural foods" is the designation used for foods that contain no chemical additives, such as preservatives, emulsifiers, and antioxidants. Relatively few of the specific chemical substances normally present in foods have been evaluated toxicologically. ". . . it is toxicologically axiomatic that if almost any one of this myriad of chemical substances were tested in experimental animals by today's standards of safety evaluation, it would be shown to be toxic" (1). This does not imply, however, that there would be a hazard involved in eating the food. "The 'toxicity' of a substance is its intrinsic capacity to produce injury when tested by itself. The 'hazard' of a substance is its capacity to produce injury under the circumstances of its exposure." For example, oxalic acid is a toxic substance, but its presence in spinach is not a hazard for the person eating spinach. (For more on natural toxicants in foods, see p. 384.) It would seem an easier task at present to monitor the additives to foods than to assess the hazard of naturally occurring toxicants in them; the additives are known, but it is assumed that not all of those naturally occurring have yet been identified.

"Organic foods" are grown on soils fertilized with manure or compost; they are produced without the use of pesticides (any chemical used to kill insects and rodents), herbicides (a chemical that kills weeds), or chemical fertilizers. Inorganic fertilizers are excluded. Yet there is scientific evidence (ten investigations spanning seven decades) that no difference in major nutrient value exists between organically and inorganically fertilized crops. Minor variations in minerals of plants do occur as a direct result of the mineral content of the fertilizer; organic fertilizers fall short in phosphorus content. Trace minerals are introduced into inorganic fertilizers as needed. So there appears to be little advantage, and possibly some nutritional disadvantage, in organically grown crops (6).

The world's food supply is substantially reduced each year by insects, rodents, and other pests. Although pesticides help to reduce this loss, there may be hazards to human beings in the long-term use of these chemicals because of contaminants remaining in the environment. The problem of controlling pests safely is being studied by research scientists in universities; in the U.S. Department of Agriculture; in the U.S. Department of Health, Education, and Welfare; in the Food and Agriculture Organization; and in the World Health Organization.

The "health foods" designation implies that those particular foods have certain health-giving benefits that other foods do not have. That has yet to be proven.

Summary

An adequate diet is one that provides all of the essential nutrients in sufficient quantities for a given individual. Some sort of guide facilitates achieving an adequate diet. The Daily Food Guide is a practical and effective tool. Other guides include the RDA, the Dietary Nutrient Guide, nutrition labeling as a guide, and indexes of the nutritive quality of foods.

After considering daily nutrient needs, there ultimately must be a menu and a plan for the purchase of food by individuals, families, or institutions that prepare meals. Such a plan at four cost levels has been prepared by the Consumer and Food Economics Institute, USDA.

Knowledge of nutrition facilitates the selection of an adequate diet. An achievement within the past decade was the establishment in 1968 of the Society for Nutrition Education in the United States; its "over-all goal is to promote nutritional well-being for all people—through education, communication and education-related research."

Despite all of the facilities for obtaining sound nutrition information, fallacies exist. They originate in some instances because of lack of information, fear, misconceptions, superstitions, or a desire for financial gain by unscrupulous persons.

Three categories of foods without official definition or regulation are the "natural foods," "organic foods," and "health foods." Natural foods are those which contain no chemical additives, such as preservatives, emulsifiers, and antioxidants. Organic foods are grown on soils fertilized with manure or compost; they are produced without the use of pesticides, herbicides, or chemical fertilizers. The health foods designation implies that those particular foods have certain health-giving benefits that other foods do not have. That implication has yet to be proven.

Study Questions and Activities

1. Milk has been described as nature's "most nearly perfect food." What are its shortcomings?
2. Keep a food record for several days. Check to see whether it meets the minimum number of daily servings from each food group as recommended in the Daily Food Guide.
3. Plan a week's menu for a family (your own family or an imaginary one). Select the appropriate cost level, use the corresponding table in the Appendix to figure out the amounts of each category of food needed, consider the family's food preferences, and use local prices to compute cost. In planning the menu, make sure that each member of the family has the minimum number of servings daily from each food group.

References

Guides for Selecting an Adequate Diet and Plans for Food Budgets

1. Aykroyd, W. R. (1964). *Legumes in Human Nutrition*. Rome: Food and Agr. Organ., p. 14.
2. Balsley, M. (1977). Soon to come: 1978 Recommended Dietary Allowances. *J. Am. Dietet. Assoc.*, **71**: 149.
3. Brink, M. F., M. Balsley, and E. W. Speckman (1969). Nutritional value of milk compared with filled and imitation milks. *Am. J. Clin. Nutrition*, **22**: 168.
4. *Family Food Budgeting for Good Meals and Good Nutrition* (1976). Home and Garden Bull. No. 94. Washington, D.C.: U.S. Dept. Agr. pp. 1–14.
5. Guthrie, H. A. (1977). Concept of a nutritious food. *J. Am. Dietet. Assoc.*, **71**: 14.
6. Pennington, J. A. (1976). *Dietary Nutrient Guide*. Westport, Conn.: Avi Publishing Co., Inc.
7. Peterkin, B., J. Nichols, and C. Cromwell (1975). *Nutrition Labeling, Tools for its use*. Agr. Information Bull. No. 382. Washington, D.C.: U.S. Dept. Agr. pp. 1–57.
8. Rubini, M. E. (1960). Filled milk and artificial milk substitutes. *Am. J. Clin. Nutrition*, **22**: 163.
9. Wittmer, A. J., A. W. Sorenson, B. W. Wyse, and R. G. Hansen (1977). Nutrient density-evaluation of nutritional attributes of foods, *J. Nutrition Educ.*, **9**: 26.

Nutrition Education and Fallacies About Foods and Nutrition

1. Coon, J. M. (1973). Toxicology of natural food chemicals: A perspective. In *Toxicants Occurring Naturally in Foods*. 2nd ed. Washington, D.C.: Comm. on Food Protection, National Academy Sciences, p. 573.
2. Hill, M. M. (1966). Nutrition education basic to good eating habits for all. *Food and Nutrition News*. U.S. Dept. Agr., **37**: 1.
3. Jalso, S. B., M. B. Burns, and J. M. Rivers (1965). Nutritional beliefs and practices. *J. Am. Dietet. Assoc.*, **47**: 263.
4. New, P. K., and R. P. Priest (1967). Food and thought: A sociologic study of food cultists. *J. Am. Dietet. Assoc.*, **51**: 13.
5. Nickoff, A. (1969). Changing food habits. *J. Nutrition Educ.*, **1**: 10.
6. Packard, V. S., Jr. (1976). *Processed Foods and the Consumer*. Minneapolis: University of Minnesota Press, p. 175.
7. Ritchie, J. A. S. (1967). *Learning Better Nutrition*. FAO Nutritional Studies No. 20. Rome: Food and Agr. Organ., p. 32.

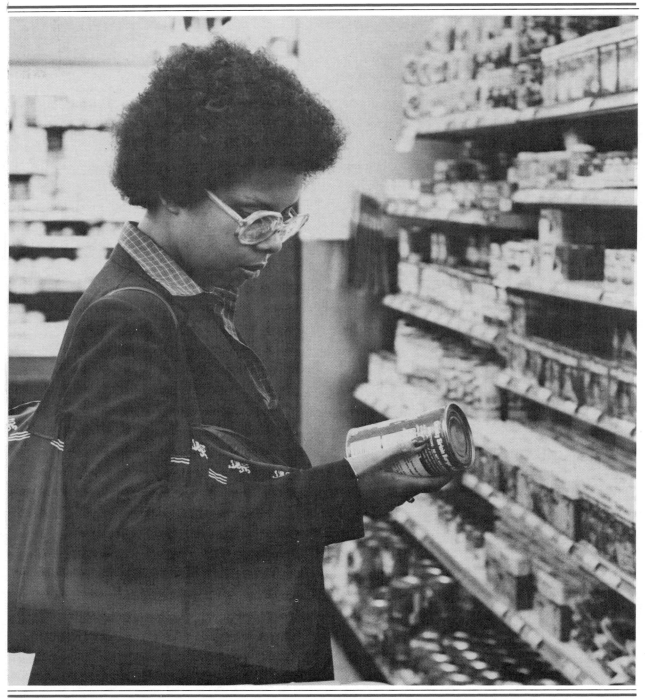

Many packaged foods in the market today have nutritional information given on the label. Good shoppers examine these labels.

Chapter 17

Foods in the Marketplace

Abbreviations

BHA: hydroxyanisole
BHT: butylated hydroxy toluene
CMS: Consumer and Marketing Service
DES: diethylstilbestrol
FAO: Food and Agriculture Organization
FDA: Food and Drug Administration
FTC: Federal Trade Commission
GRAS: generally recognized as safe
HTST: high temperature, short time

IAEA: International Atomic Energy Commission
PER: protein efficiency ratio
PHS: Public Health Service
ppb: parts per billion
USDA: United States Department of Agriculture
U.S.RDA: United States Recommended Daily
    Allowances
WHO: World Health Organization

Introduction

The foods in the grocery store of today have passed through a complex industrial network before arriving there. Even fresh fruit, fresh vegetables, and eggs have been sorted according to size and quality; fruits and vegetables are often transported across the country in trucks, freight cars, or cargo planes especially equipped with temperature and humidity controls to preserve the freshness of the produce. In the market there are fresh foods, preserved foods, and prepared foods—all of which are under surveillance to help assure their safety for use by the consumer.

Methods of Food Preservation

All methods of food preservation are intended to prevent or delay microbial spoilage and to slow down undesirable changes (darkening of cut surfaces, formation of soft spots, and the development of off flavors) caused by food enzymes, as well as damage by worms, bugs, weevils, fruit flies, and moths (the cuts made by these creatures serve as openings for microorganisms to reach the inner tissues).

Until the early part of the nineteenth century, foods were largely preserved by drying, pickling, or salting. The development of canning at that time is credited to the Frenchman Nicolas Appert, who devised this process for the armies of Napoleon. He referred to the food sealed in a complex arrangement of glass and corks as the "sealing of the seasons." During the twentieth century, other methods of preservation were developed: freezing, dehydration, freeze-drying, and irradiation.

To highlight the progress that has been made in the preservation of food, the food inventories of two historic voyages are presented: Columbus' trip to the New World in 1492, and the 2405-mile submerged voyage of the nuclear-powered submarine U.S.S. Skate across the North Pole in 1958 (Table 17.1)

Heat Preservation

Pasteurization is a preservation process that uses temperatures below the boiling point. Some of the spoilage organisms survive in pasteurized foods but not the pathogens. Pasteurized foods must usually be refrigerated. In the case of milk pasteurized by the holding process, the product is quickly brought to 63°C (145°F) and held there for 30 minutes. In high-temperature, short-time pasteurization (HTST), the milk is brought to a temperature of at least 72°C (161°F) and held there

372

for no less than 15 seconds. With both methods the milk is cooled at once. In the United States the holding system of pasteurization prevailed in both small and large plants until about 1940, when there was a rapid shift to the high-temperature, short-time procedure. The shift was due to the development of sensitive, reliable, control systems in the HTST equipment. Other foods and beverages are pasteurized to extend their keeping quality. Among them are dried fruits, fruit juices, wines, and beers.

Canning is the process of heating foods in hermetically sealed containers. The products are "commercially sterile," which means that all pathogenic and toxin-forming organisms have been destroyed, as well as those that cause spoilage. Canned foods usually have a shelf life of about two years.

The process of exhaustion, used in canning, helps to preserve the original color and flavor of a product. After filling the can, air and other gases are removed by heating the can, by filling the head space with steam, or by sealing the can in a vacuum chamber. The container is then permanently sealed and subjected to the temperature required to obtain a commercially sterile product. More than 8 billion cans of food were processed in 1970 in the United States, including fruits, fruit juices, vegetables, and fish.

Drying Preservation

Drying, dehydration, and freeze-drying are methods of preservation by the removal of water; microbial growth and chemical reactions can occur only when sufficient water is available. Drying is the removal of water by natural means, such as the sun and dry wind. Dried products have a moisture content of from 8 to 12 percent. Dehydration is the removal of water by special equipment that accelerates the process and reduces the moisture content to 4 to 6 percent. Freeze-drying, also called sublimation or lyophilization, is the removal of water from foods in the frozen state. Freeze-drying is accomplished by applying a controlled amount of heat to the frozen product (held in the range of $-10°$ to $-25°C$) under a high vacuum to speed up the removal of ice in the form of water vapor. The vapor is collected on refrigerator plates within the chamber or by mechanical or steam vacuum systems.

Drying This has been a means of preserving foods for thousands of years. Some foods, such as grains, dry naturally in the sun. Care is taken, however, to check the moisture level of grains and other products that dry naturally, such as soybeans and peanuts, before they are stored because of the possible invasion by molds if the moisture content is above certain safe levels, which vary with the product and time of storage, ranging between 11 and 14 percent (1). Sun drying is still used for apricots, dates, figs, raisins, and prunes. When animal products, such as meat or fish, are dried in the sun, salt is added because it draws moisture out of the tissue cells, thus preventing spoilage. Spoilage of raw flesh foods is caused by the action of naturally occurring enzymes and by microorganisms that are introduced when the raw products are prepared for drying. Moisture is needed for the enzymes and microbes to act. Flesh foods provide an ideal environment for microbes because they are high in water content, rich in nitrogenous compounds, and have a favorable pH medium.

Dehydration The purpose of dehydration is to remove virtually all of the water from a food without changing its color, flavor, or texture. Dehydration is used for eggs, potatoes, fruits, citrus fruit juices, and soups, but the most widely known dehydrated food is probably skim milk powder.

The United States armed forces often use dehydrated foods for complete meals (8), including such dishes as scrambled eggs, sliced beef and brown gravy, sliced pork, beef hash, beef and noodles, spaghetti with meat and tomato sauce,

373

Table 17.1 Food Lists for Pioneer Voyages

	Niña, Pinta, Santa Marie	U.S.S. Skate
Milk group	Cheese	Milk (fresh, dried, evaporated) Cheese (canned) Butter Cream (dried, stabilized) Ice cream paste
Meat group	Salt meat (beef and pork) Salt fish (barreled sardines and anchovies) (fishing tackle)	Pork cuts (frozen) Prefried bacon, pullman hams, brown-and-serve sausage (canned) Beef, boneless (fresh, frozen, canned, corned, dehydrated) Veal, boneless (frozen) Liver, prefabricated (frozen) Luncheon meats (fresh, canned) Chile con carne (dehydrated) Poultry (chicken cuts, frozen; turkey legs, canned) Fish (frozen, canned, dehydrated) Eggs (fresh, frozen, dried)
Vegetable–fruit group	Chickpeas Lentils Beans Rice Raisins Almonds Garlic	Potatoes (fresh, canned, dehydrated granules, dehydrated diced) Cabbage, string beans, peppers, onions (dehydrated) Peas (dehydrofrozen) Beans (dried) Other vegetables and fruit (fresh, frozen, canned, dried) Tomato juice, concentrated (canned) Orange, grapefruit juice (dehydrated crystals) Lemon, concentrated (frozen) Apples, pie style (dehydrated) Applesauce (instant) Soups: potato, onion, vegetable (dehydrated) Soup bases Jellies, jams (canned) Sauces (canned) Peanut butter

Table 17.1 — Continued

	Ninã, Pinta, Santa Marie	U.S.S. Skate
Bread–cereal group	Flour (salted at milling) Biscuits (well-seasoned)	Flour Flour mixes: bread, rolls, doughnut, cake, pancake Oatmeal Cornmeal Breakfast cereal, assorted Bread (fresh) Brown bread (canned) Cookies Macaroni, spaghetti, noodles Crackers
Other foods	Olive oil Honey Wine Vinegar	Shortening (hydrogenated) Salad oil Dessert powders Ketchup, chili sauce Pickles, olives Vinegar Sugar, syrups Candies Spices, condiments Coffee (ground, instant) Tea Cocoa

From *Power to Produce. The Yearbook of Agriculture.* Washington, D.C.: U.S. Dept. Agr., 1960, p. 453.

corn, peas, rice, and fruit cocktail. By adding hot or cold water to these precooked, dehydrated foods, they are ready to eat.

Freeze-Drying In this process, the frozen water (ice crystals) in food tissues vaporizes and condenses and is thus removed without passing through the liquid stage (water). Freeze-dried foods are preferable in many ways to dehydrated foods: they retain their natural shape, are less altered chemically, and are more readily reconstituted with water. Popular freeze-dried foods include orange juice and other citrus drinks, coffee, tea, crabmeat, shrimp, and meat. Many foods processed by this method serve as ingredients in other products, such as chicken in dry soup mixes and fruit in processed dry cereals (5). The abundance of membranes in plant and animal tissues imposes an impediment to the movement of water vapor, causing major limitations to the drying rate, which increases cost of production as a consequence (6).

375

Freezing Preservation

Freezing preserves food only by retarding (not eliminating, as in canning) microbial growth and enzyme action. Freezing converts liquid water to the solid state, thus making it unavailable for microbial growth and chemical reactions. The process may damage the tissue of the product somewhat, so that when it is thawed microbial growth is encouraged. Most raw foods contain enzymes, which are not inactivated by freezing alone. Therefore vegetables are blanched (scalded or steamed) before freezing. Otherwise, the product will develop a poor color, texture, and flavor due to enzyme action. Fruits, because of their higher acid content (which helps limit enzyme action), do not need to be blanched. Oxidation, which can cause light-colored fruits to become dark, can be prevented by adding an antioxidant (vitamin C is often used).

The storage temperature of frozen foods determines how long they can be kept. Vegetables, fruits, meats, and fish (properly packaged and frozen) can be preserved for 6 to 10 months when stored at $-12°C$ (10°F), whereas most foods can be kept up to 2 or 3 years at $-18°C$ (0°F). However, at temperatures of only $-9°$ to $-7°C$ (16° to 19°F) the quality can be retained for a few days, weeks, or perhaps months, depending upon the product (8).

Frozen foods generally retain most of their original nutritive value. Blanching causes the loss of some vitamin C, small amounts of other water-soluble vitamins, and some minerals. Without blanching, however, the oxidative changes would produce much greater losses of vitamin C.

In 1975, more than 23,000 million pounds of frozen foods were produced in the United States, including vegetables, fruits, juices, and drinks, meat, poultry, seafood, and prepared foods (11). Prepared foods, such as pies, cakes, macaroni and cheese, and breaded fish sticks, accounted for the largest category of foods, followed by juices and drinks.

Preservation by Irradiation

The research and development of food preservation by irradiation resulted from efforts to find peaceful uses for atomic energy following World War II. *Radiation* preservation is being studied in numerous laboratories of the world, and there are products on the market in some countries but not in the United States. Before irradiated foods can be sold on the commercial market, their wholesomeness as judged by toxicity and nutritional adequacy tests with animals and man must be established under the requirements of the 1958 Food Additives Amendment to the Federal Food, Drug, and Cosmetic Act.

The irradiation process is sometimes referred to as "cold sterilization" because the microorganisms in the food are destroyed or inactivated by nuclear ionization rather than by heat. In heat sterilization a food must be held at about 116°C (240°F) for an hour or more to produce a sterile product, whereas in irradiation there is only a small rise in temperature (not more than 10°C [50°F]) for a very short time (9).

Two sources of radiation are being tested for food preservation: radioactive isotopes or gamma rays and radiation produced by machines or electron sources. The U.S. Army Radiation Laboratory at Natick, Massachusetts, uses cobalt-60 gamma radiation in its experimental irradiation studies. Doses of radiation used on foods are expressed by a unit called the rad, which represents 100 ergs of energy per gram of irradiated material.

Small or medium doses of *ionizing radiation* may be more practical for immediate application to food preservation than a large dose. Small doses of radiation (less than 100,000 rads) have been used successfully to deinfest flour and spices, to prevent sprouting in stored potatoes (Fig. 17.1), and to delay the ripening of fruit (Table 17.2). The same treatment can be used to destroy the *Trichinella spiralis* organism in pork that causes trichinosis (4). Medium doses of radiation (about 100,000 to 1 million rads), now referred to as "pasteurization" or "radiopasteurization," have extended the shelf life of certain refrigerated foods. Meats have been preserved five times as long when treated with 100,000 to 500,000 rads. Fruits treated with 100,000 to 150,000 rads and then vacuum-packed and stored at refrigerator temperature were quite acceptable for 4 or 5 months.

Because many countries would like to use radiation to preserve or process foods (7), a joint committee has been formed with representatives of the Food and Agriculture Organization (FAO), the International Atomic Energy Agency (IAEA), and the World Health Organization (WHO) to try to influence legislation in various countries on the control of production and the use of irradiated foods (2, 3). The committee met for the first time in 1964, at which time it issued general principles governing the production and use of irradiated foods. The committee established three categories

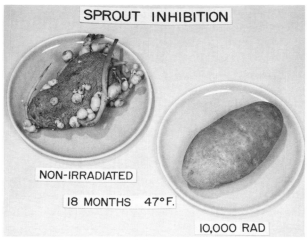

Fig. 17.1 After being stored for 18 months at 8.3°C (47°C), an untreated pungo potato (left) is compared with one exposed to 10,000 rads of radiation. (U.S. Army Photograph. Courtesy U.S. Army Radiation Laboratory, Natick, Massachusetts.)

Table 17.2 The Use and Effect of Varying Levels of Ionizing Radiation on Food and Related Products

Level of ionizing radiation	Use	Effect on finished product
Small exposure (less than 100,000)	Prevents sprouting of potatoes, destroys insects in flour and spices, and delays ripening of fruit.	Products not sterile, but there is little or no effect on the flavor or color of foods.
Medium exposure or "pasteurization" (about 100,000 to 1 million rads)	Extends the shelf life of meats, fish, fruits, and vegetables under refrigeration.	Products not completely sterile, but there is little or no effect on the flavor or color of foods.
Large exposure or "sterilization" (several million rads)	Sterilizes foods so that they can be stored as canned foods when properly packaged.	Products completely sterile, but this process often causes marked off flavors and changes in color and texture.

Adapted from Modern food processing, in *Food. The Yearbook of Agriculture*. Washington, D.C.: U.S. Dept. Agr., 1959, p. 421.

of acceptance: unconditional acceptance, where adequate biological data, including the results of long-term toxicological investigations were available to establish safety; conditional acceptance, where the criteria for unconditional acceptance were not satisfactorily met, and the requirements for further investigations were specified; and temporary acceptance, where additional evidence was asked to be submitted within a stated period (usually three to five years).

In some instances the committee cannot make a decision because the evidence submitted is inadequate or unsuitable. However, if the available evidence on an irradiated food indicates a potential health hazard, the committee's decision will be nonacceptance.

Unconditional acceptance has been given to the irradiation of stored wheat and ground wheat products to control insect infestation, of potatoes to control sprouting during storage, and of chicken to prolong storage life and reduce the number of pathogenic microorganisms in eviscerated chicken stored below 10°C. Other foods are being evaluated by the Joint FAO/IAEA/WHO Expert Committee (3).

The possible use of radiation preservation is especially important in tropical and subtropical areas, where the temperature is high and the humidity is often excessive. In India, for example, 15 to 50 percent of the food production is often lost because of spoilage (10).

Food Additives

A food additive—broadly defined—is any substance used in or around food that may become a component of the food. Some are introduced specifically for the purpose of improving the nutritive value, taste, texture, or shelf life of the product; these are intentional additives. Others enter food as residues after some stage of production or manufacture and are known as incidental additives.

Intentional Additives

To Improve Nutritive Value When the incidences of deficiency symptoms or dietary inadequacies of an essential nutrient have been found to be high among segments of the population in the United States, interested scientists and scientific groups have recommended the enrichment or fortification of various foods (4). As a result, a number of nutrients have been added to food products in the United States. Enrichment means an improvement of nutritional quality; originally it meant the addition of thiamin, riboflavin, niacin, and iron to white flour, white bread, and certain cereal grains from which some of these nutrients had been removed during processing. Fortification (although sometimes used interchangeably with enrichment) means the addition of nutrients that either do not occur naturally in the food or occur in relatively small amounts.

The addition of iodine to salt, beginning in 1924, was the first essential nutrient to be added to a staple food (see p. 297). Fortification of margarine began in 1941. (The fortification of salt and margarine are optional.) The enrichment of white flour, white bread, and certain cereal grains (cornmeal, corn grits, and rice) also began in 1941. Standards of identity for enriched white flour, white bread, and other cereal grain products were adopted. (The standard of identity is the official designation of the constituents and the amount of each that must be included in a product. The establishment of standards of identity is a function of the FDA.) Proposals for new standards are published from time to time in the *Federal Register*. There is an opportunity for interested parties, such as food processors and consumers, to study the proposals and to recommend changes. Sometimes public hearings are held.

The FDA's standards for fortification include:

1. Iodine added to salt: 0.5 to 1 part in 10,000.

2. Vitamin D added to milk: 400 USP units per quart of fluid milk or large can of evaporated milk (1²/₃ cups).

3. Vitamin A added to margarine: 15,000 USP units per pound (the year-round average for butter).

4. Enrichment levels prescribed by federal standards of identity for flour and other cereal products are listed in Table 17.3.

Thirty-five states, as of October 1977, had cereal enrichment laws in effect. However, wherever products labeled "enriched" are sold, whether in a state with an enrichment law or not, the federally specified nutrient levels must be present in those products.

To Improve Quality of Products For processed foods to be acceptable in keeping quality, flavor, and standard characteristics, the addition of certain chemicals is necessary (16). Preparing foods of good flavor and texture and keeping them in that condition throughout the time span between preparation and consumption makes the use of certain ingredients (additives) essential.

The Food Additives Amendment (1958) of the Federal Food, Drug, and Cosmetic Act of 1938 states that chemicals for use in processing food must be proved by the industry to be safe for that purpose *before* they can be sold. The manufacturer or promoter of a new food additive must test it for safety on animals and submit the results to the Food and Drug Administration. If

Table 17.3 Enrichment Levels in Mg per Lb of Finished Product

Cereal	Thiamin	Ribo-flavin	Niacin	Iron	Calcium
Enriched flour					
enriched bromated flour	2.9	1.8	24	13.0–16.5	(960)
Enriched self-rising flour	2.9	1.8	24	13.0–16.5	(960)
Enriched bread, rolls, and buns	1.8	1.1	15	8.0–12.5	(600)
Enriched corn meals,					
enriched corn grits	2.0–3.0	1.2–1.8	16–24	13.0–26.0	(500–750)
Enriched self-rising cornmeals	2.0–3.0	1.2–1.8	16–24	13.0–26.0	(500–1750)
Enriched rice[a]	2.0–4.0	1.2–2.4[b]	16–32	13.0–26.0	(500–1000)
Enriched macaroni products,					
enriched noodle products	4.0–5.0	1.7–2.2	27–34	13.0–16.5	(500–625)
Enriched farina[c]	2.0–2.5	1.2–1.5	16–20	13.0[d]	(500)[d]

When two figures are shown, they indicate the minimum-maximum levels. Figures in parentheses indicate that the use of the ingredient is optional.

[a] A proposal to revise the enriched rice standard would (a) provide for enrichment of coated rice (a product currently excluded from the standard); (b) delete present ranges, substituting single-level requirements based on the maximum now permitted; (c) provide for riboflavin as an optional ingredient; and (d) delete the provision for vitamin D as an optional ingredient.

[b] The riboflavin requirement was stayed many years ago.

[c] Nutritional quality guidelines have been proposed for fortified hot breakfast cereals, including farina.

[d] Minimum value, no maximum level stipulated.

Personal communication from Donald F. Miller, nutritionist, Division of Consumer Studies, Food and Drug Administration, Public Health Service, Dept. Health, Educ., and Welfare, Washington, D.C., 1977.

that agency is satisfied as to the safety of the additive, it will issue a regulation specifying the amount that may be used, the foods in which it may be used, and any other necessary conditions. If the safety of the additive is not established, its use will be prohibited.

The use of chemical additives in meat and poultry and their products is regulated according to the Federal Meat Inspection Act of 1907 as amended by the Federal Wholesome Meat Act of 1967 and the Wholesome Poultry Products Act of 1968 (19). Under these acts, chemical additives may be used in meat or meat products only with the approval of the U.S. Department of Agriculture.

Some of the additives used in food processing follow.

Antioxidants prevent undesirable changes caused by oxidation, such as rancidity of fats, oils, and foods that contain fat; discoloration of meat and meat products; and enzymatic darkening of fruits and vegetables. Some of the most widely used antioxidants are butylated hydroxyanisole (BHA); butylated hydroxy toluene (BHT); and propyl gallate.

Buffers, acids, bases, and neutralizing agents affect the degree of acidity or alkalinity, which is important in many classes of processed foods. For example:

The acid ingredient acts on the leavening agent in baked goods, and releases the gas which causes rising. The taste of many soft drinks is due largely to an organic acid. Acidity of churning cream must be controlled for flavor and keeping quality of the butter. Acids contribute flavor to confectionery and help to prevent a "grainy" texture. Buffers and neutralizing agents are chemicals added to control acidity or alkalinity, just as acids and alkalies may be added directly. Some common chemicals in this class are ammonium bicarbonate, calcium carbonate, potassium acid tartarate, sodium aluminum phosphate, and tartaric acid (7).

Coloring matter is added to improve the appearance and acceptability of a food. The Color Additive Amendment (enacted in 1960) to the Federal Food, Drug, and Cosmetic Act of 1938 "regulates the listing and certification of colors which are to be used in foods, drugs, and cosmetics, and in addition provides for testing both existing colors and new colors for safety" (8).

Emulsifiers are added to bakery products to increase the volume and to promote uniformity and fineness of the grain; to dairy products to achieve greater smoothness; and to confectionery goods to promote their homogeneity and shelf life. Among the common emulsifiers are lecithin (phosphatidyl choline) and the mono- and diglycerides. Chemists sometimes call the emulsifiers "surfactants," which is short for "surface active agents"; emulsifiers bind fat and water and do so at the interface between the two.

Stabilizers and thickeners are used to promote smoothness in confectionery goods, ice cream, and other frozen desserts; uniformity of color, flavor, and viscosity of chocolate milk; and "body" in artificially sweetened beverages. Stabilizing and thickening agents include pectins, vegetable gums (carob bean, guar), gelatin, and agar-agar.

Flavoring agents are added to enhance the taste of such products as soft drinks, bakery and confectionery goods, and ice cream. Synthetic flavors are produced by such chemicals as amyl acetate, benzaldehyde, and ethyl butyrate; natural flavors are the essential oils and spices.

Preservatives are added to extend the life of a product by delaying or preventing spoilage caused by mold, bacteria, or yeast. In bread, mold and rope inhibitors (antimycotic agents) are used. Those permitted include sodium and calcium propionate, sodium diacetate, acetic acid, lactic acid, and monocalcium phosphate. Sorbic acid and sodium and potassium sorbates are antimycotic agents for cheeses.

Some preservatives are used to prevent physical or chemical changes affecting flavor, color, and texture. In dairy products, sodium, calcium, and potassium salts of citric, tartaric, metaphosphoric, and pyrophosphoric acids are used. Sugar serves as a preservative for jams and jellies, vinegar for pickles, and salt for meat and fish.

Generally Recognized as Safe (GRAS) The 1958 Food Additives Amendment to the Food, Drug, and Cosmetic Act of 1938 called for prior approval by the FDA of new commercially added food ingredients. Those petitioning the use of food additives were required to present to the FDA evidence of the usefulness and of the harmlessness of the ingredients when used as proposed. Substances in common use at that time were exempted from the regulation and were known as "generally recognized as safe" (GRAS) substances. The 1958 amendment specified that the decision as to food safety should be determined by "experts qualified by training and experience" to do so. In 1970, FDA began a full-scale reevaluation of GRAS substances; by October 1977, 229 substances had been reviewed (17).

Many GRAS substances occur as a normal constituent of foods widely consumed. For example, *mannitol* is present in small amounts in olives, beets, and celery; *caprylic acid* is found in coconut and palm nut oils and butterfat; traces of tin are widespread in fish and vegetables (17).

The Delaney Clause of the 1958 Amendment states explicitly that "no additive shall be deemed to be safe if it is found to induce cancer when ingested by man or animal." This clause has influenced the decision on a number of ingredients, such as cyclamates, saccharin, and the use of nitrates in pork products (17). Delay in implementation of the imposed ban was sought and obtained for saccharin and is being sought for the nitrates.

Incidental Additives

Pesticide Residues Pesticides, which include insecticides, fungicides, and rodenticides, reduce the loss of crops and food and yield a higher quality product. The label on the pesticide container is required by law (Federal Insecticide, Fungicide, and Rodenticide Act of 1947) to list the ingredients, to give instructions for using the pesticide, and to give a precautionary statement about its safety. All pesticides intended for shipment in interstate commerce must be registered with the U.S. Secretary of Agriculture. In order for a pesticide to be registered, the manufacturer must show that it can be used as directed on a specific food crop without leaving an illegal residue (an amount exceeding the "tolerance" level established by the government). The law also covers products for home use to control insects, rodents, molds, mildew, and bacteria.

Another related measure is the 1954 Pesticide Chemicals Amendment to the Federal Food, Drug, and Cosmetic Act of 1938. This law provided for the establishment of safety standards for the human consumption of pesticides. If the Department of Agriculture was convinced that a given pesticide was useful, it certified that fact to the FDA and prepared a statement indicating the amount of residue permitted to remain on the crop from the proposed use. The FDA determined if the tolerance data submitted by the industry complied with the tolerances established. If so, the product was approved for registration by the Department of Agriculture and for use by consumers. The FDA had established tolerance levels for pesticides until 1970, when it became the responsibility of the Tolerances Division of the Environmental Protection Agency.

Feed Utilization Residues Antibiotics and the hormone *diethylstilbestrol* (DES) are fed to animals to improve their feed utilization. It is required by law that no residue of these substances be present in the meat when it is consumed.

Radioactive Contamination *Radioactivity* can enter food and water from naturally occurring *radioactive isotopes*, from radioactive fallout due to nuclear weapon explosions, and from occasional emissions from nuclear-powered generator plants (3). At the present time, the major

381

source of environmental radioactivity is that from naturally occurring radioisotopes, which are concentrated rather uniformly around the world (9). They are present in the earth's surface and in cosmic rays. The two major contaminants of food come from natural sources — potassium-40 and carbon-14. Each has a long radioactive physical half-life, 220 million and 5760 years, respectively. (The physical half-life is the length of time required for one-half of the mass of a radioactive substance to decay, that is, spontaneously transform itself into another substance through radiation emissions). The long radioactive half-life of potassium-40 and carbon-14 makes them potentially hazardous. However, the danger from carbon-14 is lessened somewhat because it is absorbed into the body in small amounts, and the danger of potassium-40 is reduced by the relatively rapid rate with which it leaves the body; potassium-40 remains in the body for only a few months (1).

After a nuclear explosion, radioactive particles fall back to the earth's surface. Contaminated plants and water may be ingested by humans and animals; humans may also consume radioactive elements through the milk or meat of animals. Some of these elements are absorbed by the body, and some are excreted in the feces.

The radioactive elements that enter the food supply due to nuclear explosions are primarily strontium-90, cesium-137, iodine-131, and carbon-14. Strontium-90 has a physical half-life of 28 years. It belongs to the same chemical group as calcium; like calcium, it is deposited in the bones and teeth, where it remains for a number of years. The radiation of strontium-90 has a detrimental effect not only on the bones but also on the bone-forming and blood-forming cells in the bone cavity. Strontium-90 is absorbed by the intestinal mucosa in much the same way as is calcium (2). However, when both are present, calcium is absorbed in preference to strontium (see p. 267). The major source of strontium-90 in the diet is milk, although vegetables also contain a significant amount. Cesium-137, like potassium-40,

is distributed widely throughout the body, particularly in the soft tissues. Its *physical half-life* is the same as that of strontium-90 (28 years), but it has a much shorter biological half-life (about 140 days), and so it is potentially much less harmful. (The biological half-life is the time required for the body to excrete one-half of the amount ingested.) Iodine-131 has a short physical half-life (eight days). Although milk is the principal source, fresh foods also contain iodine-131. This radioactive element tends to concentrate in the thyroid gland, and this occurs primarily in children between birth and one year when the gland is small and the consumption of milk is high. The excessive concentration of radioactive elements poses the danger of eventual cancer. Those that concentrate in certain tissues or organs, such as strontium-90 in the bones and iodine-131 in the thyroid gland, pose a greater danger than cesium-137 or potassium-40, which are distributed throughout the body.

Several government agencies periodically test the concentration of radionuclides in the food supply — the Atomic Energy Commission, the U.S. Department of Agriculture, the Food and Drug Administration, and the U.S. Public Health Service. The last agency maintains 63 milk sampling stations throughout the United States, the Canal Zone, and Puerto Rico (14). The Federal Radiation Council of the Environmental Protection Agency stipulates the levels of radiocontamination beyond which remedial action is necessary.

Mercury Contamination The first known cases of human poisoning from consuming methylmercury were reported in Japan in 1953 on the Island of Kyushu around Minamata Bay, where contaminated fish were eaten (13). In 1964, a similar outbreak occurred at Niigata, Japan, along the Agano River. Between 1953 and 1970, there were 168 illnesses and 52 deaths from methylmercury poisoning in Japan. The methylmercury came from industrial waste that had been discharged into the bay and river. Metallic mercury

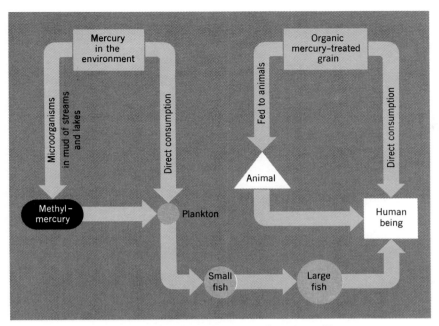

Fig. 17.2 The pathways by which human beings can be poisoned by mercury from food.

is converted to methylmercury by bacteria *(methanobacterium omelanskii)* living in the bottom mud of bays, rivers, and streams (5). The pathways of human mercury poisoning from food contamination, either directly or indirectly, are illustrated in Fig. 17.2.

Symptoms usually appear in the human several weeks after the ingestion of a toxic dose, but they may not appear until months or even years afterward. The disease, called Minamata disease, is characterized by a burning or tingling sensation of the extremities, mouth, lips, and tongue; loss of vision, difficulty in articulating words, and swallowing; some loss of hearing; weakness and fatigue; an inability to read, write, or recall; emotional instability; ataxia, stupor, coma; and death (6).

A suggested limit on the weekly intake of mercury—a total of 0.3 mg per person (0.005 mg per kg of body weight), of which no more than 0.2

mg (0.0033 mg per kg of body weight) should be methylmercury—was established by the Joint FAO/WHO Expert Committee on Food Additives. The committee recognizes that the existing levels of methylmercury in the food of some fish-eating populations will exceed 0.2 mg per person per week and urges that all possible steps be taken to lower this amount (15).

In 1969, three New Mexican children in one family suffered severe brain damage after the family had eaten meat from hogs that had been fed grain (intended for seed purposes) that had been treated with organic mercury. Although the entire family ate the same meat, only the children suffered severe brain damage (5, 10).

Organic mercury compounds were responsible for the poisonings cited. Metallic mercury is toxic only if its vapor is inhaled. Some inorganic mercurial compounds have medicinal uses. (11, 12).

383

Toxicants Occurring Naturally in Foods

Toxicants occurring naturally in foods are "chiefly the natural components of plant and animal tissues as produced during normal growth, various other substances derived from the animals' feed or the soil or aquatic environment in which the plants or fish grew, and compounds produced by or as a result of microbial contamination of food materials" (18); they are substances that occur in foods without man's intervention. Some of the more common ones will be discussed here.

Solanine, a chemical which occurs in potatoes, particularly the green areas found in potatoes exposed to the sun or to bright artificial light, is poisonous if eaten in sufficient amounts. In humans, an oral dose of around 2.8 mg of solanine per kilogram of body-weight was found to cause drowsiness and labored breathing (dyspnea), whereas higher amounts caused vomiting and diarrhea (20). The normal range of solanine in good market potatoes is about 3 to 6 mg per 100 g; 20 mg per 100 g is considered to be the maximum safe level (18). Solanine, because it is an insoluble substance, is not lost in the cooking water, nor is it inactivated by heat. As a safeguard, green-colored portions of potatoes should be discarded.

Fungus toxins (mycotoxins) have caused human suffering and loss of life. At present, the most feared mycotoxin is aflatoxin, discovered (1960–1961) in peanut meal containing the mold *aspergillus flavus* (18, 21). This black mold occurs in grains stored with a moisture content that is too high, that is, above 15 percent. Aflatoxin is fluorescent, which facilitates its detection in contaminated products. The FDA has set a maximum limit of 15 parts per billion (ppb) of the toxin in a product (15 lb of the toxin in one billion lb of grain). The FDA seizes and destroys products exceeding the maximum limit for aflatoxin in the product.

Mold-damaged (black-rotted) sweet potatoes were found to cause toxic symptoms in farm animals consuming them; the animals developed an accumulation of fluid in the lungs (lung edema) and died of apparent asphyxia (22). (The toxins are ipomeamarone, upomeamaronol, and others.) A preliminary survey of sweet potatoes available in markets demonstrated that those with blemishes in the peeling and discoloration contained toxins. Normal boiling or baking does not eliminate the toxins. Even though no reports of human intoxication due to sweet potatoes has been recorded, it is important to select only sound, unblemished, sweet potatoes for human or animal use (21).

Food-Borne Diseases

For the unwitting consumer, food-borne diseases are far too common. Bacterial food infections, bacterial food poisoning, and parasitic infestations are types of food-borne diseases.

Bacterial Food Infection

Food infection results from the ingestion of food containing large numbers of bacteria. The bacteria multiply in the intestine, causing symptoms to appear 12 to 24 hours after the contaminated food is eaten.

Salmonellosis Raw meat, poultry, eggs, and dairy products are the most common carriers of *Salmonella*; animals used for food harbor the organism. The organism multiplies readily in custards and egg dishes; contaminated cake mixes and bakery goods have caused outbreaks of the infection. Careless and unsanitary handling of food is also a cause of the infection.

Shigellosis (bacillary dysentery) The source of the bacteria of the genus *Shigella* is human feces and transmission by unsanitary practices resulting in contamination of food. The infection may be mild (as is often the case in adults) or extremely severe (as often occurs in children).

384

Clostridium Perfringens Food Infection *Clostridium perfringens*, the organism that causes gas gangrene in wounds, ordinarily is present in the intestinal tract, and in the numbers present causes no problem. However, when a food contaminated with the bacterium is eaten, illness occurs. The bacteria are destroyed by heat, but the spores survive (boiling) as long as five hours. Slow cooking of foods, especially meat and meat dishes, allows the organism to multiply; thorough cooking of these products and refrigeration are deterrents to *Clostridium perfringens* food infection. Outbreaks are usually traced to banquets, picnics, or meals served to large gatherings of people.

Brucellosis The microorganism *Brucella* is the cause of brucellosis (undulant fever) in man; the organism is transmitted in the milk of cows and goats. The boiling or pasteurization of milk destroys the organism.

The incidence of human brucellosis increased in 1975 over 1974. Sixty percent of the cases occurred in people working in the meat processing industry. Persons handling infected meat who have cuts or scratches on the skin are susceptible to infection. In 1975, 24 cases (8 percent of the total) were attributed to the ingestion of unpasteurized dairy products (8 to milk consumed by farm families and 16 to foreign dairy products, either raw milk or cheese) (3).

Bacterial Food Poisoning

Food poisoning results from the ingestion of food containing the toxin produced by a contaminating bacteria. The symptoms, which usually appear soon after the food is eaten (within one to six hours), are caused by the toxin.

Staphylococcal Food Poisoning *Staphylococcus* is a toxin-producing bacterium; it is the most common cause of bacterial food poisoning in the United States (3). The source of contamination may be the food handler whose nose, throat, or hands are carriers of the organism. *Staphylococci* are present in the air and in infected wounds and abrasions of the skin. Foods that are common sources of the organism are custards, cream fillings in pastries and cream puffs, cream sauces, mayonnaise, chicken and turkey salads, potato salad, croquettes, ham, ground beef stews, poultry dressing, fish, ice cream, and casserole combinations. The food contaminated with the toxin usually tastes, smells, and appears as usual; the victim has no forewarning.

Botulism Botulism is caused by the ingestion of any food that contains the toxin produced by the gas-forming, anaerobic organism *Clostridium botulinum*. Inadequately processed home-canned foods have most often been the cause of botulism, especially low- and medium-acid foods, such as string beans, sweet corn, beets, or even low-acid tomatoes. Sometimes commercially canned foods are also found to contain the toxin. The effect of the toxin may vary from slight discomfort with nausea and dizziness to death with paralysis of the respiratory passages (1). (Procedures for safe home canning are available from the U.S. Department of Agriculture or from one's own County Agricultural Extension Office.) The following precautions should be taken against botulism: (a) all canned foods that appear in any way to be spoiled should be rejected; (b) any canned food that exhibits pressure in the container (a bulging lid) should not be eaten; and (c) all home-canned vegetables should be boiled ten minutes before they are tasted or used.

Parasitic Infestations of Food

Many protozoa and helminths (worms) enter the body by way of food eaten and reside in the colon where they cause injury to the mucosal lining. Some parasites move from the intestine to the liver, the lungs, and even the brain (2).

Entamoeba histolytica causes amebic dysentery.

The source of the infection is human feces; the mode of transmission is by the oral route — the ingestion of food or water containing cysts of the parasite, contaminated by unsanitary practices (such as failure to wash hands) of food handlers who are carriers. The parasite lodges in the intestine but also moves to the liver, lungs, and even the brain.

Trichinella spiralis is a minute roundworm found in the muscle of pork, particularly in animals fed uncooked garbage. The eating of raw or partially cooked pork infested with the parasite is the mode of transmission. The parasite multiplies in the intestine and moves into the diaphragm and muscle tissue. Muscular pain, chills, and weakness are symptoms of trichinosis. *Trichinella spiralis* is destroyed by cooking pork to the well-done stage, until no pink color remains. The recommended internal temperature for cooked pork is 77°C (170°F).

Consumer Protection

Consumer-protection laws exist at the local, state, and federal levels. Some of the federal agencies that act to protect and serve the consumer are the Food and Drug Administration, the Federal Trade Commission, the U.S. Public Health Service, and the Consumer and Marketing Service of the U.S. Department of Agriculture (5).

Food and Drug Administration (FDA)

This agency came into existence by that name in 1931. Since January 1, 1907, when the Food and Drug Act of 1906 became effective, activities similar to those performed by the FDA had been carried on under different organizational titles.

FDA's activities are directed mainly toward protecting the public health of the Nation by insuring that foods are safe, pure, and wholesome; drugs are safe and effective; cosmetics are harmless; therapeutic devices are safe and effective; products are honestly and informatively labeled and packaged (5).

Field activities to enforce the laws under the jurisdiction of the FDA are carried out within 10 regions by laboratories and administrative offices located in 17 major cities. A limitation to the FDA enforcement capability is that the agency has authority only over those products that pass in interstate commerce. Products produced and sold within a state do not fall within the jurisdiction of the FDA.

The Bureau of Foods of the FDA conducts research and develops standards and policy on the composition, quality, nutrition, and safety of foods, food additives, colors, and cosmetics; conducts research designed to improve the detection, prevention, and control of contamination that may be responsible for illness or injury conveyed by foods, colors, and cosmetics; plans, coordinates, and evaluates FDA's surveillance and compliance programs relating to foods, colors, and cosmetics; reviews industry petitions and recommends the promulgation of regulations for food standards and to permit the safe use of color additives and food additives; and collects and interprets data on nutrition, food additives, and environmental factors affecting the total chemical insult posed by food additives (5).

Nutrition Labeling The White House Conference on Food, Nutrition, and Health in 1969 recommended that the labels on foods should give information on the nutritive value of the contents. The recommendation was studied jointly by professional groups, manufacturers, consumers, and the FDA; proposals were published in 1972, and public reaction to them was solicited. In 1973, the final regulations were published* with the stipulation that there be full compliance in 1976.

In the case of many foods, this practice is voluntary. However, if a product has been fortified with certain nutrients, or if a nutritional claim

---

* *Federal Register,* **38:** 2131 (No. 13, January 19), 1973.

has been made on the label or in advertising of a product, labeling is mandatory.

Standards for Labeling. The FDA developed the United States Recommended Daily Allowances (U.S. RDA) to be used as the standard for nutrition labeling. The standards now in use are for adults and children four years of age and over. Standards have been established for infants to one year of age, children one to three years, and pregnant and lactating women also; implementation of the standards for these three special groups has been delayed pending further investigation (4).

Format for Labeling. The label must adhere to a specified format. The information required and the sequence of listing are as follows:

1. Serving size.
2. Number of servings per container.
3. Caloric content per serving.
4. Number of grams of protein per serving.
5. Number of grams of carbohydrate per serving.
6. Number of grams of fat per serving.
7. Percentage of U.S. RDA for protein, vitamins A and C, thiamin, riboflavin, niacin, calcium, and iron.

Percentages of the U.S. RDA are given in increments of 2 percent, that is, 2, 4, 6, 8, up to 10 percent; of 5 percent, that is, 10, 15, 20, up to 50 percent; and of 10 percent above 50 percent, that is, 50, 60, 70, and so forth.

Protein is listed both in terms of number of grams per serving and as a percentage of the U.S. RDA (see p. 34). The U.S. RDA for protein varies according to the quality (expressed as the Protein Efficiency Ratio [PER]) of the total protein in a product (see p. 106 for discussion of PER). If the PER is equal to or greater than that of casein, the U.S. RDA is 45 g; if the PER is less than that of casein, the U.S. RDA is 65 g. Optional information that may be on the label follows:

1. The percentage of the U.S. RDA per serving for any of the following vitamins and minerals: vitamin D, vitamin E, vitamin B-6, folic acid, vitamin B-12, biotin, pantothenic acid, phosphorus, iodine, magnesium, zinc, and copper.
2. The percentage of kilocalories that comes from fat, the amounts of polyunsaturated fat, saturated fat, and cholesterol per serving.
3. The amount of sodium per serving of food.
4. Nutrition information for a serving of food cooked or prepared in combination with other foods according to directions given on the label.

Federal Trade Commission (FTC)

This agency is empowered to protect the consumer by preventing food advertisements that are false or deceptive or that promote a food that may be injurious to health or that is claimed to prevent or treat a disease, and by regulating the packaging or labeling of certain products to prevent deception and facilitate price comparisons.

Public Health Service (PHS)

One of the major functions of this agency is to identify and to prevent health hazards in food. Toward this end it may establish model sanitary codes and ordinances for milk, food service establishments, food and beverage vending machines, poultry processing, ice manufacturing, and the fish-smoking industry. The PHS also conducts and supports research on the epidemiology of food-borne diseases, food microbiology, radionuclides in foods, and pesticide residue analysis of food. The PHS offers technical and consultative services on food sanitation problems to state and local governments.

Consumer and Marketing Service (CMS) USDA

This agency is responsible for establishing standards for the wholesomeness of meat, poultry, and egg products that are imported, exported, or that move in interstate commerce. The CMS also inspects these products and maintains surveillance over their processing to assure truthful

387

labeling and to prevent adulteration and deception. The CMS has also established a classification system for grading most of the important farm commodities according to quality. The grading of some produce is mandatory, but in most cases it is voluntary.

The grading of meat is elective with the packer. If the decision is to grade, the USDA system may be used or the packer's own system. Factors determining quality of beef, veal, and lamb (USDA system) are firmness of the lean, amount of marbling (dispersion of fat among the muscle fibers), and maturity of the animal. Pork is graded only as acceptable and unacceptable. That which is unacceptable is soft and watery. In the retail market, the consumer will find no grade designations on pork, but beef, veal, and lamb may have the grade appearing on the cut. The USDA grades for beef, veal, and lamb are given in Table 17.4.

Poultry is a general term used for chicken, turkey, duck, goose, and guinea. Grades for poultry (USDA) are U.S. Grade A, U.S. Grade B, and U.S. Grade C. The only one of the three grades to appear in the retail market, as a rule, is U.S. Grade A; birds of this grade are good in formation and meatiness, have a well-developed layer of fat in the skin, and a skin virtually free of defects.

The grading of fish for the market comes under the direction of the U.S. Department of the Interior. Grade A is used for the top or best quality; Grade B for good quality; and Grade C is used for fish of somewhat lower quality but a wholesome food.

The USDA directs the grading of shell eggs using three designations: U.S. Grade AA or Fresh Fancy Quality, U.S. Grade A, and U.S. Grade B. Condition of the shell, size of the air cell, and lack of defects in the yolk and the centering of it are taken into consideration in the grading process.

Vegetables and fruits are available in the market—fresh, frozen, canned, and dehydrated—throughout the year. There are USDA grades for fresh vegetables and fruits with at least two designations for each vegetable or fruit. For frozen and canned vegetables, three grades have been established on a national basis: U.S. Grade A or Fancy is the top quality based on color, tenderness, and freedom from blemishes; the other two grades are U.S. Grade B or Extra Standard and U.S. Grade C or Standard. There are also three grades for frozen and canned fruits. The top grade U.S. Grade A or Fancy is characterized by fruit of excellent color, uniform size, optimum ripeness, and few or no blemishes; the other two grades are U.S. Grade B or Choice and U.S. Grade C or Standard. The federal government has established grades for dried fruits; however, they are used very little.

Summary

The foods in the grocery store of today have passed through a complex industrial network before arriving there. In the market there are fresh foods, preserved foods, and prepared foods—all of which are under government surveillance to help ensure their safety for use by the consumer.

The market has foods preserved by heat treatment (pasteurization and canning), foods preserved by drying, and by the specialized processes of dehydration and freeze-drying. Also in the market are frozen foods. Frozen prepared foods, such as pies, cakes, macaroni and cheese, and

Table 17.4 USDA Grades for Beef, Veal, and Lamb

Beef	Veal	Lamb
Prime	Prime	Prime
Choice	Choice	Choice
Good	Good	Good
	Standard	
Commercial	Utility	Utility
Utility	Cull	Cull
Cutter		
Canner		

breaded fish sticks, accounted for the largest sale category of frozen products in 1975, followed by juices and drinks. Foods preserved by irradiation are not on the market in the United States.

Food additives may be intentional, added to the food to improve the nutritive value or the keeping quality, flavor, or other characteristics. Some of the intentional additives are closely regulated by the FDA; others are generally recognized as safe (GRAS) and may be added to the food without restriction. Then there are the incidental additives that are in the food unintentionally as residues; pesticide residues and food utilization residues are causing the most concern at this time. Another is mercury contamination.

Toxicants occur naturally in foods. Solanine is a toxicant found in potatoes; it occurs in the green portion that develops on exposure of the tuber to the sun. Aflatoxin, a mycotoxin, is found in grains, legumes, and peanuts stored without sufficient drying. The most common bacterial food infection in the United States is salmonellosis, and the most deadly food poisoning is botulism.

In the United States there are federal agencies that function to protect the consumer. They are the Food and Drug Administration, the Federal Trade Commission, the U.S. Public Health Service, and the Consumer and Marketing Service of the U.S. Department of Agriculture.

Glossary

Ataxia: failure of muscular coordination.
caprilic acid: see p. 66.
diethylstilbestrol: a synthetic estrogenic (produces sexual receptivity in the female) compound.
erg: a unit of work.
ionizing radiation: emission of atoms; among the types of ionizing radiation are x-rays, alpha particles, and high-speed electrons

mannitol: alcohol derived from mannose.
radiation: see ionizing radiation.
radioactive isotopes (radioisotopes): see p. 11.
radioactivity: the spontaneous disintigration of certain unstable atoms, caused by changes in the nucleus of the atom transforming it into a different one with the emission of one or more types of ionizing radiation, such as alpha particles, beta particles, or gamma rays.

Study Questions and Activities

1. What are some of the advantages of freeze-dried foods? Of frozen foods? What are the disadvantages of these methods of food preservation?
2. Explain how food is preserved by irradiation.
3. Name three products that have been fortified with nutritional additives.
4. What radioactive elements enter the food supply from nuclear explosions? From natural background radiation?
5. What retail food products will be affected by the proposals for nutrition labeling?

References

Methods of Food Preservation

1. Golumbic, C. and M. M. Kulik (1969). In *Aflatoxin*, edited by L. A. Goldblatt. New York: Academic Press, p. 312.
2. Joint FAO/IAEA/WHO Expert Committee (1966). *The Technical Basis for Legislation on Irradiated Food*. WHO Tech. Rept. Series 316. Geneva: World Health Organ., pp. 1–37.
3. Joint FAO/IAEA/WHO Expert Committee (1977). *Wholesomeness of Irradiated Food*. Tech. Rept. Series 604. Geneva: World Health Organ., p. 24.
4. Kraybill, H. F. (1958). Nutritional and biochemical aspects of foods preserved by ionizing radiation. *J. Home Econ.*, **50:** 695.
5. Liebman, H. L. (1977). Recent departures in volume freeze-drying, from L.-R. Ray, Glimpses into

389

the Fundamental Aspects of Freeze-Drying. In *International Symposium on Freeze-Drying of Biological Products*, edited by V. J. Cabasso and R. H. Regamey. Basel: S. Karger, p. 19.

6. Meryman, H. T. (1977). Historical recollections of freeze-drying. In *International Symposium on Freeze-Drying of Biological Products. Develop. Biol. Stand.*, **36:** 29.

7. Pizer, V. (1970). *Preserving Food with Atomic Energy*. Oak Ridge, Tenn.: U.S. Atomic Energy Commission.

8. Potter, N. N. (1968). *Food Science*. Westport, Conn.: Avi Publishing Co., p. 149.

9. Ryer, R., III (1956). Influence of radiation preservation of foods on military feeding. *Food Technol.*, **10:** 516.

10. Sreenivasan, A. (1972). Food irradiation: A survey. *Indian J. Nutrition and Dietet.*, **9:** 91.

11. *Statistical Abstracts of the United States, 97th Annual Ed.* (1976). Washington, D.C.: Bureau of Census, Social and Economics Statistics Adm., U.S. Dept. Commerce.

Food Additives

1. Brill, A. B. and R. E. Johnston (1970). Exposure of man to radiation. In *Late Effects of Radiation*, edited by R. J. M. Fry, D. Grahn, M. L. Griem, and J. H. Rust. New York: Van Nostrand Reinhold.

2. Comar, C. L. and J. C. Thompson, Jr. (1973). Radioactivity in foods. In *Modern Nutrition in Health and Disease*, 5th ed., edited by R. S. Goodhart and M. E. Shils. Philadelphia: Lea and Febiger, p. 442.

3. Committee on Food Protection, National Research Council (1973). *Radionuclides in Foods*. Washington, D.C.: National Academy Sciences, p. 95.

4. Committee on Food Standards and Fortification Policy, National Research Council and American Medical Association (1974). *Proposed Fortification Policy for Cereal-Grain Products*. Washington, D.C.: National Academy Sciences.

5. Curly, A., V. A. Sedlak, E. F. Girling, R. E. Hawk, W. F. Barthel, P. E. Pierce, and W. H. Likosky (1971). Organic mercury identified as the cause of poisoning in humans and hogs. *Science*, **172:** 65.

6. Eyl, T. B. (1971). Methylmercury poisoning in fish and human beings. *Clin. Toxicol.*, **4:** 291.

7. *Facts for Consumers, Food Additives*. FDA Publ. No. 10. Washington, D.C.: U.S. Dept. Health, Educ., and Welfare.

8. Food and Nutrition Board (1971). *Food Colors*. Washington, D.C.: National Research Council.

9. Gillette, R. (1972). Radiation standards: The last word or at least a definitive one. *Science*, **178:** 966.

10. Goldwater, L. J. (1971). Mercury in the environment. *Sci. Am.*, **224:** 15.

11. Hammond, A. L. (1971). Mercury in the environment: Natural and human factors. *Science*, **171:** 788.

12. Lu, F. C., P. E. Berteau, and D. J. Clegg (1972). The toxicity of mercury in man and animals. In *Mercury Contamination in Man and His Environment*. Tech. Rept. Series 137. Vienna: International Atomic Energy Agency, p. 67.

13. Matsumoto, H., G. Koya, and T. Takouchi (1965). Fatal Minamata disease. A neuropathological study of two cases of intrauterine intoxication by a methylmercury compound. *J. Neuropath. Exp. Neurol.*, **24:** 563.

14. Milk surveillance. November 1969 (1970). *Radiol. Health Data and Repts.*, **11:** 141.

15. Olcott, H. S. (1972). Mercury, DDT, and PCBs in aquatic food resources. *J. Nutrition Educ.*, **4:** 156.

16. Packard, V. S., Jr. (1976). *Processed Foods and the Consumer*. Minneapolis: University of Minnesota Press, p. 43.

17. Select Committee on GRAS Substances, Fed. Am. Soc. Exptl. Biol. (1977). Evaluation of health aspects of GRAS food ingredients: Lessons learned and questions unanswered. *Federation Proc.*, **37:** 2519.

18. Strong, F. M. (1976). Toxicants occurring naturally in food. In *Present Knowledge in Nutrition*, 4th ed., edited by D. M. Hegsted, Chm., and Editorial Comm. Washington, D.C.: The Nutrition Foundation, Inc., p. 516.

19. *The Use of Chemicals in Food Production, Proc-*

essing, Storage, and Distribution (1973). Washington, D.C.: National Academy Sciences.

20. Whitaker, J. R. and R. E. Feeney (1973). Enzyme inhibitors in foods. In *Toxicants Occurring Naturally in Foods*, 2nd ed., edited by Comm. on Food Protection, National Research Council. Washington, D.C.: National Academy Sciences.

21. Wilson, B. J. and A. W. Hayes (1973). Microbial toxins. In *Toxicants Occurring Naturally in Foods*, 2nd ed., edited by Comm. on Food Protection, National Research Council. Washington, D.C.: National Academy Sciences.

22. Wilson, B. J., D. T. C. Yang, and M. R. Boyd (1970). Toxicity of mold-damaged sweet potatoes (Impomoea balalas). *Nature*, **227**: 521.

Food-Borne Diseases and Consumer Protection

1. The deadliest poison (1975). *Nutrition Today*, **10**: 4.

2. Faust, E. C., P. R. Russell, and R. C. Jang (1970). *Craig and Faust's Clinical Parasitology*. 8th ed. Philadelphia: Lea and Febiger.

3. Food poisoning notes (1976). *Morbidity and Mortality Weekly Report*. Sept. 24. Atlanta, Ga.: Center for Disease Control, Public Health Service, U.S. Dept. Health, Educ., and Welfare.

4. Stephenson, M. (1975). Making food labels more informative. *FDA Consumer*, **9**: 13.

5. United States Government Manual (1977/1978). Washington, D.C.: U.S. Govt. Printing Office.

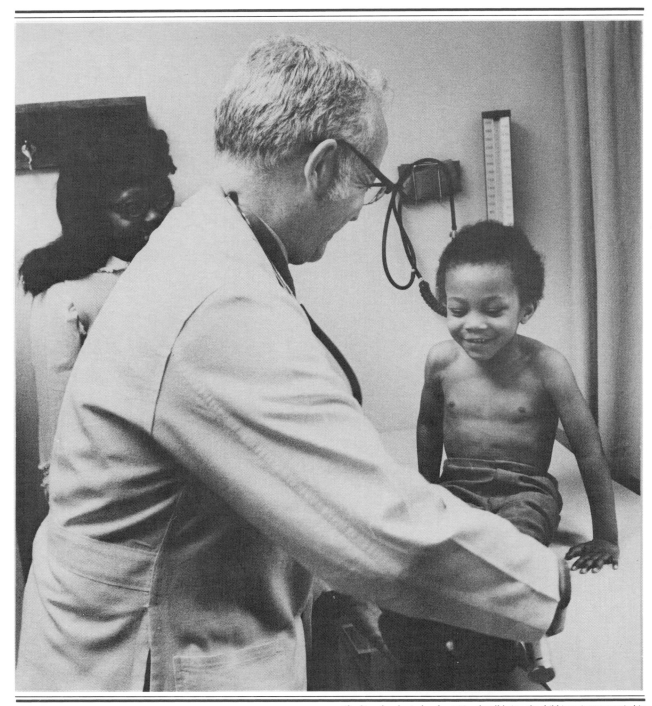

Checking the physical and nutritional well-being of a child is an investment in his future.

Chapter 18

Nutritional Status

Abbreviations

HANES: Health and Nutrition Examination
 Survey
RDA: Recommended Dietary Allowances

USDA: U.S. Department of Agriculture
WHO: World Health Organization

Introduction

One of the reasons for studying nutrition is to learn how to select a diet that will enable one to achieve and maintain a good nutritional status. A diet is judged to be adequate if those who consume it enjoy long-term health. To attain good nutrition, the food supply must be adequate, and individuals must be able to select, obtain, and consume foods that will meet their nutrient needs. In addition, the body must be able to utilize the food consumed; thus it must be free of organ dysfunctions (particularly those concerned with digestion and absorption) and nervous and emotional strain. Nutritional status represents the health of an individual as conditioned by (a) the quantity and quality of *nutrients* consumed, and (b) the body's ability to utilize these nutrients to meet its metabolic needs.

Evaluation of Nutritional Status

Objectives for Evaluation

The main purpose of most nutritional status studies is to identify individuals at risk, those persons and groups whose nutritional status ought to be improved. The findings can lead to the development of educational programs to help people improve their diets. They may also provide a basis for decisions by those who are responsible for programs relating to food production or consumption to meet people's nutritional needs at the local, state, national, or international level.

Methods of Evaluation

Because many body functions may be affected by inadequate nutrition, there is no simple procedure for assessing nutritional status. Some stages of *malnutrition* can be detected by one method, and others by another or by a combination of methods. It is easy to identify marked deficiency symptoms but difficult to detect mild symptoms. Four common methods used in evaluating nutritional status are clinical examination, biochemical analysis, physical measurements and dietary assessment. An evaluation of nutrient intake alone, however, does *not* give sufficient evidence for judging the nutritional status of individuals or population groups. Each of the techniques has unique contributions as well as inherent limitations that need to be considered in the interpretation of data.

Clinical Examination A clinical assessment of an individual's nutritional status indicates the level of health in relation to food consumption (9). Of all methods of evaluation, this one should be the most important because it takes into account the total individual. Unfortunately, this assessment is largely influenced by the observer's training and skill; experienced observers will often rate the same individual differently. However, a pretraining session for all observers before a survey will often help to increase their agreement on rating by establishing certain criteria for judgment. The clinical examination is usually made by a physician, although some-

394

times it may be made by a nurse practitioner or nutritionist. The clinical signs of nutrient deficiency used in the HANES survey (see p. 402) are presented in Appendix Table A-26.

Another shortcoming of the clinical method is that many of the symptoms that an observer may note are not specific for any one deficiency and can sometimes be caused by a nonnutritional condition. *Glossitis,* for example, can be due to an inadequate intake of niacin and/or riboflavin; it can also be due to other physiological conditions. The subjective nature of clinical evaluation limits the reliability of the information yielded.

Well-nourished persons appear to be in good physical condition and to be free from illnesses. Well-nourished children tend to have the following characteristics (20):

Sense of well-being: alert, interested in activities usual for the age; vigorous; happy.

Vitality: endurance during activity, quick recovery from fatigue; looks rested; does not fall asleep in school, sleeps well at night.

Weight: normal for height, age, and body build.

Posture: erect; arms and legs straight; abdomen pulled in; chest out.

Teeth: straight, without crowding in well-shaped jaw.

Gums: firm, pink; no signs of bleeding.

Skin: smooth, slightly moist; healthy glow; reddish-pink mucous membranes.

Eyes: clear, bright; no circles of fatigue around them.

Hair: lustrous; healthy scalp.

Muscles: well-developed; firm.

Nervous control: good attention span for his age; gets along well with others; does not cry easily; not irritable and restless.

Gastrointestinal factors: good appetite; normal, regular elimination.

Poorly nourished persons tend to be fatigued and in poor physical condition; hyperirritable and unhappy, with a strained, tense look (especially when underweight); hyperactive even if underweight and without physical endurance;

and lacking some or all of the characteristics of the well-nourished person.

Biochemical Analysis With this method, quantitative chemical analyses may be made of the blood and/or the urine. The analyses are made either for a given nutrient or for some of the *metabolites* of that nutrient. Blood analysis is an indicative measurement because blood is the body's principal medium of transport. It carries nutrients to the tissues and brings back the waste products and the nutrients' metabolites. There is an increased excretion of some nutrients or metabolites in the urine when the blood level of those nutrients is above normal and usually a diminished excretion when the blood level is low. The renal system thus helps to maintain the composition of the blood at a fairly constant state.

It is almost impossible to collect a urine specimen over a 24-hour period in survey studies; casual urine specimens (collected at any one time during the day) have been used, but they give unreliable information. Blood analyses using micromethods make a battery of determinations possible using only a finger-tip sample. Guidelines for the interpretation of blood analyses in HANES, 1971–1972 (3), are shown in Appendix Table A-25.

Anthropometric Assessment With this method, weight, height, arm circumference, and skinfold measurements are the indicators commonly used. Although the over-all pattern of growth is genetically determined, it is significantly affected by nutrition.

Weight. This is the most commonly used measure and may be the most significant one. It reflects the level of food intake much more quickly than does height. If a child at any age fails to gain weight and follow a normal growth pattern, the reason must be sought. It is particularly serious in the very young, who normally gain weight more rapidly than at any other time in life. Skinfold measurements taken together with body

395

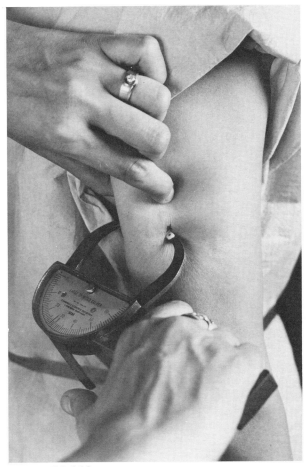

Fig. 18.1 Skinfold measurement.

ference of the mid-upper arm (as well as the skin-fold), one can estimate the size of the arm muscle. Both arm circumference and triceps skinfold are used for assessing protein-calorie malnutrition in young children.

Skinfold. Skinfold measurements enable one to estimate the amount of subcutaneous fat and thus the total amount of body fat. The amount of fat in the subcutaneous layer is directly proportional to the total body fat of adults. Skinfold measurements are made with specially designed and calibrated calipers. The two standard measurement sites are the back upper right arm halfway between the elbow and the shoulder tip (the triceps) and below the tip of the right scapula (subscapular or infrascapular). Either one or both sites are used. Fig. 18.1 shows a measurement being taken at the triceps site with a Lange skinfold caliper.

Standards for Anthropometric Assessments. Physical measurements of children are more valuable if they can be repeated at successive ages (longitudinal measurements), thus enabling one to follow the progress of growth. However, in surveys, often times only one measurement can be taken (cross-sectional measurements). Therefore it is desirable to have a standard of reference, based on the height and weight of well-nourished children, in order to evaluate a population in terms of its deviation from the standard. New growth charts have been constructed (15) for infants and children in the U.S., and they include weight, length (recumbent or upright), weight by length, and head circumference.

Also available now in the United States through HANES (see p. 402), are height and weight measurements of a representative sample of individuals 2 to 24 years of age and triceps and subscapular skinfold measurements of a representative sample 1 to 17 years (4). These data presented as the mean, median, and standard error for each age group may serve as a point of comparison for children of this country. They are presented in Appendix Tables A-17, A-18, A-19, A-20, A-21, and A-22 for height, male and female; weight,

weight give an indication of the proportion that is adipose tissue. Information on body composition is especially important in the case of children who are gaining weight above the expected rate. Therefore body weight in combination with skinfold measurement serves as a useful index of leanness–fatness; these measurements reflect energy adequacy in children and adults.

Height (Length in Infants). Height is significantly affected by heredity but not solely, for environment also has an effect.

Arm Circumference. By measuring the circum-

396

male and female; triceps, and subscapular skinfolds, respectively.

For adults, a rule of thumb about weight is that for good health, one's ideal weight at age 25 should be maintained for the rest of one's life. The Metropolitan Life Insurance Company published tables of desirable weights for men and women 25 years of age and over based on height and body frame—small, medium, and large (Appendix Tables A-14 and A-15). (If the criteria for determining the frame size had been given, the tables would be more useful.) The data are from the Body Build and Blood Pressure Study of 5 million persons made in 1959 by the Society of Actuaries. The weights suggested are those associated with lowest mortality. (These tables have been criticized because the data pertain only to persons who buy life insurance and not to the population as a whole.)

A nationwide representative sample of 13,671 adults was measured for height and weight as a part of HANES (1971–1974). These data are summarized in Appendix Table A-16, giving average weights for men and women by age group and height (2).

For adults, the reference skinfold measurements came from an earlier nationwide study, 1960 to 1962, of men and women of ages 18 to 79 years (21) Triceps and subscapular skinfolds are presented in Appendix Tables A-23 and A-24.

Dietary Surveys

Dietary surveys may be grouped according to food intake studies of individuals and those of households. Per capita food disappearance can be estimated by using agricultural production data and census figures on population.

Food Intake of Individuals

Four procedures (or combinations) may be used: recall, food intake records, diet history, and weighed food intake. Attempts are made to obtain information on the customary or habitual pattern of intake.

Recall With this method (often called the 24-hour recall), the interviewee is asked to name the kind and amount of all food consumed during the preceding 24-hour period. The amounts are estimated in common household measures or servings. The interviewer helps the interviewee to determine the amounts by showing him food models and by providing him with measuring cups and rulers.

Because the recall method entails only one day, it is preferable to select a weekday. To make sure that the selected day is representative, the individual should be questioned about his usual food practices.

One significant advantage of the recall method is that it can be widely used. The period of recall is sufficiently short to accommodate most memories. The interviewer writes down the foods and the quantities so that the interviewee's inability to read or write will not exclude a person from the survey.

The recall method was used in the HANES, 1971–1974, dietary intake phase (1, 3). Each person in the sample (10,126 persons) was interviewed about his total food and drink consumption during the day preceding the interview; the parent or other adult responsible provided information about preschool children, and for children 6 through 12 years both the parent and the child were interviewed.

Food Intake Records With this procedure, the individual writes down the kind and amount of all food eaten for a specific period of time, usually one week. This method is quite common in nutritional status studies (12) and is often used in planning nutrition education programs for college, high school, and even elementary school students.

Diet History With this method, the typical pattern of food consumption is noted over a period of time, usually by means of interviews. Burke (8), who developed this method and used it quite successfully in the Harvard prenatal studies, emphasized that the interviewer is the key person. The interviewer must be a keen observer and be familiar with the characteristic food habits of those being interviewed. The chief advantage of this method is that it probes the food practices of individuals over a period of time. The main disadvantage is that only skilled interviewers can collect the data; therefore it is more expensive than the 24-hour recall or food intake records.

Weighed Food Intake This is the most accurate of all four procedures, but it is more time-consuming, tedious, and expensive than any of the others. It requires that the individual (or a trained worker) weigh all food eaten for a specified period of time. The advantage of accuracy may be offset to some extent by the individual's tendency to change the usual diet when each food must be weighed. In controlled metabolic research studies, all food to be eaten is weighed. In these studies food samples are usually analyzed chemically.

Food Intake of Households

Food List Using this method, a member of the household (usually the homemaker) is asked to recall which foods and how much were consumed at home during a certain period. The quantities are given in weight, household measure, or retail unit. The data are collected in person by an interviewer. One advantage to this method is that it requires only one relatively short visit to the home; consequently, a higher proportion of homemakers are likely to cooperate.

Food Record Method With this method, all foods on hand at the beginning of an observation period are weighed, and this is repeated at the end. During the observation period all foods brought into the house for household use are also weighed. The homemaker is asked to keep a record of the daily menus in order to check the ac-

curacy of the entries. This method requires the interviewer to visit the home from time to time.

Although this method is quite accurate in measuring food consumption, it has several disadvantages: the family may change its usual diet somewhat, the method places a burden on the cooperating household, and there is no accounting made for food waste.

Evaluation of Food Intake Records

The method selected to assess the food intake record will depend upon the quantitative accuracy of the data collected and the use that will be made of the evaluation. If the data are not precise, it might be desirable merely to assess the meal patterns, or the number of servings from the essential food groups used in a day, utilizing a dietary score card or some modification of it.

When reliable quantitative data have been obtained, the nutrient content of the diet can be determined by using food composition tables. When a research study includes larger numbers of people, the nutritive value of their food intake can be calculated by computer (11). For precisely weighed diets, a chemical analysis may be made, as in the case of metabolic studies.

Dietary Score Cards Dietary score cards are used largely in nutrition education programs (Table 18.1). Although a score card does not give the complete nutritive contribution of each food, it encourages people to eat a variety of foods and provides a good "rule of thumb" for evaluating the food selection. A proposed Dietary Score Card is shown in Table 18.1. The quantitative scores for each food group were arbitrarily set.

A plan was devised by Myers et al. (16) for evaluating meals in a four-day food record of elementary school children. The children kept the records themselves with the help of parents, teachers, and nutritionists. The investigators described the meals as "satisfactory" or "unsatisfactory" according to the various foods eaten. For example, an unsatisfactory breakfast would con-

398

Table 18.1 A Dietary Score Card

Food	Each day you need	Score for 1 day	Your score
Dark-green or yellow fruits or vegetables (raw or cooked)	1 serving	10	
Oranges, grapefruit, tomatoes, cabbage, or other vitamin-C-rich food	1 serving	10	
Potatoes and other vegetables and fruits	2 servings	5	
Milk and milk products	Children, 3 c Adolescents, 3–4 c Adults, 2 c	20	
Meat, poultry, or fish	1 serving	15	
Meat, poultry, fish, or alternates (dry beans or peas, peanut butter)	1 serving	10	
Eggs	1 daily (at least 4 a week)	5	
Cereal (whole-grain or enriched) or 1 slice of bread	1 serving	5	
Bread (whole-grain or enriched)	1 or 2 slices at each meal	5	
Butter or fortified margarine	1 to 2 level tbsp	5	
A good breakfast, including a protein such as milk, cheese, or egg		10	
	Total	100	

sist of only one food, such as milk, fruit, or cereal (without milk), whereas a satisfactory breakfast might be made up of cereal with milk or an egg and toast. The number of unsatisfactory meals during the period studied enabled the investigators to assess the adequacy of the food intake during that time.

Food Composition Tables The use of food composition tables is the most common method for estimating the nutrient content of diets. The values listed in these tables have been obtained by laboratory analyses.

There are inherent inaccuracies in food composition tables because the nutrient content of a given food varies widely, especially with fruits and vegetables. For example, the vitamin C content of 13 different varieties of potatoes ranged from 8.2 to 17.4 mg per 100 g of fresh produce, and of 35 varieties of cabbage from 32.4 to 100.7 mg per 100 g of raw vegetables (13, 17). It should be recognized, however, that the vitamin C content of foods varies more than do most other nutrients. The variety of a product, soil composition, fertilizer, care in handling, storage, processing, and method of cooking all affect the nutrients. The compilers of food tables have had to decide on what values they believed were representative. Inevitably, different tables present somewhat different food composition values.

Nutritive Value of American Foods in Common Units, Agriculture Handbook No. 456, compiled by C. F. Adams (5) of the Agricultural Research Service of the USDA, issued in 1975, includes data on approximately 1500 foods. The weight in grams is given for each household measure, which makes it possible to compute the composition of the food on a 100-gram basis if that information is desired. Home and Garden Bulletin No. 72, *Nutritive Value of Foods*, revised in 1977, shows nutritive values for household measures of 730 commonly used foods; the weight in grams, as well as the household measure, is given for each food (6). The items of this food table, arranged in alphabetical order, are presented in Appendix Table A-3. The bulletin is designed for the use of homemakers as well as nutritionists, dietitians, physicians, and other consumers.

One of the most comprehensive food tables to be compiled, *Composition of Foods: Raw, Processed, Prepared* (Agriculture Handbook No. 8), issued in 1963 by the Agricultural Research Service of USDA, is now being revised (24). The revision is being issued in sections, each of which provides data for a major food group. Agriculture Handbook 8-1 (19) includes data on dairy and egg products and Handbook 8-2, herbs and spices (14). Forthcoming are additional sections of this most comprehensive table, which includes values for refuse, energy, proximate composition (water, protein, fat, carbohydrate, and ash), seven mineral elements (calcium, iron, magnesium, phosphorus, potassium, sodium, and zinc), nine vitamins (ascorbic acid, thiamin, riboflavin, niacin, pantothenic acid, vitamin B-6, folacin, vitamin B-12, and vitamin A), individual fatty acids, totals for saturated, monounsaturated, and polyunsaturated fatty acids, cholesterol, total phytosterols, and 18 amino acids.

Laboratory Analyses   In metabolic balance studies, where the intake of certain nutrients or energy must be determined quantitatively, a laboratory analysis must be made because it is the most accurate method. Comparisons have been made between computed and analyzed values for given diets; Table 18.2 shows a comparison of energy values. The results from the two methods are sufficiently close to give assurance that the use of food composition tables is quite satisfactory for dietary surveys and for most controlled studies (except for the specific nutrient or nutrients that may be under investigation).

Standards for Evaluating Diets   Most American diets are evaluated by comparing their nutritive content with the RDA. Because these allowances are "designed for the maintenance of good nutrition of practically all healthy people in the U.S.A.," intakes of at least two-thirds of the RDA for protein, calcium, iron, vitamin A, thiamin, riboflavin, and vitamin C have been considered adequate in earlier studies, including the USDA nationwide survey in 1965–1966 (23). The use of this criterion has been questioned because the margin of safety in the RDA for each nutrient was not defined. Failure to meet the recommended allowance for a particular nutrient does not constitute evidence of malnutrition. It is possible, however, to state that the risk of nutritional deficiency tends to increase as the nutrient intake falls below the dietary standard. Standards for

Table 18.2 A Comparison of the Energy Value of a Common Breakfast as Assessed by a Bomb Calorimeter and a Food Table

| | | Method of dietary assessment | |
| | | Bomb calorimeter assay,[a] kcal | Food table,[b] kcal |
Food	Measure		
Orange juice	1 serving (100 g)	42	48
Egg, scrambled	1 serving (100 g)	200	173
Bread (white, enriched)	2 sl (46 g)	129	126
Butter	1 tbsp (14 g)	107	102
Jelly	2 tbsp (40 g)	102	109
Milk, whole	8 oz (244 g)	181	159
		761 (3.2 MJ)	717 (3.0 MJ)

[a] R. W. Swift, et al. *Relative Dynamic Effects of High versus Low Protein Diets of Equicaloric Content*, Penn. State Univ. Agr. Expt. Sta. Bull. No. 618. University Park: Penn. State University, 1957.

[b] *Nutritive Value of American Foods*, Agr. Handbook No. 456. Washington, D.C.: U.S. Dept. Agr., 1975.

HANES dietary intake data are presented in Appendix Table A-27. Protein, calcium, vitamin A, vitamin C, thiamin, riboflavin, niacin and energy are included. The HANES standards, as compared to the RDA, are variable for energy, agreeing in some age–sex groups, higher in some, and lower in others—higher for protein; less for calcium; the same for iron, with but few exceptions; less for vitamin A; more for vitamin C; and less for thiamin, riboflavin, and niacin, except in the case of the standard for riboflavin for women, which is higher.

Food Nutrients: Quantities Available for Consumption per Capita per Day

Estimates of the yearly per capita disappearance of various foods are determined by the USDA using statistics on agricultural production, food exports and imports, inventories on hand, industrial use, feed use, and losses in distribution between farm and kitchen. Calculations are made of the nutrient content of foods available for human consumption, and then of the per capita availability of nutrients per day using population figures provided by the Bureau of the Census. These calculations give a rough estimate of the adequacy of the national food supply. The per capita national averages indicate trends in food consumption and production needs (10).

Nutritional Status and Food Consumption in the United States

Comprehensive information on the food consumption and nutritional status of the people of the United States has been provided by three extensive studies carried out since 1965. There was the Household Food Consumption Survey (1965–1966), the Ten-State Nutrition Survey (1968–1970), and the First Health and Nutrition Examination Survey (1971–1974).

The Household Food Consumption Survey (1965–1966) (7), conducted by the USDA, provided data collected by asking homemakers to

401

recall the kinds, quantities, and costs of food used at home during the 7 days preceding the interview. Approximately 15,000 households were questioned. Similar surveys had been conducted in 1936, 1942, 1948 (urban only), and 1955. It was found in the 1965–1966 survey that among both high- and low-income families, 50 percent were eating good diets, about 30 percent had fair diets, and 20 percent had poor diets. A poor diet was one that provided less than two-thirds of the RDA (1963) for protein, calcium, iron, vitamin A, thiamin, riboflavin, and vitamin C.

The Ten-State Nutrition Survey (1968–1970) (22) was conducted by the Public Health Service of the Department of Health, Education, and Welfare to determine the prevalence of malnutrition and related health problems in the United States. The ten states were California, Kentucky, Louisiana, Massachusetts, Michigan, New York (including a separate survey of New York City), South Carolina, Texas, Washington, and West Virginia. Those persons surveyed were randomly selected from districts that had the lowest average income (the bottom 25 percent) in each state, according to the 1960 census. Some of the districts had changed between 1960 and 1968, and certainly everyone who lived there was not poor. Therefore some middle- and upper-income families were included in the survey. The findings on the lower-income families are believed to be representative of lower-income families elsewhere in the country, but those on middle- and upper-income families may not be representative of middle- and upper-income families elsewhere.

The nutritional status of approximately 40,000 individuals was assessed; biochemical and dietary analyses were made on selected subgroups. The highest prevalence of unsatisfactory nutritional status was among children 10 to 16 years of age; the deficiency was more severe among males than females. A correlation was found between the educational attainment (the number of years of formal schooling) of the homemaker and the nutritional status of children below 17 years of age. As the homemaker's educational level increased, there was less evidence of nutritional inadequacies in the children.

The Health and Nutrition Examination Survey (HANES) (1971–1974) program was undertaken by the National Center for Health Statistics, Department of Health, Education, and Welfare, to establish a continuing national nutrition surveillance system under the authority of the National Health Survey Act of 1956. This system has as its objectives the measuring of nutritional status of the population of the United States and monitoring changes that may take place in this status with time. The HANES is the first program in the United States to collect information on nutritional status of a scientifically designed sample representative of the U.S. civilian, noninstitutionalized population in a broad range of ages from 1 to 74 years (4). The measurement methods used in HANES to assess nutritional status include: (a) estimations of dietary intake (kind and quantity of food consumed and its nutritional value), (b) biochemical tests made on samples of blood and urine to determine the levels of various nutrients, (c) clinical examinations made by physicians and dentists alerted to detect signs of malnutrition or conditions indicative of nutritional problems, and (d) body measurements that would indicate abnormal growth patterns as well as obesity. Some findings have been published and have been incorporated in the respective chapters of this book where the data are pertinent (protein; riboflavin, thiamin, and niacin; vitamin A; vitamin C; calcium; iron; and iodine).

Additional Information Useful in Assessing Nutritional Status

In order to interpret and use the findings from any study of nutritional status, particularly of large populations in developed and developing countries, it is important to have certain background information; the factors recommended by the WHO Committee on Nutritional Status (9) are

Table 18.3 Information Required to Assess Nutritional Status

Source of information	Nature of information obtained	Nutritional implications

1. Agricultural data
Food balance sheets
	Gross estimates of
	  agricultural production
	Agricultural methods
	Soil fertility
	Predominance of cash crops
	Overproduction of staples
	Food imports and exports
		Approximate availability of
		  food supplies to a popu-
		  lation

2. Socioeconomic data
Information on marketing,
  distribution, and storage
	Purchasing power
	Distribution and storage
	  of foodstuffs
		Unequal distribution of avail-
		  able foods among the
		  socioeconomic groups in
		  the community and within
		  the family

3. Food consumption
  patterns
Cultural–anthropological
  data
	Lack of knowledge, erroneous
	  beliefs and prejudices,
	  indifference	

4. Dietary surveys	Food consumption	Low, excessive, or unbalanced nutrient intake

5. Special studies on foods	Biological value of diets
	Presence of interfering factors
	  (e.g., goitrogens)
	Effects of food processing
		Special problems related to
		  nutrient utilization

6. Vital and health statistics	Morbidity and mortality data	Extent of risk to community Identification of high-risk groups
7. Anthropometric studies	Physical development	Effect of nutrition on physical development

8. Clinical nutritional
  surveys
	Physical signs	Deviation from health due
		  to malnutrition

9. Biochemical studies	Levels of nutrients, metabo-
	  lites, and other components
	  of body tissues and fluids
		Nutrient supplies in the body
		Impairment of biochemical
		  function

10. Additional medical
  information
	Prevalent disease patterns,
	  including infections and
	  infestations
		Interrelationships of state of
		  nutrition and disease

From *Expert Committee on Medical Assessment of Nutritional Status*, WHO Tech. Rept. Series 258. Geneva: World Health Organ., 1963, p. 7. Used by permission.

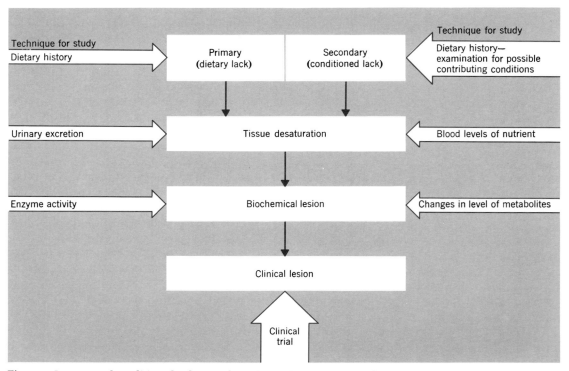

**Fig. 18.2 Sequence of conditions leading to clinical manifestations of a deficiency. (From W. N. Pearson [1962].
Biochemical appraisal of the vitamin nutritional status in man.** *J. Am. Med. Assoc.,* **180:49.) Used by permission.**

presented in Table 18.3. One important factor is a nation's own food-producing capacity and supply, which can avert serious food shortages and human suffering.

Estimates of the quantity and nutritional value of food consumed by families and individuals should be available for use by those working with the people to improve their eating practices and those concerned with food supply. Vital statistics are important also; they draw attention to the morbidity and mortality of various groups. It was such data that drew attention to the weanling child in the developing countries; it was found that the high death rate of children from one to four years of age was mainly due to undernutrition.

Infections and parasite infestations negate the effects of a good diet. As background information, it must be determined if the community and the

home are assuming responsibility for problems of sanitation.

Pearson (18) has outlined a sequence of changes that take place from the body's normal condition to the appearance of clinical symptoms of malnutrition. First the body's stores of a nutrient are depleted, resulting in "tissue desaturation"; this may be reflected in the lower blood level or urinary excretion of the nutrient or its metabolites. As the deficiency becomes greater, metabolic changes take place; biochemical deviations from the normal will be reflected in measurements of diminished enzyme activities in the blood or in the level of metabolites in the urine. As the deficiency becomes more severe, there will be functional impairment of the organs and finally anatomical lesions that characterize clinical symptoms of the deficiency disease

(Fig. 18.2). The deficiency disease may be due to dietary lack (the primary cause) or to poor absorption, impaired transport of the nutrient by the blood and other body fluids, or impaired utilization of the nutrient by the tissues (secondary causes).

Dietary intake studies are an essential part of any complete nutritional status survey. If low dietary intakes of a specific nutrient are found in conjunction with biochemical and clinical signs of a deficiency, the dietary data confirm the diagnosis. Such agreement is not always found, however. A diet that induces deficiency symptoms in some persons may not do so in others because individuals vary considerably in their daily need for a given nutrient, as well as in their body stores of that nutrient. In addition, the nutrient intake from dietary assessments tends to reflect current consumption whereas the biochemical and clinical information reflects the nutrient pattern of intake over a long period of time. Therefore efforts must be directed toward eliciting dietary information that would represent the habitual nutrient intake of the individual or group over an extended period.

Summary

Methods for the evaluation of nutritional status are clinical examination, biochemical analysis, physical measurement, and dietary assessment. Essential in any complete nutrition survey is the determination of food intake. Dietary surveys may be conducted on an individual or household basis. For the measures of nutritional status and the nutritive value of the dietary intake (obtained by computation using food composition tables), standards of reference are used for interpretation of the findings.

An annual estimate is made by USDA of the quantity of nutrients available for human consumption per capita per day. These data are valuable as indicators of trends in production and nutrient availability for human use.

Information on food consumption and nutritional status has been provided by three surveys done since 1965: the Household Food Consumption Survey (1965–1966), the Ten-State Nutrition Survey (1968–1970), and the First Health and Nutrition Examination Survey (1971–1974).

Glossary

anthropometry: the science that deals with the measurement of the size, weight, and proportions of the human body.

glossitis: see p. 234.

health: a state of complete physical, mental, and social well-being, and not merely the absence of disease and infirmity.

malnutrition: an over-all term for poor nourishment; it may be due to an inadequate diet or to some defect in metabolism that prevents the body from using the nutrients properly.

metabolite: see p. 197

nutrient: see p. 11

Study Questions and Activities

1. Is it possible to assess the nutritional status of a group by determining their dietary habits? Justify your answer.
2. Of what practical value are the findings from a nutritional status survey?
3. Try to recall what foods you ate yesterday and how much of each. What are the advantages and disadvantages of the recall method for obtaining dietary information? Of the food record method? Of the diet history method? Of the weighed food intake method?
4. Compare your own height, weight, and skinfold (triceps) with the appropriate reference table.
5. Do an experiment with a friend: Ask the person to keep a record of food eaten for one day. Then, the next day, after you have collected the record, surprise the friend by asking for a recall of all food eaten the day before.

405

References

1. Abraham, S., M. D. Carroll, C. M. Dresser, and C. L. Johnson (1977). *Dietary Intake Findings, United States, 1971–1974.* DHEW Publ. No (HRA) 77-1647. Hyattsville, Md.: Natl. Center for Health Stat., U.S. Dept. Health, Educ., and Welfare.

2. Abraham, S., C. L. Johnson, and M. F. Najjar (1977). *Weight by Height and Age of Adults 18–74 Years: United States, 1971–1974.* Advanced Data. Washington, D.C.: Natl. Center for Health Stat., U.S. Dept. Health, Educ., and Welfare.

3. Abraham, S., F. W. Lowenstein, and C. L. Johnson (1974). *Preliminary Findings of the First Health and Nutrition Examination Survey, United States, 1971–1972. Dietary Intakes and Biochemical Findings.* DHEW Publ. No. (HRA) 74-1219-1. Rockville, Md.: Natl. Center for Health Stat., U.S. Dept. Health, Educ., and Welfare.

4. Abraham, S., F. W. Lowenstein, and D. E. O'Connell (1975). *Preliminary Findings of the First Health and Nutrition Examination Survey, United States, 1971–1972. Anthropometric and Clinical Findings.* DHEW Publ. No. (HRA) 75-1229. Rockville, Md.: Natl. Center for Health Stat., U.S. Dept. Health, Educ., and Welfare.

5. Adams, C. F. (1975). *Nutritive Value of American Foods.* Agriculture Handbook No. 456. Washington, D.C.: U.S. Dept. Agr.

6. Adams, C. F. and M. Richardson (1977). *Nutritive Value of Foods.* Revised. Home and Garden Bulletin No. 72. Washington, D.C.: U.S. Dept. Agr.

7. Adelson, S. F. and B. B. Peterkin (1968). Quality of diets in U.S. households in Spring 1965. *Family Econ. Rev.,* March, ARS 62-5.

8. Burke, B. S. (1947). The dietary history as a tool in research. *J. Am. Dietet. Assoc.,* **23:** 1041.

9. *Expert Committee on Medical Assessment of Nutritional Status Report* (1963). WHO Tech. Rept. Series 258. Geneva: World Health Organ. p. 7.

10. Friend, B. (1970). Nutritional review. *National Food Situation,* NFS-134. Washington, D.C.: U.S. Dept. Agr., p. 21.

11. Hertzler, A. A. and L. W. Hoover (1977). Development of food tables and use of computers. *J. Am. Dietet. Assoc.,* **70:** 20.

12. Kelsay, J. L. (1969). A compendium of nutritional status studies and dietary evaluation studies conducted in the United States, 1959–1967. *J. Nutrition,* **99:** Suppl. 1, Part 2.

13. Leichsenring, J. M. and L. M. Norris (1951). *Factors Influencing the Nutritive Value of Potatoes.* Univ. of Minnesota Agr. Expt. Sta. Tech. Bull. No. 196. St. Paul: Univ. of Minnesota.

14. Marsh, A. C., M. K. Moss, and E. W. Murphy (1977). *Composition of Foods, Spices and Herbs, Raw, Processed, Prepared.* Revised. Agriculture Handbook No. 8-2. Washington, D.C.: U.S. Dept. Agr.

15. National Center for Health Statistics (1976). NCHS Growth Charts, 1976. *Monthly Vital Statistics Report,* **25:** p. 1-21, June 22, 1976.

16. Myers, M. L., S. C. O'Brien, J. A. Mabel, and F. J. Stare (1968). A nutrition study of school children in a depressed urban district. *J. Am. Dietet. Assoc.,* **53:** 226.

17. Patton, M. B. and M. E. Green (1954). *Cabbage: Factors Affecting Vitamin Values and Palatability.* Ohio Agr. Exp. Sta. Bull. No. 742. Wooster: Ohio Agricultural Experiment Station.

18. Pearson, W. N. (1966). Assessment of nutritional status: Biochemical methods. In *Nutrition: A Comprehensive Treatise,* Vol. 3, edited by G. H. Beaton and E. W. McHenry. New York: Academic Press, p. 265.

19. Posati, L. P. and M. L. Orr (1976). *Composition of Foods, Dairy and Egg Products: Raw, Processed, and Prepared.* Revised. Agriculture Handbook No. 8-1. Washington, D.C.: U.S. Dept. Agr., Agricultural Research Service.

20. Robinson, C. H. and M. R. Lawler (1977). *Normal and Therapeutic Nutrition.* 15th ed. New York: Macmillan Publ. Co., p. 314.

21. Stoudt, H. W., A. Damon, and R. M. McFarland (1965). *Skinfolds, Body Girths, Biacromial Di-*

ameter, and Selected Anthropometric Indices of Adults. Series 11, No. 35. Washington, D.C.: Natl. Center for Health Stat., U.S. Dept. Health, Educ., and Welfare.

22. *Ten-State Nutrition Survey, 1968–1970* (1973). DHEW Publ. No. (HSM) 72-8134. Atlanta, Ga.: Health Services and Mental Health Administration, U.S. Dept. Health, Educ., and Welfare.

23. *U.S. Department of Agriculture Household Food Consumption Survey 1965–1966* (1969). Dietary Levels of Households in the United States, Spring 1965. Rept. No. 6.

24. Watts, B. K. and A. L. Merrill (1963). *Composition of Foods: Raw, Processed, Prepared.* Agriculture Handbook No. 8. Washington, D.C.: U.S. Dept. Agr.

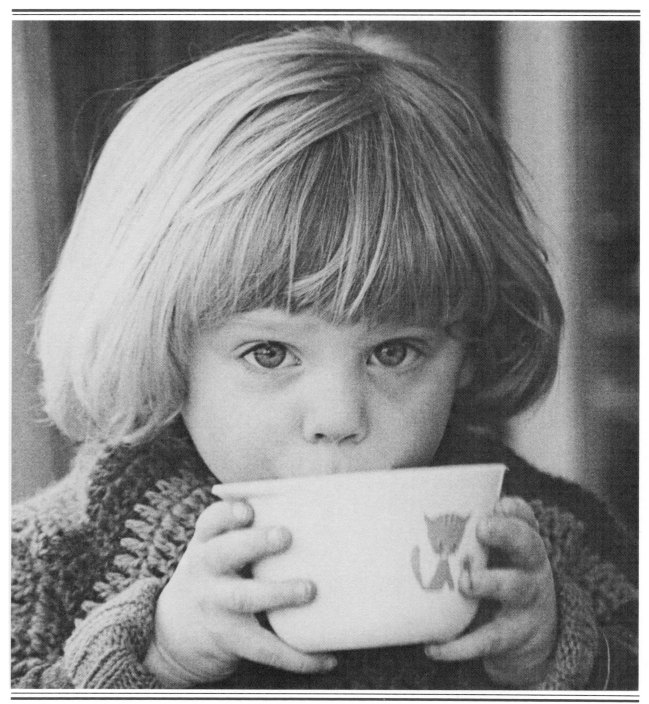

The preschool child enjoys looking about at his environment more than he does eating his food.

Abbreviations

AAP: American Academy of Pediatrics
AMA: American Medical Association
FAO/WHO: Food and Agriculture Organization/
World Health Organization

FNS: Food and Nutrition Service
RDA: Recommended Dietary Allowances
USDA: United States Department of Agriculture
WIC: Women, Infants, and Children

The Human Life Cycle

The human being goes through distinct phases and transitions during the life cycle: from conception through the embryonic and fetal stages, from birth through infancy and childhood, from adolescence to young adulthood, and from the middle years to late adulthood or old age.

The remarkable processes of *growth* and *development* begin at conception, and after about two decades, the mature human body evolves. Three principal agents participate in these processes: *genes* to direct the shaping of the fertilized egg cell, or ovum; *hormones* to control many chemical reactions within the cell; and *nutrients*, including water and oxygen, to supply raw materials for cell growth. Other biological and environmental factors influence the course of progress through this phase of the life cycle.

Growth does not cease when physical maturity is attained in adulthood; it continues into old age. The term "aging" describes the process of gradual and progressive changes which take place over the entire adult life span. The aging patterns vary in rate and degree; some individuals show signs of aging faster than do others.

Biological Landmarks

Certain biological landmarks are associated with each successive phase of the human life cycle, as shown in Table 19.1. Although the stages are distinct, the dividing lines between phases are hazy and imprecise.

The spread of chronological ages at which the transitions occur shows the increasing variability as people get older. For example, the age at onset of old age may vary by plus or minus ten years, which is indicative that aging brings about wide individual variability. Chronological age (age timed after birth), however, is not the same as biological or physiological age. Biological age is a measure of the degree of physical maturity attained by the individual. Skeletal age (bone age), for example, is commonly used as an index of physiological maturity. It is assessed by taking X-ray photographs of selected bones, such as the hand and wrist of children; these X-rays are then compared with standards. Biological age, though more difficult to define, is a better index of human physical development, endurance, and mental capabilities.

Biological and environmental factors influence the kinds and amounts of nutrients needed by the individual at all ages and stages within the life cycle. Therefore at any point in the life span, the nutritional health of a person will reflect the cumulative effects of the impact of many diverse factors. Genes, hormones, and environment (such as nutrients, drugs, toxins, bacteria, virus, and radiation) interact from the moment life begins to old age. These factors direct and control the intricate processes of growth, development, and maintenance throughout the life span.

410

Table 19.1 Biological Landmarks for Different Periods in the Life Cycle

Biological landmarks	Average chronological age at onset period[a]	Period
Conception		Embryonic
		Fetal
Birth	9 months ± 2 weeks	Newborn
		Infancy
		Childhood
Puberty	12 years ± 2 years	Adolescence
Fertility	19 years ± 3 years	Young adulthood (Maturity)
Climacterium	45 years ± 5 years	Middle adulthood (Middle age)
Old Age	70 years ± 10 years	Late adulthood (Senescence)

[a] Note increasing variability in chronological age at onset of various periods of chronological age. Adapted from E. J. Stieglitz, *The Second Forty Years*. 1st ed. New York: J. B. Lippincott Co. (1946), p. 56.

The best provision for well-being in any period of life is to arrive at that point in good nutritional and physical status. The well-born infant is sturdier throughout infancy than the baby poorly born; the sturdy infant has stores to give impetus to growth in the preschool years. The child who is in excellent nutrition will have stores to be drawn upon during the rapid growth at puberty. The well-nourished mother can nourish her fetus well; therefore, the best insurance for a healthy infant is a mother who is healthy and well nourished throughout her entire life, as well as during the period of pregnancy itself. (11)

Fetal Period: First Nine Months

The most critical and rapid period of growth occurs in the first nine months in *utero* (inside the uterus) during the human life cycle. In all mammals, fetal life begins as a single cell, which multiplies several billion times before birth.

Fetal Growth and Development

Life *in utero* may be divided into three distinct phases based on characteristic stages of fetal development: the implantation or "ovular"; the differentiation or "embryonic"; and the growth phase or "fetal" (8).

Implantation (First Two Weeks of Gestation) Following fertilization, the ovum travels from the fallopian tube (or oviduct) toward the *uterus*. At this time, the developing ovum derives its nourishment from the secretion of glands lining the oviduct. After it reaches the uterus, the actively dividing cell mass attaches itself to the endometrium (lining of the uterus), and nourishes on the fluid and nutrients from the endometrium. Once implanted, rapid cell proliferation takes place, and the placenta and fetal membrane begin to form as the embryo develops inside the cell mass.

411

Differentiation (Between the Second and Eighth Weeks of Gestation) During the first week after implantation, the nutrients stored in the endometrical cells (glycogen, proteins, lipids, and some minerals) provide the only source of nourishment for the growing embryo. The same reserves supply a large share of nutrients until approximately the twelfth week of pregnancy. Gross structural changes have taken place, and in the eight-week embryo, cells have started to specialize. For example, liver cells can be distinguished from the cells of the heart. Differentiation is a particularly vulnerable phase, and fetal development may be impaired permanently by serious virus infection, such as rubella, or by the use of certain drugs.

Growth Phase (from the Eighth Week to the Ninth Month) By the ninth week of uterine life, the embryo has become a fetus with recognizable human features. During this growth period, organ tissues and the total fetal weight increase notably.

Functions of the Placenta The *placenta* is a double structure derived in part from the maternal tissue and in part from the embryo. At maturity (time of birth), the human placenta is round and flat with a diameter of about 18 cm (7 in.), and a thickness of 2.54 cm (1 in.), and weighs about 2.2 lb (1 kg). At delivery, the placenta becomes detached from the uterus and is called the afterbirth.

The umbilical cord links the fetus to the placenta, and within this cord and the placenta are blood vessels. There is no direct circulatory connection between the fetus and the mother, but in the placenta the two independent systems are brought closely together. Nutrients and oxygen are transported from the mother to the fetus and vice versa by crossing a "placental barrier." The fetal side of the placenta is equipped with a tremendous number of villi containing blood capillaries.

The welfare of the fetus depends upon certain preciseness in the kinds and amounts of substances that are transported across the placental membrane. The permeability of the placental membrane varies according to the materials that must raverse it. Water, oxygen, and certain electrolytes, such as sodium, potassium, and chloride ions, diffuse readily through the placental membrane. Other compounds may require a carrier substance to cross the barrier. Another basic mechanism involves the *active transport system* that requires expenditure of metabolic energy; this is used when concentrations of substances are higher in fetal than in maternal blood. The distribution of substances between the fetal and maternal plasma (Table 19.2) reflects (a) the different mechanisms that operate in the transport of substances across the placenta, and (b) the speed of transfer of a particular substance and its physiological function in the fetus. As summarized in Table 19.3, those materials that pass through the placenta most readily are the most essential; those that provide nutrition and affect growth follow next. Those that pass through the placenta more slowly are primarily of immunological importance (protecting the infant in the early months of his life) (2).

The placenta cannot discriminate between drugs that are harmful and those that are innocuous to the fetus. Anesthetics, tranquilizers, hypnotics, sedatives, and most antibiotics are transmitted into the fetal circulation. Sodium thiopental, a short-acting anesthetic, reaches equilibrium on both sides of the placenta in about three minutes. Tranquilizers, hypnotics, and sedatives pass through a little less rapidly. Since the majority of all drugs pass through the placenta, the pregnant woman should be extremely cautious about taking drugs of any kind without her doctor's permission (3).

The placenta not only provides a medium of exchange between the mother and the fetus, but it also functions as the lungs, the liver, and the kidneys. It stores important substances, such as glycogen, and synthesizes important hormones. The placental hormones help induce certain metabolic changes that are essential for fetal sur-

412

Table 19.2 The Distribution of Substances Between Fetal and Maternal Plasma

Higher in fetal plasma	About equal	Higher in maternal plasma
Amino acids	Sodium	Total proteins
Nonprotein nitrogen	Chloride	Alpha and beta globulins
Creatinine	Creatine	Fibrinogen
Total phosphorus	Urea	Total lipids
Inorganic phosphorus	Uric acid	Phospholipids
Fructose	Magnesium	Fatty acids
Lactate		Glucose
Serum iron		Cholesterol
Calcium		Vitamin A
Thiamin chloride		Vitamin E
Pyridoxine		
Riboflavin		
Vitamin C		

From E. W. Page, Physiology and biochemistry of the placenta. In J. P. Greenhill, *Obstetrics*. 13th ed. Philadelphia: W. B. Saunders Co., 1965, p. 140. Used by permission.

19.3 Classification of Placental Transfer

Class of substances	Rates of transfer	Examples
Essential to fetal life and homeostasis	mg per second	oxygen, water, electrolytes
Primarily for nutrition	mg per minute	dextrose, amino acids, vitamins
Growth-modifying factors	mg per hour	steroids, protein hormones
Primarily of immunological importance	mg per day	plasma proteins

From N. J. Eastman and L. M. Hellman, *Williams Obstetrics*. 13th ed., 1966. Courtesy of Appleton-Century-Crofts, Publishing Division of Prentice-Hall, Inc., Englewood Cliffs, N.J.

vival and well-being (see section on Pregnancy, p. 451). Because of the diversified role of the placenta in growth and development of the fetus, one admonishment goes (9):

> "Don't make mirth
> of the afterbirth!"

Nutrient Needs of the Fetus

At the end of the first trimester, the fetus is still very small and measures about 9 cm in length. During the next two trimesters, substantial changes occur in length and weight. The greatest change in length takes place in the second trimester, and in weight, during the third trimester. At five lunar months the fetus weighs about 300 g; at birth it weighs about 3000 g (about 6½ lb). Beginning with the third lunar month, the fetus grows in length at about 4 or 5 cm per day (12).

Increasing amounts of nutrients are needed as fetal growth gains momentum. The nutrient supply to the growing fetus depends upon (a) the quantity and composition of maternal blood reaching the placenta, and (b) the integrity and capability of the placenta to concentrate, synthesize, and transport essential nutrients from the maternal to the fetal side (7). Although the nutritional requirements for infants are reasonably well known, the needs of the growing human fetus have not been defined.

Maternal Nutrition and Fetal Growth

Many studies with experimental animals, the rat in particular, suggest that inadequate maternal nutrition during pregnancy leads to stunted growth *in utero* and impaired development of the fetal brain (6, 13, 14). Similar experiments involving dietary manipulations that may harm the fetus cannot be done in humans because of problems relating to ethics and methodology.

Low-Birth-Weight Infants Birth weight serves as a useful index of fetal growth. The term "low birth weight" refers to infants who weigh 2500 g (5½ lb) or less at birth. There are essentially three broad groups of small babies: preterm infants who are born before 37 weeks of gestation, full-term infants who are gestationally mature but are conceived small, and mature full-term infants (or small-for-dates) whose growth *in utero* has been retarded. Low birth weight contributes significantly to perinatal (fetal period and first 30 days after birth) and infant mortality in both developed and less developed countries (6). There are also reports of physical and behavioral abnormalities in small-for-dates infants

(13). Intrauterine growth retardation implies that some factors limited normal growth during a full-term pregnancy. These factors may be related to either the incapability of the mother to supply nutrients to the fetus or the inability of the fetal placenta to draw sustenance from the mother. Evidence is accumulating that indicates that the environment *in utero* may have as great an influence as the genetic endowment in determining the size of the infant at birth (6). In experimental animals, maternal restriction in either energy or protein intake during pregnancy reduced the birth weight of the offspring (14). Variations in intrauterine growth as reflected in birth weight of human infants have been related to several factors including maternal nutrition during acute starvation, multiple births, maternal age and size, and smoking (1, 6, 10). Recent studies of pregnant women in rural Guatemalan villages showed a rise in mean birth weight of infants with maternal energy supplementation during pregnancy; protein supplements, however, had no significant effect on birth weight (4, 5). (See section on Diet and Pregnancy, p. 451.)

The First Year

At no other time in life is food so important as during the first year. The kind, amount, and sanitation of the food as well as the manner of feeding are all important. The nutrient requirements are high per unit of body weight because of rapid growth (38).

In a healthy full-term infant the pattern of growth varies during the first year, but the rate of growth is greatest at the outset. During the first 3 months, the baby may gain about 28 g (1 oz) a day or about 910 g (2 lb) a month. After that, the pace slows to a gain of approximately 455 g (about 1 lb) a month. By 1 year of age, the birth weight has almost tripled. The baby's length also increases most rapidly at the beginning; during the first 3 months, the baby gains about 20 percent of the birth length, and by the end of the first

414

year, the total length is about one and one-half times the birth length.

In addition to growing normally, a well baby is alert, responds to attention, and is curious about the environment. The skin of well babies is smooth, the eyes bright, body movements are according to the muscular development, and coordination is appropriate to the age. They eat well, sleep well, and cry little.

Breast-Feeding versus Bottle-Feeding

Incidence of Breast-Feeding Although the natural food for infants is human milk, either by choice or by necessity, it is not the universal infant food. Between 1946 and 1966, there was a trend in the United States toward less breast-feeding. National surveys of hospitals made at 10-year intervals have shown that the percentage of mothers who were breast-feeding their babies when they left the hospital was as follows: in 1946, 38 percent [4]; in 1956, 21 percent [40]; and in 1966, 18 percent [37], but in 1977, it was 40 percent [13].

In the developing countries, breast-feeding is almost universal in rural areas, but in the cities it is diminishing; this is especially true among well-to-do mothers but also among lower-class women as well [20]. Jelliffe [30], who worked for many years in tropical countries, believes that the decline in breast-feeding among the urban poor may be due to the separation of the working mother from her child, but also—even more important—to "the example of economic 'superiors' who are successfully bottle-feeding their infants." and to the advertising of bottle-feeding directed to mothers [15].

In the United States, by contrast, it is the well-educated and upper-class mothers who tend to breast-feed their infants [45]. It was found that breast-feeding was initiated in 68 percent of 95 infants from middle- and upper-middle-class families in the Denver area and that it was continued beyond 2 months in the case of 25 percent of the infants [5]. In Rochester, Minnesota, 41 percent of the 383 mothers who cooperated in a child-feeding practices survey carried out by the Well Child Clinic of the Mayo Clinic breast-fed their infants for varying periods of time. Physicians' wives comprised 20.1 percent of the entire group and 27.1 percent of those who breast-fed their babies [22]. In a study done in Honolulu, one-fifth of 147 mothers of low income and one-third of 135 mothers of moderate income breast-fed their infants [9]. A resurgence in interest in breast-feeding has been noted among the more educated sections of the population in the United States, Australia, the United Kingdom, and Norway over the past decade [32].

Relative Merits The nutritional merits of breast-versus bottle-feeding are still being debated [10]. Where the formula has been properly selected and prepared, as it was in a study carried out in Boston in 1949 [48], in rural Sweden in 1960 [33], and in Kuala Lumpur, Malaysia, in 1971 [11], few differences were noted in the well-being of breast-fed and bottle-fed infants. However, in the Boston and Sweden studies, there were fewer infections in the breast-fed than in the bottle-fed infants. Besides preventing exposure to environmental contamination, breast-feeding is associated with a lower incidence of infection because human milk has a higher concentration of *immunoglobulin* A (which is synthesized in the mammary gland) than cows' milk; this substance counteracts viruses and bacteria. Also, human milk promotes the formation of a bifidobacteria flora in the infant's intestine that is antagonistic to certain pathogens [36].

Since 1961, it has been known that infants can absorb antibodies that are present in human milk. Infants whose mothers had an elevated concentration (high serum titer) of poliomyelitis antibodies demonstrated resistance to the disease when they were given an orally administered vaccine

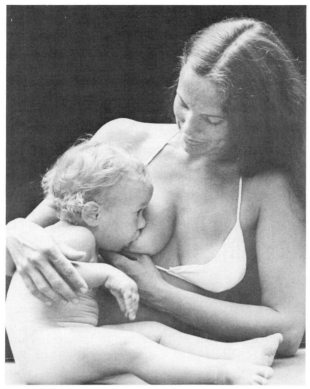

Fig. 19.1 Breast feeding can promote a warm, secure and loving relationship between mother and baby. (Hans Namuth/ Photo Researchers.)

better relationship with her baby through bottle-feeding. The many factors involved in the psychological differences between breast and bottle feeding need further study (42). Results from research conducted in 1963 showed that "warmth and nervous stability of the mother" are more important to the baby's emotional health than whether it is breast- or bottle-fed (25). The Committee on Nutrition of the American Academy of Pediatrics (AAP) reaffirms its recommendations for encouraging breast-feeding in the U.S. for mothers who can and wish to adopt it (2).

Supplying the Required Nutrients

Milk, of course, is the most important food for young infants. The composition of milk varies somewhat according to the species. Here, human and cows' milk will be discussed, although other milks are sometimes given to infants. In comparison with cows' milk, human milk contains more lactose, iron, vitamin C, and vitamin A per unit of volume, but less protein, calcium, phosphorus, riboflavin, and thiamin; the fat content of the two milks is about the same (Appendix Table A-8 and Fig. 19.2). It is believed that each milk is adapted to provide the best nourishment for the young of each species.

that causes attenuated cases of the disease. Another finding is that the stools of breast-fed babies contain significant amounts of an antibody (that originates in breast milk) to pathogenic strains of *Escherichia coli* (34); this organism causes diarrhea, especially in children (14).

If breast-feeding promotes a warm, secure, and loving relationship between the mother and her baby (Fig. 19.1), it is the more desirable method of feeding. However, if the mother resents being confined at home or having to take her baby with her wherever she goes (which would be necessary if she were breast-feeding the baby), this resentment might be transmitted (unconsciously) to the baby. This mother might be able to develop a

Energy Need The energy allowances recommended for infants are based on the general energy consumption of infants who are thriving well (44). A newborn full-term baby increases his daily energy intake per unit of body weight until sometime between the first and sixth months. At that time he is consuming around 117 kcal (490 kJ) per kg. Toward the end of the first year, the energy intake per unit of weight begins to decline and this continues throughout childhood. The Recommended Dietary Allowance (RDA) for energy during the first 6 months is 117 kcal (490 kJ) per kg of body weight, or 702 kcal (2937 kJ) daily; between 6 and 12 months of age the recommendation is 108 kcal (452 kJ) per kg

416

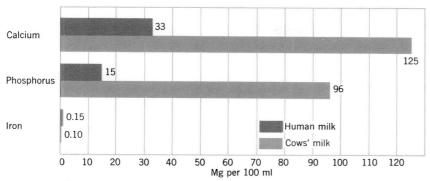

Fig. 19.2 Calcium, phosphorus, and iron content of human and cow's milk. (Adapted from Macy, I. G. and H. J. Kelly (1961). Human and cow's milk in infant nutrition. *In Milk: The Mammary Gland and Its Secretion*, Vol. 2, edited by S. K. Kon and A. T. Cowie, New York: Academic Press, p. 268.)

of body weight or 972 kcal (4067 kJ) daily. These allowances cover the estimated energy needs for the following (38): basal metabolism, 55 kcal (230 kJ) per kg; growth, about 35 kcal (146 kJ) per kg; normal activity, from 10 to 25 kcal (42–105 kJ) per kg of body weight.

The energy consumption of formula-fed babies appears to depend upon the concentration of the formula. In a study of 27 male infants during the first 112 days of life, those who were given a formula providing 67 kcal (280 kJ) per 100 ml drank more than those who were given a formula that had 133 kcal (556 kJ) per 100 ml. Even though the former group consumed more formula, their total energy intake was less (Fig. 19.3) (14). Most formulas provide about 67 kcal (280 kJ) per 100 ml, whereas human milk contains 75 kcal (314 kJ) per 100 ml.

Carbohydrates Lactose is the carbohydrate in all milks. The quantity in cows' milk is about 70 percent of that in human milk. Lactose provides 29 percent of the total energy in cows' milk and 38 percent of the total energy in human milk.

Most commercially prepared infant formulas provide about 40 to 50 percent of the energy value as carbohydrates. If this amount should exceed 50 percent, it is possible that the intes-

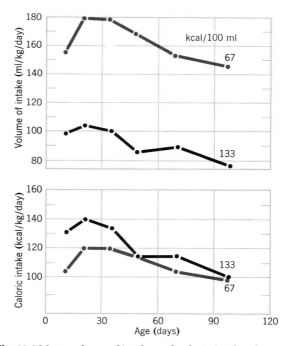

Fig. 19.3 Mean volume of intake and caloric intake of a group of normal male infants fed *ad libitum* a formula providing 67 kcal/100 ml (colored lines) and another group given a formula providing 133 kcal/100 ml (black lines). (From Fomon, S. J. (1971). A pediatrician looks at early nutrition. *Bull. New York Acad. Med.*, 47: 573, Data from Fomon, S. J., et al. (1969). Relationship between formula concentration and rate of growth of normal infants. *J. Nutrition*, 98: 241. Used by permission.)

417

tinal mucosal cells might not be able to hydrolyze all of the disaccharides due to the lack of enough disaccharidase enzymes. When these carbohydrates are not hydrolyzed and absorbed, their presence exerts an osmotic effect, causing water to enter the intestine; the result is diarrhea. In the case of insufficient lactase, lactose will accumulate in the intestine; bacteria will then act upon it and produce carbon dioxide and lactic acid, which irritate the colon and will aggravate any diarrhea.

The sugars commonly used in formulas are sucrose (cane or beet) and corn syrup. Lactose, the sugar that occurs naturally in milk, is the least sweet of all the common sugars. It would be the best sugar for infant formulas, but it is expensive. Combinations of maltose and dextrin have been used in infant formulas; these mixtures are not as sweet as either sucrose or corn syrup.

When cows' milk is used, it is generally modified to make the important nutrients comparable in concentration to that of human milk; it is usually diluted because it has a higher concentration of proteins and minerals than human milk has. The nitrogenous end products of protein metabolism and the excess of minerals (especially phosphorus) to be eliminated may cause an overload on the excretory capacity of the infant's kidneys. By diluting the milk, its energy value is reduced. Sugar is sometimes added to increase the caloric value of the formula; otherwise the infant's stomach capacity may not be able to accommodate enough of the formula to meet the energy need. As other foods—cereals, fruits, and vegetables—are included in the diet, the sugar added to the formula can gradually be decreased. No sugar should be added to these other foods, for young children are developing their tastes at this time.

Water It is sometimes forgotten that infants need water. The amount required depends upon how much is lost in regulating the body temperature and how much is needed by the kidneys for waste disposal. Water is also needed for growth and for fecal excretion, but this is only a small amount. Babies should be given more fluids when the weather is hot (21) because body temperature control takes priority over everything else. Without additional water in hot weather, there will be less water for urine formation. A more concentrated urine is not good for infants; the excretory capacity of their kidneys is not as efficient as that of adults.

Infants require about 150 ml of water a day per kg of body weight. In relation to energy intake, the baby needs about 1.5 ml of water per kilocalorie of food. Babies get most of the water they need from milk and fruit juices, but they should be offered water between meals, especially in hot weather.

Protein Cows' milk contains about three times as much protein as human milk does. The proteins in both milks are casein (which is in the curd) and lactalbumin (which is in the whey). Lactalbumin and casein are contained in human milk in about equal amounts (Appendix Table A-8); in cows' milk, however, casein predominates. It has been demonstrated that the proteins of cows' milk and human milk are equally effective with respect to nitrogen retention in infants (14).

Raw cows' milk tends to produce large, firm curds in the infant's stomach. However, diluting the milk with water, heat treatment, acidification, and homogenization all help to promote the formation of softer curds.

The estimated requirements of infants for the essential amino acids are presented in Table 19.4. Two studies were utilized by the Food and Agriculture Organization (FAO/WHO) World Health Organization Committee on Energy and Protein Requirements (12) in arriving at their estimates: Holt and Snyderman (see Table 19.4) determined the maximal individual requirement of amino acids to achieve normal growth; Fomon and Filer calculated the intake of amino acids by infants fed a variety of formulas at levels to maintain good growth in all infants studied. The com-

418

Table 19.4 Estimated Amino Acid Requirements of Infants

Amino acid	Estimated requirements			
	Holt and Snyderman[a] (mg per kg per day)	Fomon and Filer[b] (mg per kg per day)	Composite of lower values (mg per kg per day)	Suggested pattern[c] (mg per g of protein)
Histidine	34	28	28	14
Isoleucine	119	70	70	35
Leucine	229	161	161	80
Lysine	103	161	103	52
Methionine and cystine	45 + cys	58[d]	58	29
Phenylalanine and tyrosine	90 + tyr	125[d]	125	63
Threonine	87	116	87	44
Tryptophan	22	17	17	8.5
Valine	105	93	93	47

[a] These requirements were estimated when the amino acids were fed or incorporated in basal formulas. The values represent estimates of maximal individual requirements to achieve normal growth.

[b] These values represent the calculated intakes of amino acids when the formulas were fed in amounts sufficient to maintain good growth in all the infants studied; the amino acids were not varied independently.

[c] Based on a recommended level of intake of 2 g of protein per kg of body weight per day, this is the average of suggested levels for infants up to 6 months of age.

[d] The values for cystine and tyrosine were estimated according to the methionine/cystine and phenylalanine/tyrosine ratios in human milk.

From *Energy and Protein Requirements*, FAO Nutrition Meetings Rept. Series 52, and WHO Tech. Rept. Series 522. Rome: Food and Agr. Organ., 1973, p. 55.

mittee selected from the two sets of data the lower value for each amino acid, establishing a pattern for amino acids considered to be adequate for infants up to 6 months of age.

An infant appears to need a larger amount of essential amino acids per unit of body weight than does an older child or adult because it must build much more new tissue; infants also need histidine, which is not required by older children or adults (26, 29). On a histidine-free diet young babies (under 2 months) not only failed to gain enough weight, but they developed a scaly rash that cleared up shortly after histidine was reincorporated into their diet. It is not yet understood precisely why infants need histidine.

The RDA (44) for protein for infants during the first 12 months is 1.9 g per 100 kcal of energy intake. Per kilogram of body weight, the allowances are: birth to 6 months, 2.2 g; and 6 to 12 months, 2.0 g.

Fat The total quantity of fat in human and cows' milk is 4.5 and 3.7 g per 100 ml, respectively. However, the kinds of fatty acids differ substantially. Cows' milk contains proportionately more saturated fatty acids, whereas human milk contains proportionately more polyunsaturated fatty acids (human milk has about five times as much linoleic acid as does cows' milk).

Symptoms of linoleic acid deficiency in infants include dryness of the skin with desquamation, thickening, and eventual chafing; these in-

419

fants also show a slow rate of growth. These symptoms disappeared when the infants were given linoleic acid in the amount of at least 1 percent of their energy intake (19). It has been recommended that linoleic acid supply 3 percent of the energy value in an infant's formula; in human milk it provides about 6 percent.

Minerals

Calcium Cows' milk contains almost four times the amount of calcium as does human milk per unit of volume (Fig. 19.2 and Appendix Table A-8). Consequently a breast-fed baby receives about 60 mg of calcium per kg of body weight each day, whereas one given a typical cows' milk formula receives about 170 mg calcium per kg of body weight. However, although the percentage of calcium retained is higher for human than for cows' milk (66 percent versus 35 to 50 percent, respectively), the total retention is higher for cows' milk. The RDA for formula-fed babies is as follows: birth to 6 months, 360 mg; and 6 to 12 months, 540 mg.

Iron Both human and cows' milk contain very little iron (Fig. 19.2). Fortunately, full-term infants whose mothers had adequate stores of iron are born with enough iron to provide for the first 3 months of life. However, because premature infants do not receive the iron transfer that usually takes place during the last weeks of pregnancy, they often show symptoms of anemia before the end of the first 3 months of life. Because the infant's body uses iron frugally, at 1 year 70 percent of the total body iron is still of transplacental origin. This information came from a study in which pregnant women were given transfusions of blood in which the red cells contained radioactive iron; thus it could be traced and later identified and measured quantitatively in the blood of the infant in comparison with its total blood iron (8, 47).

At birth the infant has about 80 mg of iron per

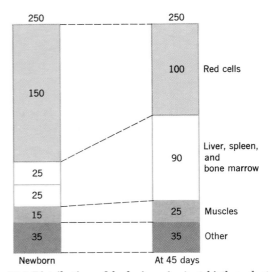

Fig. 19.4 Distribution of body iron (mg) at birth and at 45 days. (From Sjolin, S., and L. Wranne (1968). Iron requirements during infancy and childhood. In *Occurrence, Causes and Prevention of Nutritional Anemias*, edited by G. Blix, Uppsala, Sweden: Almquist and Wiksells, p. 149. Used by permission.)

kg of body weight (8). The hemoglobin level at birth is relatively high—around 22 g per 100 ml—but it decreases to approximately 10.5 to 11.5 g per 100 ml at about 3 months of age. Iron shifts from the red blood cells to the storage depots between birth and 45 days, as shown in Fig. 19.4. This shift may be a physiological adjustment to bring the hemoglobin level closer to what is considered normal for the infant. No appreciable amount of iron is excreted from the body. Premature infants need to receive more dietary iron than do full-term ones since they are born with far less hemoglobin and storage iron.

The RDA for infants is based upon the amount of dietary iron needed to maintain an optimal hemoglobin level. Clinical studies of infants and children show that when they retain approximately 0.8 to 1.0 mg per day of iron, their normal hemoglobin levels are maintained.

In 1969, an FAO/WHO Joint Expert Group on Vitamin and Mineral Requirements (50) recom-

420

Table 19.5 Daily Recommended Intakes for Iron[a]

	Age, years	Type of diet		
		Animal foods below 10% of kilocalories, mg	Animal foods 10–25% of kilocalories, mg	Animal foods over 25% of kilocalories, mg
Infants	0–1/3	[b]	[b]	[b]
	1/3–1	10	7	5
Children	1–12	10	7	5
Boys	13–16	18	12	9
Girls	13–16	24	18	12

[a] Since the absorption of iron from mixed diets varies according to the proportion of foods of animal origin and soybeans in the diet, daily recommended intakes are given for three types of diet: diets with foods of animal origin and soybeans that contribute less than 10 percent, 10–25 percent, and more than 25 percent of the total energy intake.

[b] Breast feeding is assumed to be adequate.

From requirements of ascorbic acids, vitamin D, vitamin B12, Folte, and Iron. WHO technical Report Series 452, Geneva: World Health Organ 1970, pg 54.

mended that iron intakes should vary according to the proportion of foods of animal origin and soybeans in the diet. Since iron is better absorbed from these two sources than from others, less is needed (24). The recommended intakes for children up to 16 years of age are presented in Table 19.5.

Consumption studies reveal a mean intake of iron by infants that is generally below the RDA. In the Denver longitudinal studies of 59 infants, the median iron intake during the first year was 0.83 mg per kg of body weight, or approximately 6.6 mg, daily. Since the infants' blood analysis and rate of growth indicated that was sufficient (6), it can be seen that a low-iron diet does not necessarily produce iron-deficiency anemia.

Before 1959, it was believed that the infant could absorb very little dietary iron until he was 4 to 6 months of age. However, the Swedish investigators Garby and Sjölin (16), using a label-tracer technique, showed that infants below 3 months of age absorbed iron at a faster rate than at any other age. Iron in milk and in cereal seem

to be well utilized during the earliest months (41).

The American Medical Association AMA Committee on Iron Deficiency has concluded that there is a high incidence of iron-deficiency anemia among infants, but the exact extent has not yet been determined (27). In general, iron-deficiency anemia in children is defined as a hemoglobin level of less than 10 to 10.8 g per 100 ml of blood (28, 35, 43). Using this criterion, it was found that among 46 infants of less than 1 year of age from poor families in New York City, 41 percent had anemia (23). The incidence among infants admitted for all causes to hospitals in the larger cities of the United States was 30 percent (41). However, among 1-year-old children from well-to-do families in Denver, only 2 out of 59 had anemia (6). In view of these findings, Beal, Meyers, and McCammon (6) "make a plea for continued and more complete investigations of dietary iron, iron absorption, and iron metabolism in infants before undertaking nationwide supplementation of infant diets."

The WHO is very much concerned about iron-

421

deficiency anemia (7), which is estimated to be as high as 50 to 90 percent in the developing countries. One of its major causes is loss of blood from hookworms and other intestinal parasites. The AMA Committee on Iron Deficiency (27) indicated that because of the high incidence of iron deficiency, even among American infants, there is justification for administering iron prophylactically in amounts not exceeding 5 to 15 mg daily. The Committee on Nutrition of the ACP (1) believes that certain foods should be fortified with iron to supply the needed intake.

Iodine The breast-fed infant whose mother is adequately nourished receives sufficient iodine. If the infant consumes 850 ml of human milk a day, he may get between 60 and 120 μg of iodine. The RDA for the first 6 months is 35 μg; and between 6 and 12 months, 45 μg. The infrequency of iodine deficiency in infants seems to indicate that cows' milk and prepared formulas also provide sufficient iodine.

It may be necessary to add iodine to soy-milk formulas. Several investigators have reported the development of goiter in infants who ingested a soy-containing commercial formula. When iodine was subsequently added to the mixture, the problem was corrected (14).

Sodium Requirements for sodium during the first year of life are estimated to be 4 to 8 mEq daily (14). A breast-fed infant who consumes 150 to 200 ml per kg of body weight per day would have an intake of 1.0 to 1.4 mEq per kg of body weight (for a 3-month-old baby, this would be about 5.5 to 7.5 mEq daily). An infant who consumes undiluted cows' milk would receive about three or four times as much sodium.

Other Minerals The RDA for phosphorus is less than for calcium during the first year (but not at any other age). Milk, the baby's principal food, contains less phosphorus than calcium. The recommendations for magnesium and zinc are given in Table 3.1.

Vitamins

Vitamin A Milk contains both the preformed vitamin A and carotenoid pigments. Human milk contains more of the preformed vitamin than of the carotenoids, whereas cows' milk has about the same proportion of each.

The RDA during the first 6 months is 1400 IU of vitamin A activity per day, and from 6 to 12 months 2000 IU per day. This calculation was made by taking the vitamin A value of 100 ml of human milk (170 IU) and assuming that the infant consumes 850 ml per day. Fomon (14) believes that it is "unlikely that any normal infant in North America [who receives] an otherwise adequate diet will benefit from supplementary administration of vitamin A" and warns against the hazard of overdosage. (The symptoms of vitamin A toxicity are discussed in Chapter 9.)

In many countries, however, there is a serious vitamin A deficiency. In an effort to reduce this deficiency among infants and preschool children in India, 1785 of them were experimentally given a massive dose of vitamin A once a year (49). In a 2-year trial study, it was found that 300,000 IU of the vitamin in an oil base sustained the children's levels of serum vitamin A within normal range for up to 6 months and reduced the prevalence of vitamin A deficiency symptoms.

Vitamin D Physicians routinely recommend a supplemental source of vitamin D for both breast-fed and bottle-fed infants beginning soon after birth and continuing throughout childhood.

The vitamin D requirement for infants and children is defined as the amount that, together with enough calcium and phosphorus in a well-balanced diet, will permit normal growth and mineralization of the bones and teeth. Because of rapid growth, infants and young children need proportionately more vitamin D than older children do. A daily intake of 135 IU will prevent rickets in infants, but better growth will be achieved with 400 IU (the RDA). Increasing the

422

intake to 600 IU per day does not seem to improve the infant's rate of growth or calcium utilization accordingly (46). Care should be taken not to give an infant excessive amounts of vitamin D (for a discussion of its toxic effects, see Chapter 9).

In the United States, reconstituted evaporated milk, most commercially prepared infant formulas, and most fresh whole milk are fortified to provide 400 IU of vitamin D per quart. With the addition of vitamin D to milk, infantile rickets has largely been eliminated.

Reports from Scotland, South Africa, the Philippines, Israel, Ethiopia, and Algeria indicate that rickets is a common public health problem in those countries (3, 31). Figure 19.5 shows the bowing of the legs and the dwarfing effect of rickets.

Vitamin E The newborn baby has very little vitamin E in its tissues because little passes through the placenta. Human milk, however, has a relatively high vitamin E content—about 6.6 IU per liter (the RDA is 4 IU daily for infants up to 6 months of age, and 5 IU daily for those 6 to 12 months of age). Although cows' milk contains only about 1.0 IU per liter, infants seem to thrive on formulas made from it without a vitamin E supplement.

Vitamin K Between the second and sixth day of life, infants show a low prothrombin level in the blood (hypoprothrombinemia). By the second week, however, the prothrombin level becomes normal, because by this time the intestinal flora is fully developed and capable of producing vitamin K. (The infant is born with a sterile intestinal tract.) Since human milk is generally lower in vitamin K than is cows' milk, it is not surprising that hemorrhagic disease is more common among breast-fed babies (18).

Thiamin The amount of thiamin in the diet of the mother seems to be the major factor affecting the quantity in human milk. Human milk has about 0.016 mg of thiamin per 100 ml as com-

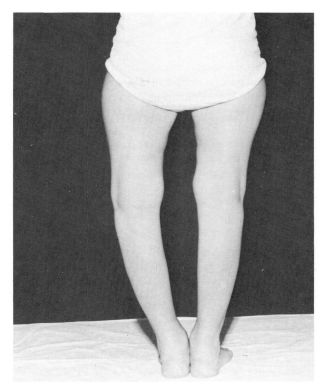

Fig. 19.5 Bowed legs in adults result from rickets in childhood. (Armed Forces Institute of Pathology.)

pared with 0.04 mg per 100 ml in cows' milk. The RDA for thiamin is: from birth to 6 months, 0.3 mg; and from 6 to 12 months, 0.5 mg. If the human milk intake is about 850 ml per day, it will provide 0.14 mg. The consumption of cereals and other foods increases the thiamin intake.

Riboflavin The amount of riboflavin in human milk is also directly related to the riboflavin content of the mother's diet. (On days when mothers have eaten liver, there has been a higher concentration of riboflavin in their milk.) Human milk contains about 0.6 mg per 1000 kcal (4184 kJ), which is about one-fifth the amount in cows' milk. The degree of utilization of riboflavin from the two milks is not known.

The daily RDA is 0.4 mg for babies up to 6

423

months of age, and 0.6 mg for those between 6 and 12 months.

Niacin Human milk contains an average of 1.47 mg of niacin and 220 mg of tryptophan per liter (which is a niacin equivalent of around 0.5 per 100 ml, or 7 niacin equivalents per 1000 kcal [4184 kJ]). The RDA for infants is 5 mg of niacin per day up through 5 months of age, and 8 mg per day for 6 to 12 months of age. When infants have been fed a diet without niacin, their needs were met by 6 niacin equivalents derived from tryptophan.

Vitamin B-6 The infant is born with a substantial amount of vitamin B-6. During the first month of lactation, human milk contains between 0.01 to 0.02 mg per liter, but then it increases to 0.1 mg per liter. The need for vitamin B-6 is related to protein intake. The average concentration of vitamin B-6 in human milk appears to be adequate for metabolizing its low protein content (11 g per liter). In cows' milk, both the level of protein (33 g per liter) and that of vitamin B-6 (about 0.6 mg per liter) are higher than in human milk, but the quantitative ratio between the vitamin and the protein is satisfactory. The RDA for the first 6 months is 0.3 mg per day, and for 6 to 12 months, 0.4 mg per day.

Folacin and Vitamin B-12 The RDA for both folacin and vitamin B-12 are approximately equivalent to the daily intake of each of these vitamins in breast milk (Table 3.1).

Vitamin C The vitamin C content of human milk depends upon the mother's diet, but it generally exceeds that of cows' milk. Commercial processes, including pasteurization, evaporation, and drying, tend to inactivate the vitamin C content so that little remains in formula milk. Vitamin C (often in the form of orange juice) is usually recommended for both the bottle-fed and breast-fed baby soon after birth.

The RDA for infants up to 12 months of age is 35 mg of vitamin C daily (approximately the amount supplied by 850 ml of human milk in the United States).

Infant Formulas

The Committee on Nutrition of the ACP (2) has recommended nutrient levels for infant formulas; these are shown in Table 19.6 with the corresponding RDA. The minimum levels of nutrients per 100 kcal reflect the composition of human milk and are least likely to result in any undesirable nutrient interactions. These standards apply to formulas prepared for healthy infants from birth (2.5 to 4.0 kg body weight) to 12 months of age (8 to 10 kg). The committee further recommends that a formula should contain the nutrients at the levels proposed before it can be labeled "infant formula." These standards may also be used as guidelines for preparing formulas for infants with specific nutritional problems, such as malabsorption and low birth weight. The footnotes of Table 19.6 give further specifications. Most of the proposed minimum levels of nutrients per 100 kcal of formula meet or exceed the RDA for infants.

Feeding the Baby

The manner in which a baby is fed affects his emotional development. For example, if he is fed when he experiences hunger, he will develop trust for the person who feeds him. Since hunger is one of the baby's first frustrations, receiving food is one of his first satisfactions. In years past, mothers were instructed to use a rigid feeding schedule, which meant feeding the baby at regular times, whether he had to be awakened from a sound sleep or left to cry until the specified hour for eating. Now the accepted practice is self-regulation, in which the baby generally determines his own mealtimes. Mothers eventually learn to distinguish the special hunger cry. It should be cautioned, however, that too much permissiveness (that is, feeding the baby whenever

424

Table 19.6 RDA of Infants and Proposed Nutrient Levels of Infant Formulas per 100 kcal (0.8 MJ)

	RDA[a]		1974 Recommendations[b]	
	0–6 months	6–12 months	Minimum	Maximum
Protein, g	1.9	1.9	1.8[c]	4.5[c]
Fat, g			3.3	6.0[d]
percent kcal			30	54
Essential fatty acid				
Linoleate, g			300	
percent kcal			3	
Fat-soluble vitamins				
A, IU	200 (55 μg)[e]	200 (40 μg)	250 (75 μg)	750 (225 μg)
D, IU	55	40	40	100
E, IU	0.6	0.5	3 (with 0.7 IU/g linoleic acid)	
K, μg			4	
Water-soluble vitamins				
Thiamin, μg	70	50	40	
Riboflavin, μg	90	60	60	
Niacin, μg	115	82	250	
B$_6$, μg	60	40	35 (with 15 μg/g of protein in formula)	
B$_{12}$, μg	0.04	0.03	0.15	
Ascorbic acid, mg	5	4	8	
Minerals				
Calcium, mg	50	55[f]	50	
Phosphorus, mg	35	40[f]	25	
Iron, mg	1.42	1.54	0.15[g]	
Magnesium, mg	9	9	6	
Iodine, μg	5	5	5	
Zinc, mg	0.4	0.5	0.5	
Sodium, mEq			6[h]	17[h]
Potassium, mEq			14[h]	34[h]
Chloride, mEq			11[h]	29[h]

[a] 1974 RDA expressed as allowance per 100 kcal.

[b] Committee on Nutrition of the American Academy of Pediatrics recommendations. *Pediatrics*, **57**, 1976, p. 281.

[c] For proteins with a protein efficiency ratio (PER) of at least 100 percent that of casein. Level should be correspondingly increased if PER is less than 100 percent of casein; no protein with PER less than 70 percent should be used.

[d] This maximum fat level will still ensure sufficient carbohydrate and fat to avoid ketosis or acidosis from excess fat.

[e] Values in parentheses represent retinol equivalents.

[f] Calcium to phosphorus ratio must be no less than 1:1 and no more than 2:0.

[g] Lower level found in human milk; iron must be in a form that would be available to the body.

[h] Milliequivalents for 670 kcal per liter (20 kcal per oz) of formula.

he cries) can be as bad as too much rigidity. During the first few weeks of life, infants who are regulating themselves tend to want to eat at intervals of less than four hours; these intervals gradually lengthen so that by the end of the first year three meals a day are usually enough (22).

Adding Solid Foods

The transition from an all-liquid diet to one that includes solids takes place gradually. Although the first solid food given is often cereal (a thin gruel), applesauce or mashed banana are also good to start with. Later, other pureed fruits and vegetables are added: infants generally seem to like fruits quite well. New foods should be introduced in tiny portions. Although the infant will typically reject each new food, repeated trials will eventually bring success. It is good practice to offer a variety of fruits and vegetables in order to accustom the child to liking many rather than only a few foods. At a later time protein foods and simple desserts can be added. Before he is 1 year of age, the child will be able to eat chopped foods (39).

When to add solid foods to the baby's diet is an individual matter; it depends upon the maturity, appetite, and digestion, but there is no special virtue in doing this before he reaches 3 months of age. The total nutrient intake of 50 infants at the age of 3, 5, 7, 9, 11, and 13 weeks was studied in a university community. It was found that those whose diet included solid foods had about the same energy intake as those who received only milk. However, those who ate solid foods ingested more vitamin A, thiamin, and iron. But these solid food nutrients only augmented an already adequate diet, as judged by the RDA (17).

The Preschool Child

Between the ages of 2 and 6, children grow at a slower rate than during their first year. They may gain only 1.8 to 2.3 kg (4 or 5 lb) per year, whereas the infant may gain that much in a couple of months. The preschool child grows relatively more in height and becomes taller and thinner. The arms and legs become longer in proportion to his trunk; the short infant neck becomes longer; and his head, which at birth accounted for about one-fourth of his total length, grows more slowly and thus constitutes a smaller fraction of his total height (Fig. 19.6). The well-nourished preschool child is sturdily built, has an alert appearance, bright eyes, clear skin, and happy disposition. He is busy exploring his environment and establishing himself as an individual in it.

Since the nutrient needs of each child depend upon the rate of growth and activity, the following discussion sets forth only general principles.

Nutrient Needs of Children Between 1 and 6 Years of Age

The best index of an adequate energy intake for preschool children is a weight gain, not according to standard weight tables, but according to each child's own individual rate. It is important that he gain weight continuously (6, 7, 10, 14).

The relative magnitude of the components of the energy requirement per kilogram of body weight decreases during the preschool years. When children weigh about 13 to 20 kg (28 to 44 lb), their basal metabolism and their energy need for growth per kilogram of body weight both diminish. The RDA for energy is about 100 kcal (418 kJ) per kg of body weight per day (1300 kcal, or 5439 kJ daily) for 1-to-3-year-olds, and 90 kcal (376 kJ) per kg of body weight per day (1800 kcal, or 7531 kJ daily) for 4-to-6-year-olds.

The RDA for protein is 23 g daily for children between 1 and 3 years of age, and 30 g for those between 4 and 6.

The requirement for minerals also depends upon the growth rate. Between the ages of 1 and 8, the daily retention of calcium for skeletal growth has been estimated to be between 75 and

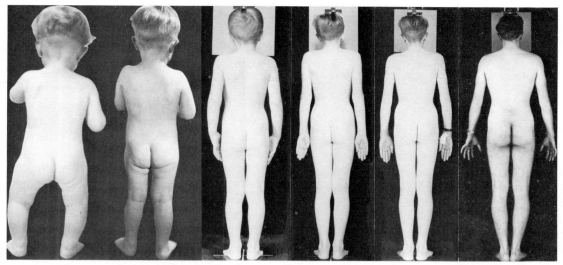

Fig. 19.6 A boy at various ages, showing the change in his proportions. From left to right, he is 15 months, 30 months, 6, 11, 14, and 18 years of age. (Reprinted from Growth Diagnosis, by L. Bayer and N. Bayley, by permission of The University of Chicago Press. Copyright © 1959 by the University of Chicago Press.)

150 mg daily. To assure this retention, the RDA is 800 mg daily for children between 1 and 6 years of age.

A group of 28 children between the ages of 3 and 5 in Vellore, India, who were accustomed to a low intake of dietary calcium (about 200 mg daily) were found to be storing calcium on this intake; they retained about 33 percent of it (about 66 mg), whereas the average daily retention is 79 mg (1). Few studies have been done on the need for calcium by children living in tropical areas. It is possible that, in addition to their lifetime adaptation to a low intake of calcium, the tropical sun (which activates the vitamin D precursor in skin) has increased the efficiency of the use of their intake.

The RDA for iron is 15 mg daily for children between 1 and 3 and 10 mg for those between 4 and 6. This recommendation allows a retention of at least 0.2 mg daily. To obtain this amount, iron-rich foods must be included in the diet. (See Table 14.4 for the iron content of foods.)

An iron intake of somewhat less than the recommended 10 mg daily may not lower the hemoglobin level. In a study of 40 Nebraska preschool children (half of whom were from well-to-do families and half from poor families), although only five met the RDA (the authors used the 1963 RDA of 8 mg), their mean hemoglobin value was normal — 12 g per 100 ml (8).

Studies of preschool children from low-income families have showed hemoglobin levels ranging from low to normal. Among 460 such children studied in Washington, D.C., about half had hemoglobin levels below 10.5 g per 100 ml, which indicates an anemic condition (5).

The preschool child's need for an intake of vitamins has not been extensively investigated. The Nebraska study of 40 preschool children revealed that their most serious lack was in vitamins A and C. It was found that the children from poorer families had more adequate vitamin intakes from their diet than did the children from wealthier families. However, because 65 percent of the

427

latter group was taking vitamin supplements (as compared with only 25 percent of the former group), the total vitamin intake was greater among those from well-to-do families (8).

The RDA for vitamins and the other minerals is presented in Table 3.1.

Eating Habits of the Preschool Child

Children of this age vary in their eating habits from day to day and from meal to meal. Their preferences for certain foods as well as quantities are often quite unpredictable. In nursery schools it has been found that allowing some choice of food is desirable. When children were permitted to choose between two vegetables, they ate more and had fewer eating problems.

During the preschool years children have definite food likes and dislikes. Of course, there are significant individual differences but, as Lowenberg (11) pointed out, these children tend to prefer foods that are mild-flavored; that have a soft, jellylike texture; and that are lukewarm in temperature. Colorful foods tend to have a special appeal. Finger foods are also popular: fresh carrots and rutabagas prepared as raw sticks were preferred to the same vegetables cooked. Among a group of Minnesota children, meats, fruits, and sweets were the most popular foods, whereas vegetables were the least popular (4).

In a unique study of taste sensitivity for sweetness, sourness, saltiness, and bitterness among 25 nursery-school children, it was found that those who were highly sensitive to one taste sensation were also quite sensitive to the other three. Those with the lowest taste sensitivity tended to accept more foods (9).

The food likes and dislikes of the parents tend to affect the eating habits of the child. This influence may be indirect because the foods disliked by the parents are generally not served at home (2). Similarly, in an Ohio study (13), the foods disliked by both parents were, with few exceptions, either unfamiliar to or disliked by the child.

Other factors also affect the child's eating habits. Foods should be served in small portions, taking into consideration his food preferences, appetite, and physical and emotional well-being at the time. The atmosphere during mealtime should be pleasant: if the children eat with the family, the conversation should be friendly and cordial; the chair on which they sit, the table from which they eat, and the utensils used should be the right size to make eating easy and comfortable for them.

The preschool child is more interested in his environment than in his food—a total change from babyhood. The mother who understands this will not be alarmed. Refusing to eat is sometimes used by the preschool child as a weapon to command attention from concerned adults. Parents should never try to force children to eat if they do not want to, for it can lead to unpleasant associations with food, which can last for many years. When children are sufficiently hungry, they will eat.

Daily Foods

Foods that should be included in the daily diet of the preschool child are listed in Table 19.7.

Some Nutritional Concerns

Iron-deficiency anemia is considered one of the most prevalent nutritional disorders among infants and children in the U.S., particularly those between 6 and 24 months of age. The incidence is also high in preschool children from low-income families (15). The relative frequency of iron-deficiency anemia may be attributed to (a) a lack of knowledge by professional workers and parents regarding good food sources of iron for infants and children, (b) possible insufficient iron stores in infants born to mothers with marginal iron status, and/or (c) an erroneous belief among many health professionals that before 2 to 3 months of age, iron absorption is inefficient; healthy young infants do absorb iron efficiently.

Obesity from excessive weight gain during in-

428

Table 19.7 Daily Foods for the Preschool Child

Food	Amount[a]	Comments
Milk	2 to 3 cups	Some preschool children cannot drink this much. If the child does not, let him drink what he wants and try to use more in cooking.
Meat, fish, or poultry	1 serving	Occasionally, cheese may be substituted for a serving of meat. (For an average serving at this age, nutritionists sometimes estimate about 1 level tablespoon of meat per year of age. But put on his plate only what you think he will eat.)
Eggs	1	
Potatoes	1 serving	1 tbsp per year of age is an average serving for children 2 to 5 years of age.
Vegetables	1 or 3 servings (1 serving of green or yellow, 1 serving raw)	Suggestions: Carrots Cabbage Lettuce Spinach Squash Green peas Green beans Broccoli Green peppers Tomatoes Celery about 1 level tablespoon per year of age is an average serving.
Fruits	2 servings	For vitamin C one of these fruits should be a medium orange or ½ grapefruit, ¼ cantaloupe, 10 strawberries, or 1 medium tomato.
Cereal	1 serving	Whole-grain or enriched.
Bread	2 or 3 slices	Whole-grain or enriched.
Butter or fortified margarine	2 tbsp	
Vitamin D supplement	400 IU (especially when child cannot be in the sunshine)	

[a] It is better to serve less than the child will probably eat and let him ask for a second helping if he wants it.

This food plan was worked out by Miriam E. Lowenberg, who followed carefully the food intake of preschool children for years, where she was in charge of the feeding.

429

fancy may increase the chance of developing obesity in childhood and later life (see Chapter 8). Evidence continues to accumulate indicating that prevention of obesity should start in infancy.

Dental caries is another widespread nutrition-related disorder among children in the United States. The incidence of this dental disease may be reduced by (a) ingestion of appropriate amounts of fluoride (see Chapter 14), (b) a decreased consumption of refined sugar, especially in the form of sticky candy (see Chapter 4), and (c) good oral hygiene and regular dental check-ups.

Federal Food Programs

The Food and Nutrition Service of the U.S. Department of Agriculture (USDA) administers several food programs to safeguard the health and well-being of infants and children in this country.

The Child Nutrition Programs include (a) the National School Lunch Program authorized by the National School Lunch Act of 1946, and (b) the School Breakfast Program, the special Milk Program, and the Special Food Service Program, all of which were authorized by the Child Nutrition Act of 1966 (3). Guidelines are specified for participation in these programs (see pp. 434–435).

The Special Supplemental Food Program for Women, Infants, and Children (WIC) provides special nutritious food supplements to low-income pregnant and lactating women, infants, and children up to 4 years of age who are nutritional risks (12). This program was authorized by a September 1972 amendment to the Child Nutrition Act of 1966. Under this program infants below 1 year of age are allowed iron-fortified formula, iron-fortified cereals, and fruit juices. Children 1 to 4 years and women are provided milk, iron-fortified cereals and fruit juices. These food packages are intended to correct known nutritional inadequacies of iron and vitamins A and C in the diets of low-income individuals in the United States.

The Elementary-School Child

Measurements reveal that children in the United States are generally becoming taller and heavier than their predecessors. Since 1880 children of the same chronological age have shown a marked increase in body size. For those 6 to 11 years of age cross-sectional data show a 10 percent increase in height and a 15 to 30 percent increase in weight (13). One of the causes of this trend is undoubtedly improved nutrition; other causes include improved housing and sanitary conditions, increased immunization against disease, and better medical care.

Both boys and girls grow at a fairly steady rate during the elementary-school years (Fig. 19.7). Findings from a study done during 1963–1965 of 7119 American children, 6 to 11 years of age, indicated an annual increase in mean height for girls of 6.0 cm (2.36 in) and for boys 5.4 cm (2.13 in) (13). The yearly increment in mean weight for both boys and girls is less regular than for height. The increment for girls between ages 6 and 7 is about 2.8 kg (6.2 lb) and between ages 10 and 11, 6.5 kg (14.3 lb). For boys the increments for those same ages are about 2.6 kg (5.7 lb) and 4.6 kg (10.1 lb), respectively. (See Appendix Tables A-19 and A-20.)

It is easiest to judge the adequacy of an individual child's energy intake by observing his pattern of growth. If his growth rate seems to be normal and if he has firm muscles that are sufficiently padded with fat, it can be concluded that his energy needs are being met. In the case of most healthy children, if there is enough wholesome food available, their appetites will be a fairly reliable index of their energy requirements.

Two extensive studies have been made of the nutritional needs and status of children. Macy and her coworkers in Detroit measured the intake and excretion of 18 chemical substances in children 4 to 12 years of age (18). In a Southern Regional Experiment Station project (19), an investigation was made of the preadolescent girl's

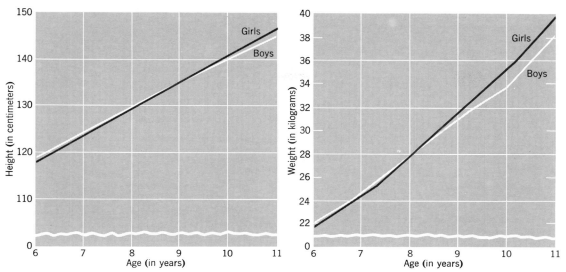

Fig. 19.7 Mean heights and weights for U.S. children, 6-11 years of age, by sex and age. (From Hamill, P. V. V., F. E. Johnson, and W. Grams, *Height and Weight of Children, United States*, Vital and Health Statistics, Series 11. No. 104 Rockville, Md.: U.S. Dept. Health, Education and Welfare, National Center for Health Statistics, 1970, pp. 3 and 4.)

need for energy (24), protein (1, 17), amino acids (1, 22), fat (37), calcium, phosphorus, magnesium (34), cobalt, copper, manganese, molybdenum (11, 32), zinc (10, 32), sulfur (39), vitamin A and carotene (23), thiamin (4), riboflavin (3), niacin (20, 25), vitamin B-12 (12), vitamin C (33), pantothenic acid, and folic acid (31). The findings from these and other studies are reflected in the RDA for children (Table 3.1).

Values for the minimum requirement for eight essential amino acids were suggested by Nakagawa and his coworkers in Japan (27) for boys 10 to 12 years of age. They found that these same minimum requirements were also suitable for girls (8 to 13 years of age), although they did not study the girls' need for each separate amino acid (28). In making their determination, the investigators prepared an amino acid mixture and then withdrew, one by one, each amino acid until a negative nitrogen balance was induced. In replacing each amino acid, the least amount required to maintain a positive nitrogen balance was held to be the minimal need. The removal of both arginine and

histidine did not induce a negative balance. Nakagawa's findings for boys are summarized in Table 19.8, together with other research on girls from 7 to 9 years of age. The wide variation among findings on the amino acid needs of individuals makes it difficult to express representative values at this time (15).

Adequacy of Food Intake

Dietary studies of school children throughout the United States have been made by both government agencies and private institutions. There are excellent summaries of these studies: one for the period, 1947 to 1958 (21); another for 1957 to 1967 (16); a review of vitamin and mineral studies for the years 1950 to 1968 (8); and abstracts from the U.S. Senate Hearings on Nutrition and Human Needs (29).

Studies of children from relatively poor homes show a high incidence of inadequate diets. In an investigation of 642 economically disadvantaged New York City school children in the mid-1960s,

431

Table 19.8 Estimates of the Minimum Daily Amino Acid Requirements of Boys and Girls

Amino acid	Boys (10–12 years)[a] mg/kg	Girls (7–9 years)[b] mg/kg
Isoleucine	30	24
Leucine	45	45
Lysine	60	29
Methionine	27[c]	21[c]
Phenylalanine	27	28
Threonine	35	20
Tryptophan	3.7	4.9
Valine	33	31

[a] From I. Nakagawa et al., (1963). Amino acid requirements of children, *J. Nutrition* 80, 310. Used by permission. These values are tentatively defined as minimum.
[b] From R. P. Abernathy et al. (1968). Effects of several levels of dietary protein and amino acids on nitrogen balance of preadolescent girls, *Am. J. Clin. Nutrition,* **19:** 412. Used by permission. These values are the lowest level of the acid supplied by an experimental diet that supported positive nitrogen retention.
[c] Methionine and cystine.

Table 19.9 Meal Score Ratings of 322 Boston School Children

Meal	Satisfactory[a] (percent)	Relatively satisfactory[b] (percent)	Unsatisfactory[c] (percent)
Breakfast	45	28	27
Lunch	40	27	33
Dinner	58	28	14

[a] Four out of four meals satisfactory.
[b] Three out of four meals satisfactory.
[c] Two or less out of four meals satisfactory.
From M. L. Myers et al. (1968). A nutrition study of school children in a depressed urban district. I. Dietary findings, *J. Am. Dietet. Assoc.* **53** 229. Used by permission.

73 percent had diets that were judged to be poor (5). (A diet was considered poor in this particular study if it supplied less than one-half of the RDA for protein, calcium, phosphorus, iron, vitamin A, thiamin, riboflavin, niacin, and vitamin C.)

The diets of 322 Boston school children from a depressed area were evaluated (26); it was found that the boys had poorer eating habits than the girls; that the diets of black children were nutritionally inferior to those of whites; and that the children's eating habits became worse as they grew older—for the boys the turning point was 10 years of age and for the girls 11 years of age.

The meals of the Boston school children were rated as "satisfactory" or "unsatisfactory" according to the foods eaten. Breakfast was judged to be unsatisfactory if it consisted of cereal alone (no milk), unsatisfactory nonbreakfast-type foods (such as a candy bar or cake), milk alone, fruit alone, or no food at all. Lunch was considered unsatisfactory if it consisted of only a sandwich; only fruit; only milk; only cake, cookies, candy, or potato chips; or no food at all. An unsatisfactory dinner would consist of only animal protein, only vegetable protein, only pasta or cereal, only milk, only snack-type foods, or no food at all. The children's lunches were rated as unsatisfactory more often than their other two meals. The children brought their lunches because food was not served at school and the children were not permitted to leave the grounds at noontime (see Table 19.9).

Meals of School Children

Breakfast Poor Breakfasts. Studies made in the mid-1950s of the breakfast habits of children showed that many were eating either inadequate breakfasts or none at all (21, 30, 35, 36). By contrast, a late 1960s survey made in a poor urban area showed that 45 percent of the 322 children sampled were having "satisfactory" breakfasts and 28 percent "relatively satisfactory" breakfasts (26). A surprisingly large number of the 400 Syracuse, New York, children (9) who participated in a nutritional status study had eaten breakfast before they arrived at the laboratory. The mean percentages of those who had eaten breakfast were 96, 93, and 59 for the three schools studied (the last of which is in an economically poor area). In an Iowa study of 2045 adolescents (14), the investigators found that a substantial minority had not eaten breakfast. In these studies (done in the 1960s) only a minority of children were eating poor breakfasts or none at all, whereas various studies reported that it had been a majority in the 1950s (21).

Protein eaten at breakfast (or other meal) causes the blood glucose to remain above the fasting level (a base or low level following an overnight fast) longer (2, 6, 30, 38). When the blood glucose is low, some people experience sensations of hunger and weakness. It was found that the blood glucose of young men and women who had consumed about 22 to 25 g of protein at breakfast remained above the fasting level for 3½ to 4 hours. Meals that are low in protein but high in either carbohydrate or fat will raise the blood glucose above the fasting level for only 2 or 3 hours, respectively.

Good Breakfasts. Any foods can be served for breakfast if they are wholesome and nutritious. Generally the morning meal should provide one-fourth or one-fifth of the day's total nutritional requirements (with lunch and dinner each supplying one-third and snacks the remainder.

Under the Child Nutrition Act of 1966 a program was initiated to provide breakfast at school in needy areas and for children who travel a long distance to school (40). Under this program breakfasts must consist of at least the following (7):

1. One cup of fluid whole milk, served as a beverage or on cereal or both.

2. One-half cup of fruit, or full-strength fruit or vegetable juice.

3. One slice of whole-grain or enriched bread; or an equivalent serving of cornbread, biscuits, rolls, muffins, etc., made of whole-grain or enriched meal or flour; or ¾ cup of whole-grain cereal or enriched or fortified cereal; or an equivalent quantity of any combination of these foods.

The breakfasts may also include such protein-rich foods as an egg; or a 28-g (1 oz) serving of meat, poultry, or fish; or 28 g (1 oz) of cheese; or 2 tablespoons of peanut butter; or an equivalent amount of any combination of these foods.

Lunch School Lunches. A child's lunch at school ought to supply about one-third of his nutritional needs for the day. If only a partial meal is served, it should supplement the nutrients provided by the rest of the day's diet. At school, children should not be given the same foods they receive in abundance at home, but the meal should be at least as good as they would have had at home. Those who are locally responsible for providing school lunches ought to be familiar with the prevailing food habits of the children's families, ought to take into consideration the children's food likes and dislikes, and ought to arrange for children to participate in some of the meal planning. If this could be done, the children's eating habits and enjoyment of the meals would be substantially improved. Children are sensitive to the quality of food preparation and the manner of serving. They like food simply cooked, attractively served, and in suitable portions. It is sometimes helpful to take children into the school kitchen to see the food being prepared. Such first-hand experience often whets disinterested appetites so that the children will accept certain disliked foods. It should always be remembered that the school lunch is for the child and not the child for the school lunch. The lunch program will be successful if it is built around the child's needs and interests (Fig. 19.8).

The school lunch also affords unique educational opportunities. In connection with the school lunch program, children can be taught good health habits, table manners, and nutrition; lunchroom practices can be related to classroom discussion and guidance in an integrated program.

In September 1977, proposed changes in the National School Lunch Program were announced. These proposals by the U.S. Department of Agriculture represent the most significant changes in meal patterns since the initiation of the program

433

Table 19.10 School Lunch Pattern Requirements—Amounts of Foods Listed by Food Components to Serve Children of Various Ages

Food components	Preschool children		Elementary school children		Secondary school
	Group I (1 and 2 years)	Group II (3, 4, and 5 years)	Group III (6, 7, and 8 years)	Group IV (9, 10, and 11 years)	Boys and girls Group V (12 years and over)
MEAT AND MEAT ALTERNATES[1]					
Meat—a serving (edible portion as served) of cooked lean meat, poultry, or fish, OR Meat Alternates:	1 ounce equivalent[2]	1½ ounces equivalent	1½ ounces equivalent	2 ounces equivalent	3 ounces equivalent
Cheese	1 ounce equivalent[2]	1½ ounces equivalent	1½ ounces equivalent	2 ounces equivalent	3 ounces equivalent
The following meat alternates[3] may be used to meet only ½ of the meat/meat alternate requirement:					
Eggs (1 large egg may replace 1 ounce cooked lean meat.)	1 egg[4]	¾ egg	¾ egg	1 egg	1½ eggs
Cooked Dry Beans or Peas (½ cup may replace 1 ounce cooked lean meat.)[5]	¼ cup	⅜ cup	⅜ cup	½ cup	¾ cup
Peanut Butter (2 tablespoons may replace 1 ounce cooked lean meat.)	1 tablespoon	1½ tablespoons	1½ tablespoons	2 tablespoons	3 tablespoons
VEGETABLES AND FRUITS[5] Two or more servings consisting of vegetables or fruits or both. A serving of full strength vegetable or fruit juice can be counted to meet not more than ½ of the total requirement.	½ cup	½ cup	½ cup	¾ cup	¾ cup

	5 slices or alternates/week	8 slices or alternates/week	8 slices or alternates/week	8 slices or alternates/week	10 slices or alternates/week
BREAD AND BREAD ALTERNATES[6] A serving (1 slice) of enriched or whole-grain bread; OR a serving of biscuits, rolls, muffins, etc., made with whole-grain or enriched meal or flour;[7] OR a serving (½ cup) of cooked enriched or whole-grain rice, macaroni, or noodle products.[8]	5 slices or alternates/week	8 slices or alternates/week	8 slices or alternates/week	8 slices or alternates/week	10 slices or alternates/week
MILK, FLUID An option to fluid whole milk or flavored milk must be offered.[9]	½ cup	¾ cup	¾ cup	½ pint	½ pint

NOTES:

[1] Meat and Meat Alternates must be served in a main dish, or in a main dish and one other menu item.

[2] Equivalents will be determined and published in guidance materials by FNS/USDA.

[3] Eggs, cooked dry beans or peas, and peanut butter may be combined with one-half of the quantity requirements for meat, poultry, fish or cheese to meet the total Meat/Meat Alternate requirement, or they may be used in equal quantities in combination with one another to meet the total Meat/Meat Alternate requirement. For example, for Group IV children, 2 tablespoons of peanut butter may be supplemented with 1 hard cooked egg to meet the total Meat/Meat Alternate component.

[4] For Group I children an egg may be served to meet the total Meat/Meat Alternate requirement.

[5] Cooked dry beans or dry peas may be used as part of the Meat Alternate or as part of the Vegetable/Fruit component, but not as both food components in the same meal.

[6] One-half or more slices of bread or an equivalent amount of bread alternate must be served with each lunch with the total requirement being served during a five day period. Schools serving lunch 6 or 7 days per week should increase this specified quantity for the five day period by approximately 20% (1/5) for each additional day.

[7] Bread Alternates and serving sizes will be published in guidance materials by FNS/USDA.

[8] Enriched macaroni products with fortified protein as defined in Appendix A, March 1974, may be used as part of a Meat Alternate or as a Bread Alternate, but not as both food components in the same meal.

[9] Unflavored fluid lowfat milk, skim milk, or buttermilk must be available to students, in addition to whole milk, or any flavored milk. From Federal Register, Vol. 42, No. 175, September 9, 1977 on Proposed Rules. National School Lunch Program, U.S. Department of Agriculture, Food and Nutrition Service.

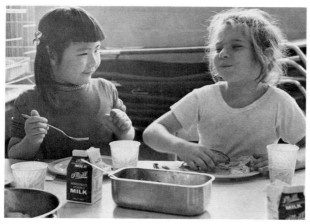

Fig. 19.8 School lunch. (Alice Kandell/Rapho-Photo Researchers.)

in 1946. The proposed lunch patterns define minimum food portion for five age groups (Table 19.10): I. 1–2 years; II. 3–5 years; III. 6–8 years; IV. 9–11 years; and V. 12 years and older. Portion sizes offered would be adjusted according to age group, and these are the first attempts toward reducing plate waste. Other changes in the meal pattern are indicated in Table 19.10. A pilot test of these proposals was scheduled from January through April of 1978.

Dinner A good evening meal, like breakfast and lunch, is essential to assure an adequate food intake for the day.

Snacks Most children eat snacks. The adolescents in the Berkeley longitudinal study (14) ate about four times a day. There seemed to be little relationship between the frequency of eating and the nutritive value of their diet except that when they ate less than three times a day, their food intake was less adequate. The Iowa adolescents (15) snacked after school, at bedtime, or while they were studying. Some good snack foods are

fruit, whole-grain or enriched bread or crackers, cheese, and milk.

Good Diets for School Children

There are government publications that provide helpful suggestions on adequate diets for children. The following are sample 1-day meals for children of different ages:

FOR A 10-YEAR-OLD
  BREAKFAST
      Tomato juice ($^3/_4$ c)
      Hot whole wheat cereal ($^2/_3$ c) with milk ($^1/_2$ c)
      Toast (2 sl) with butter or fortified margarine (2 tsp)
      Milk (1 c)
  LUNCH
  (If served at school or at home)
      Creamed eggs ($^3/_4$ c)
      Green beans ($^1/_2$ c) with butter or fortified margarine (1 tsp)
      Oatmeal muffins (2) with butter or fortified margarine (2 tsp)
      Milk (1 c)
  (If brought from home)
      Sandwich: peanut butter and grated raw carrot (or chopped dried fruit) on buttered whole-grain or enriched bread
      Supplemented at school by:
      Orange (1)
      Milk soup (1 c) or cocoa (1 c)
  DINNER
      Meat loaf (1 serving)
      Scalloped potatoes ($^2/_3$ c)
      Coleslaw with red and green peppers ($^1/_2$ c)
      Whole wheat or enriched bread (2 sl) with butter or fortified margarine (2 tsp)
      Applesauce ($^1/_2$ c)
      Molasses cookies (2 thin)
      Milk (1 c)
  SNACKS
      Fruit
      Milk
      Graham crackers

436

Summary

The nutritional needs of an individual at any given age and stage of the life cycle are influenced by a variety of biological factors (such as genes and hormones) and environmental factors (such as nutrients, drugs, toxins, bacteria, virus, and radiation). Socioeconomic and psychological conditions also affect greatly the nutritional requirements.

During periods of rapid growth, increased amounts of energy and nutrients are needed for tissue synthesis. These critical phases include the first nine months *in utero* (fetal period), the first year after birth (infancy), the transition stage between childhood and adulthood (adolescence), and in pregnancy and lactation. Because of the increased nutrient requirements, individuals during these periods are highly vulnerable to nutritional inadequacies.

In utero the rapidly growing fetus depends upon the nutrient supply from the maternal blood that reaches the placenta and the integrity and capability of the placenta to transport these nutrients to the fetus. Intrauterine malnutrition may lead to low-birth-weight mature infants. These small-for-dates babies contribute significantly to perinatal and infant mortality. The well-nourished mother nourishes her fetus well. Therefore, the best insurance for a healthy infant has been a mother who is healthy and well nourished throughout her entire life, as well as during the period of pregnancy.

During the first year, the nutrient needs are high per unit of body weight, particularly in early infancy. Human milk and/or modified cows' milk serves as one of the most important sources of several nutrients to support the rapid growth of healthy babies. The dietary pattern is adjusted in both the quality and variety of foods offered to meet the needs of the individual growing infant. As the child gets older and grows in body size, the total nutrient needs increase, but the requirements based on body weight decline.

Glossary

active transport: the movement of substances (particularly electrolyte ions) across cell membranes, usually against a concentration gradient. Unlike diffusion or osmosis, active transport requires the expenditure of metabolic energy.

development: generally denotes the series of changes by which the individual embryo becomes a mature organism. For example, the replacement of skeletal cartilage by calcified bone in the growing child.

gene: one of the units of heredity arranged in a definite fashion along a chromosome.

growth: generally denotes the increases in physical size of the human body as a whole, or any of its dimensions, parts, or tissues which begin at conception and continue through the life cycle.

hormone: a secretion produced in the body (chiefly by the endocrine glands) that is carried in the bloodstream to other parts of the body; each hormone has a specific effect on cells, tissues, and organs.

Nutrient: see p. 11.

placenta: a spongy structure that grows on the wall of the uterus during pregnancy and through which the fetus is nourished.

uterus: a hollow muscular organ in the female pelvis; it holds the growing fetus.

Study Questions

1. Why is the nutritional status of the mother before and during pregnancy important to the fetus?
2. What is the role of the placenta in nourishing the growing fetus?
3. Obtain a diagram with some details showing a fetus connected by the umbilical cord to the placenta and examine the relationship between the maternal and fetal circulations. Note how nutrient exchange takes place.
4. Why is it more important for the infant to have an adequate diet than the older child or adult?

437

5. What are some ways in which solid foods could be successfully introduced to the infant?

6. Examine the labels on bottles of multiple vitamin preparations that are intended for infants or young children and compare their potencies with the RDA for those age groups. Do they need these supplements? Give reasons to support your answer.

7. Examine the label on a commercial infant formula and compare the nutrients supplied with the RDA. What additional nutrients are included in the formula? Do healthy infants need them? Give reasons to support your answer.

8. Visit a day care center for preschool children during mealtime. What foods were offered and what serving sizes were given to each child? Compare the kinds and amounts of foods eaten by three or more children. Give some reasons for the similarities and/or differences in the observed eating patterns. Describe the environment during mealtime.

9. What is a good index of the adequacy of a child's energy intake?

10. Why is it advisable to have a protein-rich food at breakfast?

11. Visit a school lunch program during lunch time. Check the adequacy of the menu against the standard set up for a complete lunch by the National School Lunch Program. Compare the kinds and amounts of foods that were eaten by the elementary school children. What similarities and differences in eating habits did you observe? Why are eating patterns different? Similar?

References

Fetal Period

1. Bergner, L., and M. W. Susser (1970). Low birth weight and prenatal nutrition: An interpretative review. *Pediatrics*, **46:** 946.

2. Ferreira, A. S. (1969). *Prenatal Environment*. Springfield, Ill.: Charles C Thomas, p. 117.

3. Hytten, F. E., and I. Leitch (1971). *The Physiology of Human Pregnancy*. Oxford, England: Blackwell Scientific Publications.

4. Lechtig, A., J.-P. Habicht, H. Delgado, R. E. Klein, C. Yarbrough, and R. Martorell (1975). Effect of food supplementation during pregnancy on birth weight. *Pediatrics*, **56:** 508.

5. Lechtig, A., C. Yarbrough, H. Delgado, J.-P. Habicht, R. Martorell, and R. E. Klein (1975). Influence of maternal nutrition on birth weight. *Am. J. Clin. Nutrition*, **28:** 1223.

6. *Maternal Nutrition and the Course of Pregnancy* (1970). Washington, D.C.: Natl. Acad. Sci.–Natl. Research Council.

7. Metcoff, J. (1976). Maternal nutrition and fetal growth. In *Textbook of Paediatric Nutrition*, edited by D. S. McLaren and D. Burman. Edinburgh: Churchill Livingstone, p. 19.

8. Nesbitt, K. E. L., Jr. (1966). Prenatal development. In *Human Development*, edited by F. Falkner. Philadelphia: W. B. Saunders Co., p. 123.

9. Page, E. W. (1957). Transfer of materials across the human placenta. *Am. J. Obstet. Gynecol.*, **74:** 705.

10. Rush, D., Z. Stein, G. Christakis, and M. Susser (1974). The Prenatal Project: The first 20 months of operation. In *Nutrition and Fetal Development*, edited by M. Winick. New York: John Wiley and Sons, p. 95.

11. Stearns, G. (1958). Nutritional state of the mother prior to conception. *J. Am. Med. Assoc.*, **168:** 1655.

12. Watson, E. H., and G. H. Lowrey (1962). *Growth and Development of Children*. 4th ed. Chicago: Year Book Medical Publishers, p. 43.

13. Winick, M. (1976). *Malnutrition and Brain Development*. New York: Oxford University Press.

14. Winick, M., J. A. Brasel, and P. Rosso (1972). Nutrition and cell growth. In *Nutrition and Development*, edited by M. Winick. New York: John Wiley and Sons, p. 49.

The First Year

1. American Academy of Pediatrics, Committee on Nutrition (1969). Iron balance and requirements in infancy. *Pediatrics*, **43:** 134.

2. American Academy of Pediatrics, Committee on

Nutrition. Commentary on breast-feeding and infant formulas, including proposed standards for formulas (1976). *Pediatrics,* 57: 278.

3. Arneil, G. C. (1969). The return of infantile rickets to Britain. In *World Review of Nutrition and Dietetics,* Vol. 10, edited by G. H. Bourne. White Plains, N.Y.: Phiebig, p. 239.

4. Bain, K. (1948). The incidence of breast feeding in hospitals in the United States. *Pediatrics,* 2: 313.

5. Beal, V. A. (1969). Breast- and formula-feeding of infants. *J. Am. Dietet. Assoc.,* 55: 31.

6. Beal, V. A., A. J. Meyers, and R. W. McCammon (1962). Iron intake, hemoglobin, and physical growth during the first two years of life. *Pediatrics,* 30: 518.

7. Blood, the stream of life (1968). *World Health,* June, p. 28.

8. Bothwell, T. H., and C. A. Finch (1962). *Iron Metabolism.* Boston: Little, Brown, p. 313.

9. Brown, M. L., and S. F. Adelson (1969). Infant feeding practices among low and middle income families in Honolulu. *Trop. Geogr. Med.,* 21: 53.

10. Chaudhuri, K. C. (1961). Nutritional disorders in childhood. II, Biochemical study. *Indian J. Pediatrics,* 28: 411.

11. Dugdale, A. E. (1971). The effect of the type of feeding on weight gain and illnesses in infants. *Brit. J. Nutrition,* 26: 423.

12. *Energy and Protein Requirements* (1973). FAO Nutrition Meetings Rept. Series 52, and WHO Tech. Rept. Series 522. Rome: Food and Agr. Organ.

13. Filer, L. J., Jr. (1977). Relationship of nutrition to lactation in newborn development. In *Nutritional Impacts on Women,* edited by K. S. Moghissi and T. N. Evans, Hagerstown, Md.: Harper and Row, publishers.

14. Fomon, S. J. (1974). *Infant Nutrition.* 2nd ed. Philadelphia: W. B. Saunders Co., pp. 29, 484.

15. Fomon, S. J., and M. C. Egan (1972). Part 1. Improving the nutrition of those most vulnerable to hunger and malnutrition. 1. Infants, children, and adolescents. In *U.S. Nutrition Policies in the Seventies,* edited by J. Mayer. San Francisco: W. H. Freeman and Co., p. 13.

16. Garby, L., and S. Sjölin (1959). Absorption of labelled iron in infants less than three months old. *Acta Paediat.,* 48: Suppl. 117, 24.

17. Guthrie, H. A. (1966). Effect of early feeding of solid foods on nutritive intake of infants. *Pediatrics,* 38: 879.

18. György, P. (1971). The uniqueness of human milk. Biochemical aspects. *Am. J. Clin. Nutrition,* 24: 970.

19. Hansen, A. E., H. F. Wiese, A. N. Boelsche, M. E. Haggard, D. J. D. Adam, and H. Davis (1963). Role of linoleic acid in infant nutrition. *Pediatrics,* 31: 171.

20. Harfouche, J. K. (1971). The importance of breast-feeding. Monograph No. 10. *J. Trop. Pediatrics,* 16: 133.

21. Harper, P. A. (1962). *Preventive Pediatrics.* New York: Appleton-Century-Crofts, p. 245.

22. Harris, L. E., and J. C. M. Chan (1969). Infant feeding practices. *Am. J. Diseases Children,* 117: 483.

23. Haughton, J. G. (1963). Nutritional anemia of infancy and childhood. *Am. J. Public Health,* 53: 1121.

24. Heinrich, H. C. (1970). Intestinal iron absorption in man. In *Iron Deficiency,* edited by L. Hallberg, H. G. Harwerth, and A. Vannotti. New York: Academic Press, p. 253.

25. Heinstein, M. I. (1963). Influence of breast feeding on children's behavior. *Children,* 10: 93.

26. Holt, L. E., Jr. (1968). Some problems in dietary amino acid requirements. *Am. J. Clin. Nutrition,* 21: 367.

27. Iron deficiency in the United States (1968). *J. Am. Med. Assoc.,* 203: 119.

28. *Iron Deficiency Anaemia* (1959). WHO Tech. Rept. Series 182. Geneva: World Health Organ., p. 4.

29. Irwin, M. I., and D. M. Hegsted (1971). Amino acid requirements of man. *J. Nutrition,* 101: 541.

30. Jelliffe, D. B. (1967). The significance of breast feeding in tropical countries. In *Proceedings of the Seventh International Congress of Nutrition,* Vol. 4. New York: Pergamon Press, p. 555.

31. Jelliffe, D. B. (1968). *Infant Nutrition in the Sub-*

tropics and Tropics. Geneva: World Health Organ., p. 83.

32. Jelliffe, D. B. (1976). World trends in infant feeding. *Am. J. Clin. Nutrition,* **29:** 1227.

33. Koss, A. (1969). Breast feeding in mothers today. *Nutrition Abstr. and Rev.,* **39:** 539.

34. Kenny, J. F., M. I. Boesman, and R. H. Michaels (1967), Bacterial and viral coprantibodies in breast fed infants. *Pediatrics,* **39:** 202.

35. *Manual for Nutrition Surveys,* 2nd ed. (1963), Bethesda, Md.: National Institutes of Health, p. 235.

36. Mata, L. J., and R. G. Wyatt (1971). The uniqueness of human milk. Host resistance to infection. *Am. J. Clin. Nutrition,* **24:** 976.

37. Maternal and child health (1968). *Children,* **15:** 81.

38. McCallister, J., and J. F. Fitzgerald (1974). Infant feeding. *J. Indiana State Med. Assoc.,* **67:** 252.

39. *Medical Evaluation of the Special Supplemental Food Program for Women, Infants and Children* (1976). Select Committee on Nutrition and Human Needs, U.S. Senate. Washington, D.C.: U.S. Govt. Printing Office.

40. Meyer, H. F. (1958). Breast feeding in the United States. *Pediatrics,* **22:** 116.

41. Moore, C. V., and R. Dubach (1962). Iron. In *Mineral Metabolism,* Vol. 2, Pt. B., edited by C. L. Comar and F. Bonner. New York: Academic Press, p. 325.

42. Newton, N. (1971). Psychologic differences between breast and bottle feeding. *Am. J. Clin. Nutrition,* **24:** 993.

43. *Nutritional Anaemias* (1968). WHO Tech. Rept. Series 405. Geneva: World Health Organ., p. 9.

44. *Recommended Dietary Allowances, Eighth Edition* (1974). Natl. Acad. Sci.-Natl. Research Council. Washington, D.C.: Natl. Research Council.

45. Robertson, W. O. (1961). Breast feeding practices: Some implications of regional variations. *Am. J. Public Health,* **51:** 1035.

46. Slyker, F., B. M. Hamil, M. W. Poole, T. B. Cooley, and I. G. Macy (1937). Relationship between vitamin D intake and linear growth in infants. *Proc. Soc. Exp. Biol. Med.,* **37:** 499.

47. Smith, C. A., et al. (1955). Persistence and utilization of maternal iron for blood formation during infancy. *J. Clin. Invest.,* **35:** 1391.

48. Stevenson, S. S. (1949). Comparison of breast and artificial feeding. *J. Am. Dietet. Assoc.,* **25:** 752.

49. Swaninathan, M. C., T. P. Susheela, and B. V. S. Thimmayamma (1970). Field prophylactic trial with a single annual oral massive dose of vitamin A. *Am. J. Clin. Nutrition,* **23:** 119.

50. Vitamin and mineral requirements (1969). *FAO Nutrition Newsletter,* **7:** 42.

The Preschool Child

1. Begum, A., and S. M. Pereira (1969). Calcium balance studies on children accustomed to low calcium intakes. *Brit. J. Nutrition,* **23:** 905.

2. Bryan, M. S., and M. E. Lowenberg (1958). The father's influence on young children's food preferences. *J. Am. Dietet. Assoc.,* **34:** 30.

3. Child Nutrition Programs. *Dairy Council Digest,* **45:** No. 1 (January–February) 1974. Chicago: National Dairy Council.

4. Dierks, E. C., and L. M. Morse (1965). Food habits and nutrient intakes of preschool children. *J. Am. Dietet. Assoc.,* **47:** 292.

5. Gutelius, M. F. (1969). The problem of iron deficiency anemia in preschool Negro children. *Am. J. Public Health,* **59:** 290.

6. Jelliffe, D. B. (1968). *Infant Nutrition in the Subtropics and Tropics.* Geneva: World Health Organ., p. 86.

7. Jelliffe, D. B. (1968). The preschool child as a biocultural transition. *J. Trop. Pediatrics,* **14:** 217.

8. Kerrey, E., S. Crispin, H. M. Fox, and C. Kies (1968). Nutritional status of preschool children. I. Dietary and biochemical findings. *Am. J. Clin. Nutrition,* **21:** 1274.

9. Korslund, M. K., and E. S. Eppright (1969). Taste sensitivity and eating: Behavior of preschool children. *J. Am. Dietet. Assoc.,* **59:** 168.

10. Latham, M. (1965). *Human Nutrition in Tropical Africa.* Rome: Food and Agr. Organ., p. 45.

11. Lowenberg, M. E. (1948). Food preferences of young children. *J. Am. Dietet. Assoc.,* **24:** 430.

12. Medical Evaluation of the special supplemental food programs for women, children and infants, (1976), Select Committee on Nutrition and Human Needs, U. S. Senate, Washington, D.C., U.S. Government Printing Office.

13. Metheny, N. Y., F. E. Hunt, M. B. Patton, and H. Heye (1962). I. Nutritional sufficiency findings and family marketing practices. II. Factors in food acceptance. *J. Home Econ.,* **54:** 297, 303.

14. Nicholls, L., H. M. Sinclair, and D. B. Jelliffe (1961). *Tropical Nutrition and Dietetics.* London: Baillière, Tindall, and Cox, p. 166.

15. Owen, G. M., K. M. Kram, P. J. Garry, J. E. Lowe, Jr., and A. H. Lubin (1974). A study of nutritional status of preschool children in the United States, 1968–1970. *Pediatrics,* **53:** 579.

The Elementary School Child

1. Abernathy, R. P., M. Spiers, R. W. Engel, and M. E. Moore (1966). Effects of several levels of dietary protein and amino acids in nitrogen balance of pre-adolescent girls. *Am. J. Clin. Nutrition,* **19:** 407.

2. Addison, V. W., W. W. Tuttle, K. Daum, and R. Larsen (1953). Effect of amount and type of protein in breakfast on blood sugar levels. *J. Am. Dietet. Assoc.,* **29:** 674.

3. Boyden, R. E., and S. E. Erikson (1965). Metabolic patterns in preadolescent children. XVI. Riboflavin utilization in relation to nitrogen intake. *J. Nutrition,* **86:** 82.

4. Boyden, R. E., and S. E. Erikson (1966). Metabolic patterns in preadolescent children. Thiamin utilization in relation to nitrogen intake. *Am. J. Clin. Nutrition,* **19:** 398.

5. Christakis, G., A. Miridjanian, I. Nath., H. S. Khurana, C. Cowell, M. Archer, O. Frank, H. Ziffer H. Baker, and G. James (1968). A nutritional epidemiologic investigation of 642 New York City children. *Am. J. Clin. Nutrition,* **21:** 107.

6. Clayton, M. M., and S. W. Randall (1955). Blood changes following breakfasts of different types. *J. Am. Dietet. Assoc.,* **31:** 876.

7. *Closing the Nutrition Gap* (1968). Washington, D.C.: U.S. Govt. Printing Office.

8. Davis, T. R. A., S. N. Gershoff, and D. F. Gamble (1969). Review of studies of vitamin and mineral nutrition in the United States (1950–1968). *J. Nutrition Educ.,* **1:** Suppl. 1, 41.

9. Dibble, M. V., M. Brin, E. McMullen, A. Peel, and N. Chen (1965). Some preliminary biochemical findings in junior high school children in Syracuse and Onondaga County, New York. *Am. J. Clin. Nutrition,* **17:** 218.

10. Engel, R. W., R. F. Miller, and N. O. Price (1966). Metabolic patterns in preadolescent children. XIII. Zinc balance. In *Zinc Metabolism,* edited by A. S. Prasad. Springfield, Ill.: Charles C Thomas, p. 336.

11. Engel, R. W., N. O. Price, and R. F. Miller (1967). Copper, manganese, cobalt, molybdenum balance in preadolescent girls. *J. Nutrition,* **92:** 197.

12. Feeley, R. M., and E. Z. Moyer (1961). Metabolic patterns in preadolescent children. VI. Vitamin B$_{12}$ intake and urinary excretions. *J. Nutrition,* **75:** 447.

13. Hamill, P. V. V., F. E. Johnston, and W. Grams (1970). *Height and Weight of Children, United States.* Vital and Health Statistics, Series 11, No. 104. Rockville, Md.: U.S. Dept. Health, Education, and Welfare, National Center for Health Statistics, p. 14.

14. Hodges, R. E., and W. A. Krehl (1965). Nutritional status of teenagers in Iowa. *Am. J. Clin. Nutrition,* **17:** 200.

15. Irwin, M. I., and D. M. Hegsted (1971). Amino acid requirements of man. *J. Nutrition,* **101:** 541.

16. Kelsay, J. L. (1969). A compendium of nutritional status studies and dietary evaluation studies conducted in the United States, 1957–1967. *J. Nutrition,* **99:** Suppl. 1, Pt. 2.

17. Korslund, M. K., E. V. Leung, C. R. Meiners, M. G. Crews, J. Taper, R. P. Abernathy, and S. J. Ritchey (1976). The effects of sweat nitrogen losses in evaluating protein utilization by preadolescent children. *Am. J. Clin. Nutrition* **29:** 600.

441

18. Macy, I. G. (1942). *Nutrition and Chemical Growth in Childhood*, Vol. 1, *Evaluation*. Springfield, Ill., Charles C. Thomas, p. 85.

19. *Metabolic Patterns in Preadolescent Children. X. Description of 1962 Study* (1964). Southern Cooperative Series Bull. No. 64. Agr. Expt. Sta. of Georgia, Kentucky, Louisiana, South Carolina, Tennessee, Texas, Virginia, and the Agr. Res. Service (U.S. Dept. Agr.). Blacksburg, Va.: Virginia Polytechnic Institute and State University.

20. Miller, J., and R. P. Abernathy (1965). Metabolic patterns in preadolescent children. XIV. Excretion of niacin or tryptophan metabolites by girls fed controlled diets supplemented with nicotinamide. *J. Nutrition*, **86:** 309.

21. Morgan, A. F., ed. (1959). *Nutritional Status U.S.A.* Univ. of Calif. Agr. Expt. Sta. Bull. No. 769. Berkeley, Calif.: Univ. of California Agricultural Experiment Station.

22. Moore, M. E., and S. J. Ritchey (1966). Serum levels and urinary excretion of amino acids in preadolescent girls on two levels of protein intake. *Am. J. Clin. Nutrition*, **19:** 390.

23. Moschette, D. S. (1962). *Metabolic Patterns in Preadolescent Children. Blood Serum, Vitamin A, and Carotene Studies of Preadolescent Children.* Louisiana Agr. Expt. Sta. Bull. No. 552. Baton Rouge, La.: Louisiana Agricultural Experiment Station.

24. Moschette, D. S., S. T. Ehrlich, C. W. Bedell, and B. R. Farthing (1967). Prediction of metabolizable energy in preadolescent children. *J. Nutrition*, **91:** 348.

25. Moyer, E. Z., G. A. Goldsmith, O. N. Miller, and J. Miller (1963). Metabolic patterns in preadolescent children. VII. Intake of niacin and tryptophan and excretion of niacin or tryptophan metabolites. *J. Nutrition*, **79:** 423.

26. Myers, M. L., S. C. O'Brien, J. A. Mabel, and F. J. Stare (1968). A nutrition study of school children in a depressed urban district. I. Dietary findings. *J. Am. Dietet. Assoc.*, **53:** 226.

27. Nakagawa, I., T. Takahashi, T. Suzuki, and K. Kobayashi (1963). Amino acid requirements of children: minimal needs of tryptophan, arginine, and histidine based on nitrogen balance method. *J. Nutrition*, **80:** 305.

28. Nakagawa, I., T. Takahashi, T. Suzuki, and K. Kobayashi (1965). Amino acid requirements of children: quantitative amino acid requirements of girls based on nitrogen balance method. *J. Nutrition*, **86:** 333.

29. *Nutrition and Human Needs*, Pt. 3 (1969). The National Nutrition Survey. Washington, D.C.: U.S. Govt. Printing Office, p. 1077.

30. Orent-Keiles, E., and L. F. Hellman (1949). *The Breakfast Meal in Relation to Blood-sugar Values.* U.S. Dept. Agr. Cir. No. 827. Washington, D.C.: U.S. Dept. Agr.

31. Pace, J. K., L. B. Stier, D. D. Taylor, and P. S. Goodman (1961). Metabolic patterns in preadolescent children. V. Intake and urinary excretion of pantothenic acid and of folic acid. *J. Nutrition*, **74:** 345.

32. Price, N. O., G. E. Bunce, and R. W. Engel (1970). Copper, manganese, and zinc balances in preadolescent girls. *Am. J. Clin. Nutrition*, **23:** 258.

33. Ritchey, S. J. (1965). Metabolic patterns in preadolescent children. XV. Ascorbic acid intake, urinary excretion, and serum concentration. *Am. J. Clin. Nutrition*, **17:** 78.

34. Schofield, F. A., and E. Morrell (1960). Calcium, phosphorus, and magnesium. *Federation Proc.*, **19:** 1014.

35. Spurling, D., M. Krause, N. Callaghan, and R. L. Huenemann (1954). Poor food habits are everybody's concern. *J. Home Econ.*, **46:** 713.

36. Steele, B. F., M. M. Clayton, and R. E. Tucker (1952). Role of breakfast and of between-meal foods in adolescents' nutrient intake. *J. Am. Dietet. Assoc.*, **28:** 1054.

37. Stier, L. B., D. D. Taylor, J. K. Pace, and J. N. Eisen (1961). Metabolic patterns in preadolescent children. IV. Fat intake and excretion. *J. Nutrition*, **73:** 347.

38. Thornton, R., and S. M. Horvath (1965). Blood sugar levels after eating and after omitting breakfast. *J. Am. Dietet. Assoc.*, **47:** 474.

39. Wright, J. B., P. C. Martin, M. L. Skellenger, and D. S. Moschette (1960). Metabolic patterns in preadolescent children. III. Sulfur balance on three levels of nitrogen intake. *J. Nutrition,* **72:** 314.

40. 1969 marked new era in child nutrition (1970). Agr. Marketing, **15:** 3.

443

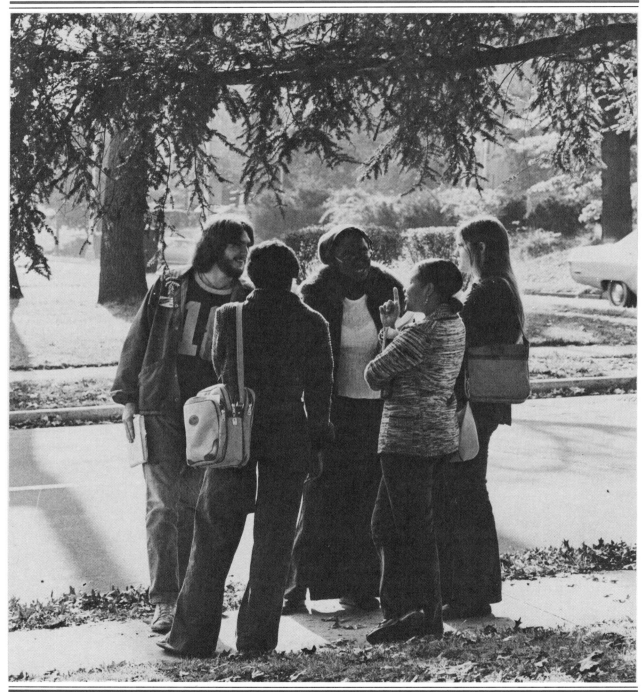

Growing into adulthood.

Chapter 20

Nutrition During the Life Cycle II

Adolescence and Young Adulthood

Adolescence is a period of "growing up" or growing toward adulthood. It is a transition stage from childhood to adulthood and covers nearly a decade with no sharply defined beginning or end. Its biological landmark is "*puberty*," during which sexual development takes place, and it terminates with the attainment of the capacity for sexual reproduction. *Menarche*, or the onset of menstrual function in girls, also marks puberty. The ability to reproduce follows some time after the first menstrual period. Extensive changes in hormonal secretions stimulate the dramatic growth spurt which occurs concomitantly with the development of female and male characteristics. Behavioral changes also characterize this particular phase of the life cycle.

As puberty ends, adulthood begins and growth continues at a decreased rate; new cells are formed just to replace those that are destroyed or lost. Adulthood, therefore, may be described as the time a steady state of body cell population is finally attained. For a healthy young woman, the menstrual cycle is well-established and the reproductive system is fully matured, and now she is well-equipped for childbearing. Fertility or the ability to reproduce offspring is the biological landmark of this period.

Chronologically, young adulthood in America is not clearly defined, although the age interval from 25 to 45 years has been suggested. Census data refer to the youth of America as those who are neither adults nor children; they are between 14 and 24 years of age. One in 5, or 42.4 million Americans, belong to youth (25).

The Adolescent

Growth and Maturation During Adolescence

Physical growth basically takes place during the first 18 years of life. If growth is expressed as a rate, it moves with decelerating velocity from birth until the time of the adolescent spurt; then the rate accelerates. During adolescence a substantial amount of new tissue is built. For girls the adolescent growth spurt may begin at any age from 8 to 13 years, and for boys it comes about 2 years later. Between the ages of 8 and 14, girls may double their body weight; boys may do so between 10 and 17 (5). Adolescent girls gain proportionately more fat than lean tissue and maintain this ratio throughout the growth period. The boys, on the other hand, deposit less fat and more lean mass (1).

Adolescents must adjust not only to their sudden increase in size, but to the appearance of secondary sex characteristics. Physiologically these changes are related. It is well established that the administration of androgens (male sex hormones) to prepubertal boys will produce a growth spurt similar to that which occurs at puberty. During puberty, of course, the secretion of testosterone (a male sex hormone) begins. On the basis of some experimental work, Cheek (1) postulates that the secretion of testosterone (as measured by the excretion of an end product in the urine) parallels the rate of growth.

For the adolescent, a problem may arise if he is quite different from his peers in size and shape. Boys often want to be larger, for early maturation may give them an advantage in athletics and in leadership roles. Girls often want to be physically more mature, for it may enhance their status with girls and increase their popularity with boys.

Tanner (20) believes that the chief factor determining the initiation of puberty is genetic; he cites as evidence the correlation between the age of menarche of mothers and daughters. On the other hand, there has been a trend toward earlier menarche in different countries whose peoples have improved their nutrition and health during the past 50 years (Table 20.1).

The Views of Adolescents

About Their Body Build Huenemann and co-workers (9, 12) surveyed 1000 adolescents in an

446

entire grade of the public high school system in Berkeley, California. They were all keenly interested in their size and shape, but most were dissatisfied with their dimensions.

In a study of senior high school students in a well-to-do Boston suburb, the girls generally wanted to weigh less while the boys generally wanted to weigh more (except for the obese boys) (4). Their concern was clear because of the frequency with which they weighed themselves: 24 percent of the girls and 16 percent of the boys weighed themselves every day, and 33 percent of the girls and 31 percent of the boys weighed themselves once a week. In another study of Boston senior-high-school girls (3), only 15 percent were found to be obese by triceps skinfold measurements but 30 percent of them were on reducing diets. Among the girls in the Berkeley longitudinal study (ninth through twelfth grades), 43 percent of those in the ninth grade, 49 percent of those in the tenth, and 56 percent of those in the twelfth grade believed they were fat, although only 25 percent were classified as truly obese (Fig. 20.1).

In general, high-school boys seem to want to be taller, whereas girls appear to be satisfied with their height or want to be a little shorter.

About Food In the Berkeley longitudinal study, students were asked: "What foods should be eaten every day for health?" The majority mentioned fruits, vegetables, meat, and milk; a smaller percentage said bread and cereals (Table 20.2). About 10 percent felt that sugar was necessary for their health (12).

One hundred and twenty-two students were asked to keep a daily record of their food intake for one complete week at four different periods. They were also asked to rate their diets as "poor," "fair," "good," or "excellent." Some of the students (the ninth grade girls and all of the twelfth grade students) assessed their diets realistically: in this group, those who rated their diets "good" or "excellent" actually ingested more nutrients

Table 20.1 Average Age of Menarche in Different Countries at Different Periods of Time

Country	Age, in years		
	1850	1900	1950
Norway	17.0	15.5	13.5
Finland		16.0	13.5
United States		14.5	13.0
England			13.5

From P. A. Harper, *Preventive Pediatrics*, 1962. Courtesy of Appleton-Century-Crofts, Publishing Division of Prentice-Hall, Inc., Englewood Cliffs, N.J.

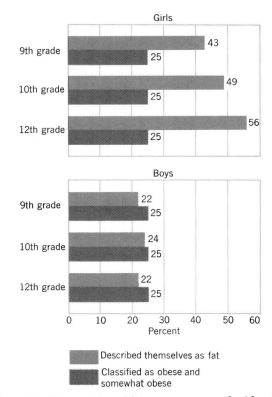

Fig. 20.1 Self-perception of fatness as compared with actual fatness. (From Huenemann, R. L., et al. (1966). A longitudinal study of gross body composition and body conformation and their association with food and activity in a teenage population, *Am. J. Clin. Nutrition*, 18: 332. Used by permission.)

Table 20.2 Percentage of Ninth and Eleventh Grade Students Who Mentioned the Following Foods When Asked: "What Foods Should be Eaten Every Day for Health?"

Food	Boys		Girls	
	9th grade (465)[a]	11th grade (426)	9th grade (519)	11th grade (425)
Fruits and vegetables	83.4	84.3	90.2	94.6
Meat	81.5	84.5	86.3	93.2
Milk	66.5	69.0	76.7	82.8
Grains	35.9	42.5	56.1	58.6
Sugars	9.5	9.4	10.0	10.8
Liquids	6.7	4.9	6.4	4.7
Fats	5.8	4.0	6.7	3.8
Vitamin supplements	0.6	2.4	0.6	1.4

[a] Numbers in parentheses indicate the number of students questioned.
From R. L. Huenemann et al., A longitudinal study of gross body composition and body conformation and their association with food and activity in a teenage population. *Am. J. Clin. Nutrition*, **18**: 329, (1966). Used by permission.

that reached at least two-thirds of the RDA than did those who rated their diets "poor" or "fair" (8).

Nutrient Needs and Intakes of Adolescents

Nutrient Requirements

The nutrient needs during adolescence are conditioned by the profound biological changes that characterize this period. Marked variations exist among individuals at the onset of the growth spurt and maturation. There are three characteristics that influence directly the nutritional requirements and vulnerability of the adolescent (10): (a) body mass nearly doubles during the adolescent spurt; (b) energy and protein needs are closely related to the growth spurt, thus the

amounts needed are at their peak in the life cycle (except during pregnancy and lactation); and (c) the increased rate of tissue synthesis raises the demand for energy to carry out the process, and the adolescent becomes highly sensitive to caloric restriction.

Very limited research studies have been conducted on the actual nutrient needs of adolescents. Many of the RDA values are at best, judgments and deductions drawn from studies of preadolescents and young adults.

The RDA for adolescents are presented in Table 20.3 under two age categories for girls and boys: 11–14 years and 15–18 years. Nutritional recommendations by sex begins at age 11 in the RDA table, and this separation recognizes gender and growth as important factors influencing nutrient needs. The age categories, however, do not reflect accurately the physiological events that characterize adolescence. For example, girls enter puberty at an earlier age than do boys (average of 13 years for girls, 15 years for boys), undergo the growth spurt sooner, and reach full physical growth at least two years earlier than boys do.

The energy needs of adolescents are difficult to estimate because of the wide variations among individuals in growth patterns, body build, and levels of activity. Chronological age or calendar age is not a reliable predictor of the total energy requirements. The increased demand for energy during the adolescent growth spurt is recognized (Table 20.3) and reflected in a significant reduction in the energy allowance after physical maturity is reached (Table 3.1).

Protein requirements, like energy and other nutrient needs, are greatly influenced by the growth pattern. Synthesis of tissue protein is at its height during the growth spurt and then diminishes as growth slows down. The suggested protein allowances per kilogram of body weight per day are 1.0 g for 11–14 years and 0.9 g for 15–18 years old.

Allowances for the vitamins during adolescence are based on fragmentary information. To meet growth and tissue needs, increased amounts of several vitamins are recommended (Table 20.3).

Table 20.3 RDA for Adolescents

Nutrient		Boys		Girls	
		11–14	15–18	11–14	15–18
Energy	kcal	2800	3000	2400	2100
Protein	g	44	54	44	48
Vitamin A	IU	5000	5000	4000	4000
Vitamin D	IU	400	400	400	400
Vitamin E	IU	12	15	12	12
Ascorbic Acid	mg	45	45	45	45
Folacin	mg	0.4	0.4	0.4	0.4
Vitamin B_{12}	μg	3	3	3	3
Niacin	mg	18	20	16	14
Riboflavin	mg	1.5	1.8	1.3	1.4
Thiamin	mg	1.4	1.5	1.2	1.1
Vitamin B_6	mg	1.6	2.0	1.6	2.0
Calcium	g	1.2	1.2	1.2	1.2
Phosphorus	g	1.2	1.2	1.2	1.2
Iodine	μg	130	150	115	115
Iron	mg	18	18	18	18
Magnesium	mg	350	400	300	300
Zinc	mg	15	15	15	15

From *Recommended Dietary Allowances, Eighth Edition.* Washington, D.C.: Natl. Acad. Sciences, 1974.

Balance studies are used to estimate calcium requirements, and results show that calcium absorption and retention are increased during the growth spurt (17). The calcium allowance of 1.2 g per day for both girls and boys takes into consideration the increased demands for adequate skeletal mineralization during the period of accelerated growth.

During adolescence, significant amounts of iron are needed for the rapid growth in muscle tissues, the increase in blood volume and respiratory enzymes, and the maintenance of adequate iron stores. In addition, puberty brings about menstruation in girls with its concomitant blood and iron losses. The recommended allowance for adolescent girls and boys is 18 mg of iron per day.

Other essential mineral elements have diverse functions that relate directly or indirectly to growth (19). They form part of many enzyme systems that catalyze metabolic reactions. Others assist in strengthening bones and teeth. In addition, they help in preserving the integrity of body cells. Therefore several macro- and micro-elements are essential for growth and development in adolescence.

Eating Patterns

Adolescents are notorious for their poor eating habits, and studies have shown that they generally consume the least satisfactory diets of all age groups in the United States (16). National surveys have shown that adolescent girls have poorer diets than their male peers do (11, 16, 22, 23, 24). The dietary habits of an adolescent usually reflect patterns developed in early childhood. Both family and school food-related practices influence greatly the eating behavior of the adolescent.

Some Nutritional Concerns of Adolescents

Obesity is a common nutritional problem in adolescents, especially among girls, and puberty is the most difficult time in life to shed excess body fat. During this critical period, the entire physiological mechanism is geared to promote growth, and any attempt to reverse its course may encounter resistance. Underactivity or low energy expenditure is often directly responsible for adolescent obesity (see Chapter 8), and prevention is better than treatment. For the obese teenager, a sensible weight-reduction program should place more emphasis on increased energy output than on food restriction at a stressful period in life. Establishment of regular physical activity and moderate dietary practices consistent with adequate growth would prepare the adolescent for attaining and maintaining desirable weight throughout adulthood (see Nutrition and Physical Activity, p. 460).

Overemphasis on slimness among teenage girls

449

may also lead to another health hazard. When adolescents, including those who are slim by nature, become obsessed by "dieting" to excessive degrees, a severe emotional and psychological disorder, *anorexia nervosa*, can occur (see Chapter 8). This condition requires prompt medical attention.

Adolescent pregnancy leads to extra demands for nutrients, and therefore increases the vulnerability of the individual toward nutritional deprivation. Girls who become pregnant before the age of 17 years are considered high biological and psychological risks (15). In the exceptionally young prospective mothers age 14 years and younger, it is difficult to distinguish adverse effects due to physical immaturity from those due to unfavorable socioeconomic and psychological conditions (21).

Because they are still growing and developing, pregnant teenagers require more energy and nutrients than any other group of women. A few studies have shown that foods selected by pregnant adolescents generally resemble those of their nonpregnant peers (13, 14). Diets consumed are usually low in calcium, iron, and vitamin A value. Caloric restriction imposed to control weight gain during pregnancy reduces significantly the mean dietary intakes of the essential nutrients (7). It is now recognized that the outcome of pregnancy may be improved by higher energy intakes than those previously considered adequate. The NRC Committee on Maternal Nutrition recommends a desirable average weight gain of 11 kg (24 lb) during pregnancy (15).

Nontraditional eating patterns are part of today's counterculture movements among adolescents and young adults (6). The most common unconventional dietary practices include vegetarian, "health," "natural," or "organic" eating styles. Many of these individuals are raising questions concerning established eating patterns and their wholesomeness. Do we need meat in our diet? Is milk the best source of calcium? Will an all-vegetarian diet cause illness? What are the effects of food additives on our health? As

they seek for answers to these and other questions, they try different diets. Some individuals experiment with a no-meat, no-processed food diets; others may adopt an all-vegetarian diet supplemented with dairy products and/or eggs. In some instances, however, meat is omitted from the diet for economic reasons; meat such as beef and pork are expensive food items. These types of meal patterns, especially the strict vegetarian diet (no foods from animal sources whatsoever), will require careful planning in order to provide adequate amounts of all the required nutrients (18) (see Chapter 7).

Teenage male athletes are notorious for their bizarre dietary practices to meet weight requirements for certain sports. Many adolescents may compromise their health and well-being by adopting hazardous practices (2). For example, weight reduction by restricting food and fluid intakes is a common way to lose weight rapidly. The practice of water deprivation shortly before an athletic event is potentially dangerous. It may be responsible for many tragic accidents such as collapse and even death during the stress of a game performance. Severe caloric restriction including total fasting or starvation may have adverse effects on the health of the teenage athlete. The young athlete needs careful guidance and counsel on nutritional practices that are compatible with good health and physical fitness (see Nutrition and Physical Activity p. 460).

The Young Adult

Nutritional Requirements

Early in young adulthood, physical maturation is completed and most body systems are well-established and functioning at optimum efficiency. The average body size attained in terms of stature and body weight is described by a set of standards. There are, however, limitations in the existing height–weight tables or standards (see Chapter 18).

Compared with other age groups, more basic information is available on the actual nutrient requirements of adults. The RDA for young women and men are given for age 19–22 years. The next older age grouping of 23–50 years extends beyond the arbitrary limits of young adulthood set at 25 to 45 years.

For ages 19 to 22 years, the allowances for most nutrients remain high, except for significant reductions in calcium and phosphorus needs of both sexes (Table 3.1). Protein requirements per kilogram of body weight drop from 0.9 g daily for the younger age group to 0.8 g daily for adults. Requirements for iron and magnesium decrease for young men but not for young women. Beyond age 22, energy allowances are reduced progressively, and the needs for calorie-related nutrients (thiamin, riboflavin, niacin) also diminish.

Pregnancy and Lactation

Throughout the life cycle, there are critical periods that deserve special attention to achieve and maintain optimum health. Pregnancy and lactation represent such stages when nutrient demands increase the vulnerability of childbearing women to nutritional inadequacies.

Pregnancy

Pregnancy is a normal physiological process, "an integrated maternal-cum-fetal system undergoing progressive change. In order that the growth of the product of conception may be safeguarded even under conditions of environmental stress, change in ordinary physiological functions is not merely normal, but necessary" (16).

During pregnancy the maternal body is protected by powerful physiological safeguards in the form of extensive adjustments in metabolism (14). These metabolic adjustments are widespread and varied and complex in nature. Many changes occur early in pregnancy in preparation for increased fetal demands during the later stages of gestation (see p. 411, Fetal Growth). For example, maternal storage of fat increases in midpregnancy to meet the energy needs for fetal growth and lactation.

Concentrations of most nutrients and metabolites in the blood fall progressively during pregnancy—most of the amino acids, glucose, vitamins C, B-6, B-12, and folic acid; some constituent levels increase—serum total lipids, triglyceride, cholesterol, and phospholipids (19).

Many body functions are altered in pregnancy (14). Cardiac output rises steadily, and blood flow increases with the kidneys and the skin as major targets. The increased blood flow promotes efficient elimination of soluble waste materials through the kidneys; heat is dissipated through the skin. Often times, pregnant women complain of the heat and usually can tolerate the cold better than a warm surrounding temperature. Gastric motility and muscle tone of the gastrointestinal tract are reduced, and these changes contribute to constipation. Intestinal absorption is improved for some nutrients such as iron. Total body water increases considerably, and most, if not all, of the water gained is lost six to eight weeks after delivery. These and many other metabolic adjustments are undoubtedly related to the extensive hormonal changes associated with the reproductive period. *Homeostatic controls* in the body are reset, but the precise mechanisms involved in these metabolic adjustments are poorly understood. Therefore in healthy pregnant women clinical and laboratory indices of *nutritional status* must be interpreted on the basis of standard values obtained for pregnant women rather than on values from nonpregnant individuals (19).

Diet and Pregnancy

If a woman remains healthy during pregnancy, gives birth to a healthy, full-term baby, is capable of satisfactory lactation, and shows normal recovery, then her diet, by definition, is nutritionally adequate (14). Survey studies of pregnant women examined associations between nutrient intakes and clinical information, such as pattern of weight gain during pregnancy, condition of the mother during gestation, labor, and delivery, and the condition of the infant at birth.

Results of dietary and clinical investigations of pregnant women are contradictory. Pioneering studies of Ebbs and her coworkers in Toronto (8) and by Burke and her collaborators (6) in Boston showed that the nutritive quality of the prenatal diet frequently affects the course of pregnancy and the condition of the infant at birth. At the prenatal clinic of the Boston Lying-in Hospital, women with good or excellent diets (31 cases) suffered fewer complications and less difficulties during pregnancy and labor than did women with poor diets; almost all of their babies (94 percent) rated good or superior in physical condition. Ebbs et al. and later groups of investigators (7, 18) confirmed the findings of Burke and coworkers.

Other studies, however, failed to demonstrate any positive association between improved dietary intake and successful outcome of pregnancy. Based on rigorously designed surveys, both the Vanderbilt group in Tennessee (20) and the Aberdeen group in Scotland (28) obtained predominantly negative results. Thomson and his Aberdeen coworkers concluded in 1959 that "the diets of pregnant women can vary widely, in quantity as well as in quality, without clinically obvious impairment of the reproductive process. But although the importance of diet in pregnancy is usually inconspicuous in terms of the individual mother and child, the same is not necessarily true in terms of large populations."

Wartime observations in Leningrad, Russia and in Holland during World War II are often cited as evidence of the adverse effects of maternal malnutrition on pregnancy performance (21). Periods of acute starvation or semistarvation were associated with a significant drop in fertility rate, birth weight, and *perinatal* survival. Considerable economic, environmental, and psychological stresses characterized wartime, and these factors undoubtedly contributed to the decline in reproductive efficiency of the women.

Several factors complicate studies of diet and pregnancy outcome. The effects of diet during pregnancy cannot be isolated from those that arise from unfavorable socioeconomic circumstances (poor living conditions, lack of medical care and good hygiene, and limited education). The size of the nutritional reserves of prospective mothers may also modify the course of pregnancy. Unusual psychological and physiological stresses may have adverse effects on reproductive performance, and these conditions often accompany adolescent pregnancy (see p. 450). Many of these factors cannot be controlled in studies of human population groups.

Experimental animals, particularly the rat, are used in studies of dietary influences on pregnancy. Recent investigations have shown that dietary restriction of either energy or protein during pregnancy profoundly affects maternal metabolic adjustments and fetal growth and development (21). Similar experiments involving dietary manipulations that may harm the fetus cannot be used in human studies because of ethical considerations and methodological problems.

There still is much to be learned regarding the precise role of diet during pregnancy. Current knowledge indicates that the chances for successful childbearing are improved greatly if women consumed adequate diets from infancy to maturity. Favorable living circumstances would also contribute significantly to increased reproductive efficiency by providing opportunities for regular medical and health care, and education.

Nutritional Requirements During Pregnancy

Energy Needs and Weight Gain   An adequate intake of energy during pregnancy is critical to meet the extra demands for (a) the formation of new tissues in the mother and fetus, (b) the elevation of metabolism incurred by increments of

Table 20.4 Components of Weight Gained During Normal Pregnancy[a,b]

	Increase in weight (g) up to:			
	10 weeks	20 weeks	30 weeks	40 weeks
Fetus	5	300	1500	3300
Placenta	20	170	430	650
Amniotic fluid	30	250	600	800
Uterus	135	585	810	900
Mammary gland	34	180	360	405
Maternal blood	100	600	1300	1250
Not accounted for	326	1915	3500	5195
Observed total gain	650	4000	8500	12,500

[a] Modified from Hytten, F. E., and I. Leitch (1964). *The Physiology of Human Pregnancy.* Oxford, England: Blackwell Scientific Publications.
[b] Values are for well-fed Scottish women with a gain of 12.5 kg during pregnancy.
From *Nutrition in Pregnancy and Lactation,* WHO Tech. Rept. Series 302. Geneva: World Health Organ., 1965, p. 21.

new tissues, and (c) moving additional body mass associated with physical activity (5). Some investigators believe that the extra cost of physical effort during pregnancy is minimal and may be offset by a reduction in physical activity, especially in the third trimester (9, 14). Because of the wide variability in the energy expenditures of pregnant women, the adequacy of energy intake is judged by a satisfactory pattern of weight gain during gestation.

Although physicians advise different weight gains during pregnancy, the Committee on Maternal Nutrition (21) recommends an average gain of 11 kg (24 lb), whereas the British group suggests 12.5 kg (27.5 lb). The pattern of weight gain during normal pregnancy is shown in Table 20.4. Weight gains associated with the fetal (fetus, placenta, *amniotic fluid*) and the maternal compartments (uterus, mammary gland, blood) vary with the different stages of pregnancy. In the early phase of pregnancy, the weight increments of the various components are minimal. At 20 weeks of gestation, most of the gain reflects increases in the maternal components. In the final phase, the predominant gain involves the fetal compartment.

At 40 weeks, approximately 1 kg of the unexplained gain of about 5 kg may be water and the rest is assumed to be fat. These extra fat deposits may serve to subsidize lactation.

A slow, steady weight gain reflects normal progress of the mother and fetus. The approximate pattern of weight gain is as follows: about 0.9 kg (2 lb) for the first 10 weeks, about 5 kg (10 lb) by 20 weeks, 9 kg (20 lb) in 30 weeks, and 11 to 14 kg (25 to 30 lb) at term.

If the pregnant woman is slightly overweight or obese, weight gain must be carefully monitored by adjusting both intake and expenditure of energy. Efforts should be made to promote increments of nonfatty tissue while minimizing further deposition of fat. The Committee on Maternal Nutrition questions the advisability of imposing weight reduction measures during pregnancy (21). Family planning should give obese women the opportunity to attain desirable weight before conception. Underweight women who become pregnant also need careful nutritional guidance to achieve satisfactory weight gain.

The size of the baby is affected both by the mother's weight gain during pregnancy and by

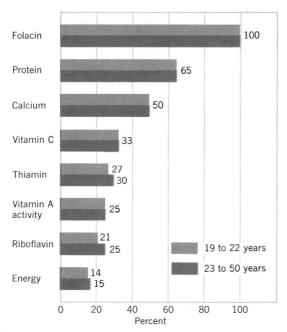

Fig. 20.2 Percentage increase in the Recommended Dietary Allowances for women during pregnancy above the usual allowances for women. (Adapted from *Recommended Dietary Allowances, Eighth Edition*, Natl. Acad. Sci.—Natl. Research Council. Washington, D.C.: Natl. Research Council, 1974.)

her pregravid weight (4). It has been found that the average weight of a baby born to a woman who gains less than 4.5 kg (10 lb) during pregnancy will weigh about 0.45 kg (1 lb) less than a baby born to a woman who gains 18.0 kg (40 lb) (21). In a study of Scottish women, Hytten and Leitch found that short women gave birth to babies who were about 8 percent lighter than those of tall women, and underweight women gave birth to babies who were about 8 percent lighter than those of overweight women. Women who were both short and light gave birth to babies who were about 14 percent lighter than those of tall and heavy women (23).

The recommended allowance for energy (26) is an additional 300 kcal (1260 kJ) a day during pregnancy over the usual allowance for non-pregnant women. This increase represents 14 percent for the 19-to-22-year group and 15 percent for those 23 years and older. The increments for energy are much less than those for most nutrients (Fig. 20.2). Consequently, the diet for a pregnant woman must be planned carefully to include foods of *high-nutrient density*.

Protein   The need for protein during pregnancy is greatly increased (see Table 3.1). About 950 g of protein accumulates in the mother's body during pregnancy, most of which is added during the last 6 months (an increment of 5 g per day). The RDA is an additional 30 g of protein daily over the normal allowance, or a total of 76 g daily.

Calcium   At birth the baby's body has about 22 g of calcium, most of which is deposited during the last month. The fetus accumulates calcium at about 50 mg per day during the third month; 120 mg daily during the seventh month, and 450 mg per day during the last month.

The daily dietary needs for calcium have been determined by balance studies. For women who are in a state of good nutrition before pregnancy, the RDA is 400 mg per day more than the usual allowance, or a daily total of 1200 mg (26). During pregnancy more calcium is retained than is believed to be needed by the fetal and maternal tissues. Such storage is important, for during lactation the diet often does not supply enough calcium to meet that requirement. Women who have been undernourished before pregnancy should try to increase their intake of calcium, protein, and other nutrients throughout pregnancy.

The bodies of women accustomed to a low intake of calcium (400 mg daily) attempt to adjust to it. When the need is greatest (during the last 6 months of pregnancy) they use the mineral more efficiently: absorption from the intestine is increased and excretion in the urine is decreased (27).

454

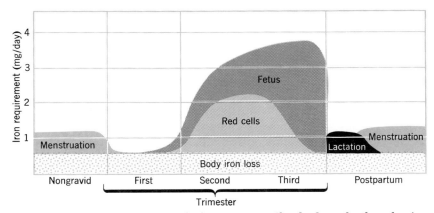

Fig. 20.3 Daily iron requirements during pregnancy (for the fetus, for the enlarging red cell mass, and for that which is being excreted) and during lactation. (Courtesy Bothwell, T. H., and C. A. Finch (1962). *Iron Metabolism.* Boston: Little, Brown, p. 309.)

Iron Pregnancy requires substantial amounts of iron, especially during the last six months (Fig. 20.3). For the last stage of pregnancy, the iron requirements may reach about 4 mg per day. In addition to iron that is required for the fetus and the increased red cell mass, extra iron is needed to replace that which is being excreted (Table 20.5). To satisfy these needs, about 3.5 mg of iron should be absorbed each day (2).

The average adult woman has about 300 mg of iron stored in her body (11), and this amount is not enough to meet the additional needs for fetal development and to cover losses during delivery. Normally, iron absorption is approximately 10 percent of the dietary intake. With pregnancy, however, the efficiency of iron absorption increases progressively and reaches a peak of 25 percent in the third trimester (10). The average American diet supplies about 6 mg of iron per 1000 kcal, and the pregnant woman consumes 13 to 14 mg of iron daily (21). Even with the increased efficiency in iron absorption, diet alone will not provide enough iron to satisfy the needs of normal pregnant women. The RDA of 18 + mg of iron during pregnancy cannot be met by dietary sources alone (see Chapter 14 on micronutrients). Supplementation of the diet with 30 to

Table 20.5 Iron Requirements During the Second and Third Trimesters

Needs	Trimester	
	Second	Third
	mg	mg
Excretion	55	55
Red cell mass increase	133	67
Fetus	75	200
Total	263	322

Data from T. H. Bothwell and C. A. Finch, (1962). *Iron Metabolism* (Boston: Little, Brown) p. 308. Copyright © 1962 by Little, Brown and Company. Used by permission.

60 mg of elemental iron is recommended for the last six months of pregnancy and simple ferrous salts are often used (21).

Other minerals Additional amounts of phosphorus, iodine, magnesium, and zinc are recommended during pregnancy.

Vitamins Although the need for vitamins during pregnancy has not been studied as thor-

455

oughly as has the need for protein and minerals, undoubtedly the requirement for vitamins too is increased (Table 3.1). The RDA for folacin during pregnancy is increased 100 percent over the nonpregnant values (Fig. 20.2). There is widespread interest in folacin deficiency and its possible relationship to megaloblastic anemia (21, 24) and to a variety of complications during pregnancy (1). Although megaloblastic anemia of pregnancy due to folate deficiency is not common in the U.S., it is believed that folic acid supplements would reduce the incidence of this type of nutritional anemia, especially in high-risk groups such as the low socioeconomic class and those with multiple pregnancies. The relationship between folate deficiency and obstetric complications is still not clear.

Vitamins and mineral supplements are often routinely prescribed for pregnancy or lactation or both. Their value is questionable, with the exception of iron and possibly folacin supplements (25). These supplements are not necessary if the pregnant woman consumes an adequate diet, is healthy, and does not show a specific clinical sign of need for additional nutrients.

Lactation

The amount of nutrients needed by the mother depends primarily upon the quantity of milk secreted; this capacity is a highly individual characteristic. The secretion of milk may be diminished (or even suppressed completely) by such emotional factors as excitement, fear, or anxiety. Another factor that affects secretion is "demand." The breast must be completely emptied at each nursing in order to maintain secretion. If the infant does not take it all, the residual portion must be removed by hand (or pump) in order to assure continued secretion.

In establishing an RDA, it is assumed that the mother will secrete about 850 ml of milk per day. Actually the amount varies considerably from one woman to another. On the average, the mother who is able to nurse her infant secretes about one-half a liter of milk a day during the first week or two; this amount increases to as much as one liter a day by the fifth month.

The first milk secreted is colostrum. It is light yellow in color and contains more protein and minerals and less fat and sugar than milk. Colostrum is an excellent food but, insofar as is known, contains nothing that is indispensable to the newborn. Gradually the composition of the milk changes so that after about 10 days the milk is called "mature" milk to differentiate it from colostrum.

Nutritional Needs

The RDA for lactation are in Table 3.1, and the percentage increments in the allowances are shown in Fig. 20.4.

Energy The RDA is an additional 500 kcal (2092 kJ) above the normal allowance. Since the average energy value of human milk is 70 kcal (293 kJ) per 100 ml, and since the secretion averages 850 ml daily, approximately 600 kcal (2510 kJ) is secreted in milk. An assessment of human requirements during lactation indicates that probably the physiological process of forming milk requires only a limited expenditure of energy.

British investigators (29) found that the daily energy need during lactation was an additional 600 kcal (2510 kJ). The diets (weighed during a 7-day period, between the sixth and seventeenth week postpartum) of 23 lactating mothers were about 600 kcal (2510 kJ) per day more than the diets of 32 nonlactating mothers. The average energy value of the milk secreted (estimated from the weight gain of the babies) was approximately 600 kcal (2510 kJ) per day. Both groups (the lactating and nonlactating) were losing weight. It was assumed that they were losing the fat that they had accumulated during pregnancy. The maternal fat stores that accumulate during pregnancy provide additional energy sources to help meet the

456

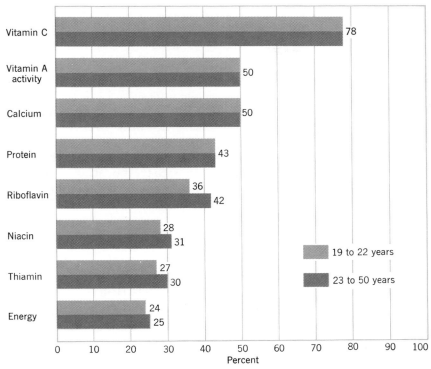

Fig. 20.4 Percentage increase in the Recommended Dietary Allowances for women during lactation above the usual allowances for women. (Adapted from *Recommended Dietary Allowances, Eighth Edition,* Natl. Acad. Sci.—Natl. Research Council. Washington, D.C.: Natl. Research Council, 1974.)

high energy cost of lactation for the first three months. A mother who does not breast feed her baby will have to adjust her energy intake in order to reattain her body weight before pregnancy. A recent study (22) showed that a weight loss of about 3 kg over three months was achieved by a group of nonlactating mothers through conscious restriction of food intake to an average of 2000 kcal (8368 kJ). In the breast feeding group, a similar weight loss occurred at an average intake of 2900 kcal (12,133 kJ).

Protein The RDA for protein during lactation is 10 g a day less than the allowance during pregnancy and 20 g a day more than the ordinary al-

lowance (Table 3.1). This recommendation was made by assuming that the average daily secretion is 850 ml (with an upper limit of 1200 ml). Since human milk contains about 1.1 g of protein per 100 ml, it was estimated that the mother at the upper limit of milk production needed about 15 g daily. In order to allow for the varying quality of protein in the diet, this figure was raised to 20 g a day. Another method of computing the additional protein needed during lactation is to consider the efficiency of converting food protein into milk protein. Hytten and Thomson (15) have suggested an 80 percent efficiency; thus, to produce 15 g of milk protein a day, about 20 g of food protein per day is needed.

There is some evidence that an adequate intake

457

of protein during pregnancy (about 75 g daily) and lactation (about 65 g daily) will help the production of milk (15). It has also been observed that lactating Indian women who have a low protein intake (below 34.4 g per day) also have less protein in their milk. However, except when the intake is very low to begin with, increased protein consumption will not alter the composition of the milk (13).

Mineral Elements and Vitamins Additional amounts of calcium are particularly important during lactation, and the intake must be adjusted to individual milk secretion. Some lactating mothers with a high milk yield may lose as much as 1 g of calcium per day through the milk, and they would require increased dietary calcium. The estimated calcium content of human milk is 250 mg per day during early lactation and about 300 mg after 3 months of lactation (12).

The RDA for iron during lactation of 18 mg per day is the same as for all women of reproductive age. Between 1 and 1.5 mg of iron is secreted in human milk per day. Assuming that about 10 percent of the dietary iron is absorbed, 18 mg per day should be adequate. Diets, however, must be carefully planned to include foods high in iron as well as foods that would help increase iron absorption, such as meat (animal protein) and citrus fruits (vitamin C).

The quantity of vitamins needed by the mother depends upon the amount of milk secreted. Human milk has a mean vitamin A activity of about 190 IU per 100 ml. Assuming that the secretion is 850 ml daily, the output of vitamin A in the milk would be about 1600 IU. To help ensure a high level of vitamin A in the milk, the RDA for vitamin A activity is 6000 IU daily, or 2000 IU more than the normal allowance.

Based on very little research, the recommended intake per day is 400 IU. The vitamin D content of milk does not seem to be especially affected by diet. However, in general the amounts of the different vitamins in the mother's diet greatly influence their concentrations in her milk. Available information shows that the composition of breast milk is not constant. It varies from mother to mother, with the stage of lactation, and with some constitutents in the mother's diet (30).

Fluid Intake When milk secretion is insufficient, mothers are often advised to drink large amounts of fluids to increase the milk supply. Thirst is commonly experienced by mothers when breast feeding their babies and intakes of fluids (water, tea, and coffee) to satisfy the needs would be adequate. Studies have shown that forcing increased quantities of fluids will neither increase the quantity of milk produced nor improve its quality (17).

Recommended Dietary Pattern in Pregnancy and Lactation

Ideally the following foods should be eaten each day during pregnancy and lactation:

1. Milk: 1 quart of whole or skim milk fortified with 400 IU of vitamin D.

2. Lean meat, poultry, or fish: 1 liberal serving of about 4 oz (115 g) or 2 small servings, 2 oz each (60 g).

3. Egg: 1 each day.

4. Fruits and vegetables: 5 or more servings which should include citrus fruit or other good source of vitamin C, 1 serving each day; dark-green or deep-yellow vegetable, 1 serving each day; other fruits and vegetables, 3 or more servings each day. (One serving of fruit and vegetable is equal to $\frac{1}{2}$ cup cooked, canned, frozen, or $\frac{1}{2}$ cup of vegetable or fruit juice, or 1 medium fresh fruit or vegetable.)

5. Bread and cereals: whole-grain or enriched, 4 servings daily. (One serving is equal to 1 regular slice of bread, or one-half cup cooked cereal, or three-fourths cup dry cereal.)

6. Additional foods including either more of the foods from the groups listed above or other preferred foods. Amounts of these extra foods must be adjusted to meet energy needs of the

458

individual to promote satisfactory weight gain during pregnancy. In lactation, caloric intake will depend upon the energy demands for milk production and for extra activity associated with the care of the infant. After breast feeding, the mother must readjust food intake downwards to maintain desirable body weight.

Every effort must be made to include at least one good source of iron in the daily diet during pregnancy. These foods are organ meats (liver, heart, kidney), dark-green leafy vegetables (greens, spinach), eggs, oysters and clams, dried beans (navy and pinto), raisins and dried apricots, whole-grain or enriched cereals.

Liquid intake (water, coffee, tea) must be adequate and the use of iodized rather than non-iodized salt is recommended.

The pregnant woman should consult her physician at an early date about her dietary needs. Many chemical compounds ingested by a lactating mother either intentionally or unintentionally are excreted in her milk in varying amounts and forms. Because of possible potential hazards for the nursing baby, mothers while breast-feeding are advised against the use of the following drugs: any drug or chemical in excessive amounts, oral contraceptives, *diuretics, atropine, reserpine, anticoagulants, steroids, hallucinogens,* bromides, radioactive preparations, morphine and its derivatives, *anthraquinones,* and *antimetabolites* (3).

Oral Contraceptives and Nutrient Requirements

Oral contraceptives are widely used by women of childbearing age in the United States and other developed countries. Several types of hormonal contraceptive preparations are available, and the most commonly used variety consists of combinations of different *estrogens* and *progestogens.* They are administered in varying dosage, sequence, frequency, and duration.

A wide range of metabolic effects has been attributed to the use of hormonal contraceptives (1) and these effects, in turn, may alter nutrient requirements. These metabolic disturbances are reflected in changes in the concentrations of nutrients and their metabolites or enzymes in the blood, urine, and tissues. Some of these changes, however, may represent metabolic adaptations to these contraceptive drugs (4).

Hormonal contraception has been associated with alterations in the metabolism of all the nutrients—carbohydrate, lipid, protein, vitamins, minerals, and water (1, 2, 3, 5). *Glucose tolerance* is impaired; serum concentrations of *triglyceride, cholesterol, phospholipids,* and *lecithin* are elevated; and serum concentrations of albumin and several amino acids are reduced while the globulins rise. Roe (4) summarized some of the metabolic effects of the drugs on vitamins and minerals (Table 20.6).

Table 20.6 Nutritional Aberrations Attributed to Contraceptive Steroids

Nutrient	Effect
Folacin	Serum level decreased
	Erythrocyte level decreased
	Megaloblastic anemia (rare)
Vitamin B_{12}	Serum level decreased
Riboflavin	Erythrocyte level decreased
	Glossitis (rare)
Vitamin B_6	Disturbed tryptophan metabolism
	Depression
Ascorbic acid	Leukocyte content decreased
	Platelet level decreased
Vitamin A	Plasma level increased
Iron	Serum level increased
	*TIBC increased
Copper	Plasma copper increased
	Ceruloplasmin increased
Zinc	Plasma zinc decreased

Adapted from D. Roe, Nutrition and the contraceptive pill. In *Nutritional Disorders of American Women,* edited by M. Winick, (New York: John Wiley and Sons, 1977) p. 44.
* Total iron-binding composition (blood).

459

The use of oral contraceptives increases nutrient requirements by (a) decreasing absorption, (b) increasing urinary excretion, and/or (c) mobilizing tissue stores of nutrients. The mechanisms involved in these changes are not known. It is believed that users of oral contraceptives are nutritionally vulnerable when their nutritional status is marginal or poor.

Some women on hormonal contraceptives gain weight, whereas others show no significant weight changes. The gain in weight may be related to retention of either fluid or nitrogen.

The interaction between hormonal contraceptives and nutrition is complicated by the differences in composition and mode of administration of these drugs. It is also possible that metabolic adaptations occur with prolonged use of these preparations. The long-term nutritional and health consequences of the metabolic changes need to be assessed.

Based on the available information, supplementation with vitamins and minerals will depend upon the nutritional state of the oral contraceptive user. If nutritional status is marginal, the use of appropriate supplements, particularly folacin, is advocated. *Fortification* of foods such as breakfast cereals has also been suggested as a possible preventive measure against adverse metabolic effects of oral contraceptives (5).

Nutrition and Physical Activity

Good habits of nutrition and physical activity or exercise contribute significantly to the attainment and maintenance of optimum health throughout the life cycle. The active nature of young children has not changed, but this inclination needs to be nurtured from late childhood through adolescence and extended to late adulthood. A sensible program of eating and exercise must be started at an early age and continued throughout life with appropriate adjustments as age advances and needs, interests, and capabilities change.

The health benefits from a regular exercise program are many and varied. Physical activity brings about physiological adaptations for achieving and maintaining optimum physical fitness. These special adaptations allow the body to increase cardiac output, and acquire muscular strength (6). Body composition may be modified by exercise so that the ratio of lean tissues to body fat is increased. In a group of sedentary middle-aged men, a vigorous walking program for 20 weeks improved cardiovascular function significantly; total body weight and percentage of body fat were reduced slightly (12). Older men in their seventies who have maintained a lifelong program of intensive physical exercise showed a higher lean mass than nonactive men in their sixties, and these two age groups exhibited similar muscle strength (8). During periods of physical training, athletes gained more lean tissues at the expense of body fat, but when physical training diminished, enhanced fat deposition occurred (11).

Because of the predominant contribution of physical activity to the total energy expenditure, a regular exercise program has a significant role in controlling body weight. Prolonged periods of inactivity have been associated with the development of obesity, a major health hazard (see Chapter 8). There also is the possibility that regular physical activity involving significant improvement in cardiovascular function may help reduce the risk of coronary heart disease.

Fuel for Muscular Work Carbohydrate and fat are the major sources of fuel for the working skeletal muscles. Their percentage of contribution is related to the intensity and duration of the physical activity (2, 3, 4). For light to moderate exercise, carbohydrate and fat each contributes about half of the muscle energy; with prolonged work at the same level of intensity, increasing amounts of fat are used. During strenuous exercise, the oxygen supply becomes limited, and carbohydrate serves as the dominant source of fuel for muscular work.

At high rates of energy expenditure, muscle *glycogen* is used preferentially for work, particularly in endurance events lasting for 30 minutes or more. Studies have shown that physical performance improves with increased stores of muscle glycogen (3, 4). The glycogen reserves are built up by a process called glycogen loading. A week before an endurance event, muscle glycogen is exhausted by a combined regimen of vigorous exercise and a diet high in protein and fat but low in carbohydrate for three or four days. After depletion, glycogen reserves are replenished to amounts exceeding normal levels by consuming a high carbohydrate diet, while keeping activity relatively low. This dietary regimen, however, may have adverse effects on physical performance and health (5, 10) and expert advice is necessary.

Diets During Athletic Training The athlete in training needs the usual well-balanced diet with calories adjusted to meet the high demands for energy. Optimum fluid intake is also essential during periods of increased physical exertion. Intakes of sodium from salt (sodium chloride) also need to be carefully monitored so that losses of this important mineral through sweat can be adequately replaced (see Chapter 15). Excessive intakes of salt, however, must be avoided because water requirement is increased, which leads to fluid retention and subsequent impairment of physical performance. This type of dietary pattern should contribute significantly to maximum physical performance during competition.

As energy intake is increased by the consumption of nutritionally adequate diets, intakes of protein and essential vitamins and minerals are also increased concomitantly. Therefore supplementary sources of these nutrients are not necessary during physical training and conditioning. There is no evidence that massive doses of protein, vitamins, and/or minerals will improve athletic performance (9). Excessive intakes of water-soluble vitamins are wasteful, and daily supplements of large quantities of fat-soluble vitamin A may be harmful (see Chapters 9, 10, 11, and 12).

Diet Before and During Competition Considerable controversy exists regarding the types of food that should be eaten before competition, and bizarre eating practices are common. A suggested sensible diet before competition (13) should emphasize light, balanced meals that are high in carbohydrate but limited in protein and fat. Meals must be eaten at regular intervals approximately three hours before the event to allow proper digestion and absorption. Optimum fluid intake is essential to prevent dehydration. In addition to water, fruit juices and noncarbonated fruit-flavored drinks are recommended. Food preferences of the athlete should be considered in planning the meals to help make the individual a winner. Fluids and electrolyte replacements are the main dietary concerns during competition, particularly in prolonged athletic events.

Dehydration and Starvation For some sports, such as wrestling, "making weight" to lower range classifications is a frequent practice. Weight loss is accomplished by severely restricted intakes of fluids and food, and by using thermal (examples: steam rooms, saunas, and rubber suits) and exercise procedures. Most of the weight loss occurs a few days or a day before the official "weigh-in" (a specified time interval immediately preceding the competition). Dehydration through sweating is the method most frequently selected for rapid weight loss, and this approach upsets both the fluid and electrolyte balance (see Chapter 15).

Dehydration and starvation, used singly or in combination, are generally associated with impaired body functions and reduced muscular per-

461

formance (1). In the classic Minnesota study of conscientious objectors on a semistarvation regimen, a loss of 25 percent of the body weight diminished work performance, endurance, and strength of the large skeletal muscles (7). For the adolescent athlete, normal growth and development may be adversely affected by these weight-loss procedures.

The potential hazards created by the methods used to "make weight" by wrestlers have been recognized, and the American College of Sports Medicine (1) issued guidelines for a sound weight loss program which include the following:

1. Assess the body composition of each wrestler several weeks before the competitive season. Individuals with body fat below 5 percent of the certified body weight should receive medical clearance before they are allowed to compete.

2. Emphasize that the daily caloric needs should be supplied by a well-balanced diet and estimated on the basis of age, body size, and level of physical activity.

3. Discourage the practice of fluid deprivation and dehydration by (a) educating coaches and wrestlers on the health hazards associated with such practices, and (b) prohibiting the single or combined use of rubber suits, hot boxes, sauna, steam rooms, diuretics, and laxatives to "make weight."

Summary

Extensive physiological and behavioral changes occur during adolescence which influence greatly the nutritional needs. Accelerated physical growth and maturation in adolescence increase the demands for energy and essential nutrients. The increased rate of tissue synthesis requires additional energy input, and the teenager becomes highly vulnerable to energy deficits. Teenage girls tend to become obsessed by "dieting" for slimness, and teenage male athletes adopt dangerous dietary practices to meet weight classification for certain sports. These individuals need careful nutritional guidance on controlling body weight.

When physical growth and maturation are completed in early adulthood, most of the body systems are functioning at optimum efficiency. The healthy young woman becomes fully equipped for pregnancy.

Pregnancy is associated with extensive metabolic adjustments that serve as physiological safeguards to protect the maternal body and the developing fetus. Extra energy and nutrients are needed for the increased synthesis of maternal and fetal tissues. Both intake and expenditure of energy must be carefully adjusted to promote a satisfactory pattern of weight gain. If a mother does not breast-feed her baby, she will need to readjust her energy intake and output to achieve and maintain desirable weight. The amounts of nutrients needed during lactation will depend upon the volume of milk produced by the mother. The use of oral contraceptives may alter the nutrient requirements.

For optimum physical performance, the athlete needs a well-balanced normal diet with calories adjusted to meet the high demands for energy. As the energy intake is increased, intakes of protein and essential vitamins and minerals also increase. Therefore extra nutrients from supplements are not necessary during physical conditioning and training. Optimum intakes of water and salt (sodium chloride) are also essential during strenuous physical activity.

Glossary

amniotic fluid: the fluid secreted by the amnion (innermost membrane enclosing the developing fetus); it immerses the fetus and thereby cushions it against injury.

anorexia nervosa: a serious nervous condition in which

an individual loses appetite, eats little food, and becomes greatly emaciated.

anthraquinone: a yellow substance from a coal tar product.

anticoagulant: any substance that inhibits the blood-clotting mechanism.

antimetabolite: a substance bearing a close structural resemblance to one required for normal physiological functioning, and exerting its desired effect perhaps by replacing or interfering with the utilization of the essential metabolite.

atropine: an alkaloid from belladonna used in a variety of conditions; actions include relaxation of smooth muscles and increased heart rate.

cholesterol: see p. 79.

diuretic: a substance that promotes the excretion of urine; diuretic drugs are used chiefly to rid the body of excess fluid.

estrogen: a general name for the principal female sex hormones.

fortification: see p. 378.

glucose tolerance: see p. 308.

glycogen: see p. 49.

hallucinogen: an agent that produces hallucinations or false sensory perceptions.

high-nutrient density: a high proportion of a specific nutrient to total kilocalories in a given amount of food.

homeostasis: keeping constant body conditions.

homeostatic controls: mechanisms that regulate homeostasis.

lecithin: a phospholipid found in many animal tissues.

menarche: the establishment of menstrual function.

nutritional status: health of an individual as influenced by the quality of foods eaten and the ability of the body to utilize these foods to meet its needs.

obesity: the accumulation of body fat beyond the amount needed for good health.

perinatal: fetal period and first 30 days after birth.

phospholipid: see p. 70.

progestogen: substances that induce changes in the lining of the uterus preparatory to gestation.

puberty: the period between the time of appearance of secondary sex characteristics and the completion of body growth.

reserpine: an active alkaloid from Rauwolfia species,

used as an antihypertensive, tranquilizer, and sedative.

steroid: a group name for compounds that resemble cholesterol chemically.

triglyceride (fat): see p. 80.

Study Questions and Activities

1. Why do adolescent girls generally have poorer food habits than do their male peers? How does your eating pattern compare with that of the adolescent girl (or boy, if you are a male)?

2. Compare the energy and nutrient needs of adolescent girls with those of boys. Give reasons for the similarities and differences.

3. What weight reduction practices are common among adolescent girls and boys? Are they nutritionally and medically acceptable? Give reasons to support your answer. Why do adolescents need expert nutritional guidance in matters relating to weight reduction?

4. Give reasons why an adolescent who becomes pregnant before 17 years of age may have serious nutritional problems.

5. Plan a day's menu for a pregnant adolescent of average weight who has a limited income. If she chooses to nurse her baby for about three months, what foods and how much should she include in her diet? When she stops breast-feeding her baby, what adjustments should she make in her eating pattern and why?

6. Are vitamin and mineral supplements necessary for healthy pregnant women? Give reasons to support your answer.

7. How do the nutritional requirements of young adults differ from those of adolescents? Give reasons for the differences.

References

Adolescence

1. Cheek, D. B. (1968). *Human Growth.* Philadelphia: Lea and Febiger, p. 544.

2. Consolazio, C. F. (1976). Physical activity and

463

performance of the adolescent. In *Nutrient Requirements in Adolescence*, edited by J. I. McKigney and H. N. Munro. Cambridge: The Massachusetts Institute of Technology Press. p. 203.

3. Dwyer, J. T., J. J. Feldman, and J. Mayer (1964). Adolescent dieters: Who are they? *Am. J. Clin. Nutrition*, **20**: 1045.

4. Dwyer, J. T., J. J. Feldman, C. C. Seltzer, and J. Mayer (1969). Adolescent attitudes toward weight and appearance. *J. Nutrition Educ.*, **1**: 14.

5. Falkner, F. (1962). Some physical growth standards for white North American children. *Pediatrics*, **29**: 467.

6. Frankle, R. T., and F. K. Heussenstamm (1974). Food zealotry and youth. New dilemmas for professionals. *Am. J. Publ. Health*, **64**: 11.

7. Garcia, P. A., W. D. Brewer, and C. W. Merritt (1973). Nutritional status of adolescent primigravidae: I. Dietary characteristics during pregnancy and postpartum. *Iowa State J. Research*, **48**: 193.

8. Hampton, M. C., R. L. Huenemann, L. R. Shapiro, and B. W. Mitchell (1967). Caloric and nutrient intakes of teen-agers. *J. Am. Dietet. Assoc.*, **50**: 385.

9. Hampton, M. C., R. L. Huenemann, L. R. Shapiro, B. W. Mitchell, and A. R. Behnke (1966). A longitudinal study of gross body composition and body conformation and their association with food and activity in a teen-age population. Anthropometric evaluation of body fluid. *Am. J. Clin. Nutrition*, **19**: 422.

10. Heald, F. P., and L. M. Roeder (1976). Nutrition of the school child and adolescent. In *Textbook of Paediatric Nutrition*, edited by D. S. McLaren and D. Burman. Edinburgh: Churchill Livingstone, p. 76.

11. Hodges, R. E., and W. A. Krehl (1965). Nutritional status of teenagers in Iowa. *Am. J. Clin. Nutrition*, **17**: 200.

12. Huenemann, R. L., L. R. Shapiro, M. C. Hampton, and B. W. Mitchell (1966). A longitudinal study of gross body composition and body conformation and their association with food and activity in a teen-age population. *Am. J. Clin. Nutrition*, **18**: 325.

13. King, J. C., S. H. Cohenour, D. H. Calloway, and H. N. Jacobson (1972). Assessment of nutritional status of teenage pregnant girls: I. Nutrient intake and pregnancy. *Am. J. Clin. Nutrition*, **24**: 916.

14. McGanity, W. J., H. M. Little, A. Fogelman, L. Jennings, E. Calhoun, and E. B. Dawson (1969). Pregnancy in the adolescent: I. Preliminary summary of health status. *Am. J. Obstet. Gynecol.*, **103**: 773.

15. *Maternal Nutrition and the Course of Pregnancy* (1970). Washington, D.C.: Natl. Acad. Sci.–Natl. Resarch Council.

16. Morgan, A. F., ed. (1959). *Nutritional Status U.S.A.* Univ. of Calif. Agr. Expt. Sta. Bull. No. 769. Berkeley, Calif.: Univ. of California Agricultural Experiment Station.

17. Olson, M. A., and G. Stearns (1959). Calcium intake of children and adults. *Federation Proc.*, **18**: 1076.

18. Raper, N. R., and M. M. Hill (1974). Vegetarian diets. *Nutrition Rev.*, **32**: Suppl. No. 1: 29.

19. *Recommended Dietary Allowances, Eighth Edition* (1974). Natl. Acad. Sci.–Natl. Research Council. Washington, D.C.: Natl. Research Council.

20. Tanner, J. M. (1962). *Growth at Adolescence.* 2nd ed. Oxford, England: Blackwell Scientific Publications.

21. Thomson, A. M. (1976). Pregnancy in adolescence. In *Nutrient Requirements in Adolescence*, edited by J. I. McKigney and H. N. Munro. Cambridge: The Massachusetts Institute of Technology Press, p. 245.

22. U.S. Department of Agriculture (1972). *Food and Nutrient Intake of Individuals in the U.S. Spring, 1965.* Household Food Consumption Survey 1965–1966, Report No. 17. Washington, D.C.: U.S. Government Printing Office.

23. U.S. Department of Health, Education, and Welfare. *Dietary Intake Findings, United States, 1971–1974*, DHEW Publication No. (HRA) 77-

1647, Series 11-No. 202. Hyattsville, Md.: Natl. Center for Health Stat.

24. U.S. Department of Health, Education, and Welfare. Ten-State Nutrition Survey, 1968–1970. V. Dietary and Highlights. DHEW Publication No. (HSM) 72-8133. Atlanta, Ga., Health Services and Mental Health Adm.

25. *We The Youth of America.* Social and Economic Statistics Administration, Bureau of the Census, June 1973. Washington, D.C.: U.S. Depart. Commerce.

Pregnancy and Lactation

1. Alperin, J. B., M. E. Haggard, and W. J. McGanity (1969). Folic acid, pregnancy, and abruptic placentae. *Am. J. Clin. Nutrition,* **22:** 1354.

2. American Medical Association Committee on Iron Deficiency (1968). Iron deficiency in the United States. *J. Am. Med. Assoc.,* **203:** 407.

3. Arena, J. M. (1970). Contamination of the ideal food. *Nutrition Today,* 5,: 2.

4. Beal, V. A. (1971). Nutritional studies during pregnancy. II. Dietary intake, maternal weight gain, and size of infant. *J. Am. Dietet. Assoc.,* **58:** 321.

5. Blackburn, M. L., and D. H. Calloway (1974). Energy expenditure of pregnant adolescents. *J. Am. Dietet. Assoc.,* **65:** 24.

6. Burke, B. S., V. A. Beal, S. B. Kirkwood, and H. C. Stuart (1943). The influence of nutrition during pregnancy upon the condition of the infant at birth. *J. Nutrition,* **26:** 569.

7. Dieckmann, W. J., D. F. Turner, E. J. Meiller, L. J. Savage, A. J. Hill, M. F. Straube, R. E. Pottinger, and L. M. Rynkiewicz (1951). Observations on protein intake and the health of the mother and baby. 1. Clinical and laboratory findings. 2. Food intake. *J. Am. Dietet. Assoc.,* **27:** 1046.

8. Ebbs, J. F., F. F. Tisdall, and W. A. Scott (1941). Influence of prenatal diet on mother and child. *J. Nutrition,* **22:** 515.

9. Emerson, K., Jr., B. N. Saxena, and E. L. Poindexter (1972). Caloric cost of normal pregnancy. *Obstet. and Gynecol.,* **40:** 786.

10. Finch, C. A. (1969). Iron-deficiency anemia. *Am. J. Clin. Nutrition,* **22:** 512.

11. Finch, C. A., and E. R. Monsen (1972). Iron nutrition and the fortification of food with iron. *J. Am. Med. Assoc.,* **219:** 1462.

12. Food and Agriculture Organization/World Health Organization (1962). *Calcium requirements.* WHO Tech. Rept. Ser. 230, Geneva: World Health Organ.

13. Gunther, M. (1968). Diet and milk secretion in women. *Proc. Nutrition Soc.* (Cambridge), **27:** 77.

14. Hytten, F. E., and I. Leitch (1971). *The Physiology of Human Pregnancy.* Oxford, England: Blackwell Scientific Publications.

15. Hytten, F. E., and A. M. Thomson (1961). Nutrition of the lactating woman. In *Milk: The Mammary Gland and Its Secretion,* Vol. 2, edited by S. K. Kon and A. T. Cowie. New York: Academic Press, p. 35.

16. Hytten, F. E., and A. M. Thomson (1970). Maternal physiological adjustments. In *Maternal Nutrition and the Course of Pregnancy.* Washington, D.C.: National Academy of Sciences, p. 41.

17. Illingworth, R. S., and B. Kilpatrick (1953). Lactation and fluid intake. *Lancet,* **2:** 1175.

18. Jeans, P. C., M. B. Smith, and G. Stearns (1955). Incidence of prematurity in relation to maternal nutrition. *J. Am. Dietet. Assoc.,* **31:** 576.

19. *Laboratory Indices of Nutritional Status in Pregnancy* (1977). Summary Report. Committee on Nutrition of the Mother and Preschool Child. Washington, D.C.: Natl. Acad. Sci.–Natl. Research Council.

20. McGanity, W. J., E. B. Bridgforth, and W. J. Darby (1958). Vanderbilt Cooperative Study of Maternal and Infant Nutrition. XII. Effect of reproductive cycle on nutritional status and requirements. In *Nutrition in Pregnancy.* Symposium 4. Council on Foods and Nutrition. Chicago: American Medical Association.

21. *Maternal Nutrition and the Course of Pregnancy* (1970). Washington, D.C.: Natl. Acad. Sci.–Natl. Research Council.

22. Naismith, D. J., and C. D. Ritchie (1975). The effect of breast-feeding and artificial feeding on body-weights, skinfold measurements, and food intakes of forty-two primiparous women. *Proc. Nutrition Soc.*, (Cambridge) **34**: 116A.

23. *Nutrition in Pregnancy and Lactation* (1965). WHO Tech. Rept. Series 302. Geneva: World Health Organ., p. 14.

24. *Nutritional Anemias* (1972). WHO Tech. Rpt. Series 503. Geneva: World Health Organ.

25. Pitkin, R. M. (1977). Nutrition during pregnancy: The clinical approach. In *Nutritional Disorders of American Women*, edited by M. Winick. New York: John Wiley and Sons, p. 27.

26. *Recommended Dietary Allowances, Eighth Edition* (1974). Natl. Acad. Sci.–Natl. Research Council Publ. Washington, D.C.: Natl. Research Council.

27. Shenolikar, I. S. (1970). Absorption of dietary calcium in pregnancy. *Am. J. Clin. Nutrition*, **23**: 63.

28. Thomson, A. M. (1959). 3. Diet in relation to the course and outcome of pregnancy. *Brit. J. Nutrition*, **13**: 509.

29. Thomson, A. M., F. E. Hytten, and W. Z. Billewicz (1970). The energy cost of human lactation. *Brit. J. Nutrition*, **24**: 565.

30. Widdowson, E. (1977). Nutrition and lactation. In *Nutritional Disorders of American Women*, edited by M. Winick. New York: John Wiley and Sons, p. 67.

Oral Contraceptives and Nutrient Requirements

1. Belsey, M. A. (1977). Hormonal contraception and nutrition. In *Nutritional Impacts on Women*, edited by K. S. Moghissi and T. N. Evans. Hagerstown, Md.: Harper and Row, Publishers, Chap. 14, p. 189.

2. Prasad, A. S., K. Y. Lei, D. Oberleas, K. S. Moghissi, and J. C. Stryker (1975). Effect of oral contraceptive agents on nutrients: II. Vitamins. *Am. J. Clin. Nutrition*, **28**: 385.

3. Prasad, A. S., D. Oberleas, K. Y. Kei, K. S. Mog-
hissi, and J. C. Stryler (1975). Effect of oral contraceptive agents on nutrients: I. Minerals. *Am. J. Clin. Nutrition*, **28**: 377.

4. Roe, D. (1977). Nutrition and the contraceptive pill. In *Nutritional Disorders of American Women*, edited by M. Winick. New York: John Wiley and Sons, p. 37.

5. Smith, J. L., G. A. Goldsmith, and J. D. Lawrence (1975). Effects of oral contraceptive steroids on vitamin and lipid levels in serum. *Am. J. Clin. Nutrition*, **28**: 371.

Nutrition and Physical Activity

1. American College of Sports Medicine Position Stand on Weight Loss in Wrestlers (1976). *Sports Med. Bull.*, **11**: 2.

2. Astrand, P. (1967). Diet and athletic performance. *Federation Proc.*, **26**: 1772.

3. Astrand, P. (1968). Something old and something new . . . very new. *Nutrition Today*, **3**: 9.

4. Astrand, P. (1973). Nutrition and physical performance. In *World Review of Nutrition and Dietetics*, Vol. 16, edited by M. Rechcigl. Washington: S. Karger, pp. 59–79.

5. Diet, exercise and endurance (1972). *Nutrition Rev.*, **30**: 86.

6. Guyton, A. C. (1976). *Textbook of Medical Physiology*. 5th ed. Philadelphia: W. B. Saunders Company. Chapters 1 and 29.

7. Keys, A. L., J. Brozek, A. Henschel, O. Mickelsen, and H. L. Taylor (1950). *The Biology of Human Starvation*. Minneapolis: U. of Minn. Press, Vol. 1, pp. 718–748.

8. Kuta, I., J. Parízkova, and J. Dýcka (1970). Muscle strength and lean body mass in old men of different physical activity. *J. Appl. Physiol.*, **29**: 168.

9. Mayer, J., and B. Bullen (1960). Nutrition and athletic performances. *Physiol. Rev.*, **40**: 369.

10. Mirkin, G. (1973). Carbohydrate loading: A dangerous practice. Letter to the editor. *J. Am. Med. Assoc.*, **223**: 1511.

11. Pařizková, J. (1965). Physical activity and body

composition. In *Human Body Composition*, Vol. VII, edited by J. Brozek. New York: Pergamon Press, p. 161.

12. Pollock, M. L., H. S. Miller, Jr., R. Janeway, A. C. Linnerud, B. Robertson, and R. Valentino (1971).

Effects of walking on body composition and cardiovascular function of middle-aged men. *J. Appl. Physiol.*, **30:** 126.

13. Smith, N. J. (1976). *Food for Sport*. California: Bull Publishing Co.

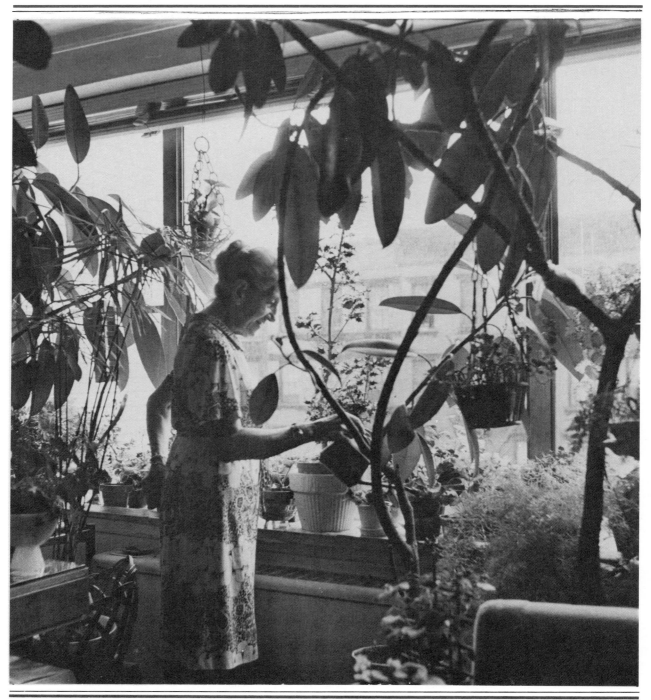

Good nutrition helps older persons maintain their health and vitality so that they can enjoy a wide range of interests and hobbies.

Chapter 21

Nutrition During the Life Cycle III

Middle Age and Old Age

What Is Middle Age?

Chronologically, middle age is a nebulous term. Some view middle age loosely as the period between youth and old age. Sociologists consider the age interval from 40 to 65 as the middle years. Demographers and government statisticians use the age limits of 45 and 64. Psychologically, it is whatever one wants it to be: Some are middle-aged in outlook at 30 or 35, whereas others are young in spirit at 65 or older. According to the 1970 Census, two of every ten Americans are between 45 and 65 years. The middle-aged represent 20 percent of the population, or 42 million people.

Middle age portrays a new transition phase in the life cycle that has evolved from dramatic changes in the modern social systems (24) and from the marked increase in longevity. Middle adulthood is often viewed as the "prime of life." It also signifies a period of added pressures that are economic, social, and cultural in nature. The middle-aged generally bear the heavy responsibilities of caring for both the young and the old (7).

Biological Changes

One of the biological landmarks of middle age is the *climacterium*, a period when endocrine, somatic, and psychic changes may occur in varying degrees. Menopause—the cessation of menstrual flow—is a part of the climacterium; it marks the end of the woman's reproductive potential. During aging, the ovaries undergo atrophic changes and *estrogen* production declines (12). Menopause and other manifestations of the climacterium have little psychological significance for most women (23).

Other endocrine changes occur during the aging process, but the pattern is not uniform (17). The delicate balance in hormonal secretions may no longer be maintained with advancing years, and body adaptive mechanisms fail. These hormonal imbalances affect profoundly many metabolic processes of the body.

After age 40, men and women lose bone tissue, with women showing greater rates of loss. The rate of bone loss per decade in women is 8 percent compared with 3 percent in men (21). Skeletal bone loss may result in debilitating clinical disorders in middle and advanced age.

Changes in the relative proportions of adipose tissue and lean body mass occur as people age (9, 44). With advancing age, body fat increases progressively and lean body mass declines (Table 21.1). These trends in body composition favor the development of *obesity* in older people, which in turn increases the risk of coronary heart disease. In the U.S., heart disease is the leading cause of death in middle age and old age (Table 21.2). The death rate from this disease is higher for males than for females. Cancer and stroke rank second

Table 21.1 Mean Values for Body Weight, Lean Body Mass (LBM), and Body Fat of Adults in Different Age Groups

Age	Number of subjects	Weight, kg	LBM, kg	Fat kg	Fat percent
		Men			
25	585	73	59	14	19
45	881	76	56	20	26
55	835	74	52	22	30
65–70	234	73	47	26	35
		Women			
25	267	59	40	19	33
45	391	67	39	28	42
55	373	70	39	31	44
65–70	144	69	35	34	49

Source: G. B. Forbes and J. C. Reina (1970). Adult lean body mass declines with age: Some longitudinal observations. *Metabolism*, **19**: 658. Data were based on estimated lean body mass with ^{40}K counting. Mean values were based on measurements of many individuals for each age group at one time interval (cross-sectional data).

Table 21.2 Death Rates per 100,000 Population for the Three Leading Causes of Death at Ages 45–64 and 65 and Over, by Sex: United States, 1974

Cause of death	45–64 years		65 years and older		45–64 years, both sexes	65 years and older, both sexes
	Women	Men	Women	Men		
Heart disease	195	591	2,159	3,081	385	2,538
Malignancies (cancer)	261	338	723	1,293	298	957
Cerebrovascular diseases (mainly stroke)	56.2	73.1	791.8	810.7	64.3	799.5

Accidents rank fourth among the causes of death for the middle-aged (45–64 years) of both sexes; cirrhosis of the liver and diabetes rank fifth and sixth, respectively. For 65 years and older, pneumonia and diabetes rank fourth and fifth. Other major causes of death in later life include accidents, emphysema, and cirrhosis of the liver.

Source: From Pocket Data Book U.S.A. (1976), 5th ed. National Center for Health Statistics. Washington, D.C.: U.S. Dept. Commerce, 1976, page 74.

and third, respectively, among the major causes of death in these age groups. The incidence of *diabetes mellitus* is also high in both sexes 45 years and older. Other physiological changes that occur during aging are described under the section of Old Age.

Energy and Nutrient Needs

Healthy middle-aged individuals need the same assortment of nutrients as younger persons, but the amounts required may vary because of changes associated with the aging process. The middle-aged are exposed to a barrage of stress-inducing experiences that are physiological, social, and psychological in nature. The effects of these stress factors are interrelated, and they often affect the nutritional status both by influencing the intake of food and by impairing the utilization of ingested nutrients.

Energy, Carbohydrate, and Fat An adult's total energy needs generally decline with age, largely because of a decrease in *basal metabolism* and in physical activity (20, 43). The gradual decline in basal metabolism (18, 26) may reflect the loss

in functioning body cells as age increases (34). Because of these age-related changes, the FAO/WHO Committee on Energy and Protein Requirements (8) suggested that the average energy requirements be decreased from the recommendations for the 20 to 39 year age group, 5 percent between 40 and 49 years, 10 percent from 50 to 59 years, 20 percent from 60 to 69 years; for age 70 and older 30 percent.

For mature adults engaged in light occupation in the U.S., the RDA for energy are specified for two age categories: 23–50 years and 51 years and older (29). The allowances for the 58-kg woman are 2000 kcal (8368 kJ) at ages 23 to 50 years and 1800 kcal (7531 kJ) for 51 years and above. For the 70-kg man, the corresponding values are 2700 (11,297 kJ) and 2400 kcal (10,042 kJ), respectively. Because of the large individual variations, the energy allowances must be adjusted for body size and physical activity pattern of each person. Obesity and its potential hazards of diseases may be averted by continuous and conscious effort toward achieving and maintaining desirable body weight throughout adulthood.

There is evidence indicating that glucose tolerance declines progressively with age (3), and

471

diabetes is highly prevalent among older adults. Some investigators believe that the mature-onset diabetes reflects a physiological adaptation to the aging process, whereas others support the view that it is a pathological change.

Although carbohydrates are essential dietary constituents, no quantitative requirements at any age have been suggested. The average American diet supplies about 46 percent of the total energy as carbohydrates.

Fat provides an average of 42 percent of the total energy in the U.S. diet. No quantitative requirements have been specified for this nutrient.

Excessive intakes of fat or sucrose and a low intake of dietary "fiber" are among the risk factors suggested in heart disease (29). Obesity and high blood levels of cholesterol and/or triglycerides have also been implicated. Considerable controversy continues to exist on the role of dietary fat and carbohydrate in the development of coronary heart disease (see Chapter 5).

Protein Many diverse factors affect intake and utilization of protein, and these influences contribute greatly to individual variations in protein needs. These factors include dietary protein quality and quantity; protein: energy intake ratio; age, sex, genetic endowment, and health status of the individual; and socioeconomic conditions. Thus nitrogen balance studies of older persons have yielded variable and inconclusive results (42).

For nearly all healthy individuals in the U.S., the protein allowance is 0.8 g of mixed protein per kg of body weight per day. The allowances for both age categories 23–50 years and 51 years and older are 46 g per day for a 58-kg woman and 56 g for a 70-kg man. It is possible, however, that "cummulative stresses of life in a competitive society" may increase nutritional needs (29) and the middle-age group would be particularly vulnerable.

Mineral Elements Several mineral elements are essential for good nutrition in humans at all ages. The RDA include the macrominerals calcium, phosphorus and magnesium, and the microminerals iron, iodine and zinc. The requirements of the other essential microminerals have not yet been established (29). Calcium and iron are less widely distributed in foods than are other mineral elements, and older people tend to select diets that are often inadequate in these two nutrients.

Aging implies impaired adaptation. During menopause, calcium absorption may fail to keep up with increasing demands. As calcium absorption falls with age and bone resorption rises, osteoporosis develops (25). In *osteoporosis*, the total bone mass is reduced, but its chemical composition remains unchanged (normal calcium to protein ratios). It is a major bone disorder found in about 25 percent of postmenopausal women. The incidence tends to be four times greater in women than in men (2). Osteoporosis is a poorly understood syndrome of middle age. Inactivity and immobility, hormonal (estrogen) deficiency, and dietary inadequacy have been suggested as possible factors that contribute to its development.

The RDA for calcium is 0.8 g daily for adult women and men (29). Although there is a lack of agreement among research workers, recent evidence has been interpreted to suggest that a minimum daily intake of 1 g of calcium daily is needed to maintain normal bone density in older individuals (2).

Iron-deficiency anemia is prevalent among older individuals in the U.S., especially those with limited income (15, 41). The frequency of chronic illness increases with age, and this may have adverse effects on the absorption and/or utilization of ingested iron. In addition, low dietary intakes of iron may result from (a) reduced food intake because of poor appetite, (b) poor food selection because of lack of nutrition knowledge and/or insufficient money, and (c) poor food habits.

The RDA for adult women before menopause is 18 mg of iron daily (29). After menopause, women are relieved of iron loss through the menstrual blood flow, which averages about 0.5 mg per day; some women lose as much as 1.5 mg of iron daily. After 50 years of age, the RDA for women is the same as that for adult men, that is, 10 mg of iron per day.

Vitamins Aging *per se* does not increase the requirements for vitamins (42). Older individuals who are clinically healthy and who subsist on nutritionally adequate diets seldom show evidence of vitamin deficiencies.

For the two older age categories, 23–50 years and 51+ years, the RDA are the same as those specified for younger adults, except for thiamin, riboflavin, and niacin. The allowances of these three vitamins are based on the energy intake, and recommended amounts decrease as energy needs decline with age. When the energy allowance falls below 2000 kcal (8368 kJ) for women over 50 years, the Food and Nutrition Board suggests that 1.0 mg per day of thiamin should be the minimum intake (29).

What Is Old Age?

Grow old along with me!
The best is yet to be,
The last of life, for which the first was made.
—Robert Browning, "Rabbi Ben Ezra"

Old age is a period in the human life cycle that is marked by a high degree of variability among individuals. The elderly, according to Butler (7), "are as diverse as in other periods of life, and their patterns of aging show useful constructive participation to disinterest, from the prevailing stereotype of aging to rich forms of creativity. . . . This period of life is characterized by complex changes that are multiple, occur rapidly and have profound effects. Some people are overwhelmed. Others can come to accept or substitute for the loss of loved ones, prestige, social status and adverse physiological changes."

Physiological indices vary widely in old people, therefore, chronological age (calendar age) is a misleading measure of their physical health,

mental capacity, and endurance. Ages 60–65 were arbitrarily chosen as the beginning of late adulthood, primarily to identify a point for retirement and for eligibility for services and financial benefits for the elderly. Age 65 has become the reference point by which to distinguish the old from the middle-aged. Gerontologists (scientists who study the aging process) divide old age into (a) early old age, 65 to 74 years, and (b) advanced age, 75 years and older.

The Elderly American

Concern for the nutrition of the elderly has understandably increased because the percentage of Americans over the age of 65 has risen substantially. In 1900, there were about 3 million persons 65 years of age and over (4 percent of the total population), whereas in 1970 there were about 20 million (or about one out of every ten Americans). It is the fastest growing minority group in this country. The percentage of people age 65 to 69 years is getting smaller, whereas that for age 75 years and older continues to grow (Fig. 21.1).

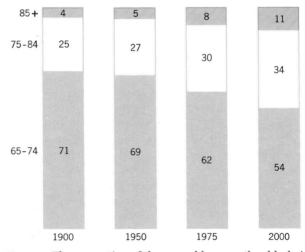

Fig. 21.1 The proportion of the very old among the elderly is increasing. (From *Our Future Selves*, U.S. Dept. Health, Education, and Welfare, Public Health Service, National Institutes of Health DHEW Publication No. 77-1096, p. 9.)

473

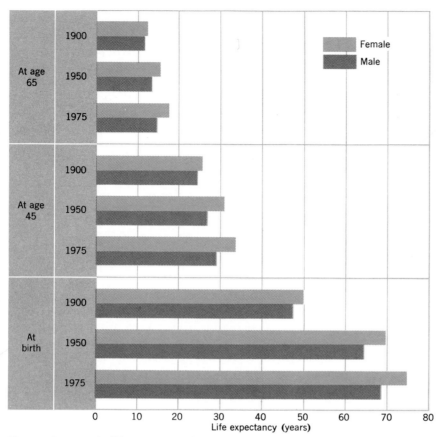

Fig. 21.2 Increase in life expectancy for women and men. (From *1961 White House Conference On Aging Chart Book*. Washington, D.C.: U.S. Govt. Printing Office, p. 9.)

The proportion of elderly persons 75 years and over has increased from 29 percent in 1900 to 38 percent in 1970. Elderly women outnumber elderly men. Ninety-five percent of older people live in the community (6). Of these noninstitutionalized elderly, 14 percent have no chronic ailments and 65 percent have chronic conditions that do not interfere with their mobility. An increasing proportion of the elderly, particularly women (they outlive men), are economically deprived.

It is predicted that by 1975 life expectancy at birth will have increased by 45 to 50 percent over what it was in 1900. Figure 21.2 shows the life expectancy for women and men in 1900, 1950, and 1975 at three ages: birth, 45 years, and 65 years. This increase in life expectancy reflects improved technology, sanitation, housing, medical care, and nutrition. More people can hope to reach the age of 60 today than was possible at the turn of the century, but life expectancy after 60 is little more than it was 150 or 200 years ago (see Figs. 21.3 and 21.4).

Biological Changes During Aging

Aging is recognized as an inevitable process characterized by progressive deterioration (21).

474

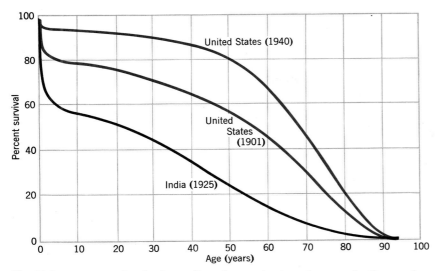

Fig. 21.3 Percentage of males born alive who survive to a given age for the populations indicated (modified from A. Comfort, 1964). (From Curtis, H. J. (1966). *Biological Mechanisms of Aging.* Courtesy of Charles C Thomas, Publisher, Springfield, Illinois.)

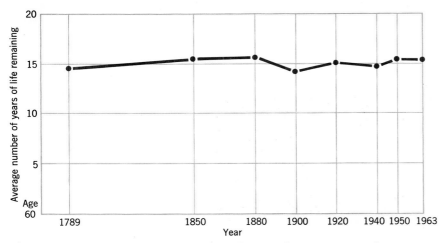

Fig. 21.4 Life expectancy of a white male in the United States at age 60 from 1789 to 1963. (Source: *Vital Statistics of the United States,* 1963, Vol, 2, Section 5, Life Table 5.5. From S. Bakerman, ed., *Aging Life Processes,* 1967. Courtesy of Charles C Thomas, Publisher, Springfield, Illinois.)

475

Since the process is affected by the stresses of life, it is difficult for investigators to separate clearly the effects of aging from those of other causes. The process occurs at different rates among individuals.

Some changes are obvious, for example, those that occur in the skin. Old skin is less elastic than young. The *collagen* fibers of the skin's connective tissue are less elastic. Therefore wrinkles that occur in frowning, squinting, or smiling do not smooth out as quickly with advancing age. There is also decreased elasticity in the connective tissue of the arteries, and in studies of the aorta, it has been observed that there is a thickening of the wall due to the formation of new collagenous connective tissue. These two changes help to produce increased pressure within the blood vascular system.

Certain histological changes take place in the heart muscle with aging: after the age of 60 the fibers decrease in size and the nuclei become larger. The heart's functional capacity also changes: the resting cardiac output (amount of blood pumped by the heart) decreases.

Few studies have been made of changes in the organs of the digestive system. The mucous lining of the stomach becomes thinner. There is also a change in the cells of some of the gastric glands (from specialized to simple), which, it is believed, may account for the achlorhydria (lack of hydrochloric acid) of the gastric secretion frequently observed in older people (4). Without sufficient acid, *pepsinogen* cannot be converted to the protein-digesting *enzyme* pepsin, nor can bacteria that may have entered the stomach be destroyed, both of these factors may contribute to indigestion. It is believed that with advancing age there is some atrophy (wasting) of the smooth muscle of the mucosa in both the small and large intestine.

In general, with advancing age there is a gradual loss of functioning cells in the muscle and nerve tissue. However, the cells of the skin, hair, gastrointestinal tract lining, and liver retain their capacity to divide and reproduce themselves (34). Certain tests can indicate the extent of physiological retrogression. One test is of *vital capacity*, which tends to decrease with age; another is of blood pressure, which often increases with age; and another is of muscular strength, which decreases with age (5).

Skeletal bone loss occurs with aging and may have serious consequences among the elderly (see section on Mineral Elements under Middle Age). Old people, especially women, are highly vulnerable to fracture risk (2). A significant proportion of all women over 60 years old suffer from osteoporosis (loss of bone substance; see Fig. 21.5). Rapid loss of alveolar bone (tooth-bearing bone) often accompanies osteoporosis, and this condition ultimately leads to loss of teeth. In the

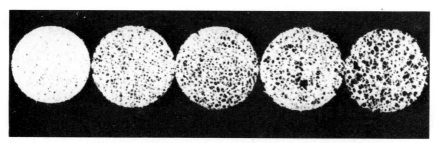

Fig. 21.5 Bone disks removed from the center of the first lumbar vertebra, illustrating five degrees of vertebral bone density. The very dense bone at the extreme left is from a young man. The porous bone at the extreme right is from an osteoporotic individual. (Reprinted from *Bone*, 3rd ed., by F. C. McLean and M. R. Urist, by permission of the University of Chicago Press. Copyright © 1968 by the University of Chicago Press.)

U.S., over 50 percent of the population have lost all their teeth by age 60 years. The role of nutrition in the development of periodontal disease (disease of the supporting structure of the teeth) is not clearly understood.

Changes in body composition with age and the health hazards of obesity in later years have been described in the section on Middle Age. Obesity in the elderly presents additional health problems: it places extra strain on bones and joints, thus aggravating the tendency toward *arthritis* and other *rheumatic diseases.*

Nutrition and Food of the Elderly

Although the requirement for energy decreases with age, the need for nutrients does not change for healthy older individuals (see section under Middle Age). In fact, the RDA per 1000 kcal show that the needs for protein, calcium, and vitamins A, C, B-6, and B-12 are higher at age 51 years and older than for the young age groups (Table 21.3). Therefore the reduced needs for energy by the elderly would require a carefully selected assortment of foods with *high-nutrient density.*

Nutrition surveys at the national level have provided information on the dietary intake and nutritional status of the elderly in the United States. The 1965–1966 Household Food Consumption Survey by the U.S. Department of Agriculture indicated that mean intakes of energy and nutrients decreased with age (38). Diets of women 65 years and older tended to supply more nutrients in amounts below the RDA than diets of men of the same age or younger women. Mean intakes of calcium were inadequate for both older women and men.

From the Ten-State Survey in 1968–1970 by the U.S. Department of Health, Education, and Welfare, information was obtained on low-income population groups in ten states (41). Among the elderly, iron deficiency was prevalent in both sexes. Obesity was the most common nutritional disorder observed in black and white older women.

Table 21.3 Recommended Dietary Allowances per 1000 kcal for Three Age Ranges of Men

Nutrient	Age range		
	19–22	23–50	51 and over
Protein, g	18	21	23
Vitamin A activity, IU	1667	1852	2083
Vitamin C, mg	15	17	19
Niacin, mg	7	7	7
Riboflavin, mg	0.6	0.6	0.6
Thiamin, mg	0.5	0.5	0.5
Vitamin B-6, mg	0.7	0.7	0.8
Vitamin B-12, μg	1.0	1.1	1.3
Calcium, mg	267	296	333
Iron, mg	3	4	4

Computed from *Recommended Dietary Allowances. Eighth Edition* (1974). Washington, D.C.: Natl. Research Council.

Recently, the *nutritional status* of the U.S. population ages 1 to 74 years was assessed during the first Health and Nutrition Examination Survey (HANES) in 1971–1974 (40). Observations were made on a scientifically designed sample which represented the noninstitutionalized civilian population in the United States. Individuals 65 years and older reported mean intakes of calories that were below the HANES dietary standards (39). Mean intakes for protein, calcium, and iron failed to meet the standards, especially for the elderly Negro women. Clinical signs of nutrient deficiencies were not frequently encountered. It is possible, however, that malnutrition is widespread at the subclinical (unapparent) level among the elderly.

Several dietary studies have shown that the elderly use vitamin and/or mineral supplements (20, 35, 38). In many instances, these supplements were taken based on a physician's recommendation. A high proportion of supplement users reported diets that met the recommended intakes of nutrients. For individuals who failed to meet the dietary allowances, some used preparations that covered all dietary inadequacies;

others took mixtures with some, but not all, of the essential nutrients that were low in the diet, whereas others consumed the wrong supplement.

Other factors are important in the nutrition of elderly persons besides the amount of nutritious foods ingested. Food habits, preferences, and prejudices are not easily changed (15). A longitudinal study of 35 Iowa women during aging showed that dietary patterns are maintained, except for a decrease in fat consumption (10). These women, ages 29 to 88 years, consumed their usual diets during the study periods and kept records of their weighed food intakes for either 7 or 10 days. Dietary data were taken at four different periods between 1948 and 1966. The reduced intake of fat with advancing years may have resulted from (a) a decrease in fat tolerance due to physiological changes associated with aging such as a diminished digestive capacity, (b) efforts to control body weight, (c) a change in food pattern brought about by the increased publicity on dietary fat intake, or (d) combined influences of these and other unidentified factors.

Limited income for food is another problem for many older persons. As of 1971, 33.6 percent of all heads of households in the lowest-fifth income group in the United States was 65 years of age or over (37). Two federal government programs are available to help needy persons secure additional food: the Food Stamp Program and the Family Food Donation Program, both administered by the U.S. Department of Agriculture (11).

Since eating is traditionally a social occasion, it is not surprising that persons living alone tend to have less adequate diets than do married couples (27, 28). And when these persons are able to eat with a family and share communal life for part of the day, they eat more than when they are alone. In a food intake study of 155 older persons in Cincinnati, those who had eaten a meal at a senior center or had had a meal delivered to their home in the preceding 24 hours tended to have a more nutritious diet than those who prepared their own food at home (16).

In September 1973, projects under the Nutrition Program for Older Americans started serving meals for the elderly in congregate settings. This meal program was authorized by Title VII of the Older Americans Act of 1965, as amended. At least one hot meal each day is offered five days a week, and it supplies one-third of the RDA. The participants dine together at meal sites where they are given the opportunity to use a variety of health-related and other supportive services (1).

The elderly who can live quite well in their own homes but cannot prepare food for themselves may benefit from the home-delivered meals or "Meals on Wheels" program (13, 22, 36). Under this program, a hot noontime meal is delivered, and sometimes either a cold supper or breakfast. This program began in the United States in 1954; by 1970, there were more than 80 "Meals on Wheels" groups operating. In 1971, there were 350 home-delivered meal programs of various types in the United States (14).

Diet and Longevity

Experimental work with animals has demonstrated that the type and amount of food consumed, as well as the manner of feeding, all affect *longevity*. In his laboratory at Columbia University, Sherman (33) found that when more calcium, riboflavin, and vitamin A were added to diets that were already adequate for growth and reproduction in white rats, the animals showed increased growth, a prolonged reproductive period, and an increased lifespan.

The lifespan of animals can also be increased by limiting their energy intake. At Cornell University, McCay (19) prepared diets for animals that were high in all food essentials but low in energy value. Animals that received this diet grew slowly, matured late, and outlived those who ate an adequate diet *ad libitum*. Recently, Ross (30) demonstrated that the age at which dietary restriction of the rats begins is an important determinant of longevity. When imposed later in life, life expectancy decreased. In later studies, Ross and colleagues (31, 32) examined the influence of dietary self-selection on lifespan. When allowed to choose freely from three different diets, the rats selected combinations that maximized the incidence of degenerative disease and minimized their life span. Such studies with animal models point to the influence of diet on life processes, but it is not known precisely how these findings might relate to human longevity.

Summary

During the entire adult lifespan, gradual and progressive changes occur as part of the aging process. Certain body structures change, and the functional capacity of different organ systems decline. After age 40, men and women tend to lose bone tissues; body fat increases progressively and lean mass declines. Energy expenditure for basal metabolism and physical activity decreases with age. Middle-aged people often lapse into a sedentary lifestyle while retaining the same eating habits—a condition that favors the development of obesity. Obesity is a major health hazard in the U.S. Continuous and conscious effort is needed by the individual to achieve and maintain desirable body weight throughout adulthood. A sensible program of eating and regular physical exercise is essential for controlling body weight. The kinds of nutrients needed by middle-aged individuals are the same as those for younger adults; amounts, however, may increase because of stress factors that often plague this particular age group.

In old age, the needs of healthy individuals for energy is reduced but not for the essential nutrients. Factors that contribute to nutritional deficiencies in older people include: questionable eating habits and food preferences, limited income, lack of nutrition knowledge, loneliness, physical disabilities, and chronic illness. Community programs are helping improve the nutritional health status of the elderly through group or home-delivered meals, nutrition education, medical and dental care, and recreation.

Glossary

arthritis: inflammation of a joint.

basal metabolism: see p. 132

climacterium: combined phenomena accompanying cessation of the reproductive function in the female or the normal diminution of sexual activity in the male.

collagen: see p. 101

diabetes (mellitus): see p. 60.

enzyme: see p. 28.

estrogen: see p. 463.

high-nutrient density: high nutrient to energy content in foods.

longevity: the condition or quality of being long-lived.

nutritional status: see p. 463.

obesity: see p. 144.

osteoporosis: see p. 268.

pepsinogen: the inactive precursor of pepsin, produced by the chief cells of the stomach and converted to pepsin under acid conditions.

rheumatic disease: a disease marked by inflammation of the connective tissue structures of the body, especially the muscles and joints, and by pain in these parts.

vital capacity: the volume of air a person can forcibly expire from the lungs after a maximal inspiration.

Study Questions and Activities

1. Compare the nutritional needs of healthy middle-aged and elderly individuals with those of younger adults. Give reasons for the similarities and differences.

2. Describe the current food pattern of your mother, father, and grandparents. Why do they eat as they do? Are their diets nutritionally adequate? Give reasons to support your answers.

3. Visit a senior citizen center or a congregate meal site during mealtime. How many participants were present? How many males? Females? Approximately what proportion of the group is average in body weight? Overweight? Underweight? What factors contribute to the differences in body weights among the elderly? What was the day's menu? Observe several participants, and compare their food

choices and intakes. Give possible reasons for differences and similarities in eating patterns. Also note the mealtime atmosphere and how it may contribute to or detract from the consumption of the meal offered. What similar programs do you have in your community?

References

Middle Age and Old Age

1. Administration on Aging Fact Sheet: *National Nutrition Program for Older Americans* (April 1976). DHEW Publication No. (OHD) 76-20230. Washington, D.C.: Dept Health Educ. and Welfare.

2. Albanese, A. A., H. H. Edelson, E. J. Lorenze, M. L. Woodhull, and E. H. Wein (1975). Problems of bone health in the elderly. *New York State J. Med.*, **75:** 326.

3. Andres, R. (1972). Aging and carbohydrate metabolism. In *Nutrition in Old Age*, edited by L. A. Carlson. Symposia of the Swedish Nutrition Fdn. X. Uppsala: Almquist and Wiksell, p. 24.

4. Andrew, W. (1971). *The Anatomy of Aging in Man and Animals*. New York; Grune and Stratton.

5. Bourliere, F. (1970). *The Assessment of Biological Age in Man*. Public Health Papers No. 37. Geneva: World Health Organ., p. 39.

6. Brotman, H. B. (1974). The fastest growing minority: The aging. *Am. J. Publ. Health*, **64:** 249.

7. Butler, R. N. (1975). *Why Survive? Being Old in America*. New York: Harper and Row, Publishers.

8. *Energy and Protein Requirements* (1973). FAO Nutrition Meetings Rept. Series 52, and WHO Tech. Rept. Series 522. Rome: Food and Agr. Organ.

9. Forbes, G. B., and J. C. Reina (1970). Adult lean body mass declines with age: Some longitudinal observations. *Metabolism*, **19:** 653.

10. Garcia, P. A., G. E. Battese, and W. D. Brewer (1975). Longitudinal study of age and cohort influences on dietary patterns. *J. Gerontol.*, **30:** 349.

11. Getting a program started (1969). *Agr. Marketing*, **14:** 11.

12. Guyton, A. C. (1976). *Textbook of Medical Physiology*. 5th ed. Philadelphia: W. B. Saunders Company, p. 1098.

13.. *Home-Delivered Meals for the Ill, Handicapped, and Elderly* (1965). Report by the Committee on Guidelines for the Project. New York: National Council on the Aging, Inc.

14. *Home Delivered Meals—A National Directory* (1971). Publ. No. SRA-AOA 1964–1971. Washingtion. D.C.: U.S. Dept. Health, Educ. and Welfare, Administration on Aging.

15. Howell, S. C., and M. B. Loeb (1969). Nutrition and Aging. A Monograph for Practitioners. *The Gerontologist*, **9.**

16. Joering, E. (1971). Nutrient contribution of a meal program for senior citizens. *J. Am. Dietet. Assoc.*, **59:** 129.

17. Leathem, J. H. (1977). Endocrine changes with age. In *Epidemiology of Aging*, edited by A. M. Ostfeld and D. C. Gibson. Public Health Service, Publ. No. (NIH) 77-711, Washington D.C., U.S. Dept. Health Educ. and Welfare, p. 177.

18. Leverton, R., A. Biester, I. Pesek, L. Burrill, M. Mangel, and D. C. Cederquist (1957). Changes with age in basal metabolic rate of adult women. *Federation Proc.*, **16:** 390.

19. McCay, C. M., M. F. Crowell, and L. A. Maynard (1935). The effect of retarded growth upon the length of life span and upon the ultimate body size. *J. Nutrition*, **10:** 63.

20. McGandy, R. B., C. H. Barrows, Jr., A. Spanias, A. Meredith, J. L. Stone, and A. H. Norris (1966). Nutrient intakes and energy expenditure in men of different ages. *J. Gerontol.*, **21:** 581.

21. Masoro, E. (1977). Other physiologic changes with age. In *Epidemiology of Aging*, edited by A. M. Ostfeld and D. C. Gibson. Public Health Service, Publ. No. (NIH) 77-711, Washington D.C., U.S. Dept. Health, Educ. and Welfare, p. 137.

22. Meals on wheels (1969). *Agr. Marketing*, **14:** 8.

23. Neugarten, B. L. (1968). The awareness of middle age. In *Middle Age and Aging*, edited by B. L. Neugarten. Chicago, Ill., The University of Chicago Press, p. 93.

24. Neugarten, B. L., and J. W. Moore (1968). The

changing age-status system. In *Middle Age and Aging*, edited by B. L. Neugarten. Chicago, Ill., The University of Chicago Press, p. 5.

25. Nordin, B. E. C., J. Aaron, J. C. Gallagher, and A. Horsman (1972). Calcium and bone metabolism in old age. In *Nutrition and Old Age*, edited by L. A. Carlson. Symposia of the Swedish Fdn. X. Uppsala: Almquist and Wiksell, p. 77.

26. Norris, A. H., T. Lundy, and N. W. Shock (1963). Trends in selected indices of body composition in men between the ages 30 and 80 years. *Ann. New York Acad. Sci.*, **110:** 589.

27. Pearson, R. C. M. (1968) Feeding the elderly in their own homes: Meeting the need. *Proc. Nutrition Soc.* (Cambridge), **27:** 37.

28. Pelcovits, J. (1972) Nutrition to meet the human needs of older Americans. *J. Am. Dietet. Assoc.*, **60:** 297.

29. *Recommended Dietary Allowances, Eighth Edition* (1974). Natl. Acad. Sci.–Natl. Research Council, Washington, D.C.: Natl. Research Council.

30. Ross, M. H. (1972). Length of life and caloric intake. *Am. J. Clin. Nutrition*, **25:** 834.

31. Ross, M. H. (1977). Dietary behavior and longevity. *Nutrition Rev.*, **35:** 257.

32. Ross, M. H., and G. Brass (1975). Food preference and length of life. *Science*, **190:** 165.

33. Sherman, H. C. (1952). *Chemistry of Food and Nutrition*. 8th ed. New York: Macmillan, p. 275.

34. Shock, N. W. (1970). Physiologic aspects of aging. *J. Am. Dietet. Assoc.*, **56:** 491.

35. Steinkamp, R. C., N. L. Cohen, and H. E. Walsh (1965). Resurvey of an aging population — fourteen years follow-up. The San Mateo nutrition study. *J. Am. Dietet. Assoc.*, **46:** 103.

36. Todhunter, E. N., and D. M. Watkin (1971). *Nutrition*. 1971 White House Conference on Aging. Washington, D.C.: U.S. Govt. Printing Office.

37. U.S. Bureau of the Census (1972). *Money Income in 1971 of Families and Persons in the United States*. Series P60, No. 85. Washington, D.C.: U.S. Dept. Commerce, Social and Econ. Stat. Admin.

38. U.S. Department of Agriculture (1972). *Food and Nutrient Intake of Individuals in the U.S., Spring, 1965.* Household Food Consumption Survey 1965–1966. Report No. 17. Washington, D.C.: U.S. Government Printing Office.

39. U.S. Department of Health, Education, and Welfare (1977). *Dietary Intake Findings, United States, 1971–1974.* DHEW Publication No. (HRA) 77--1647. Hyattsville, Md.: Natl. Center for Health Stat.

40. U.S. Department of Health, Education, and Welfare. *Preliminary Findings of the First Health and Nutrition Examination Survey, United States, 1971–1972: Dietary Intake and Biochemical Findings.* DHEW Publication No. (HRA) 74-1219-1. Rockville, Md.: Natl. Center for Health Stat.

41. U.S. Department of Health, Education, and Welfare (1972). *Ten-State Nutrition Survey, 1968–1970.* V. Dietary and Highlights. DHEW Publication No. (HSM) 72-8133. Atlanta, Ga.: Center for Disease Control.

42. Watkin, D. M. (1973). Nutrition for the aging and the aged. In *Modern Nutrition in Health and Disease*, 5th ed., edited by R. S. Goodhart and M. E. Shils. Philadelphia: Lea and Febiger, p. 681.

43. Wessel, J. A., A. Small, W. D. Van Huss, D. J. Anderson, and D. C. Cederquist (1968). Age and physiological responses to exercise in women 20–69 years of age. *J. Gerontol.*, **23:** 269.

44. Young, C. M., J. Blondin, R. Tensuan, and J. H. Fryer (1963). Body composition studies of "older" women, thirty to seventy years of age. *Ann. New York Acad. Sci.*, **110:** 589.

481

Glossary

absorption: the passage of the end products of digestion through the walls of the digestive tract.

acclimatize: the process of becoming adjusted to a new environment.

acetylcholine: a chemical compound normally present in many parts of the body, essential to the conveying of nerve impulses.

acrolein: a volatile, irritating liquid — acrylic aldehyde, CH_2–CH–CHO that results from overheating fat; it is a decomposition product of glycerol.

actin: a major protein in voluntary muscle.

action potential: the electrical energy of a stimulated membrane, produced by the flow of ions across the membrane with the change in its permeability on stimulation.

activate: to render a substance such as an inactive substance capable of exerting its proper effect.

activated amino acid: an amino acid that is to be at-tached to molecules of transfer RNA; the transfer is an energy-requiring process carried out by a set of spontaneous reactions during which the amino acid becomes linked to intermediate products.

activation of enzymes: some enzymes, in order to function, require a metal (such as magnesium), or a non-metal, or both, attached to them, either loosely or tightly; others function independently.

active transport: the movement of substances (particularly electrolyte ions) across cell membranes, usually against a concentration gradient. Unlike diffusion or osmosis, active transport requires the expenditure of metabolic energy.

adenosine triphosphate (ATP): a compound that consists of one molecule each of adenine (a purine) and ribose (a 5-carbon sugar) and three molecules of phosphoric acid; it is required for energy transfer and the phosphorylation of compounds.

aerobic: a chemical reaction involving sufficient O_2.

aldosterone: an electrolyte-regulating hormone secreted by the adrenal cortex.

amine: an organic compound containing nitrogen; derivative of ammonia (NH_3)

amino acid residue: that portion of an amino acid that is present in a peptide; the amino acid minus the atoms that are removed from it in the process of linking it to other amino acids by means of peptide bonds.

amino acids: any one of a class of organic compounds, containing an amino (NH-2) and a carboxyl (COOH) group, that form the chief constituent of protein.

amniotic fluid: the fluid secreted by the amnion (innermost membrane enclosing the developing fetus); it immerses the fetus and thereby cushions it against injury.

amphetamine: a drug (alpha-methylphenethylamine) used to reduce appetite, also reduces nasal congestion, increases blood pressure, stimulates central nervous system.

amphoteric: descriptive of a compound that has at least one group that can act as an acid and one group that can act as a base.

anaerobic: a chemical reaction in the absence of O_2.

analog: a chemical compound with a structure similar to that of another but differing from it in some respect.

anemia: reduction in number of erythrocytes per cu mm; the quantity of hemoglobin or the volume of packed red cells per 100 ml of blood.

anemia, folic acid deficiency: failure of the synthesis and maturation of the red blood cells, with formation of megaloblasts (large immature red cells). See p. 245 for discussion.

anemia, iron-deficiency: microcytic (red cells, small in size), hypochromic (hemoglobin level, low) caused by deficiency of iron in the diet, blood loss, inadequate absorption.

anemia, pernicious: low red cell count; macrocytic (larger than normal) red cells; caused by a lack of intrinsic factor in gastric juice and consequently failure to absorb vitamin B-12. See p. 248 for discussion.

angiotensin: a polypeptide present in blood which stimulates the secretion of aldosterone by the adrenal cortex.

anion: a negatively charged ion.

anorexia: loss or lack of appetite for food.

anorexia nervosa: a serious nervous condition in which individual loses the appetite, eats little food, and becomes greatly emaciated.

anorexigenic: an agent that diminishes appetite.

antagonist: a substance that exerts a nullifying or opposing effect to another substance.

anthraquinone: a yellow substance from a coal tar product.

anthropometry: the science that deals with the measurement of the size, weight, and proportions of the human body.

antibody: a protein of the globulin type that is formed in an animal organism in response to the administration of an antigen and is capable of combining specifically with that antigen.

anticoagulant: any substance that inhibits the blood clotting mechanism.

antigen: any substance not normally present in the body, which when introduced into it stimulates the production of a protein (antibody) which reacts specifically with it.

antimetabolite: a substance bearing a close structural resemblance to one required for normal physiological functioning, and exerting its desired effect perhaps by replacing or interfering with the utilization of the essential metabolite.

antineuritic: a substance effective against neuritis.

antioxidant: a substance that prevents or retards oxidation in another substance; for example, vitamin E prevents autoxidation of unsaturated fatty acids.

antivitamin: a substance that interferes with the metabolism or synthesis of a vitamin.

aqueous emulsion: solution of a liquid soluble in fat and fat solvents (such as vitamin A) in water; the combination is made possible by use of an emulsifying agent (see emulsifying agent).

arachidonic acid: a 20-carbon atom fatty acid with four double bonds; in the body it is synthesized from the essential fatty acid linoleic acid.

ariboflavinosis: a deficiency of riboflavin.

arthritis: inflammation of a joint.

atherosclerosis: a condition in which the inner walls of the arteries have been thickened by deposits of plaques of material, including cholesterol.

484

atropine: an alkaloid from belladonna used in a variety of conditions; actions include relaxation of smooth muscles, increased heart rate.

availability: in nutrition, free to be absorbed from the intestine into the blood.

basal metabolic rate: the basal metabolism expressed as kilocalories per unit of body size (square meter of body surface: weight to the three-fourths power $W^{3/4}$).

basal metabolism: the energy expenditure of the body at rest, under comfortable environmental conditions, and in the postabsorptive state (12 hours after the ingestion of food).

beriberi: a deficiency disease caused by an insufficient intake of thiamin and characterized by polyneuritis, edema (in some cases), emaciation, and cardiac disturbances (enlargement of the heart and an unusually rapid heartbeat).

bicarbonate ion: the prefix "bi" indicates the presence of hydrogen; the bicarbonate ion is ($^-HCO_3$).

bile acids: glycocholic and taurocholic acid, formed in the liver and secreted in the bile.

bioassay: also termed biological assay; the measurement of either the activity or the amount of a substance based on the use of living organisms; in the case of vitamin A, the rat is used.

biological value: the relative nutritional value of a protein; the amino acid composition, digestibility, and availability of the products of digestion are taken into consideration.

blood cells: also known as corpuscles; include red blood cells (erythrocytes) and white blood cells (leukocytes).

blood vascular system: vessels that transport blood throughout the body.

bolus: a mass of food entering the esophagus in one swallow.

bone, cancellous (or spongy): a porous type of bone located at the end of the long bones, surrounded by compact bone.

bone, compact: a dense type of bone; forms the outer layer of the long bones (bones of the arms, legs, and clavicle) surrounding the marrow in the shaft and the spongy bone at the end of the bone.

bone density: the mineral compactness of bone.

bone matrix: the protein groundwork in which the minerals are deposited.

brush border: minute cylindrical processes (microvilli) on the surface of a cell, greatly increasing the surface area; found in the intestinal epithelium.

buffer system: buffers are substances that tend to stabilize the pH of a solution; a buffer is a mixture of either a weak acid and its salt or a weak base combined with an acid. An acid–base pair is made up of a proton donor and a proton acceptor. For example:

$$\frac{\text{bicarbonate}, \quad HCO_3^-, \quad \text{proton (H+) acceptor}}{\text{carbonic acid} \quad H_2CO_3 \quad \text{proton (H+) donor}}$$

The pairs are called "buffer systems."

caffeine: a slightly bitter tasting substance found in coffee and tea that acts as a stimulant of the central nervous system.

calcitonin: one of two hormones responsible for fine regulation of blood calcium level; the other is the parathyroid hormone. Calcitonin, secreted by the thyroid gland, inhibits bone resorption and release of calcium to the blood, thereby lowering blood calcium.

capillary: a minute blood vessel between the arterioles (minute arteries) and venules (small veins); the interchange of material between the blood and the tissues takes place through the capillary walls.

calorimeter: the equipment used to measure the heat generated in a system. In nutrition it is an instrument for measuring the amount of heat produced by a food on oxidation or by an individual.

caprylic acid: an eight-carbon saturated fatty acid.

carbohydrases: a group of enzymes that digest disaccharides.

carbon dioxide: a colorless, odorless gas, CO_2, resulting from the oxidation of carbon; formed in the tissues and eliminated by the lungs.

caries: tooth decay.

cariogenic: conducive to decay.

carious: affected with decay.

cassava: a tropical plant of the spurge family with edible starchy roots.

catalyze: to accelerate the rate of a chemical reaction through the action of an element or compound (a catalyst) that remains unchanged during the reaction or is regenerated to its original form at the end of the reaction.

cation: an ion having a positive charge; sodium, potassium, calcium are examples of cations.

cellulose: the structural carbohydrate in plants that passes undigested through the human digestive tract.

cementum: calcified tissue covering the rest of the tooth.

chemical reaction: changes in the orbital electrons (those outside the nucleus) of an atom; the process may require energy or yield it.

chloride ion: Cl⁻.

cholesterol: a solid alcohol with fatlike properties which occurs in animal tissue.

cholic acid: a family of compounds (steroids) comprising the bile acids; they are derived from cholesterol.

chylomicron: a lipoprotein with a density of about 0.96; composed of about 1 percent protein and 99 percent total lipids.

cirrhosis of the liver: progressive destruction of the liver cells and an abnormal increase of connective tissue.

climacterium (climacteric): combined phenomena accompanying cessation of the reproductive function in the female or the normal diminution of sexual activity in the male.

coenzyme: an organic molecule required for the activation of an apoenzyme to an enzyme; the vitamin coenzymes are thiamin, riboflavin, niacin, pyridoxine, folic acid, and pantothenic acid.

cofactor: a nonprotein component that may be required by an enzyme for its activity.

collagen: a comparatively insoluble protein that is found in the skin, tendons, bones, and cartilage; it is converted to gelatin by boiling.

compound lipids: compounds (esters) of fatty acids containing groups in addition to an alcohol and fatty acid, i.e., phospholipids.

conjunctiva: delicate membrane lining the eyelids and covering the eyeballs.

conjunctival hemorrhages: hermorrhages in the membranes that line the eyelids and cover the eyeball.

corn, opaque-2: genetically developed; lysine and tryptophan contents are significantly higher than that of common corn.

corn, sugary-2, opaque-2: corn with high quality protein; has harder kernel than opaque-2, a desired quality for culinary uses.

coronary heart disease: ischemic heart disease: a cardiac disability arising from a reduction or arrest of blood supply to part of the heart muscle either by a narrowing or complete obstruction of a blood vessel.

creatine phosphokinase (creatine kinase): the enzyme that catalyzes the conversion of ADP (adenosine diphosphate, a high-energy compound that functions in many reactions in the body) and phosphocreatine (a high-energy phosphate compound occurring in muscle) to ATP (adenosine triphosphate; occurs in all cells where it represents energy storage) and creatine (a constituent of muscle).

cytoplasm: protoplasm of a cell surrounding the nucleus.

deamination: removal of an amino group from a compound.

dementia: a psychosis (mental disorder) characterized by serious mental impairment and deterioration.

dentin: the chief substance of the tooth, which surrounds the tooth pulp and is covered by enamel on the exposed part of the tooth (crown) and by cementum on the roots.

deoxyribonucleic acid (DNA): the substance that constitutes the genetic material in most organisms.

derived lipids: compounds (esters) formed from the hydrolysis of lipids, i.e., fatty acids, glycerol, cholesterol.

dermatitis: an inflammation of the skin.

development: generally denotes the series of changes by which the individual embryo becomes a mature organism. For example, the replacement of skeletal cartilage by calcified bone in the growing child.

diabetes mellitus: a disorder of carbohydrate metabolism in which the ability to oxidize and utilize carbohydrate is lost as a result of disturbances in the normal insulin mechanism; characterized by elevated blood sugar (hyperglycemia), sugar in the urine (glycosuria), excessive urination (polyuria), increased thirst (polydipsia), increased appetite (polyphagia), and general weakness.

diabetic acidosis: a relative decrease of alkali in body fluids in proportion to the content of acid.

diarrhea: rapid movement of the fecal matter through the intestine producing a frequent, watery stool.

diffusion: the movement of molecules from a region of higher to one of lower concentration.

digestion: the mechanical and chemical breakdown of food into simple substances that can be absorbed and used by the body cells.

disaccharide: a carbohydrate composed of two sugars.

diuretic: a substance that promotes the excretion of urine; diuretic drugs are used chiefly to rid the body of excess fluid.

duodenal or gastric ulcer: a defect (ulceration) of the mucous membrane of the duodenum or stomach.

duodenum: the first portion of the small intestine.

edema: an abnormal accumulation of fluid in the intercellular spaces of the body.

elastin: a major connective tissue protein of elastic structures (i.e. large blood vessels); a yellow, elastic, fibrous mucoprotein.

electrocardiogram (ECG and EKG): a tracing representing the heart's electrical action that is made by amplifying the minutely small electrical impulses normally generated by the heart.

electrolyte: any compound that, when dissolved in water separates into charged particles (ions) capable of conducting an electric current, such as sodium chloride, which dissociates into Na+ and Cl−.

electron microscope: developed in 1933 by Knoll and Ruska; available for research use about 1940; magnifies from 150,000 to 300,000 times permitting visualization of cellular structure.

emaciation: excessive leanness; a wasted condition of the body.

emulsifying agent: a substance that aids the dispersion of one liquid in another, liquids that are naturally immiscible, such as oil and water.

enamel: the calcified tissue covering the crown of a tooth.

encephalomalacia: softening of the brain; occurs in vitamin E deficient chicks.

endemic: a disease of low morbidity that persists over a long period of time in a given region.

endocrine gland: a ductless gland that produces one or more hormones and secretes them directly into the blood.

endogenous: produced within the organism.

endoplasmic reticulum: continuous system of cavities (channels) bound by a membrane that passes throughout the cytoplasm of the cell.

enteric: pertaining to the small intestine.

enzyme: a protein formed in plant and animal cells that acts as an organic catalyst in initiating or speeding up specific chemical reactions.

epidemiology: the scientific study of factors that influence the frequency and distribution of infectious diseases in humans.

epidermis: the outermost layer of the skin.

epigastric: region overlying the stomach.

epinephrine: a hormone secreted by the medulla (inner portion) of the adrenal gland; causes an increase in blood pressure, heart rate, and elevates the blood sugar level by increasing the breakdown of liver glycogen.

ergometer: an instrument for measuring amount of work done under controlled condtions.

erythroid: pertaining to the development of erythrocytes.

erythropoiesis: the production of erythrocytes.

esophagus: the hollow muscular tube extending from the mouth to the stomach.

estrogen: a general name for the principal female sex hormones.

extracellular fluid: fluid outside the cell; comprises about one-third of the total body fluid; includes tissue fluid, blood plasma, cerebrospinal fluid, fluid in the eye, and fluid of the gastrointestinal tract.

extrinsic radioiron tags: radioactive iron added to food, making it possible to identify the iron in the body.

exudative diathesis: accumulation of fluid in subcutaneous tissues, muscles, or connective tissues, caused by the escape of plasma from the capillaries.

fatty acid: organic compound composed of carbon, hydrogen, and oxygen; combines with glycerol to form fat.

femoral: pertaining to the thigh.

ferritin: an iron-containing protein; concentration in blood is a good index of amount of storage iron; serves as a storage form for iron in the liver, spleen, and other tissues.

fibrinogen: a protein in blood that through the action

of the enzyme thrombin is converted to fibrin (the insoluble protein essential to the clotting of blood).

flatulence: excessive formation of gas in the stomach or intestines.

fluid: liquid.

Food and Agriculture Organization of the United Nations (FAO): established in 1945, the FAO's main purpose is to raise the levels of nutrition and the standards of living of the people of the UN member nations. Periodic estimates are made of the food available to each country in an attempt to improve production and distribution. Its headquarters is in Rome.

Food and Nutrition Board (National Academy of Sciences – National Research Council): established in 1940, this board serves as an advisory body to the government on food and nutrition. One of its functions has been the establishment and periodic revision of the Recommended Dietary Allowances.

fortification: the addition of one or more nutrients to a food in amounts so that the total content will be larger than that contained in any natural (unprocessed) food of its class; for example, the fortification of fruit juices with vitamin C; the FDA has not established standards for fortified foods.

Framingham Heart Study: a study initiated in 1949 in the town of Framingham, Massachusetts, with over 5000 healthy men and women, all over 30 years of age, participating. The purpose of the study was to identify factors in the lives of persons which are associated with coronary heart disease. At the beginning of the study the participants were examined clinically, certain laboratory (biochemical) tests were made, and their life style assessed. These observations are repeated every two years.

gastric: pertaining to the stomach.

gastric mucosa: the membrane lining of the stomach.

gastrointestinal: pertaining to the stomach and intestinal tract.

gene: one of the units of heredity arranged in a definite fashion along a chromosome.

glossitis: an inflammation of the tongue.

gluconeogenesis (glyconeogenesis): the formation of glucose from noncarbohydrate sources, chiefly certain amino acids and the glycerol portion of the fat molecule.

glucose tolerance: the body's reaction to ingested glucose; glucose tolerance can be determined quantitatively by the glucose tolerance test in which the individual ingests 100 g of glucose (12 hours after food) and later the blood glucose level is determined at intervals. Within 2 to 2½ hours after taking the sugar, the blood glucose level returns to normal unless an abnormality exists.

gluteal: pertaining to the buttocks.

glyceride: a compound (ester) formed by the combination of glycerol and fatty acids and the loss of water from the ester linkage; according to the number of ester linkages, the compound is a mono-, di-, or triglyceride.

glycerol (glycerin): the 3-carbon alcohol from the hydrolysis of fat.

glycogen: chief carbohydrate storage material in humans and animals.

glycogenesis: the formation of glycogen from glucose.

glycogenic: of or pertaining to the formation of glycogen (the storage form of carbohydrate in humans and animals).

glycogenolysis: the breakdown of liver glycogen to glucose.

glycolipid: any lipid containing a carbohydrate.

glycolysis: the breakdown of sugars into simpler compounds; aerobic glycolysis involves sufficient O and end products are CO_2, H_2O, and ATP; anaerobic glycolysis, a reaction in the absence of O, yields lactic acid.

glycoprotein: a compound of a carbohydrate and protein.

gram (g): a metric unit of weight that is equivalent to about 1/28 of an ounce (1 oz = 28.4 g), 1/1000 of a kilogram, or 1000 milligrams.

growth: generally denotes the increases in physical size of the human body as a whole, or any of its dimensions, parts, or tissues which begin at conception and continue throughout the life cycle.

half-life, physical: time required for one-half the radioactive substance to be transformed to another substance.

hallucinogen: an agent that produces hallucinations or false sensory perceptions.

health: a state of complete physical, mental, and social well being, and not merely the absence of disease and infirmity.

hematocrit: percentage of whole blood volume that is erythrocytes.

heme: the nonprotein, iron-containing constituent of hemoglobin; the pigment portion of the hemoglobin molecule.

hemicellulose: a polysaccharide that is more soluble than cellulose.

hemochromatosis: a disorder of iron metabolism characterized by excess deposition of iron in the tissue, especially in the liver and pancreas, and by bronze pigmentation of the skin. Occurs in conditions of iron overload.

hemolysis: rupture of erythrocytes with release of hemoglobin into the plasma.

hemorrhage: escape of blood from the vessels; bleeding.

hemosiderin: an insoluble form of storage iron.

high density lipoproteins (HDL): a lipoprotein with a density of about 1.063; composed of about 50 percent protein and the rest total lipids: also called alpha cholesterol.

high-nutrient density: a high proportion of a specific nutrient to total kilocalories in a given amount of food.

histology: microscopic anatomy; deals with minute structure, composition, and function of tissues.

homeostasis: maintenance of constant physiologic conditions within the body; for example, the lungs provide oxygen as it is required by the cells; the kidneys through the processes of reabsorption and elimination help to maintain the blood composition normal.

hormone: a secretion produced in the body (chiefly by the endocrine glands) that is carried in the bloodstream to other parts of the body; each hormone has a specific effect on cells, tissues, and organs.

hydrochloric acid: a normal constituent of human gastric juice.

hydrogenation: the addition of hydrogen to a compound, especially to an unsaturated fat or fatty acid; adding hydrogen at the double bond will solidify soft fats or oils.

hydrolysis: a chemical process whereby a compound is broken down into simpler units with the uptake of water.

hydroperoxide: a strong oxidizing agent, with the general formula ROOH (in which R represents an organic group such as in C_2H_5OOH).

hydroxylation: introduction of a hydroxyl group (^-OH) into an organic compound (a carbon-containing compound).

hypertension: persistently high blood pressure.

hypochromic: pertains to a condition in which there is an abnormal decrease in the hemoglobin content of the erythrocytes.

hypoproteinemea: abnormally small amounts of total protein in the circulating blood plasma.

hypothalamus: a portion of the brain occupying the upper part of the cranium.

idiopathic: a condition of spontaneous origin; of unknown causation.

ileal resection: removal of part of the ileum section of the small intestine.

ileum: the distal section of the small intestine between the jejunum and the large intestine.

immunoglobulin: a protein of animal origin that has a known antibody activity.

insensible perspiration: perspiration that evaporates before it is perceived as fluid on the skin.

International Unit (IU): units of measure; used for vitamin A activity, vitamin D, and vitamin E.

interstitial fluid: portion of body fluid present in the interspaces of tissues.

intolerance: sensitivity or allergy to certain foods.

intracellular: inside the cells.

intrinsic factor (IF): a transferase enzyme (mucoprotein) secreted by the mucosal cells of the stomach that is required for the absorption of vitamin B-12 through the intestinal wall; a lack of the factor results in pernicious anemia.

ionic iron: pertaining to an atom of iron, as Fe^{3+} or Fe^{2+} (ferric and ferrous, respectively).

iron-binding capacity: the relative saturation of the iron-binding protein transferrin—the amount of the transferrin bound to iron in relation to the amount remaining free to combine with iron.

irradiation: exposure to radiation.

ischemic heart disease: deficiency of blood supply to the heart muscle due to obstruction or constriction of the coronary arteries.

isotonicity: the same osmotic pressure among fluids (solutions).

isotopic label: marking a compound by introducing into it an isotope of one of its constituent elements, i.e.,

489

using a form of the element with a different atomic mass. The atomic mass of carbon (C) is 12; an isotope of carbon has an atomic mass of 14, expressed in this manner ^{14}C.

jejunum: the middle section of the small intestine between the duodenum and ileum.

ketogenic: conducive to the production of ketones, products of fatty acid oxidation that eventually are broken down to carbon dioxide and water.

ketosis: the accumulation of large quantities of ketone bodies (substances synthesized by the liver as a step in the combustion of fats) in the body tissues and fluids.

kilocalorie (kcal): the quantity of heat required to raise the temperature of 1 kg of water 1°C (or more precisely, from 15°C to 16°C).

kilogram (kg): a metric unit of weight that is equivalent to 2.2 pounds, or 1000 grams.

kilojoule (kJ): a metric unit of energy that is equivalent to 0.239 kcal.

labile protein: reserve protein available in most tissues.

lactic acid: a compound formed in the body in the metabolism of carbohydrates.

lecithin: a phospholipid found in many animal tissues.

legume: the pod or fruit of peas and beans.

leguminous: adjective form of legume.

lethargy: a state of prolonged unconsciousness from which a person can be aroused but into which he or she immediately relapses.

lignin: a substance that, with cellulose, makes up the woody structure of plants; it is not a carbohydrate.

linoleic acid: the essential fatty acid; it is unsaturated; and occurs widely in plant glycerides.

lipids: substances that are diverse in chemical nature but all soluble in fat solvents (such as ethanol, ether, chloroform, benzene): lipids include fats and oils; phospholipids, glycolipids, and lipoproteins; fatty acids, alcohols [glycerol, sterols (including vitamins D and A), and carotenoids].

lipoprotein: a compound composed of a lipid and a protein.

longevity: the condition or quality of being long-lived.

low density lipoprotein (LDP): a lipoprotein with a density of about 1.006 to 1.109; composed of about 11 percent protein and 89 percent total lipids; also called beta cholesterol.

lymph: a fluid that circulates within the lymphatic vessels and is eventually added to the venous blood circulation; it arises from tissue fluid and from intestinal absorption of fatty acids; it is colorless, odorless, slightly alkaline, and slightly opalescent.

lymphatic system: all the vessels and structures that carry lymph from the tissues to the blood.

macrocyte: the largest of all types of red blood cells.

malaise: a feeling of illness or depression.

malnutrition: an all-inclusive term for poor nourishment; it may be due to an inadequate diet or to some defect in metabolism that prevents the body from using the nutrients properly.

mannitol: an alcohol derived from the 6-carbon sugar mannose.

medium-chain triglycerides (MCT): manufactured triglycerides containing fatty acids of 8 or 10 carbon atoms; for individuals with a fat malabsorption disorder.

megajoule (MJ): a metric unit of energy that is equivalent to 240 kcal.

megaloblast: a large, nucleated, embryonic type of cell; it is found in the blood in cases of pernicious anemia, vitamin B-12 deficiency, and folacin deficiency.

menarche: the establishment of menstrual function.

mEq or meq: milliequivalent; one mEq of an ion is equal to the atomic weight (mg) divided by the valence. For example, for sodium, it is $23/1 = 23$.

metabolic reactions: chemical changes that occur in a living organism; some are synthetic (the formation of new compounds) and some are degradative (the breakdown of compounds).

metabolism: all the chemical changes that take place after the nutrients are absorbed into the body.

metabolite: a substance that enters into a chemical reaction in the body, as a reacting substance, an intermediate, or final product.

metalloenzyme: an enzyme containing a metal (ion) as an integral part of its active structure; examples are cytochromes (iron, copper), carbonic anhydrase (zinc).

millet: the white seeds of the grass *Panicum miliaceum* used in parts of the world as food.

molecule: the smallest unit of a compound; for example, a molecule of water is H_2O.

monodeiodination: removal of one atom of iodine from a compound.

monosaccharide: a carbohydrate composed of one sugar.

monovalent: having a valence (the power of an atom to combine with another atom) of one. The valence of the hydrogen atom is one. Sodium (Na^+) has a valence of one; it combines with chloride (Cl^-) to form sodium chloride (NaCl).

muscular dystrophy: a group of genetically determined muscle diseases that are progressively crippling because muscles are gradually weakened and become atrophied (shrunken).

mutation: the process whereby a gene undergoes a structural change leading to a sudden and stable change in the genetic make-up of a cell or organism.

myosin: one of the two main proteins of muscle; involved with actin in the contraction of muscle fibers.

National Academy of Sciences (NAS): a scientific group, founded over a century ago, to serve science and the United States Government.

National Research Council (NRC): a scientific group, founded in 1916 by the National Academy of Sciences, to work with the major American scientific and technical societies to coordinate their efforts in the service of science and the government.

native protein: a protein in its natural state.

necrosis: death of tissue, usually as individual cells, groups of cells, or in small localized areas.

neuritis: inflammation of the peripheral nerves (which link the brain and spinal cord with the muscles, skin, organs, and other parts of the body).

neutropenia: the presence of abnormally small numbers of mature white blood cells in the granulocytic series (neutrophils).

nicotinamide-adenine dinucleotide (NAD) (formerly called diphosphopyridine nucleotide—DPN): attached as a prosthetic group (a nonprotein organic group) to a protein; it serves as a respiratory enzyme (part of an oxidative-reduction system, converting substrates to CO_2 and H_2O and the transfer of electrons removed to oxygen).

nicotinamide-adenine dinucleotide phosphate (NADP) (formerly called triphosphopyridine nucleotide [TPN]): a coenzyme that participates in oxidative-reduction processes.

nomenclature: a system of technical terms; terminology.

nonheme: iron that is not a part of the hemoglobin molecule; a designation for iron in foods of plant origin.

nonvegan: a nonvegetarian; a person who includes protein of animal origin in the diet.

nourish: to provide food or other substances necessary for life and growth.

nucleolus: present within the nucleus; has no limiting membrane; area containing ribonucleic acid.

nucleus: the part of the cell that contains the chromosomes; the control center of the cell, for both chemical reactions and reproduction; contains large quantities of DNA.

nutrient: a substance essential for the growth, maintenance, function, and reproduction of a cell or an organism.

nutritional status: health of an individual as influenced by the quality of foods eaten and the ability of the body to utilize these foods to meet its needs.

obesity: the accumulation of body fat beyond the amount needed for good health.

oral hypoglycemic agents: drugs that lower the blood sugar in mild forms of diabetes mellitus; examples are tolbutamide and chlorpropamide.

organic acid: contains one or more carboxyl groups (COOH); simple examples are formic acid (HCOOH) and oxalic acid $\begin{matrix} COOH \\ | \\ (COOH.) \end{matrix}$

organic kingdom: the animal and vegetable kingdoms.

osmotic pressure: the pressure that causes water or another solvent to move from a solution with a low concentration of solid (solute) to one having a high concentration of solute.

osteodystrophy, renal: a bone condition resulting from chronic disease of the kidneys which has symptoms of several bone disorders: osteitis fibrosa cystica (rarefication of bone, with marked activity of the bone-destroying cells); osteomalacia (a condition marked by softening of the bones due to impaired mineralization with excess accumulation of organic matrix); and osteoporosis (abnormal rarefication of bone, seen most commonly in the elderly).

osteoporosis: a disease of bone characterized by an increased porosity in the bone.

ovalbumin: an albumin found in egg whites.

oxidation: the change in an atom, a group of atoms, or a molecule that involves one or more of the following: (1) gain of oxygen, (2) loss of hydrogen, (3) loss of electrons.

oxidative phosphorylation: the process whereby adenosine triphosphate (ATP) with three phosphate groups, two of which are held by high energy bonds (designated in this manner $\sim [P - P \sim P]$), is formed from adenosine diphosphate (ADP) by the addition of phosphate.

parasites, intestinal: an organism that lives in the intestine of humans and animals, gaining its nourishment there.

parathyroid: the parathyroid glands are located on each side of the thyroid gland; their secretion, the parathyroid hormone, stimulates the release of calcium from bone and the elevation of the blood calcium level.

parenteral: administered other than by mouth; may be subcutaneously (beneath the skin), or intramuscularly (into the muscle), or intravenously (into a vein).

pectin: a class of soluble carbohydrates resistant to animal enzymes.

pellagrins: individuals suffering from pellagra.

pepsin: the protein-splitting enzyme of the gastric secretion.

pepsinogen: the inactive precursor of pepsin, produced by the chief cells of the stomach and converted to pepsin under acid conditions.

peptide: a compound that consists of two or more amino acids that are linked between the carboxyl group of one amino acid and the amino group of the other with the loss of a molecule of water.

percentile: one of the values establishing the divisions of a series of items into hundreds. For example, as in Appendix Table A-17, the divisions are 5, 10, 25, 50, 75, 90, and 95; a height that is greater than only 5 percent of all height measurements is in the fifth percentile whereas a height that is greater than 95 percent of all height measurements is in the ninety-fifth percentile.

peridontal membrane: provides the connection between the root of the tooth and its socket in the bone.

perinatal: fetal period and first 30 days after birth.

peristalsis: the wavelike movement in the lining of the digestive tract that propels the food mass along by contraction and relaxation of the muscle fibers.

peristaltic: the adjective form of peristalsis.

pernicious anemia: caused by a lack of the intrinsic factor necessary for the absorption of vitamin B-12; characterized by megaloblastic anemia and neurological symptoms.

peroxidation: oxidation to the point of forming a peroxide, a compound (oxide) which contains an $-0-0-$ group.

pharmacologic dose: usually 10 times the physiologic dose used to treat an illness or condition quite unrelated to the deficiency signs or symptoms of a nutrient.

phospholipids: fatlike substances consisting of glycerol, two fatty acids, a phosphate group, and nitrogen-containing compound, such as choline (found in the phospholipid leceithin).

phosphorylation: a chemical reaction in which a phosphate group is introduced into an organic compound.

photosynthesis: the complex chemical reaction of CO_2, H_2O, and sunlight in the chlorophyll tissues of plants to form carbohydrates.

physiologic dose: the amount of a nutrient needed or recommended to prevent signs of a deficiency in practically all healthy persons; the RDA of a nutrient.

phytate: a salt of phytic acid (a phosphorus compound occurring in outer layers of cereal grains; the calcium of the insoluble calcium phytate is unabsorbable from the intestine).

pituitary gland: an endocrine gland, located below the brain, that regulates a large portion of the endocrine activity of vertebrates.

placenta: a spongy structure that grows on the wall of the uterus during pregnancy and through which the fetus is nourished.

plasma: the fluid portion of blood in which the formed bodies (red blood cells, white blood cells, platelets) are suspended.

platelets: smallest of formed elements in the blood (others are erythrocytes and leucocytes).

492

polyneuritis: an inflammation encompassing many peripheral nerves.

polyunsaturated fatty acids: fatty acids containing two or more double bonds, such as linoleic, linolenic, and arachidonic acids.

porphyrin: a compound present in hemoglobin; a tetrapyrolle ring structure.

portal blood: the blood in the portal vein passing from the gastrointestinal tract to the liver.

portal circulation: the passage of blood from the gastrointestinal tract through the portal vein to the liver.

portal vein: the vein that carries blood from the wall of the intestine to the liver.

precursor: a compound from which another, usually more active, is formed.

progestogen: substances that induce changes in the lining of the uterus preparatory to gestation.

prothrombin activator: a complex substance that splits prothrombin (present in blood) to form thrombin, an essential step in the clotting process; when tissue is injured it releases two factors (tissue factor and tissue phospholipids) that initiate the formation of prothrombin activator; or within the circulatory system, injury to the blood can initiate the formation of the prothrombin factor.

proton: a particle of the nucleus of an atom that has a charge of plus one. A proton is a positive hydrogen ion ($H+$).

ptyalin: the starch-splitting enzyme of saliva.

puberty: the period between the time of appearance of secondary sex characteristics and the completion of body growth.

purines: the parent substance of the purine bases; adenine and guanine are the major purine bases of nucleic acids; other important purines are xanthine and uric acid.

pyridoxine: vitamin B-6.

pyrimidine: the parent substance of several nitrogenous compounds found in nucleic acids — uracil, thymine, and cytosine.

pyruvic acid: a keto acid of 3-carbon atoms; it is formed of carbohydrate in aerobic metabolism; pyruvate is the salt or ester of pyruvic acid.

radiation: the emission of particles, alpha, beta, or electrons.

radioactive isotope: a chemical element that changes into another with the emission of rays (alpha, beta, or gamma). Among the naturally radioactive elements are uranium and radium; some other elements can be made radioactive by bombardment with neutrons or deutrons or other means.

radioimmunoassay: a method for determining hormones, such as insulin, by employing a radioactive-labeled substance that reacts with the hormone under test.

radiologically: studied by the examination of X-rays.

red blood cells: also called erythrocytes or red corpuscles; when mature they consist chiefly of hemoglobin and a supporting framework.

renin: an enzyme produced by the kidney in response to diminished blood pressure; renin converts angiotensinogen, present in the blood, to angiotensin which stimulates aldosterone secretion.

rennet (or rennin): an enzyme, prepared commercially from the stomachs of calves, that coagulates milk.

reserpine: an active alkaloid from Rauwolfia species, used as an antihypertensive, tranquilizer, and sedative.

respiration: the exchange of oxygen and carbon dioxide in the lungs, between the cell and its environment, and in the metabolism of the cell.

retina: the light-sensitive portion of the eye.

retinol equivalents (RE): a unit now used to express vitamin A activity; five International Units equal one retinol equivalent.

R group: the side chain of an amino acid. Each amino acid has in common an amino group and a carboxyl group but has one group that is different in each amino acid; this group is designated the R group.

rheumatic disease: a disease marked by inflammation of the connective tissue structures of the body, especially the muscles and joints and by pain in these parts.

ribonucleic acid (RNA): a compound that occurs in three major forms, ribosomal, transfer, and messenger ribonucleic acid, all of which function in the cell in the synthesis of proteins.

ribosomes: components of the cell which contain approximately equal amounts of RNA and protein; they are the sites of protein synthesis in the cell.

ruminant: an animal that has a stomach with four complete cavities and that characteristically regurgitates undigested food from the rumen, the first stomach, and masticates it when at rest.

salivary glands: glands in the mouth that secrete saliva.

sarcoplasmic reticulum: a network of smooth-surfaced tubules surrounding the myofibrils (small contractile, threadlike structures within the cytoplasm of a muscle fiber) of a muscle, such as a skeletal or a cardiac muscle.

scurvy: a deficiency disease due to vitamin C deficiency; weakness, loss of weight, bleeding gums are among its symptoms.

selective permeability: when only certain substances are permitted to pass through the membrane, others are rejected.

seleniferous: areas in which the soil is high in the mineral selenium.

semipermeable membrane: a membrane that allows the passage of only certain solids but is freely permeable to water.

serum: the fluid obtained from blood after it has been allowed to clot.

serum cholesterol: the level of the sterol cholesterol in the blood.

serum triglyceride: the level of fat in the blood.

short chain fatty acids: those with 10 or fewer carbon atoms.

sickle cell anemia: a genetic disorder characterized by the presence of crescent-shaped red blood cells, excessive hemolysis, and active blood formation (hemopoiesis); symptoms are leg ulcers, arthritic manifestations, pain, and abnormal hemoglobin (85 percent is sickle cell hemoglobin and the remainder fetal hemoglobin).

simple lipids: compounds (esters) of fatty acids with various alcohols, i.e., fats and waxes.

simple sugars: the monosaccharides; glucose, fructose, and galactose.

sorghum: syrup from the juice of the grass plant *Sorghum vulgare*; it resembles cane syrup and contains considerable fructose and some starch and dextrin.

sprue: a chronic disease caused by the imperfect absorption of nutrients (especially fat) from the small intestine; it is characterized by diarrhea, subnormal body weight, and sensations of fatigue.

standard of identity: description of a food product in terms of kinds and amounts of ingredients established by the Food and Drug Administration.

stearic acid: a saturated fatty acid composed of 18 carbon atoms.

steroid: a group name for compounds that resemble cholesterol chemically.

sterol: an alcohol of high molecular weight, such as cholesterol and ergosterol.

sympathomimetic: an agent that produces effects similar to those of the sympathetic nervous system which goes to the heart, smooth muscle, and glands of the entire body.

syndrome: a combination of symptoms resulting from a single cause.

synthesis: the process whereby a more complex substance is produced from simpler substances by a reaction or a series of reactions.

template: a molecule that functions as a mold or pattern for the synthesis of another molecule.

thrombin: an enzyme that catalyzes the conversion of fibrinogen to fibrin.

thyroiditis: inflammation of the thyroid gland.

thyroxine: an iodine-containing hormone that is produced by the thyroid gland; it is a derivative of the amino acid tyrosine and has the chemical name tetraiodothyronine.

tocopheryl: an ester form of tocopherol; alpha-tocopheryl acetate, for example, is the ester formed from the alcohol, alpha-tocopherol, and acetic acid, splitting out a molecule of water.

tocotrienol: compounds found in nature that are factors of vitamin E, but are less effective biologically than alpha- and gamma-tocopherol.

toxemia of pregnancy: a pathologic condition occurring in pregnant women, characterized by excessive vomiting (hyperemesis, gravidum), hypertension, albuminuria, and edema.

trabeculae: calcified portion of spongy bone.

transamination: the transfer of an amino group of an amino acid to another acid, forming an amino acid.

transcellular water: a term applied to the fluid of the salivary glands, the pancreas, liver, mucus membrane of the respiratory and gastrointestinal tracts, cerebrospinal fluid, and ocular fluids.

transcribe: the process of copying the genetic information of DNA in the form of RNA.

transferrin: blood protein that binds and transports iron.

transit: the act of passing through.

transketolase: an enzyme that uses thiamin diphosphate as a coenzyme: it brings about the transfer of a 2-carbon unit from one sugar (a 2-keto sugar) to aldoses [monosaccharides with the characteristic aldehyde group (—CHO)].

triglyceride (fat): an ester composed of glycerol and three fatty acids.

tristearin: a triglyceride of stearic acid.

troponin: one of the minor proteins in muscle; myosin and actin make up about 80 percent of the proteins involved in the contraction process.

trypsin: the protein-splitting enzyme of the pancreas.

urea: one of the final products of nitrogen metabolism.

USP: United States Pharmocopeia; a legally recognized compendium of standards for drugs published by the United States Pharmacopeial Convention, Inc.

uterus: a hollow muscular organ in the female pelvis; it holds the growing fetus.

valence: a whole number indicating for any element its ability to combine with another element.

very low density lipoprotein (VLDL): a lipoprotein with a density of about 0.96 to 1.006; composed of about 7 percent protein and 93 percent total lipids; also called pre-beta cholesterol.

vital capacity: the volume of air a person can forcibly expire from the lungs after a maximal inspiration.

World Health Organization of the United Nations (WHO): the specialized agency, located in Geneva, that is concerned with health on an international level.

xanthophyll: a yellow coloring matter of plants; a carotinoid which is not a provitamin A.

xerosis: abnormal dryness.

Table and Appendixes

Unit	Multiply by
Energy:	
kilocalorie to kilojoule	4.184
kilocalorie to megajoule	0.004
kilojoule to kilocalorie	0.239
megajoule to kilocalorie	239
Length:	
centimeters to inches	0.394
centimeters to meters	0.010
foot to centimeters	30.480
foot to meter	0.305
inches to centimeters	2.540
meters to inches	39.370
Liquid Measure:	
cubic centimeter to fluid ounce	0.034
fluid ounce to cubic centimeter	29.574
liter to quart	1.057
Weight:	
grams to micrograms	1 million
grams to milligrams	1000
grams to ounces	0.035
grams to pounds	0.002
kilograms to pounds	2.2
ounces to grams	28.350
pounds to kilograms	0.454

Temperature

Conversion of Fahrenheit to Centigrade (Celsius):
  F° − 32°, multiply by 5/9
Conversion of Centigrade (Celsius) to Fahrenheit:
  C° multiply by 9/5, + 32°
  Examples:
    98.6° F or 37.0° C (body temperature)
    32° F or 0° C (freezing temperature)
    212° F or 100° C (boiling temperature)

Abbreviations for Units Commonly Used in Nutrition

kcal = kilocalorie	cc = cubic centimeter
kJ = kilojoule	qt = quart
MJ = megajoule	pt = pint
kg = kilogram	c = cup
g = gram	tbsp (T) = tablespoon
mg = milligram	tsp (t) = teaspoon
μg(mcg) = microgram	m = meter
lb = pound	cm = centimeter
oz = ounce	ft = foot
l = liter	in = inch
ml = milliliter	

Table A.1 Essential Amino Acid Content of Foods (mg per 100 grams of food, edible portion)[a]

Food	Isoleucine, mg	Leucine, mg	Lysine, mg	Methionine, mg	Phenylalanine, mg	Threonine, mg	Tryptophan mg	Valine, mg
Cereals								
Maize	350	1190	254	182	464	342	67	461
Oats	526	1012	517	234	698	462	176	711
Rice, polished	296	581	255	150	342	234	95	408
Wheat								
whole grain	426	871	374	196	589	382	142	577
germ	889	1710	1608	482	1015	1047	261	1240
flour (white)	349	644	182	140	468	246	93	386
bulgur	390	766	309	190	486	340	127	468
Starchy roots								
Cassava	46	64	67	22	41	43	19	54
Potato	76	121	96	26	80	75	33	93
Sweet potato	48	71	45	22	51	50	22	59
Taro	64	133	70	24	92	74	26	111
Yam	89	154	97	38	114	86	30	110
Dry legumes								
Beans	927	1685	1593	234	1154	878	223	1016
Chick-peas	891	1505	1376	209	1151	756	174	913
Cowpeas	895	1647	1599	273	1209	842	254	1060
Groundnuts	990	1876	1036	338	1459	764	305	1224
Lentils	1045	1847	1739	194	1266	960	231	1211
Lima beans	977	1604	1466	246	1195	823	199	1015
Peas	961	1530	1692	205	1033	914	202	1058
Soybeans								
seeds	1889	3232	2653	525	2055	1603	532	1995
soya milk	171	278	195	50	175	128	48	165
fermented	924	1517	1120	259	912	742	235	921
Nuts and seeds								
Almonds	700	1267	454	518	975	492	172	1053
Brazil nuts	474	1168	474	984	661	442	322	729
Cashews	1057	1684	942	309	873	666	378	1188
Coconut	305	524	275	150	354	265	85	424
Pecans	384	574	348	112	392	275	97	345
Pistachios	881	1523	1080	367	1088	613	225	1344
Sesame	773	1433	585	602	947	763	287	985
Sunflower seeds	635	954	536	283	662	547	202	754
Walnuts	717	1376	285	247	753	494	185	809

497

Table A.1 (continued)

Food	Isoleucine, mg	Leucine, mg	Lysine, mg	Methionine, mg	Phenylala- nine, mg	Threonine, mg	Tryptophan mg	Valine, mg
Vegetables								
Asparagus	55	96	96	28	55	60	25	79
Beans	89	164	131	31	101	92	33	116
Beets								
leaves	40	93	60	17	54	62	21	60
roots	44	80	96	34	65	60	17	44
Broccoli	186	236	218	61	177	161	46	210
Brussels sprouts	230	257	252	43	172	199	58	228
Cabbage	50	86	50	17	49	61	17	68
Carrots	33	50	44	14	31	32	8	50
Cauliflower	136	196	160	44	101	119	39	156
Eggplant	52	72	63	13	49	44	12	61
Lettuce	50	83	50	24	67	54	10	71
Onions	20	37	63	16	38	20	20	30
Peas	273	457	479	61	289	247	66	311
Pumpkin	37	52	43	9	33	27	11	48
Spinach	106	208	159	46	133	116	34	133
Tomatoes	20	30	32	7	20	25	9	24
Turnips	22	36	17	10	18	25	11	22
Fruits								
Apples	13	23	22.	3	10	14	3	15
Apricots	14	23	23	4	13	16	—[b]	19
Avocados	47	76	59	29	48	40	9	63
Bananas	32	53	46	22	44	38	13	45
Dates	66	114	81	22	74	76	—	93
Figs	36	51	48	10	28	38	10	46
Grapes	6	14	15	23	14	19	3	19
Oranges	23	22	43	12	30	12	6	31
Peaches	13	29	30	31	18	27	4	40
Persimmons	36	52	42	8	38	49	14	38
Strawberries	18	42	32	1	23	25	9	23
Meat and poultry								
Beef and veal	852	1435	1573	478	778	812	198	886
Chicken	1069	1472	1590	502	800	794	205	1018
Mutton and lamb	778	1203	1275	383	625	733	198	790
Pork	608	897	961	321	496	583	162	616
Eggs, hen								
Whole	778	1091	863	416	709	634	184	847
Yolk	820	1370	1202	364	728	753	240	998
White	571	922	739	441	662	532	176	536

Table A.1 (continued)

Food	Isoleucine, mg	Leucine, mg	Lysine, mg	Methionine, mg	Phenylala-nine, mg	Threonine, mg	Tryptophan mg	Valine, mg
Fish								
Fresh, all types	900	1445	1713	539	737	861	211	1150
Meal	3228	5424	5808	2052	2892	3180	720	3816
Milk and milk products								
Cows'								
pasteurized	219	430	248	86	239	153	50	255
evaporated	481	726	480	142	328	332	91	448
powdered	1346	2526	1848	657	1236	1073	363	1640
Goats', raw	197	353	196	50	142	164	45	242
Human	48	104	81	19	41	53	20	54
Cheese, all types	956	1864	1559	530	950	725	217	1393

[a] Data available in the original source for all other amino acids.
[b] Data not available.
From *Amino Acid Content of Foods and Biological Data on Proteins*, FAO Nutritional Studies No. 24. Rome: Food and Agr. Organ., 1970.

Table A.2 Amino Acid Content of Foods[a] (in mg/g total nitrogen)

Food	Lysine	Methionine	Cystine	Methionine and cystine	Food	Lysine	Methionine	Cystine	Methionine and cystine
Polished rice	226	133	96	229	Spinach	454	132	102	234
Wheat, whole-grain	179	94	159	253	Banana	256	125	169	294
Wheat, flour, 80-90 percent extr.	195	97	127	224	Orange	330	94	75	169
					Beef	556	169	90	249
					Chicken	497	157	82	239
Potato	299	81	37	118	Pork	625	188	88	276
Bean (dry)	450	66	53	119	Fish	569	179	71	250
Peanut	221	72	78	150	Egg, whole	436	210	152	362
Brazil nut	175	363	131	494	Milk, human	428	101	84	185
Soybean, dry	399	79	83	162					
Soya milk	348	90	101	191					
Sunflower seed	225	119	93	212					

[a] Data available in the original source for other amino acids.
From *Amino Acid Content of Foods and Biological Data on Proteins*, FAO Nutritional Studies No. 24. Rome: Food and Agr. Organ., 1970.

Table A.3 Nutritive Values of the Edible Parts of Foods (Dashs in the columns denote lack of reliable data for a

In this table of 730 commonly used foods, values are given for food energy (kilocalories) and for nutrients (protein, fat, fatty acids, total carbohydrates, calcium, phosphorus, iron, potassium, vitamin A, thiamin, riboflavin, niacin, and vitamin C) in the edible part of each food, that is, in only that portion of the weight of each food that is customarily eaten—corn without the cob, meat without bones, potatoes without the skin, European-type grapes without the seeds. If additional parts are eaten (for example, the skin of the potato), the values for certain nutrients will be somewhat greater than those shown.

For toast and for vegetables, the values given do not include fat added either during the preparation or at the table. There may be some destruction of vitamins (especially vitamin C) in fruits and vegetables when these

Item No.	Food	Approximate measure	Weight, g	Water, percent	Food energy, kcal	Protein, g	Fat, g
	Almonds, shelled:						
507	Chopped (about 130 almonds)	1 cup	130	5	775	24	70
508	Slivered, not pressed down (about 115 almonds)	1 cup	115	5	690	21	62
225	Applejuice, bottled or canned	1 cup	248	88	120	Trace	Trace
	Apples, raw, unpeeled, without cores:						
223	2¾-in. diam. (about 3 per lb with cores)	1 apple	138	84	80	Trace	1
224	3¼-in. diam. (about 2 per lb with cores)	1 apple	212	84	125	Trace	1
	Applesauce, canned:						
226	Sweetened	1 cup	255	76	230	1	Trace
227	Unsweetened	1 cup	244	89	100	Trace	Trace
232	Apricot nectar, canned	1 cup	251	85	145	1	Trace
	Apricots:						
228	Raw, without pits (about 12 per lb with pits)	3 apricots	107	85	55	1	Trace
229	Canned in heavy sirup (halves and sirup)	1 cup	258	77	220	2	Trace
	Dried:						
230	Uncooked (28 large or 37 medium halves per cup)	1 cup	130	25	340	7	1
231	Cooked, unsweetened, fruit and liquid	1 cup	250	76	215	4	1
	Asparagus, green:						
	Cooked, drained:						
	Cuts and tips, 1½- to 2-in. lengths:						
564	From raw	1 cup	145	94	30	3	Trace
565	From frozen	1 cup	180	93	40	6	Trace
	Spears, ½-in. diam. at base:						
566	From raw	4 spears	60	94	10	1	Trace
567	From frozen	4 spears	60	92	15	2	Trace

[a] Applies to products without added vitamin C. For value of products with added vitamin C, refer to label.

nutrient believed to be present in a measurable amount.)

foods have been cut or shredded. Because such losses are variable, no deduction for them has been made.

The values for meat are for cuts that have been cooked and drained and do not include the drippings. For many cuts, two sets of values are shown: meat with the fat, and meat from which the fat has been removed.

Values for thiamin, riboflavin, and niacin in white flours and white bread and rolls include the increased

enrichment levels put into effect by the Food and Drug Administration in 1974.

For the approximate measure of each food as described, the weight is given in grams (rounded to the nearest whole number); in those instances where the inedible parts have been included in the description, both the measure and the weight include those parts. Each food is identified by an item number.

Fatty acids												
Satu-rated (total), g	Unsaturated		Carbo-hydrate, g	Cal-cium, mg	Phos-phorus, mg	Iron, mg	Potas-sium, mg	Vitamin A value, IU	Thia-min, mg	Ribo-flavin, mg	Niacin, mg	Vitamin C, mg
	Oleic, g	Lino-leic, g										
5.6	47.7	12.8	25	304	655	6.1	1,005	0	.31	1.20	4.6	Trace
5.0	42.2	11.3	22	269	580	5.4	889	0	.28	1.06	4.0	Trace
—	—	—	30	15	22	1.5	250	—	.02	.05	.2	2[a]
—	—	—	20	10	14	.4	152	120	.04	.03	.1	6
—	—	—	31	15	21	.6	233	190	.06	.04	.2	8
—	—	—	61	10	13	1.3	166	100	.05	.03	.1	3[a]
—	—	—	26	10	12	1.2	190	100	.05	.02	.1	2[a]
—	—	—	37	23	30	.5	379	2,380	.03	.03	.5	36
—	—	—	14	18	25	.5	301	2,890	.03	.04	.6	11
—	—	—	57	28	39	.8	604	4,490	.05	.05	1.0	10
—	—	—	86	87	140	7.2	1,273	14,170	.01	.21	4.3	16
—	—	—	54	55	88	4.5	795	7,500	.01	.13	2.5	8
—	—	—	5	30	73	.9	265	1,310	.23	.26	2.0	38
—	—	—	6	40	115	2.2	396	1,530	.25	.23	1.8	41
—	—	—	2	13	30	.4	110	540	.10	.11	.8	16
—	—	—	2	13	40	.7	143	470	.10	.08	.7	16

(Table A.3, continued)

No. Item	Food	Approximate measure	Weight, g	Water, percent	Food energy, kcal	Protein, g	Fat, g
568	Canned, spears, ½-in. diam. at base	4 spears	80	93	15	2	Trace
	Avocados, raw, whole, without skins and seeds:						
233	California, mid- and late-winter (with skin and seed, 3⅛-in. diam.; wt., 10 oz)	1 avocado	216	74	370	5	37
234	Florida, late summer and fall (with skin and seed, 3⅝-in. diam.; wt., 1 lb)	1 avocado	304	78	390	4	33
161	Bacon (20 slices per lb, raw), broiled or fried, crisp	2 slices	15	8	85	4	8
	Bagel, 3-in. diam.:						
319	Egg	1 bagel	55	32	165	6	2
320	Water	1 bagel	55	29	165	6	1
	Baking powders for home use:						
	Sodium aluminum sulfate:						
681	With monocalcium phosphate mono-hydrate	1 tsp	3.0	2	5	Trace	Trace
682	With monocalcium phosphate mono-hydrate, calcium sulfate	1 tsp	2.9	1	5	Trace	Trace
683	Straight phosphate	1 tsp	3.8	2	5	Trace	Trace
684	Low sodium	1 tsp	4.3	2	5	Trace	Trace
235	Banana without peel (about 2.6 per lb with peel)	1 banana	119	76	100	1	Trace
236	Banana flakes	1 tbsp	6	3	20	Trace	Trace
685	Barbecue sauce	1 cup	250	81	230	4	17
321	Barley, pearled, light, uncooked	1 cup	200	11	700	16	2
	Beans:						
	Lima, immature seeds, frozen, cooked, drained:						
569	Thick-seeded types (Fordhooks)	1 cup	170	74	170	10	Trace
570	Thin-seeded types (baby limas)	1 cup	180	69	210	13	Trace
	Snap:						
	Green:						
	Cooked, drained:						
571	From raw (cuts and French style)	1 cup	125	92	30	2	Trace
	From frozen:						
572	Cuts	1 cup	135	92	35	2	Trace
573	French style	1 cup	130	92	35	2	Trace
574	Canned, drained solids (cuts)	1 cup	135	92	30	2	Trace

(Table A.3, continued)

| Fatty acids | | | | | | | | | | | | |
Satu-rated (total), g	Unsaturated Oleic, g	Lino-leic, g	Carbo-hydrate, g	Cal-cium, mg	Phos-phorus, mg	Iron, mg	Potas-sium, mg	Vitamin A value, IU	Thia-min, mg	Ribo-flavin, mg	Niacin, mg	Vitamin C, mg
—	—	—	3	15	42	1.5	133	640	.05	.08	.6	12
5.5	22.0	3.7	13	22	91	1.3	1,303	630	.24	.43	3.5	30
6.7	15.7	5.3	27	30	128	1.8	1,836	880	.33	.61	4.9	43
2.5	3.7	.7	Trace	2	34	.5	35	0	.08	.05	.8	—
.5	.9	.8	28	9	43	1.2	41	30	.14	.10	1.2	0
.2	.4	.6	30	8	41	1.2	42	0	.15	.11	1.4	0
0	0	0	1	58	87	—	5	0	0	0	0	0
0	0	0	1	183	45	—	—	0	0	0	0	0
0	0	0	1	239	359	—	6	0	0	0	0	0
0	0	0	2	207	314	—	471	0	0	0	0	0
—	—	—	26	10	31	.8	440	230	.06	.07	.8	12
—	—	—	5	2	6	.2	92	50	.01	.01	.2	Trace
2.2	4.3	10.0	20	53	50	2.0	435	900	.03	.03	.8	13
.3	.2	.8	158	32	378	4.0	320	0	.24	.10	6.2	0
—	—	—	32	34	153	2.9	724	390	.12	.09	1.7	29
—	—	—	40	63	227	4.7	709	400	.16	.09	2.2	22
—	—	—	7	63	46	.8	189	680	.09	.11	.6	15
—	—	—	8	54	43	.9	205	780	.09	.12	.5	7
—	—	—	8	49	39	1.2	177	690	.08	.10	.4	9
—	—	—	7	61	34	2.0	128	630	.04	.07	.4	5

(Table A.3, continued)

No. Item	Food	Approximate measure	Weight, g	Water, percent	Food energy, kcal	Protein, g	Fat, g
	Yellow or wax:						
	Cooked, drained:						
575	From raw (cuts and French style)	1 cup	125	93	30	2	Trace
576	From frozen (cuts)	1 cup	135	92	35	2	Trace
577	Canned, drained solids (cuts)	1 cup	135	92	30	2	Trace
	Beans, dry:						
	Common varieties as Great Northern, navy, and others:						
	Cooked, drained:						
509	Great Northern	1 cup	180	69	210	14	1
510	Pea (navy)	1 cup	190	69	225	15	1
	Canned, solids and liquid:						
	White with—						
511	Frankfurters (sliced)	1 cup	255	71	365	19	18
512	Pork and tomato sauce	1 cup	255	71	310	16	7
513	Pork and sweet sauce	1 cup	255	66	385	16	12
514	Red kidney	1 cup	255	76	230	15	1
515	Lima, cooked, drained	1 cup	190	64	260	16	1
	Bean sprouts (mung):						
578	Raw	1 cup	105	89	35	4	Trace
579	Cooked, drained	1 cup	125	91	35	4	Trace
	Beef,[a] cooked:						
	Cuts braised, simmered or pot roasted:						
162	Lean and fat (piece, 2½ by 2½ by ¾ in.)	3 oz	85	53	245	23	16
163	Lean only from item 162	2.5 oz	72	62	140	22	5
	Ground beef, broiled:						
164	Lean with 10% fat	3 oz or patty 3 by ⅝ in.	85	60	185	23	10
165	Lean with 21% fat	2.9 oz or patty 3 by ⅝ in.	82	54	235	20	17
	Roast, oven cooked, no liquid added:						
	Relatively fat, such as rib:						
166	Lean and fat (2 pieces, 4⅛ by 2¼ by ¼ in.)	3 oz	85	40	375	17	33
167	Lean only from item 166	1.8 oz	51	57	125	14	7

[a] Outer layer of fat on the cut was removed to within approximately ½ in. of the lean. Deposits of fat within the cut were not removed.

(Table A.3, continued)

Saturated (total), g	Oleic, g	Linoleic, g	Carbohydrate, g	Calcium, mg	Phosphorus, mg	Iron, mg	Potassium, mg	Vitamin A value, IU	Thiamin, mg	Riboflavin, mg	Niacin, mg	Vitamin C, mg
—	—	—	6	63	46	.8	189	290	.09	.11	.6	16
—	—	—	8	47	42	.9	221	140	.09	.11	.5	8
—	—	—	7	61	34	2.0	128	140	.04	.07	.4	7
—	—	—	38	90	266	4.9	749	0	.25	.13	1.3	0
—	—	—	40	95	281	5.1	790	0	.27	.13	1.3	0
—	—	—	32	94	303	4.8	668	330	.18	.15	3.3	Trace
2.4	2.8	.6	48	138	235	4.6	536	330	.20	.08	1.5	5
4.3	5.0	1.1	54	161	291	5.9	—	—	.15	.10	1.3	—
—	—	—	42	74	278	4.6	673	10	.13	.10	1.5	—
—	—	—	49	55	293	5.9	1,163	—	.25	.11	1.3	—
—	—	—	7	20	67	1.4	234	20	.14	.14	.8	20
—	—	—	7	21	60	1.1	195	30	.11	.13	.9	8
6.8	6.5	.4	0	10	114	2.9	184	30	.04	.18	3.6	—
2.1	1.8	.2	0	10	108	2.7	176	10	.04	.17	3.3	—
4.0	3.9	.3	0	10	196	3.0	261	20	.08	.20	5.1	—
7.0	6.7	.4	0	9	159	2.6	221	30	.07	.17	4.4	—
14.0	13.6	.8	0	8	158	2.2	189	70	.05	.13	3.1	—
3.0	2.5	.3	0	6	131	1.8	161	10	.04	.11	2.6	—

(Table A.3, continued)

Item No.	Food	Approximate measure	Weight, g	Water, percent	Food energy, kcal	Protein, g	Fat, g
	Relatively lean, such as heel of round:						
168	Lean and fat (2 pieces, 4⅛ by 2¼ by ¼ in.)	3 oz	85	62	165	25	7
169	Lean only from item 168	2.8 oz	78	65	125	24	3
	Steak:						
	Relatively fat-sirloin, broiled:						
170	Lean and fat (piece, 2½ by 2½ by ¾ in.)	3 oz	85	44	330	20	27
171	Lean only from item 170	2.0 oz	56	59	115	18	4
	Relatively lean-round, braised:						
172	Lean and fat (piece, 4⅛ by 2¼ by ½ in.)	3 oz	85	55	220	24	13
173	Lean only from item 172	2.4 oz	68	61	130	21	4
	Beef, canned:						
174	Corned beef	3 oz	85	59	185	22	10
175	Corned beef hash	1 cup	220	67	400	19	25
176	Beef, dried, chipped	2½-oz jar	71	48	145	24	4
177	Beef and vegetable stew	1 cup	245	82	220	16	11
178	Beef potpie (home recipe), baked[b] (piece, ⅓ of 9-in. diam. pie)	1 piece	210	55	515	21	30
	Beets:						
	Cooked, drained, peeled:						
580	Whole beets, 2-in. diam.	2 beets	100	91	30	1	Trace
581	Diced or sliced	1 cup	170	91	55	2	Trace
	Canned, drained solids:						
582	Whole beets, small	1 cup	160	89	60	2	Trace
583	Diced or sliced	1 cup	170	89	65	2	Trace
584	Beet greens, leaves and stems, cooked, drained	1 cup	145	94	25	2	Trace
	Beverages, alcoholic:						
686	Beer	12 fl oz	360	92	150	1	0
	Gin, rum, vodka, whisky:						
687	80-proof	1½-fl oz jigger	42	67	95	—	—
688	86-proof	1½-fl oz jigger	42	64	105	—	—
689	90-proof	1½-fl oz jigger	42	62	110	—	—

[b] Crust made with vegetable shortening and enriched flour.

(Table A.3, continued)

Saturated (total), g	Fatty acids — Unsaturated Oleic, g	Linoleic, g	Carbohydrate, g	Calcium, mg	Phosphorus, mg	Iron, mg	Potassium, mg	Vitamin A value, IU	Thiamin, mg	Riboflavin, mg	Niacin, mg	Vitamin C, mg
2.8	2.7	.2	0	11	208	3.2	279	10	.06	.19	4.5	—
1.2	1.0	.1	0	10	199	3.0	268	Trace	.06	.18	4.3	—
11.3	11.1	.6	0	9	162	2.5	220	50	.05	.15	4.0	—
1.8	1.6	.2	0	7	146	2.2	202	10	.05	.14	3.6	—
5.5	5.2	.4	0	10	213	3.0	272	20	.07	.19	4.8	—
1.7	1.5	.2	0	9	182	2.5	238	10	.05	.16	4.1	—
4.9	4.5	.2	0	17	90	3.7	—	—	.01	.20	2.9	—
11.9	10.9	.5	24	29	147	4.4	440	—	.02	.20	4.6	—
2.1	2.0	.1	0	14	287	3.6	142	—	.05	.23	2.7	0
4.9	4.5	.2	15	29	184	2.9	613	2,400	.15	.17	4.7	17
7.9	12.8	6.7	39	29	149	3.8	334	1,720	.30	.30	5.5	6
—	—	—	7	14	23	.5	208	20	.03	.04	.3	6
—	—	—	12	24	39	.9	354	30	.05	.07	.5	10
—	—	—	14	30	29	1.1	267	30	.02	.05	.2	5
—	—	—	15	32	31	1.2	284	30	.02	.05	.2	5
—	—	—	5	144	36	2.8	481	7,400	.10	.22	.4	22
0	0	0	14	18	108	Trace	90	—	.01	.11	2.2	—
0	0	0	Trace	—	—	—	1	—	—	—	—	—
0	0	0	Trace	—	—	—	1	—	—	—	—	—
0	0	0	Trace	—	—	—	1	—	—	—	—	—

(Table A.3, continued)

Item No.	Food	Approximate measure	Weight, g	Water, percent	Food energy, kcal	Protein, g	Fat, g
	Wines:						
690	Dessert	3½-fl oz glass	103	77	140	Trace	0
691	Table	3½-fl oz glass	102	86	85	Trace	0
	Beverages, carbonated, sweetened, non-alcoholic:						
692	Carbonated water	12 fl oz	366	92	115	0	0
693	Cola type	12 fl oz	369	90	145	0	0
694	Fruit-flavored sodas and Tom Collins mixer	12 fl oz	372	88	170	0	0
695	Ginger ale	12 fl oz	366	92	115	0	0
696	Root beer	12 fl oz	370	90	150	0	0
	Biscuits, baking powder, 2-in. diam. (enriched flour, vegetable shortening):						
322	From home recipe	1 biscuit	28	27	105	2	5
323	From mix	1 biscuit	28	29	90	2	3
237	Blackberries, raw	1 cup	144	85	85	2	1
238	Blueberries, raw	1 cup	145	83	90	1	1
145	Bluefish, baked with butter or margarine	3 oz	85	68	135	22	4
722	Bouillon cube, ½ in.	1 cube	4	4	5	1	Trace
369	Bran flakes (40% bran), added sugar, salt, iron, vitamins	1 cup	35	3	105	4	1
370	Bran flakes with raisins, added sugar, salt, iron, vitamins	1 cup	50	7	145	4	1
	Breads:						
325	Boston brown bread, canned, slice, 3¼ by ½ in.	1 slice	45	45	95	2	1
	Cracked-wheat bread (¾ enriched wheat flour, ¼ cracked wheat):						
326	Loaf, 1 lb	1 loaf	454	35	1,195	39	10
327	Slice (18 per loaf)	1 slice	25	35	65	2	1
	French or vienna bread, enriched:						
328	Loaf, 1 lb	1 loaf	454	31	1,315	41	14
	Slice:						
329	French (5 by 2½ by 1 in.)	1 slice	35	31	100	3	1
330	Vienna (4¾ by 4 by ½ in.)	1 slice	25	31	75	2	1
	Italian bread, enriched:						
331	Loaf, 1 lb	1 loaf	454	32	1,250	41	4
332	Slice, 4½ by 3¼ by ¾ in.	1 slice	30	32	85	3	Trace

(Table A.3, continued)

Saturated (total), g	Oleic, g	Linoleic, g	Carbohydrate, g	Calcium, mg	Phosphorus, mg	Iron, mg	Potassium, mg	Vitamin A value, IU	Thiamin, mg	Riboflavin, mg	Niacin, mg	Vitamin C, mg
0	0	0	8	8	—	—	77	—	.01	.02	.2	—
0	0	0	4	9	10	.4	94	—	Trace	.01	.1	—
0	0	0	29	—	—	—	—	0	0	0	0	0
0	0	0	37	—	—	—	—	0	0	0	0	0
0	0	0	45	—	—	—	—	0	0	0	0	0
0	0	0	29	—	—	—	0	0	0	0	0	0
0	0	0	39	—	—	—	0	0	0	0	0	0
1.2	2.0	1.2	13	34	49	.4	33	Trace	.08	.08	.7	Trace
.6	1.1	.7	15	19	65	.6	32	Trace	.09	.08	.8	Trace
—	—	—	19	46	27	1.3	245	290	.04	.06	.6	30
—	—	—	22	22	19	1.5	117	150	.04	.09	.7	20
—	—	—	0	25	244	.6	—	40	.09	.08	1.6	—
—	—	—	Trace	—	—	—	4	—	—	—	—	—
—	—	—	28	19	125	12.4	137	1,650	.41	.49	4.1	12
—	—	—	40	28	146	17.7	154	2,350	.58	.71	5.8	18
.1	.2	.2	21	41	72	.9	131	0	.06	.04	.7	0
2.2	3.0	3.9	236	399	581	9.5	608	Trace	1.52	1.13	14.4	Trace
.1	.2	.2	13	22	32	.5	34	Trace	.08	.06	.8	Trace
3.2	4.7	4.6	251	195	386	10.0	408	Trace	1.80	1.10	15.0	Trace
.2	.4	.4	19	15	30	.8	32	Trace	.14	.08	1.2	Trace
.2	.3	.3	14	11	21	.6	23	Trace	.10	.06	.8	Trace
.6	.3	1.5	256	77	349	10.0	336	0	1.80	1.10	15.0	0
Trace	Trace	.1	17	5	23	.7	22	0	.12	.07	1.0	0

Fatty acids header spans Saturated (total) and Unsaturated columns; *Unsaturated* spans Oleic and Linoleic columns.

(Table A.3, continued)

Item No.	Food	Approximate measure	Weight, g	Water, percent	Food energy, kcal	Protein, g	Fat, g
	Raisin bread, enriched:						
333	Loaf, 1 lb	1 loaf	454	35	1,190	30	13
334	Slice (18 per loaf)	1 slice	25	35	65	2	1
	Rye Bread:						
	American, light (⅔ enriched wheat flour, ⅓ rye flour):						
335	Loaf, 1 lb	1 loaf	454	36	1,100	41	5
336	Slice (4¾ by 3¾ by ⁷/₁₆ in.)	1 slice	25	36	60	2	Trace
	Pumpernickel (⅔ rye flour, ⅓ enriched wheat flour):						
337	Loaf, 1 lb	1 loaf	454	34	1,115	41	5
338	Slice (5 by 4 by ⅜ in.)	1 slice	32	34	80	3	Trace
	White bread, enriched:						
	Soft-crumb type:						
339	Loaf, 1 lb	1 loaf	454	36	1,225	39	15
340	Slice (18 per loaf)	1 slice	25	36	70	2	1
341	Slice, toasted	1 slice	22	25	70	2	1
342	Slice (22 per loaf)	1 slice	20	36	55	2	1
343	Slice, toasted	1 slice	17	25	55	2	1
344	Loaf, 1½ lb	1 loaf	680	36	1,835	59	22
345	Slice (24 per loaf)	1 slice	28	36	75	2	1
346	Slice, toasted	1 slice	24	25	75	2	1
347	Slice (28 per loaf)	1 slice	24	36	65	2	1
348	Slice, toasted	1 slice	21	25	65	2	1
349	Cubes	1 cup	30	36	80	3	1
350	Crumbs	1 cup	45	36	120	4	1
	Firm-crumb type:						
351	Loaf, 1 lb	1 loaf	454	35	1,245	41	17
352	Slice (20 per loaf)	1 slice	23	35	65	2	1
353	Slice, toasted	1 slice	20	24	65	2	1
354	Loaf, 2 lb	1 loaf	907	35	2,495	82	34
355	Slice (34 per loaf)	1 slice	27	35	75	2	1
356	Slice, toasted	1 slice	23	24	75	2	1
	Whole-wheat bread:						
	Soft-crumb type:						
357	Loaf, 1 lb	1 loaf	454	36	1,095	41	12
358	Slice (16 per loaf)	1 slice	28	36	65	3	1
359	Slice, toasted	1 slice	24	24	65	3	1

(Table A.3, continued)

Satu-rated (total), g	Unsaturated Oleic, g	Lino-leic, g	Carbo-hydrate, g	Cal-cium, mg	Phos-phorus, mg	Iron, mg	Potas-sium, mg	Vitamin A value, IU	Thia-min, mg	Ribo-flavin, mg	Niacin, mg	Vitamin C, mg
3.0	4.7	3.9	243	322	395	10.0	1,057	Trace	1.70	1.07	10.7	Trace
.2	.3	.2	13	18	22	.6	58	Trace	.09	.06	.6	Trace
.7	.5	2.2	236	340	667	9.1	658	0	1.35	.98	12.9	0
Trace	Trace	.1	13	19	37	.5	36	0	.07	.05	.7	0
.7	.5	2.4	241	381	1,039	11.8	2,059	0	1.30	.93	8.5	0
.1	Trace	.2	17	27	73	.8	145	0	.09	.07	.6	0
3.4	5.3	4.6	229	381	440	11.3	476	Trace	1.80	1.10	15.0	Trace
.2	.3	.3	13	21	24	.6	26	Trace	.10	.06	.8	Trace
.2	.3	.3	13	21	24	.6	26	Trace	.08	.06	.8	Trace
.2	.2	.2	10	17	19	.5	21	Trace	.08	.05	.7	Trace
.2	.2	.2	10	17	19	.5	21	Trace	.06	.05	.7	Trace
5.2	7.9	6.9	343	571	660	17.0	714	Trace	2.70	1.65	22.5	Trace
.2	.3	.3	14	24	27	.7	29	Trace	.11	.07	.9	Trace
.2	.3	.3	14	24	27	.7	29	Trace	.09	.07	.9	Trace
.2	.3	.2	12	20	23	.6	25	Trace	.10	.06	.8	Trace
.2	.3	.2	12	20	23	.6	25	Trace	.08	.06	.8	Trace
.2	.3	.3	15	25	29	.8	32	Trace	.12	.07	1.0	Trace
.3	.5	.5	23	38	44	1.1	47	Trace	.18	.11	1.5	Trace
3.9	5.9	5.2	228	435	463	11.3	549	Trace	1.80	1.10	15.0	Trace
.2	.3	.3	12	22	23	.6	28	Trace	.09	.06	.8	Trace
.2	.3	.3	12	22	23	.6	28	Trace	.07	.06	.8	Trace
7.7	11.8	10.4	455	871	925	22.7	1,097	Trace	3.60	2.20	30.0	Trace
.2	.3	.3	14	26	28	.7	33	Trace	.11	.06	.9	Trace
.2	.3	.3	14	26	28	.7	33	Trace	.09	.06	.9	Trace
2.2	2.9	4.2	224	381	1,152	13.6	1,161	Trace	1.37	.45	12.7	Trace
.1	.2	.2	14	24	71	.8	72	Trace	.09	.03	.8	Trace
.1	.2	.2	14	24	71	.8	72	Trace	.07	.03	.8	Trace

(Table A.3, continued)

Item No.	Food	Approximate measure	Weight, g	Water, percent	Food energy, kcal	Protein, g	Fat, g
	Firm-crumb type:						
360	Loaf, 1 lb	1 loaf	454	36	1,100	48	14
361	Slice (18 per loaf)	1 slice	25	36	60	3	1
362	Slice, toasted	1 slice	21	24	60	3	1
	Breadcrumbs (enriched):						
324	Dry, grated	1 cup	100	7	390	13	5
	Soft. See White bread (items 349-350)						
	Broccoli, cooked, drained:						
	From raw:						
587	Stalk, medium size	1 stalk	180	91	45	6	1
588	Stalks cut into ½-in. pieces	1 cup	155	91	40	5	Trace
	From frozen:						
589	Stalk, 4½ to 5 in. long	1 stalk	30	91	10	1	Trace
590	Chopped	1 cup	185	92	50	5	1
	Brussels sprouts, cooked, drained:						
591	From raw, 7-8 sprouts (1¼- to 1½-in. diam.)	1 cup	155	88	55	7	1
592	From frozen	1 cup	155	89	50	5	Trace
517	Brazil nuts, shelled (6-8 large kernels)	1 oz	28	5	185	4	19
383	Buckwheat flour, light, sifted	1 cup	98	12	340	6	1
384	Bulgur, canned, seasoned	1 cup	135	56	245	8	4
	Butter:						
	Regular (1 brick or 4 sticks per lb):						
103	Stick (½ cup)	1 stick	113	16	815	1	92
104	Tablespoon (about ⅛ stick)	1 tbsp	14	16	100	Trace	12
105	Pat (1 in. square, ⅓ in. high; 90 per lb)	1 pat	5	16	35	Trace	4
	Whipped (6 sticks or two 8-oz containers per lb)						
106	Stick (½ cup)	1 stick	76	16	540	1	61
107	Tablespoon (about ⅛ stick)	1 tbsp	9	16	65	Trace	8
108	Pat (1¼ in. square, ⅓ in. high; 120 per lb)	1 pat	4	16	25	Trace	3
60	Buttermilk	1 cup	245	90	100	8	2
	Cabbage:						
	Common varieties:						
	Raw:						
593	Coarsely shredded or sliced	1 cup	70	92	15	1	Trace
594	Finely shredded or chopped	1 cup	90	92	20	1	Trace
595	Cooked, drained	1 cup	145	94	30	2	Trace
596	Red, raw, coarsely shredded or sliced	1 cup	70	90	20	1	Trace

(Table A.3, continued)

Fatty acids												
Satu-rated *(total)*, g	Unsaturated		Carbo-hydrate, g	Cal-cium, mg	Phos-phorus, mg	Iron, mg	Potas-sium, mg	Vitamin A value, IU	Thia-min, mg	Ribo-flavin, mg	Niacin, mg	Vitamin C, mg
	Oleic, g	Lino-leic, g										
2.5	3.3	4.9	216	449	1,034	13.6	1,238	Trace	1.17	.54	12.7	Trace
.1	.2	.3	12	25	57	.8	68	Trace	.06	.03	.7	Trace
.1	.2	.3	12	25	57	.8	68	Trace	.05	.03	.7	Trace
1.0	1.6	1.4	73	122	141	3.6	152	Trace	.35	.35	4.8	Trace
—	—	—	8	158	112	1.4	481	4,500	.16	.36	1.4	162
—	—	—	7	136	96	1.2	414	3,880	.14	.31	1.2	140
—	—	—	1	12	17	.2	66	570	.02	.03	.2	22
—	—	—	9	100	104	1.3	392	4,810	.11	.22	.9	105
—	—	—	10	50	112	1.7	423	810	.12	.22	1.2	135
—	—	—	10	33	95	1.2	457	880	.12	.16	.9	126
4.8	6.2	7.1	3	53	196	1.0	203	Trace	.27	.03	.5	—
.2	.4	.4	78	11	86	1.0	314	0	.08	.04	.4	0
—	—	—	44	27	263	1.9	151	0	.08	.05	4.1	0
57.3	23.1	2.1	Trace	27	26	.2	29	3,470	.01	.04	Trace	0
7.2	2.9	.3	Trace	3	3	Trace	4	430	Trace	Trace	Trace	0
2.5	1.0	.1	Trace	1	1	Trace	1	150	Trace	Trace	Trace	0
38.2	15.4	1.4	Trace	18	17	.1	20	2,310	Trace	.03	Trace	0
4.7	1.9	.2	Trace	2	2	Trace	2	290	Trace	Trace	Trace	0
1.9	.8	.1	Trace	1	1	Trace	1	120	0	Trace	Trace	0
1.3	.5	Trace	12	285	219	.1	371	80	.08	.38	.1	2
—	—	—	4	34	20	0.3	163	90	.04	.04	.02	33
—	—	—	5	44	26	.4	210	120	.05	.05	.3	42
—	—	—	6	64	29	.4	236	190	.06	.06	.4	48
—	—	—	5	29	25	.6	188	30	.06	.04	.3	43

(Table A.3, continued)

Item No.	Food	Approximate measure	Weight, g	Water, percent	Food energy, kcal	Protein, g	Fat, g
	Savoy, raw, coarsely shredded or sliced	1 cup	70	92	15	2	Trace
598	Cabbage, celery (also called pe-tsai or wongbok), raw, 1-in. pieces	1 cup	75	95	10	1	Trace
599	Cabbage, white mustard (also called bok-choy or pakchoy), cooked, drained	1 cup	170	95	25	2	Trace
	Cakes made from cake mixes with enriched flour:[a]						
	Angelfood:						
385	Whole cake (9¾-in. diam. tube cake)	1 cake	635	34	1,645	36	1
386	Piece, 1/12 of cake	1 piece	53	34	135	3	Trace
	Coffeecake:						
387	Whole cake (7¾ by 5⅝ by 1¼ in.)	1 cake	430	30	1,385	27	41
388	Piece, 1/6 of cake	1 piece	72	30	230	5	7
	Cupcakes, made with egg, milk, 2½-in. diam.						
389	Without icing	1 cupcake	25	26	90	1	3
390	With chocolate icing	1 cupcake	36	22	130	2	5
	Devil's food with chocolate icing:						
391	Whole, 2 layer cake (8- or 9-in. diam.)	1 cake	1,107	24	3,755	49	136
392	Piece, 1/16 of cake	1 piece	69	24	235	3	8
393	Cupcake, 2½-in. diam.	1 cupcake	35	24	120	2	4
	Gingerbread:						
394	Whole cake (8-in. square)	1 cake	570	37	1,575	18	39
395	Piece, 1/9 of cake	1 piece	63	37	175	2	4
	White, 2 layer with chocolate icing:						
396	Whole cake (8- or 9-in. diam.)	1 cake	1,140	21	4,000	44	122
397	Piece, 1/16 of cake	1 piece	71	21	250	3	8
	Yellow, 2 layer with chocolate icing:						
398	Whole cake (8- or 9-in. diam.)	1 cake	1,108	26	3,735	45	125
399	Piece, 1/16 of cake	1 piece	69	26	235	3	8
	Cakes made from home recipes using enriched flour:[b]						
	Boston cream pie with custard filling:						
400	Whole cake (8-in. diam.)	1 cake	825	35	2,490	41	78

[a] Excepting for angelfood cake, cakes were made from mixes containing vegetable shortening; icings, with butter.

[b] Excepting for spongecake, vegetable shortening used for cake portion; butter, for icing. If butter or margarine used for cake portion, vitamin A values would be higher.

514

(Table A.3, continued)

Saturated *(total),* g	Oleic, g	Linoleic, g	Carbohydrate, g	Calcium, mg	Phosphorus, mg	Iron, mg	Potassium, mg	Vitamin A value, IU	Thiamin, mg	Riboflavin, mg	Niacin, mg	Vitamin C, mg
—	—	—	3	47	38	.6	188	140	.04	.06	.2	39
—	—	—	2	32	30	.5	190	110	.04	.03	.5	19
—	—	—	4	252	56	1.0	364	5,270	.07	.14	1.2	26
—	—	—	377	603	756	2.5	381	0	.37	.95	3.6	0
—	—	—	32	50	63	.2	32	0	.03	.08	.3	0
11.7	16.3	8.8	225	262	748	6.9	469	690	.82	.91	7.7	1
2.0	2.7	1.5	38	44	125	1.2	78	120	.14	.15	1.3	Trace
.8	1.2	.7	14	40	59	.3	21	40	.05	.05	.4	Trace
2.0	1.6	.6	21	47	71	.4	42	60	.05	.06	.4	Trace
50.0	44.9	17.0	645	653	1,162	16.6	1,439	1,660	1.06	1.65	10.1	1
3.1	2.8	1.1	40	41	72	1.0	90	100	.07	.10	.6	Trace
1.6	1.4	.5	20	21	37	.5	46	50	.03	.05	.3	Trace
9.7	16.6	10.0	291	513	570	8.6	1,562	Trace	.84	1.00	7.4	Trace
1.1	1.8	1.1	32	57	63	.9	173	Trace	.09	.11	.8	Trace
48.2	46.4	20.0	716	1,129	2,041	11.4	1,322	680	1.50	1.77	12.5	2
3.0	2.9	1.2	45	70	127	.7	82	40	.09	.11	.8	Trace
47.8	47.8	20.3	638	1,008	2,017	12.2	1,208	1,550	1.24	1.67	10.6	2
3.0	3.0	1.3	40	63	126	.8	75	100	.08	.10	.7	Trace
23.0	30.1	15.2	412	553	833	8.2	734[c]	1,730	1.04	1.27	9.6	2

[c] Applies to product with a sodium aluminum-sulfate type baking powder. With a low-sodium type baking power containing potassium, value would be about twice the amount shown.

(Table A.3, continued)

Item No.	Food	Approximate measure	Weight, g	Water, percent	Food energy, kcal	Protein, g	Fat, g
401	Piece, $1/12$ of cake	1 piece	69	35	210	3	6
	Fruitcake, dark:						
402	Loaf, 1-lb (7½ by 2 by 1½ in.)	1 loaf	454	18	1,720	22	69
403	Slice, $1/30$ of loaf	1 slice	15	18	55	1	2
	Plain, sheet cake:						
	Without icing:						
404	Whole cake (9-in. square)	1 cake	777	25	2,830	35	108
405	Piece, $1/9$ of cake	1 piece	86	25	315	4	12
	With uncooked white icing:						
406	Whole cake (9-in. square)	1 cake	1,096	21	4,020	37	129
407	Piece, $1/9$ of cake	1 piece	121	21	445	4	14
	Pound:[d]						
408	Loaf, 8½ by 3½ by 3¼ in.	1 loaf	565	16	2,725	31	170
409	Slice, $1/17$ of loaf	1 slice	33	16	160	2	10
	Spongecake:						
410	Whole cake (9¾-in. diam. tube cake)	1 cake	790	32	2,345	60	45
411	Piece, $1/12$ of cake	1 piece	66	32	195	5	4
	Cake icings:						
	Boiled, white:						
532	Plain	1 cup	94	18	295	1	0
533	With coconut	1 cup	166	15	605	3	13
	Uncooked:						
534	Chocolate made with milk and butter	1 cup	275	14	1,035	9	38
535	Creamy fudge from mix and water	1 cup	245	15	830	7	16
536	White	1 cup	319	11	1,200	2	21
	Candy:						
537	Caramels, plain or chocolate	1 oz	28	8	115	1	3
	Chocolate:						
538	Milk, plain	1 oz	28	1	145	2	9
540	Chocolate-coated peanuts	1 oz	28	1	160	5	12
541	Fondant, uncoated (mints, candy corn, other)	1 oz	28	8	105	Trace	1
542	Fudge, chocolate, plain	1 oz	28	8	115	1	3
543	Gum drops	1 oz	28	12	100	Trace	Trace
544	Hard	1 oz	28	1	110	0	Trace

[c] Applies to product with a sodium aluminum-sulfate type baking powder. With a low-sodium type baking powder containing potassium, value would be about twice the amount shown.

[d] Equal weights of flour, sugar, eggs, and vegetable shortening.

(Table A.3, continued)

Saturated (total), g	Fatty acids Unsaturated Oleic, g	Linoleic, g	Carbohydrate, g	Calcium, mg	Phosphorus, mg	Iron, mg	Potassium, mg	Vitamin A value, IU	Thiamin, mg	Riboflavin, mg	Niacin, mg	Vitamin C, mg
1.9	2.5	1.3	34	46	70	.7	61[c]	140	.09	.11	.8	Trace
14.4	33.5	14.8	271	327	513	11.8	2,250	540	.72	.73	4.9	2
.5	1.1	.5	9	11	17	.4	74	20	.02	.02	.2	Trace
29.5	44.4	23.9	434	497	793	8.5	614[c]	1,320	1.21	1.40	10.2	2
3.3	4.9	2.6	48	55	88	.9	68[c]	150	.13	.15	1.1	Trace
42.2	49.5	24.4	694	548	822	8.2	669[c]	2,190	1.22	1.47	10.2	2
4.7	5.5	2.7	77	61	91	.8	74[c]	240	.14	.16	1.1	Trace
42.9	73.1	39.6	273	107	418	7.9	345	1,410	.90	.99	7.3	0
2.5	4.3	2.3	16	6	24	.5	20	80	.05	.06	.4	0
13.1	15.8	5.7	427	237	885	13.4	687	3,560	1.10	1.64	7.4	Trace
1.1	1.3	.5	36	20	74	1.1	57	300	.09	.14	.6	Trace
0	0	0	75	2	2	Trace	17	0	Trace	.03	Trace	0
11.0	.9	Trace	124	10	50	.8	277	0	.02	.07	.3	0
23.4	11.7	1.0	185	165	305	3.3	536	580	.06	.28	.6	1
5.1	6.7	3.1	183	96	218	2.7	238	Trace	.05	.20	.7	Trace
12.7	5.1	.5	260	48	38	Trace	57	860	Trace	.06	Trace	Trace
1.6	1.1	.1	22	42	35	.4	54	Trace	.01	.05	.1	Trace
5.5	3.0	.3	16	65	65	.3	109	80	.02	.10	.1	Trace
4.0	4.7	2.1	11	33	84	.4	143	Trace	.10	.05	2.1	Trace
.1	.3	.1	25	4	2	.3	1	0	Trace	Trace	Trace	0
1.3	1.4	.6	21	22	24	.3	42	Trace	.01	.03	.1	Trace
—	—	—	25	2	Trace	.1	1	0	0	Trace	Trace	0
—	—	—	28	6	2	.5	1	0	0	0	0	0

(Table A.3, continued)

Item No.	Food	Approximate measure	Weight, g	Water, percent	Food energy, kcal	Protein, g	Fat, g
545	Marshmallows	1 oz	28	17	90	1	Trace
271	Cantaloup, orange-fleshed (with rind and seed cavity, 5-in. diam., 2⅓ lb)	½ melon with rind	477	91	80	2	Trace
	Carrots:						
	Raw, without crowns and tips, scraped:						
600	Whole, 7½ by 1⅛ in., or strips, 2½ to 3 in. long	1 carrot or 18 strips	72	88	30	1	Trace
601	Grated	1 cup	110	88	45	1	Trace
602	Cooked (crosswise cuts), drained	1 cup	155	91	50	1	Trace
	Canned:						
603	Sliced, drained solids	1 cup	155	91	45	1	Trace
604	Strained or junior (baby food)	1 oz (1¾ to 2 tbsp)	28	92	10	Trace	Trace
518	Cashew nuts, roasted in oil	1 cup	140	5	785	24	64
	Cauliflower:						
605	Raw, chopped	1 cup	115	91	31	3	Trace
	Cooked, drained:						
606	From raw (flower buds)	1 cup	125	93	30	3	Trace
607	From frozen (flowerets)	1 cup	180	94	30	3	Trace
	Celery, Pascal type, raw:						
608	Stalk, large outer, 8 by 1½ in., at root end	1 stalk	40	94	5	Trace	Trace
609	Pieces, diced	1 cup	120	94	20	1	Trace
	Cheese:						
	Natural:						
1	Blue	1 oz	28	42	100	6	8
2	Camembert (3 wedges per 4-oz container)	1 wedge	38	52	115	8	9
	Cheddar:						
3	Cut pieces	1 oz	28	37	115	7	9
4		1 cu in.	17.2	37	70	4	6
5	Shredded	1 cup	113	37	455	28	37
	Cottage (curd not pressed down):						
	Creamed (cottage cheese, 4% fat):						
6	Large curd	1 cup	225	79	235	28	10
7	Small curd	1 cup	210	79	220	26	9
8	Low fat (2%)	1 cup	226	79	205	31	4
9	Low fat (1%)	1 cup	226	82	165	28	2
10	Uncreamed (cottage cheese dry curd, less than ½% fat)	1 cup	145	80	125	25	1
11	Cream	1 oz	28	54	100	2	10

518

(Table A.3, continued)

| | Fatty acids | | | | | | | | | | | |
| Saturated (total), g | Unsaturated | | Carbohydrate, g | Calcium, mg | Phosphorus, mg | Iron, mg | Potassium, mg | Vitamin A value, IU | Thiamin, mg | Riboflavin, mg | Niacin, mg | Vitamin C, mg |
	Oleic, g	Linoleic, g										
—	—	—	23	5	2	.5	2	0	0	Trace	Trace	0
—	—	—	20	38	44	1.1	582	9,240	.11	.08	1.6	90
—	—	—	7	27	26	.5	246	7,930	.04	.04	.4	6
—	—	—	11	41	40	.8	375	12,100	.07	.06	.7	9
—	—	—	11	51	48	.9	344	16,280	.08	.08	.8	9
—	—	—	10	47	34	1.1	186	23,250	.03	.05	.6	3
—	—	—	2	7	6	.1	51	3,690	.01	.01	.1	1
12.9	36.8	10.2	41	53	522	5.3	650	140	.60	.35	2.5	—
—	—	—	6	29	64	1.3	339	70	.13	.12	.8	90
—	—	—	5	26	53	.9	258	80	.11	.10	.8	69
—	—	—	6	31	68	.9	373	50	.07	.09	.7	74
—	—	—	2	16	11	.1	136	110	.01	.01	.1	4
—	—	—	5	47	34	.4	409	320	.04	.04	.4	11
5.3	1.9	.2	1	150	110	.1	73	200	.01	.11	0.3	0
5.8	2.2	.2	Trace	147	132	.1	71	350	.01	.19	.2	0
6.1	2.1	.2	Trace	204	145	.2	28	300	.01	.11	Trace	0
3.7	1.3	.1	Trace	124	88	.1	17	180	Trace	.06	Trace	0
24.2	8.5	.7	1	815	579	.8	111	1,200	.03	.42	.1	0
6.4	2.4	.2	6	135	297	.3	190	370	.05	.37	.3	Trace
6.0	2.2	.2	6	126	277	.3	177	340	.04	.34	.3	Trace
2.8	1.0	.1	8	155	340	.4	217	160	.05	.42	.3	Trace
1.5	.5	.1	6	138	302	.3	193	80	.05	.37	.3	Trace
.4	.1	Trace	3	46	151	.3	47	40	.04	.21	.2	0
6.2	2.4	.2	1	23	30	.3	34	400	Trace	.06	Trace	0

(Table A.3, continued)

Item No.	Food	Approximate measure	Weight, g	Water, percent	Food energy, kcal	Protein, g	Fat, g
	Mozzarella, made with—						
12	Whole milk	1 oz	28	48	90	6	7
13	Part skim milk	1 oz	28	49	80	8	5
	Parmesan, grated:						
14	Cup, not pressed down	1 cup	100	18	455	42	30
15	Tablespoon	1 tbsp	5	18	25	2	2
16	Ounce	1 oz	28	18	130	12	9
17	Provolone	1 oz	28	41	100	7	8
	Ricotta, made with—						
	Whole milk	1 cup	246	72	1,790	28	32
19	Part skim milk	1 cup	246	74	340	28	19
20	Romano	1 oz	28	31	110	9	8
21	Swiss	1 oz	28	37	105	8	8
	Pasteurized process cheese:						
22	American	1 oz	28	39	105	6	9
23	Swiss	1 oz	28	42	95	7	7
24	Pasteurized process cheese food, American	1 oz	28	43	95	6	7
25	Pasteurized process cheese spread, American	1 oz	28	48	82	5	6
	Cherries:						
239	Sour (tart), red, pitted, canned, water pack	1 cup	244	88	105	2	Trace
240	Sweet, raw, without pits and stems	10 cherries	68	80	45	1	Trace
	Chicken, cooked:						
210	Breast, fried,[a] bones removed, ½ breast (3.3 oz with bones)	2.8 oz	79	58	160	26	5
211	Drumstick, fried,[a] bones removed (2 oz with bones)	1.3 oz	38	55	90	12	4
212	Half broiler, broiled, bones removed (10.4 oz with bones)	6.2 oz	176	71	240	42	7
213	Chicken, canned, boneless	3 oz	85	65	170	18	10
214	Chicken a la king, cooked (home recipe)	1 cup	245	68	470	27	34
215	Chicken and noodles, cooked (home recipe)	1 cup	240	71	365	22	18
	Chicken chow mein:						
216	Canned	1 cup	250	89	95	7	Trace
217	From home recipe	1 cup	250	78	255	31	10

[a] Vegetable shortening used.

520

(Table A.3, continued)

| | Fatty acids | | | | | | | | | | | |
| Satu-rated (total), g | Unsaturated | | Carbo-hydrate, g | Cal-cium, mg | Phos-phorus, mg | Iron, mg | Potas-sium, mg | Vitamin A value, IU | Thia-min, mg | Ribo-flavin, mg | Niacin, mg | Vitamin C, mg |
	Oleic, g	Lino-leic, g										
4.4	1.7	.2	1	163	117	.1	21	260	Trace	.08	Trace	0
3.1	1.2	.1	1	207	149	.1	27	180	.01	.10	Trace	0
19.1	7.7	.3	4	1,376	807	1.0	107	700	.05	.39	.3	0
1.0	.4	Trace	Trace	69	40	Trace	5	40	Trace	.02	Trace	0
5.4	2.2	.1	1	390	229	.3	30	200	.01	.11	.1	0
4.8	1.7	.1	1	214	141	.1	39	230	.01	.09	Trace	0
20.4	7.1	.7	7	509	389	.9	257	1,210	.03	.48	.3	0
12.1	4.7	.5	13	669	449	1.1	308	1,060	.05	.46	.2	0
—	—	—	1	302	215	—	—	160	—	.11	Trace	0
5.0	1.7	.2	1	272	171	Trace	31	240	.01	.10	Trace	0
5.6	2.1	.2	Trace	174	211	.1	46	340	.01	.10	Trace	0
4.5	1.7	.1	1	219	216	.2	61	230	Trace	.08	Trace	0
4.4	1.7	.1	2	163	130	.2	79	260	.01	.13	Trace	0
3.8	1.5	.1	2	159	202	.1	69	220	.01	.12	Trace	0
—	—	—	26	37	32	.7	317	1,660	.07	.05	.5	12
—	—	—	12	15	13	.3	129	70	.03	.04	.3	7
1.4	1.8	1.1	1	9	218	1.3	—	70	.04	.17	11.6	—
1.1	1.3	.9	Trace	6	89	.9	—	50	.03	.15	2.7	—
2.2	2.5	1.3	0	16	355	3.0	483	160	.09	.34	15.5	—
3.2	3.8	2.0	0	18	210	1.3	117	200	.03	.11	3.7	3
2.7	14.3	3.3	12	127	358	2.5	404	1,130	.10	.42	5.4	12
5.9	7.1	3.5	26	26	247	2.2	149	430	.05	.17	4.3	Trace
—	—	—	18	45	85	1.3	418	150	.05	.10	1.0	13
2.4	3.4	3.1	10	58	293	2.5	473	280	.08	.23	4.3	10

(Table A.3, continued)

Item No.	Food	Approximate measure	Weight, g	Water, percent	Food energy, kcal	Protein, g	Fat, g
218	Chicken potpie (home recipe), baked,[a] piece (⅓ or 9-in. diam. pie)	1 piece	232	57	545	23	31
	Turkey, roasted, flesh without skin:						
219	Dark meat, piece, 2½ by 1⅝ by ¼ in.	4 pieces	85	61	175	26	7
220	Light meat, piece, 4 by 2 by ¼ in.	2 pieces	85	62	150	28	3
	Light and dark meat:						
221	Chopped or diced	1 cup	140	61	265	44	9
222	Pieces (1 slice white meat, 4 by 2 by ¼ in. with 2 slices dark meat, 2½ by 1⅝ by ¼ in.)	3 pieces	85	61	160	27	5
179	Chili con carne with beans	1 cup	255	72	340	19	16
	Chocolate:						
697	Bitter or baking	1 oz	28	2	145	3	15
539	Semisweet, small pieces (60 per oz)	1 cup or 6-oz pkg	170	1	860	7	61
	Chocolate-flavored beverage powders (about 4 heaping tsp per oz):						
546	With nonfat dry milk	1 oz	28	2	100	5	1
547	Without milk	1 oz	28	1	100	1	1
	Chocolate-flavored sirup or topping:						
553	Thin type	1 fl oz or 2 tbsp	38	32	90	1	1
554	Fudge type	1 fl oz or 2 tbsp	38	25	125	2	5
180	Chop suey with beef and pork (home recipe)	1 cup	250	75	300	26	17
	Clams:						
146	Raw, meat only	3 oz	85	82	65	11	1
147	Canned, solids and liquid	3 oz	85	86	45	7	1
	Coconut meat, fresh:						
519	Piece, about 2 by 2 by ½ in.	1 piece	45	51	155	2	16
520	Shredded or grated, not pressed down	1 cup	80	51	275	3	28
	Collards, cooked, drained:						
610	From raw (leaves without stems)	1 cup	190	90	65	7	1
611	From frozen (chopped)	1 cup	170	90	50	5	1
	Cookies made with enriched flour:[a, b]						
	Brownies with nuts:						
	Home-prepared, 1¾ by 1¾ by ⅞ in.:						
412	From home recipe	1 brownie	20	10	95	1	6
413	From commercial recipe	1 brownie	20	11	85	1	4

[a] Crust made with vegetable shortening and enriched flour.
[b] Made with enriched flour and vegetable shortening except for macaroons, which do not contain flour or shortening.

(Table A.3, continued)

	Fatty acids											
Satu-	Unsaturated											
rated		Lino-	Carbo-	Cal-	Phos-		Potas-	Vitamin	Thia-	Ribo-		Vitamin
(total),	Oleic,	leic,	hydrate,	cium,	phorus,	Iron,	sium,	A value,	min,	flavin,	Niacin,	C,
g	g	g	g	mg	mg	mg	mg	IU	mg	mg	mg	mg
11.3	10.9	5.6	42	70	232	3.0	343	3,090	.34	.31	5.5	5
2.1	1.5	1.5	0	—	—	2.0	338	—	.03	.20	3.6	—
.9	.6	.7	0	—	—	1.0	349	—	.04	.12	9.4	—
2.5	1.7	1.8	0	11	351	2.5	514	—	.07	.25	10.8	—
1.5	1.0	1.1	0	7	213	1.5	312	—	.04	.15	6.5	—
7.5	6.8	.3	31	82	321	4.3	594	150	.08	.18	3.3	—
8.9	4.9	.4	8	22	109	1.9	235	20	.01	.07	.4	0
36.2	19.8	1.7	97	51	255	4.4	553	30	.02	.14	.9	0
.5	.3	Trace	20	167	155	.5	227	10	.04	.21	.2	1
.4	.2	Trace	25	9	48	.6	142	—	.01	.03	.1	0
.5	.3	Trace	24	6	35	.6	106	Trace	.01	.03	.2	0
3.1	1.6	.1	20	48	60	.5	107	60	.02	.08	.2	Trace
8.5	6.2	.7	13	60	248	4.8	425	600	.28	.38	5.0	33
—	—	—	2	59	138	5.2	154	90	.08	.15	1.1	8
0.2	Trace	Trace	2	47	116	3.5	119	—	.01	.09	.9	—
14.0	.9	.3	4	6	43	.8	115	0	.02	.01	.2	1
24.8	1.6	.5	8	10	76	1.4	205	0	.04	.02	.4	2
—	—	—	10	357	99	1.5	498	14,820	.21	.38	2.3	144
—	—	—	10	299	87	1.7	401	11,560	.10	.24	1.0	56
1.5	3.0	1.2	10	8	30	.4	38	40	.04	.03	.2	Trace
.9	1.4	1.3	13	9	27	.4	34	20	.03	.02	.2	Trace

523

(Table A.3, continued)

Item No.	Food	Approximate measure	Weight, g	Water, percent	Food energy, kcal	Protein, g	Fat, g
414	Frozen, with chocolate icing, 1½ by 1¾ by ⅞ in.	1 brownie	25	13	105	1	5
	Chocolate chip:						
415	Commercial, 2¼-in. diam., ⅜ in. thick	4 cookies	42	3	200	2	9
416	From home recipe, 2⅓-in. diam.	4 cookies	40	3	205	2	12
417	Fig bars, square (1⅝ by 1⅝ by ⅜ in.) or rectangular (1½ by 1¾ by ½ in.)	4 cookies	56	14	200	2	3
418	Gingersnaps, 2-in. diam., ¼ in. thick	4 cookies	28	3	90	2	2
419	Macaroons, 2¾-in. diam., ¼ in. thick	2 cookies	38	4	180	2	9
420	Oatmeal with raisins, 2⅝-in. diam., ¼ in. thick	4 cookies	52	3	235	3	8
421	Plain, prepared from commercial chilled dough, 2½-in. diam., ¼ in. thick	4 cookies	48	5	240	2	12
422	Sandwich type (chocolate or vanilla), 1¾-in. diam., ⅜ in. thick	4 cookies	40	2	200	2	9
423	Vanilla wafers, 1¾-in. diam., ¼ in thick	10 cookies	40	3	185	2	6
	Corn, sweet:						
	Cooked, drained:						
612	From raw, ear 5 by 1¾ in.	1 ear[c]	140	74	70	2	1
	From frozen:						
613	Ear, 5 in. long	1 ear[c]	229	73	120	4	1
614	Kernels	1 cup	165	77	130	5	1
	Canned:						
615	Cream style	1 cup	256	76	210	5	2
	Whole kernel:						
616	Vacuum pack	1 cup	210	76	175	5	1
617	Wet pack, drained solids	1 cup	165	76	140	4	1
	Corn flakes:						
371	Plain, added sugar, salt, iron, vitamins	1 cup	25	4	95	2	Trace
372	Sugar-coated, added salt, iron, vitamins	1 cup	40	2	155	2	Trace
	Corn (hominy) grits, degermed:						
363	Enriched	1 cup	245	87	125	3	Trace
364	Unenriched	1 cup	245	87	125	3	Trace

[c] Applies to yellow varieties; white varieties contain only a trace.
[d] Weight includes cob. Without cob, weight is 77 g for item 612, 126 g for item 613.
[e] Based on yellow varieties. For white varieties, value is trace.
[f] Value varies with the brand. Consult the label.

(Table A.3, continued)

Saturated (total), g	Fatty acids — Unsaturated — Oleic, g	Linoleic, g	Carbohydrate, g	Calcium, mg	Phosphorus, mg	Iron, mg	Potassium, mg	Vitamin A value, IU	Thiamin, mg	Riboflavin, mg	Niacin, mg	Vitamin C, mg
2.0	2.2	.7	15	10	31	.4	44	50	.03	.03	.2	Trace
2.8	2.9	2.2	29	16	48	1.0	56	50	.10	.17	.9	Trace
3.5	4.5	2.9	24	14	40	.8	47	40	.06	.06	.5	Trace
.8	1.2	.7	42	44	34	1.0	111	60	.04	.14	.9	Trace
.7	1.0	.6	22	20	13	.7	129	20	.08	.06	.7	0
—	—	—	25	10	32	.3	176	0	.02	.06	.2	0
2.0	3.3	2.0	38	11	53	1.4	192	30	.15	.10	1.0	Trace
3.0	5.2	2.9	31	17	35	0.6	23	30	.10	.08	0.9	0
2.2	3.9	2.2	28	10	96	.7	15	0	.06	.10	.7	0
—	—	—	30	16	25	.6	29	50	.10	.09	.8	0
—	—	—	16	2	69	.5	151	310[d]	.09	.08	1.1	7
—	—	—	27	4	121	1.0	291	440[d]	.18	.10	2.1	9
—	—	—	31	5	120	1.3	304	580[d]	.15	.10	2.5	8
—	—	—	51	8	143	1.5	248	840[d]	.08	.13	2.6	13
—	—	—	43	6	153	1.1	204	740[d]	.06	.13	2.3	11
—	—	—	33	8	81	.8	160	580[d]	.05	.08	1.5	7
—	—	—	21	f	9	0.6	30	1,180	.29	.35	2.9	9
—	—	—	37	1	10	1.0	27	1,880	.46	..56	4.6	14
Trace	Trace	.1	27	2	25	.7	27	Trace[e]	.10	.07	1.0	0
Trace	Trace	.1	27	2	25	.2	27	Trace[e]	.05	.02	.5	0

(Table A.3, continued)

Item No.	Food	Approximate measure	Weight, g	Water, percent	Food energy, kcal	Protein, g	Fat, g
	Cornmeal:						
424	Whole-ground, unbolted, dry form	1 cup	122	12	435	11	5
425	Bolted (nearly whole-grain), dry form	1 cup	122	12	440	11	4
	Degermed, enriched:						
426	Dry form	1 cup	138	12	500	11	2
427	Cooked	1 cup	240	88	120	3	Trace
	Degermed, unenriched:						
428	Dry form	1 cup	138	12	500	11	2
429	Cooked	1 cup	240	88	120	3	Trace
445	Corn muffins (enriched degermed cornmeal and flour), 2⅜-in. diam., 1½ in. high	1 muffin	40	33	125	3	4
373	Corn, puffed, plain, added sugar, salt, iron, vitamins	1 cup	20	4	80	2	1
374	Corn, shredded, added sugar, salt, iron, thiamin, niacin	1 cup	25	3	95	2	Trace
	Cowpeas (or blackeyed peas):						
516	Dry, cooked (with residual cooking liquid)	1 cup	250	80	190	13	1
	Immature seeds, cooked and drained:						
585	From raw	1 cup	165	72	180	13	1
586	From frozen	1 cup	170	66	220	15	1
148	Crabmeat (white or king), canned, not pressed down	1 cup	135	77	135	24	3
	Crackers:						
430	Graham, plain, 2½-in. square	2 crackers	14	6	55	1	1
431	Rye wafers, whole-grain, 1⅞ by 3½ in.	2 wafers	13	6	45	2	Trace
432	Saltines, made with enriched flour	4 crackers or 1 packet	11	4	50	1	1
241	Cranberry juice cocktail, bottled, sweetened	1 cup	253	83	165	Trace	Trace
242	Cranberry sauce, sweetened, canned, strained	1 cup	277	62	405	Trace	1
	Cream, sweet:						
26	Half-and-half (cream and milk)	1 cup	242	81	315	7	28
27		1 tbsp	15	81	20	Trace	2
28	Light, coffee, or table	1 cup	240	74	470	6	46
29		1 tbsp	15	74	30	Trace	3
	Whipping, unwhipped (volume about double when whipped):						
30	Light	1 cup	239	64	700	5	74
31		1 tbsp	15	64	45	Trace	5

ᵖ Applies to white varieties. For yellow varieties, value is 150 IU.

(Table A.3, continued)

Saturated (total), g	Fatty acids Unsaturated Oleic, g	Linoleic, g	Carbohydrate, g	Calcium, mg	Phosphorus, mg	Iron, mg	Potassium, mg	Vitamin A value, IU	Thiamin, mg	Riboflavin, mg	Niacin, mg	Vitamin C, mg
.5	1.0	2.5	90	24	312	2.9	346	620g	.46	.13	2.4	0
.5	.9	2.1	91	21	272	2.2	303	590g	.37	.10	2.3	0
.2	.4	.9	108	8	137	4.0	166	610g	.61	.36	4.8	0
Trace	.1	.2	26	2	34	1.0	38	140g	.14	.10	1.2	0
.2	.4	.9	108	8	137	1.5	166	610g	.19	.07	1.4	0
Trace	.1	.2	26	2	34	.5	38	140g	.05	.02	.2	0
1.2	1.6	.9	19	42	68	.7	54	120	.10	.10	.7	Trace
—	—	—	16	4	18	2.3	—	940	.23	.28	2.3	7
—	—	—	22	1	10	.6	—	0	.11	.05	.5	0
—	—	—	35	43	238	3.3	573	30	.40	.10	1:0	—
—	—	—	30	40	241	3.5	625	580	.50	.18	2.3	28
—	—	—	40	43	286	4.8	573	290	.68	.19	2.4	15
.6	.4	.1	1	61	246	1.1	149	—	.11	.11	2.6	—
.3	.5	.3	10	6	21	.5	55	0	.02	.08	.5	0
—	—	—	10	7	50	.5	78	0	.04	.03	.2	0
.3	.5	.4	8	2	10	.5	13	0	.05	.05	.4	0
—	—	—	42	13	8	.8	25	Trace	.03	.03	.1	81
—	—	—	104	17	11	.6	83	60	.03	.03	.1	6
17.3	7.0	.6	10	254	230	.2	314	260	.08	.36	.2	2
1.1	.4	Trace	1	16	14	Trace	19	20	.01	.02	Trace	Trace
28.8	11.7	1.0	9	231	192	.1	292	1,730	.08	.36	.1	2
1.8	.7	.1	1	14	12	Trace	18	110	Trace	.02	Trace	Trace
46.2	18.3	1.5	7	166	146	.1	231	2,690	.06	.30	.1	1
2.9	1.1	.1	Trace	10	9	Trace	15	170	Trace	.02	Trace	Trace

(Table A.3, continued)

Item No.	Food	Approximate measure	Weight, g	Water, percent	Food energy, kcal	Protein, g	Fat, g
32	Heavy	1 cup	238	58	820	5	88
33		1 tbsp	15	58	80	Trace	6
34	Whipped topping (pressurized)	1 cup	60	61	155	2	13
35		1 tbsp	3	61	10	Trace	1
36	Cream, sour	1 cup	230	71	495	7	48
37		1 tbsp	12	71	25	Trace	3
	Cream products, imitation (made with vegetable fat):						
	Sweet:						
	Creamers:						
38	Liquid (frozen)	1 cup	245	77	335	2	24
39		1 tbsp	15	77	20	Trace	1
40	Powdered	1 cup	94	2	515	5	33
41		1 tsp	2	2	10	Trace	1
	Whipped topping:						
42	Frozen	1 cup	75	50	240	1	19
43		1 tbsp	4	50	15	Trace	1
44	Powdered, made with whole milk	1 cup	80	67	150	3	10
45		1 tbsp	4	67	10	Trace	Trace
46	Pressurized	1 cup	70	60	185	1	16
47		1 tbsp	4	60	10	Trace	1
48	Sour dressing (imitation sour cream) made with nonfat dry milk	1 cup	235	75	415	8	39
49		1 tbsp	12	75	20	Trace	2
	Cucumber slices, 1/8 in. thick (large, 2 1/8-in. diam.; small, 1 3/4-in. diam.):						
618	With peel	6 large or 8 small slices	28	95	5	Trace	Trace
619	Without peel	6 1/2 large or 9 small pieces	28	96	5	Trace	Trace
86	Custard, baked	1 cup	265	77	305	14	15
620	Dandelion greens, cooked, drained	1 cup	105	90	35	2	1
	Danish pastry (enriched flour), plain without fruit or nuts:						
433	Packaged ring, 12 oz	1 ring	340	22	1,435	25	80
434	Round piece, about 4 1/4-in. diam. by 1 in.	1 pastry	65	22	275	5	15
435	Ounce	1 oz	28	22	120	2	7

[a] Vitamin A value is largely from beta-carotene used for coloring. Riboflavin value for items 40-41 apply to products with added riboflavin.

(Table A.3, continued)

Saturated (total), g	Unsaturated Oleic, g	Linoleic, g	Carbohydrate, g	Calcium, mg	Phosphorus, mg	Iron, mg	Potassium, mg	Vitamin A value, IU	Thiamin, mg	Riboflavin, mg	Niacin, mg	Vitamin C, mg
54.8	22.2	2.0	7	154	149	.1	179	3,500	.05	.26	.1	1
3.5	1.4	.1	Trace	10	9	Trace	11	220	Trace	.02	Trace	Trace
8.3	3.4	.3	7	61	54	Trace	88	550	.02	.04	Trace	0
.4	.2	Trace	Trace	3	3	Trace	4	30	Trace	Trace	Trace	0
30.0	12.1	1.1	10	268	195	.1	331	1,820	.08	.34	.2	2
1.6	.6	.1	1	14	10	Trace	17	90	Trace	.02	Trace	Trace
22.8	.3	Trace	28	23	157	.1	467	220[a]	0	0	0	0
1.4	Trace	0	2	1	10	Trace	29	10[a]	0	0	0	0
30.6	.9	Trace	52	21	397	.1	763	190[a]	0	.16[a]	0	0
.7	Trace	0	1	Trace	8	Trace	16	Trace[a]	0	Trace[a]	0	0
16.3	1.0	.2	17	5	6	.1	14	650[a]	0	0	0	0
.9	.1	Trace	1	Trace	Trace	Trace	1	30[a]	0	0	0	0
8.5	.6	.1	13	72	69	Trace	121	290[a]	.02	.09	Trace	1
.4	Trace	Trace	1	4	3	Trace	6	10[a]	Trace	Trace	Trace	Trace
13.2	1.4	.2	11	4	13	Trace	13	330[a]	0	0	0	0
.8	.1	Trace	1	Trace	1	Trace	1	20[a]	0	0	0	0
31.2	4.4	1.1	11	266	205	.1	380	20[a]	.09	.38	.2	2
1.6	.2	.1	1	14	10	Trace	19	Trace[a]	.01	.02	Trace	Trace
—	—	—	1	7	8	.3	45	70	.01	.01	.1	3
—	—	—	1	5	5	.1	45	Trace	.01	.01	.1	3
6.8	5.4	.7	29	297	310	1.1	387	930	.11	.50	.3	1
—	—	—	7	147	44	1.9	244	12,290	.14	.17	—	19
24.3	31.7	16.5	155	170	371	6.1	381	1,050	.97	1.01	8.6	Trace
4.7	6.1	3.2	30	33	71	1.2	73	200	.18	.19	1.7	Trace
2.0	2.7	1.4	13	14	31	.5	32	90	.08	.08	.7	Trace

(Table A.3, continued)

Item No.	Food	Approximate measure	Weight, g	Water, percent	Food energy, kcal	Protein, g	Fat, g
	Dates:						
243	Whole, without pits	10 dates	80	23	220	2	Trace
244	Chopped	1 cup	178	23	490	4	1
	Doughnuts, made with enriched flour:						
436	Cake type, plain, 2½-in. diam., 1 in. high	1 doughnut	25	24	100	1	5
437	Yeast-leavened, glazed, 3¾-in. diam., 1¼ in. high	1 doughnut	50	26	205	3	11
	Eggs, large (24 oz per dozen):						
	Raw:						
96	Whole, without shell	1 egg	50	75	80	6	6
97	White	1 white	33	88	15	3	Trace
98	Yolk	1 yolk	17	49	65	3	6
	Cooked:						
99	Fried in butter	1 egg	46	72	85	5	6
100	Hard-cooked, shell removed	1 egg	50	75	80	6	6
101	Poached	1 egg	50	74	80	6	6
102	Scrambled (milk added) in butter. Also omelet	1 egg	64	76	95	6	7
621	Endive, curly (including escarole), raw, small pieces	1 cup	50	93	10	1	Trace
365	Farina, quick-cooking, enriched	1 cup	245	89	105	3	Trace
109	Fats, cooking (vegetable shortenings)	1 cup	200	0	1,770	0	200
110		1 tbsp	13	0	110	0	13
111	Lard	1 cup	205	0	1,850	0	205
112		1 tbsp	13	0	115	0	13
521	Filberts (hazelnuts), chopped (about 80 kernels)	1 cup	115	6	730	14	72
149	Fish sticks, breaded, cooked, frozen (stick, 4 by 1 by ½ in.)	1 fish stick or 1 oz	28	66	50	5	3
245	Fruit cocktail, canned, in heavy sirup	1 cup	255	80	195	1	Trace
698	Gelatin, dry	1, 7-g envelope	7	13	25	6	Trace
699	Gelatin dessert prepared with gelatin dessert powder and water	1 cup	240	84	140	4	0

[a] Applies to products that do not contain di-sodium phosphate. If di-sodium phosphate is an ingredient, value is 162 mg.
[b] Value may range from less than 1 mg to about 8 mg depending on the brand. Consult the label.

(Table A.3, continued)

Fatty acids												
Satu-rated (total), g	Unsaturated		Carbo-hydrate, g	Cal-cium, mg	Phos-phorus, mg	Iron, mg	Potas-sium, mg	Vitamin A value, IU	Thia-min, mg	Ribo-flavin, mg	Niacin, mg	Vitamin C, mg
	Oleic, g	Lino-leic, g										
—	—	—	58	47	50	2.4	518	40	.07	.08	1.8	0
—	—	—	130	105	112	5.3	1,153	90	.16	.18	3.9	0
1.2	2.0	1.1	13	10	48	.4	23	20	.05	.05	.4	Trace
3.3	5.8	3.3	22	16	33	.6	34	25	.10	.10	.8	0
1.7	2.0	.6	1	28	90	1.0	65	260	.04	.15	Trace	0
0	0	0	Trace	4	4	Trace	45	0	Trace	.09	Trace	0
1.7	2.1	.6	Trace	26	86	.9	15	310	.04	.07	Trace	0
2.4	2.2	.6	1	26	80	.9	58	290	.03	.13	Trace	0
1.7	2.0	.6	1	28	90	1.0	65	260	.04	.14	Trace	0
1.7	2.0	.6	1	28	90	1.0	65	260	.04	.13	Trace	0
2.8	2.3	.6	1	47	97	.9	85	310	.04	.16	Trace	0
—	—	—	2	41	27	.9	147	1,650	.04	.07	.3	5
Trace	Trace	.1	22	147	113[a]	(b)	25	0	.12	.07	1.0	0
48.8	88.2	48.4	0	0	0	0	0	—	0	0	0	0
3.2	5.7	3.1	0	0	0	0	0	—	0	0	0	0
81.0	83.8	20.5	0	0	0	0	0	0	0	0	0	0
5.1	5.3	1.3	0	0	0	0	0	0	0	0	0	0
5.1	55.2	7.3	19	240	388	3.9	810	—	.53	—	1.0	Trace
—	—	—	2	3	47	.1	—	0	.01	.02	.5	—
—	—	—	50	23	31	1.0	411	360	.05	.03	1.0	5
0	0	0	0	—	—	—	—	—	—	—	—	—
0	0	0	34	—	—	—	—	—	—	—	—	—

(Table A.3, continued)

Item No.	Food	Approximate measure	Weight, g	Water, percent	Food energy, kcal	Protein, g	Fat, g
	Grapefruit:						
	Raw, meduim, 3¾-in. diam. (about 1 lb 1 oz):						
246	Pink or red	½ grapefruit with peel[a]	241	89	50	1	Trace
247	White	½ grapefruit with peel[a]	241	89	45	1	Trace
248	Canned, sections with sirup	1 cup	254	81	180	2	Trace
	Grapefruit juice:						
249	Raw, pink, red, or white	1 cup	246	90	95	1	Trace
	Canned, white:						
250	Unsweetened	1 cup	247	89	100	1	Trace
251	Sweetened	1 cup	250	86	135	1	Trace
	Frozen, concentrate, unsweetened:						
252	Undiluted, 6-fl oz can	1 can	207	62	300	4	1
253	Diluted with 3 parts water by volume	1 cup	247	89	100	1	Trace
254	Dehydrated crystals, prepared with water (1 lb yields about 1 gal)	1 cup	247	90	100	1	Trace
	Grapes, European type (adherent skin), raw:						
255	Thompson Seedless	10 grapes	50	81	35	Trace	Trace
256	Tokay and Emperor, seeded types	10 grapes[c]	60	81	40	Trace	Trace
	Grapejuice:						
257	Canned or bottled	1 cup	253	83	165	1	Trace
	Frozen concentrate, sweetened:						
258	Undiluted, 6-fl oz can	1 can	216	53	395	1	Trace
259	Diluted with 3 parts water by volume	1 cup	250	86	135	1	Trace
260	Grape drink, canned	1 cup	250	86	135	Trace	Trace

[a] Weight includes peel and membranes between sections. Without these parts, the weight of the edible portion is 123 g for item 246 and 118 g for item 247.

[b] For white-fleshed varieties, value is about 20 IU per cup; for red-fleshed varieties, 1080 IU.

[c] Weight includes seeds. Without seeds, weight of the edible portion is 57 g.

[d] Applies to products without added vitamin C. For value of products with added vitamin C, refer to label.

[e] Applies to product without added vitamin C. With added vitamin C, based on claim that 6 fl oz of reconstituted juice contain 45 percent or 50 percent of the U.S. RDA, value in milligrams is 108 or 120 for a 6 fl oz can (item 258), 36 or 40 for 1 cup of diluted juice (item 259).

[f] For products with added thiamin and riboflavin but without added ascorbic acid, value in milligrams would be 0.60 for thiamin, 0.80 for riboflavin, and trace for vitamin C. For products with only vitamin C added, value varies with the brand. Consult the label.

(Table A.3, continued)

| Fatty acids | | | | | | | | | | | | |
Satu-rated (total), g	Unsaturated Oleic, g	Lino-leic, g	Carbo-hydrate, g	Cal-cium, mg	Phos-phorus, mg	Iron, mg	Potas-sium, mg	Vitamin A value, IU	Thia-min, mg	Ribo-flavin, mg	Niacin, mg	Vitamin C, mg
—	—	—	13	20	20	.5	166	540	.05	.02	.2	44
—	—	—	12	19	19	.5	159	10	.05	.02	.2	44
—	—	—	45	33	36	.8	343	30	.08	.05	.5	76
—	—	—	23	22	37	.5	399	(b)	.10	.05	.5	93
—	—	—	24	20	35	1.0	400	20	.07	.05	.5	84
—	—	—	32	20	35	1.0	405	30	.08	.05	.5	78
—	—	—	72	70	124	.8	1,250	60	.29	.12	1.4	286
—	—	—	24	25	42	.2	420	20	.10	.04	.5	96
—	—	—	24	22	40	.2	412	20	.10	.05	.5	91
—	—	—	9	6	10	.2	87	50	.03	.02	.2	2
—	—	—	10	7	11	.2	99	60	.03	.02	.2	2
—	—	—	42	28	30	.8	293	—	.10	.05	.5	Trace[d]
—	—	—	100	22	32	.9	255	40	.13	.22	1.5	32[e]
—	—	—	33	8	10	.3	85	10	.05	.08	.5	10[e]
—	—	—	35	8	10	.3	88	—	.03[f]	.03[f]	.3	(f)

(Table A.3, continued)

Item No.	Food	Approximate measure	Weight, g	Water, percent	Food energy, kcal	Protein, g	Fat, g
150	Haddock, breaded, fried[a]	3 oz	85	66	140	17	5
181	Heart, beef, lean, braised	3 oz	85	61	160	27	5
548	Honey, strained or extracted	1 tbsp	21	17	65	Trace	0
272	Honeydew (with rind and seed cavity, 6½-in. diam., 5¼ lb)	¹⁄₁₀ melon with rind	226	91	50	1	Trace
	Ice cream:						
	Regular (about 11% fat):						
75	Hardened	½ gal	1,064	61	2,155	38	115
76		1 cup	133	61	270	5	14
77		3-fl-oz container	50	61	100	2	5
78	Soft serve (frozen custard)	1 cup	173	60	375	7	23
79	Rich (about 16% fat), hardened	½ gal	1,188	59	2,805	33	190
80		1 cup	148	59	350	4	24
	Ice milk:						
81	Hardened (about 4.3% fat)	½ gal	1,048	69	1,470	41	45
82		1 cup	131	69	185	5	6
83	Soft serve (about 2.6% fat)	1 cup	175	70	225	8	5
549	Jams and preserves	1 tbsp	20	29	55	Trace	Trace
550		1 packet	14	29	40	Trace	Trace
551	Jellies	1 tbsp	18	29	50	Trace	Trace
552		1 packet	14	29	40	Trace	Trace
	Kale, cooked, drained:						
622	From raw (leaves without stems and mid-ribs)	1 cup	110	88	45	5	1
623	From frozen (leaf style)	1 cup	130	91	40	4	1
	Lamb, cooked:						
	Chop, rib (cut 3 per lb with bone), broiled:						
182	Lean and fat	3.1 oz	89	43	360	18	32
183	Lean only from item 182	2 oz	57	60	120	16	6
	Leg, roasted:						
184	Lean and fat (2 pieces, 4⅛ by 2¼ by ¼ in.)	3 oz	85	54	235	22	16
185	Lean only from item 184	2.5 oz	71	62	130	20	5
	Shoulder, roasted:						
186	Lean and fat (3 pieces, 2½ by 2½ by ¼ in.)	3 oz	85	50	285	18	23

[a] Dipped in egg, milk or water, and breadcrumbs; fried in vegetable shortening.

(Table A.3, continued)

| | Fatty acids | | | | | | | | | | | |
| Satu-rated (total), g | Unsaturated | | Carbo-hydrate, g | Cal-cium, mg | Phos-phorus, mg | Iron, mg | Potas-sium, mg | Vitamin A value, IU | Thia-min, mg | Ribo-flavin, mg | Niacin, mg | Vitamin C, mg |
	Oleic, g	Lino-leic, g										
1.4	2.2	1.2	5	34	210	1.0	296	—	.03	.06	2.7	2
1.5	1.1	.6	1	5	154	5.0	197	20	.21	1.04	6.5	1
0	0	0	17	1	1	.1	11	0	Trace	.01	.1	Trace
—	—	—	11	21	24	.6	374	60	.06	.04	.9	34
71.3	28.8	2.6	254	1,406	1,075	1.0	2,052	4,340	.42	2.63	1.1	6
8.9	3.6	.3	32	176	134	.1	257	540	.05	.33	.1	1
3.4	1.4	.1	12	66	51	Trace	96	200	.02	.12	.1	Trace
13.5	5.9	.6	38	236	199	.4	338	790	.08	.45	.2	1
118.3	47.8	4.3	256	1,213	927	.8	1,771	7,200	.36	2.27	.9	5
14.7	6.0	.5	32	151	115	.1	221	900	.04	.28	.1	1
28.1	11.3	1.0	232	1,409	1,035	1.5	2,117	1,710	.61	2.78	.9	6
3.5	1.4	.1	29	176	129	.1	265	210	.08	.35	.1	1
2.9	1.2	.1	38	274	202	.3	412	180	.12	.54	.2	1
—	—	—	14	4	2	.2	18	Trace	Trace	.01	Trace	Trace
—	—	—	10	3	1	.1	12	Trace	Trace	Trace	Trace	Trace
—	—	—	13	4	1	.3	14	Trace	Trace	.01	Trace	1
—	—	—	10	3	1	.2	11	Trace	Trace	Trace	Trace	1
—	—	—	7	206	64	1.8	243	9,130	.11	.20	1.8	102
—	—	—	7	157	62	1.3	251	10,660	.08	.20	.9	49
14.8	12.1	1.2	0	8	139	1.0	200	—	.11	.19	4.1	—
2.5	2.1	.2	0	6	121	1.1	174	—	.09	.15	3.4	—
7.3	6.0	.6	0	9	177	1.4	241	—	.13	.23	4.7	—
2.1	1.8	.2	0	9	169	1.4	227	—	.12	.21	4.4	—
10.8	8.8	.9	0	9	146	1.0	206	—	.11	.20	4.0	—

(Table A.3, continued)

Item No.	Food	Approximate measure	Weight, g	Water, percent	Food energy, kcal	Protein, g	Fat, g
187	Lean only from item 186	2.3 oz	64	61	130	17	6
	Lemon juice:						
262	Raw	1 cup	244	91	60	1	Trace
263	Canned, or bottled, unsweetened	1 cup	244	92	55	1	Trace
264	Frozen, single strength, unsweetened, 6-fl oz can	1 can	183	92	40	1	Trace
	Lemonade concentrate, frozen:						
265	Undiluted, 6-fl oz can	1 can	219	49	425	Trace	Trace
266	Diluted with 4⅓ parts water by volume	1 cup	248	89	105	Trace	Trace
261	Lemon, raw, size 165, without peel and seeds (about 4 per lb with peels and seeds)	1 lemon	74	90	20	1	Trace
522	Lentils, whole, cooked	1 cup	200	72	210	16	Trace
	Lettuce, raw:						
	Butterhead, as Boston types:						
624	Head, 5-in. diam.	1 head[a]	220	95	25	2	Trace
625	Leaves	1 outer or 2 inner or 3 heart leaves	15	95	Trace	Trace	Trace
	Crisphead, as Iceberg:						
626	Head, 6-in. diam.	1 head[b]	567	96	70	5	1
627	Wedge, ¼ of head	1 wedge	135	96	20	1	Trace
628	Pieces, chopped or shredded	1 cup	55	96	5	Trace	Trace
629	Looseleaf (bunching varieties including romaine or cos), chopped or shredded pieces	1 cup	55	94	10	1	Trace
	Limejuice:						
269	Raw	1 cup	246	90	65	1	Trace
270	Canned, unsweetened	1 cup	246	90	65	1	Trace
	Limeade concentrate, frozen:						
267	Undiluted, 6-fl oz can	1 can	218	50	410	Trace	Trace
268	Diluted with 4⅓ parts water by volume	1 cup	247	89	100	Trace	Trace
188	Liver, beef, fried (slice, 6½ by 2⅜ by ⅜ in.)	3 oz	85	56	195	22	9
	Macaroni, enriched, cooked (cut lengths, elbows, shells):						
438	Firm stage (hot)	1 cup	130	64	190	7	1
	Tender stage:						

[a] Weight includes refuse of outer leaves and core. Without these parts, weight is 163 g.
[b] Weight includes core. Without core, weight is 539 g.
[e] Value varies widely.

536

(Table A.3, continued)

Saturated (total), g	Fatty acids Unsaturated Oleic, g	Linoleic, g	Carbohydrate, g	Calcium, mg	Phosphorus, mg	Iron, mg	Potassium, mg	Vitamin A value, IU	Thiamin, mg	Riboflavin, mg	Niacin, mg	Vitamin C, mg
3.6	2.3	.2	0	8	140	1.0	193	—	.10	.18	3.7	—
—	—	—	20	17	24	.5	344	50	.07	.02	.2	112
—	—	—	19	17	24	.5	344	50	.07	.02	.2	102
—	—	—	13	13	16	.5	258	40	.05	.02	.2	81
—	—	—	112	9	13	.4	153	40	.05	.06	.7	66
—	—	—	28	2	3	.1	40	10	.01	.02	.2	17
—	—	—	6	19	12	.4	102	10	.03	.01	.1	39
—	—	—	39	50	238	4.2	498	40	.14	.12	1.2	0
—	—	—	4	57	42	3.3	430	1,580	.10	.10	.5	13
—	—	—	Trace	5	4	.3	40	150	.01	.01	Trace	1
—	—	—	16	108	118	2.7	943	1,780	.32	.32	1.6	32
—	—	—	4	27	30	.7	236	450	.08	.08	.4	8
—	—	—	2	11	12	.3	96	180	.03	.03	.2	3
—	—	—	2	37	14	.8	145	1,050	.03	.04	.2	10
—	—	—	22	22	27	.5	256	20	.05	.02	.2	79
—	—	—	22	22	27	.5	256	20	.05	.02	.2	52
—	—	—	108	11	13	.2	129	Trace	.02	.02	.2	26
—	—	—	27	3	3	Trace	32	Trace	Trace	Trace	Trace	
2.5	3.5	.9	5	9	405	7.5	323	45,390[c]	.22	3.56	14.0	23
—	—	—	39	14	85	1.4	103	0	.23	.13	1.8	0

(Table A.3, continued)

Item No.	Food	Approximate measure	Weight, g	Water, percent	Food energy, kcal	Protein, g	Fat, g
439	Cold macaroni	1 cup	105	73	115	4	Trace
440	Hot macaroni	1 cup	140	73	155	5	1
	Macaroni (enriched) and cheese:						
441	Canned	1 cup	240	80	230	9	10
442	From home recipe (served hot)	1 cup	200	58	430	17	22
	Margarine:						
	Regular (1 brick or 4 sticks per lb):						
113	Stick (½ cup)	1 stick	113	16	815	1	92
114	Tablespoon (about ⅛ stick)	1 tbsp	14	16	100	Trace	12
115	Pat (1 in. square, ⅓ in. high; 90 per lb)	1 pat	5	16	35	Trace	4
116	Soft, two 8-oz containers per lb	1 container	227	16	1,635	1	184
117		1 tbsp	14	16	100	Trace	12
	Whipped (6 sticks per lb):						
118	Stick (½ cup)	1 stick	76	16	545	Trace	61
119	Tablespoon (about ⅛ stick)	1 tbsp	9	16	70	Trace	8
	Milk:						
	Fluid:						
50	Whole (3.3% fat)	1 cup	244	88	150	8	8
	Lowfat (2%):						
51	No milk solids added	1 cup	244	89	120	8	5
	Milk solids added:						
52	Label claim less than 10 g of protein per cup	1 cup	245	89	125	9	5
53	Label claim 10 or more grams of protein per cup (protein fortified)	1 cup	246	88	135	10	5
	Lowfat (1%):						
54	No milk solids added	1 cup	244	90	100	8	3
	Milk solids added:						
55	Label claim less than 10 g of protein per cup	1 cup	245	90	105	9	2
56	Label claim 10 or more grams of protein per cup (protein fortified)	1 cup	246	89	120	10	3
	Nonfat (skim):						
57	No milk solids added:	1 cup	245	91	85	8	Trace

[a] Applies to product without added vitamin A. With added vitamin A, value is 500 IU.

[b] Based on average vitamin A content of fortified margarine. Federal specifications for fortified margarine require a minimum of 15,000 IU of vitamin A per pound.

(Table A.3, continued)

Saturated (total), g	Fatty acids — Unsaturated Oleic, g	Linoleic, g	Carbohydrate, g	Calcium, mg	Phosphorus, mg	Iron, mg	Potassium, mg	Vitamin A value, IU	Thiamin, mg	Riboflavin, mg	Niacin, mg	Vitamin C, mg
—	—	—	24	8	53	.9	64	0	.15	.08	1.2	0
—	—	—	32	11	70	1.3	85	0	.20	.11	1.5	0
4.2	3.1	1.4	26	199	182	1.0	139	260	.12	.24	1.0	Trace
8.9	8.8	2.9	40	362	322	1.8	240	860	.20	.40	1.8	Trace
16.7	42.9	24.9	Trace	27	26	.2	29	3,750[b]	.01	.04	Trace	0
2.1	5.3	3.1	Trace	3	3	Trace	4	470[b]	Trace	Trace	Trace	0
.7	1.9	1.1	Trace	1	1	Trace	1	170[b]	Trace	Trace	Trace	0
32.5	71.5	65.4	Trace	53	52	.4	59	7,500[b]	.01	.08	.1	0
2.0	4.5	4.1	Trace	3	3	Trace	4	470[b]	Trace	Trace	Trace	0
11.2	28.7	16.7	Trace	18	17	.1	20	2,500[b]	Trace	.03	Trace	0
1.4	3.6	2.1	Trace	2	2	Trace	2	310[b]	Trace	Trace	Trace	0
5.1	2.1	.2	11	291	228	.1	370	310[a]	.09	.40	.2	2
2.9	1.2	.1	12	297	232	.1	377	500	.10	.40	.2	2
2.9	1.2	.1	12	313	245	.1	397	500	.10	.42	.2	2
3.0	1.2	.1	14	352	276	.1	447	500	.11	.48	.2	3
1.6	.7	.1	12	300	235	.1	381	500	.10	.41	.2	2
1.5	.6	.1	12	313	245	.1	397	500	.10	.42	.2	2
1.8	.7	.1	14	349	273	.1	444	500	.11	.47	.2	3
.3	.1	Trace	12	302	247	.1	406	500	.09	.37	.2	2

(Table A.3, continued)

Item No.	Food	Approximate measure	Weight, g	Water, percent	Food energy, kcal	Protein, g	Fat, g
	Milk solids added:						
58	Label claim less than 10 g of protein per cup	1 cup	245	90	90	9	1
59	Label claim 10 or more grams of protein per cup (protein fortified)	1 cup	246	89	100	10	1
	Canned:						
	Evaporated, unsweetened:						
61	Whole milk	1 cup	252	74	340	17	19
62	Skim milk	1 cup	255	79	200	19	1
63	Sweetened, condensed	1 cup	306	27	980	24	27
	Dried:						
64	Buttermilk	1 cup	120	3	465	41	7
	Nonfat instant:						
65	Envelope, net wt., 3.2 oz[d]	1 envelope	91	4	325	32	1
66	Cup[f]	1 cup	68	4	245	24	Trace
	Milk beverages:						
	Chocolate milk (commercial):						
67	Regular	1 cup	250	82	210	8	8
68	Lowfat (2%)	1 cup	250	84	180	8	5
69	Lowfat (1%)	1 cup	250	85	160	8	3
70	Eggnog (commercial)	1 cup	254	74	340	10	19
	Malted milk, home-prepared with 1 cup of whole milk and 2 to 3 heaping tsp of malted milk powder (about ¾ oz):						
71	Chocolate	1 cup of milk plus ¾ oz of powder	265	81	235	9	9
72	Natural	1 cup of milk plus ¾ oz of powder	265	81	235	11	10
	Shakes, thick:[g]						
73	Chocolate, container, net wt., 10.6 oz	1 container	300	72	355	9	8
74	Vanilla, container, net wt., 11 oz	1 container	313	74	350	12	9

[b] Applies to product without vitamin A added.

[c] Applies to product with added vitamin A. Without added vitamin A, value is 20 IU.

[d] Yields 1 qt of fluid milk when reconstituted according to package directions.

[e] Applies to product with added vitamin A.

[f] Weight applies to product with label claim of 1⅓ cups equal 3.2 oz.

[g] Applies to products made from thick shake mixes and that do not contain added ice cream. Products made from milk shake mixes are higher in fat and usually contain added ice cream.

(Table A.3, continued)

Saturated (total), g	Fatty acids Unsaturated Oleic, g	Linoleic, g	Carbohydrate, g	Calcium, mg	Phosphorus, mg	Iron, mg	Potassium, mg	Vitamin A value, IU	Thiamin, mg	Riboflavin, mg	Niacin, mg	Vitamin C, mg
.4	.1	Trace	12	316	255	.1	418	500	.10	.43	.2	2
.4	.1	Trace	14	352	275	.1	446	500	.11	.48	.2	3
11.6	5.3	.4	25	657	510	.5	764	610[b]	.12	.80	.5	5
.3	.1	Trace	29	738	497	.7	845	1,000[c]	.11	.79	.4	3
16.8	6.7	.7	166	868	775	.6	1,136	1,000[b]	.28	1.27	.6	8
4.3	1.7	.2	59	1,421	1,119	.4	1,910	260[b]	.47	1.90	1.1	7
.4	.1	Trace	47	1,120	896	.3	1,552	2,160[c]	.38	1.59	.8	5
.3	.1	Trace	35	837	670	.2	1,160	1,610[c]	.28	1.19	.6	4
5.3	2.2	.2	26	280	251	.6	417	300[b]	.09	.41	.3	2
3.1	1.3	.1	26	284	254	.6	422	500	.10	.42	.3	2
1.5	.7	.1	26	287	257	.6	426	500	.10	.40	.2	2
11.3	5.0	.6	34	330	278	.5	420	890	.09	.48	.3	4
5.5	—	—	29	304	265	.5	500	330	.14	.43	.7	2
6.0	—	—	27	347	307	.3	529	380	.20	.54	1.3	2
5.0	2.0	.2	63	396	378	.9	672	260	.14	.67	.4	0
5.9	2.4	.2	56	457	361	.3	572	360	.09	.61	.5	0

(Table A.3, continued)

Item No.	Food	Approximate measure	Weight, g	Water, percent	Food energy, kcal	Protein, g	Fat, g
	Milk desserts, other:						
86	Custard, baked	1 cup	265	77	305	14	15
	Puddings:						
	From home recipe:						
	Starch base:						
87	Chocolate	1 cup	260	66	385	8	12
88	Vanilla (blancmange)	1 cup	255	76	285	9	10
89	Tapioca cream	1 cup	165	72	220	8	8
	From mix (chocolate) and milk:						
90	Regular (cooked)	1 cup	260	70	320	9	8
91	Instant	1 cup	260	69	325	8	7
	Muffins made with enriched flour:						
	From home recipe:						
443	Blueberry, 2⅜-in. diam., 1½ in. high	1 muffin	40	39	110	3	4
444	Bran	1 muffin	40	35	105	3	4
445	Corn (enriched degermed cornmeal and flour), 2⅜-in. diam., 1½ in. high	1 muffin	40	33	125	3	4
446	Plain, 3-in. diam., 1½ in. high	1 muffin	40	38	120	3	4
	From mix, egg, milk:						
447	Corn, 2⅜-in. diam., 1½ in. high	1 muffin	40	30	130	3	4
630	Mushrooms, raw, sliced or chopped	1 cup	70	90	20	2	Trace
	Muskmelons, raw, with rind, without seed cavity:						
271	Cantaloup, orange-fleshed (with rind and seed cavity, 5-in. diam., 2⅓ lb)	½ melon with rind	477	91	80	2	Trace
272	Honeydew (with rind and seed cavity, 6½-in. diam., 5¼ lb)	1/10 melon with rind	226	91	50	1	Trace
631	Mustard greens, without stems and midribs, cooked, drained	1 cup	140	93	30	3	1
700	Mustard, prepared, yellow	1 tsp or individual serving pouch or cup	5	80	5	Trace	Trace
449	Noodles, chow mein, canned	1 cup	45	1	220	6	11
448	Noodles (egg noodles), enriched cooked	1 cup	160	71	200	7	2
366	Oatmeal or rolled oats	1 cup	240	87	130	5	2
375	Oats, puffed, added sugar, salt, minerals, vitamins	1 cup	25	3	100	3	1

[a] Applies to product made with yellow cornmeal.

(Table A.3, continued)

Saturated (total), g	Fatty acids Unsaturated Oleic, g	Linoleic, g	Carbohydrate, g	Calcium, mg	Phosphorus, mg	Iron, mg	Potassium, mg	Vitamin A value, IU	Thiamin, mg	Riboflavin, mg	Niacin, mg	Vitamin C, mg
6.8	5.4	.7	29	297	310	1.1	387	930	.11	.50	.3	1
7.6	3.3	.3	67	250	255	1.3	445	390	.05	.36	.3	1
6.2	2.5	.2	41	298	232	Trace	352	410	.08	.41	.3	2
4.1	2.5	.5	28	173	180	.7	223	480	.07	.30	.2	2
4.3	2.6	.2	59	265	247	.8	354	340	.05	.39	.3	2
3.6	2.2	.3	63	374	237	1.3	335	340	.08	.39	.3	2
1.1	1.4	.7	17	34	53	.6	46	90	.09	.10	.7	Trace
1.2	1.4	.8	17	57	162	1.5	172	90	.07	.10	1.7	Trace
1.2	1.6	.9	19	42	68	.7	54	120[a]	.10	.10	.7	Trace
1.0	1.7	1.0	17	42	60	.6	50	40	.09	.12	.9	Trace
1.2	1.7	.9	20	96	152	.6	44	100[a]	.08	.09	.7	Trace
—	—	—	3	4	81	.6	290	Trace	.07	.32	2.9	2
—	—	—	20	38	44	1.1	682	9,240	.11	.08	1.6	90
—	—	—	11	21	24	.6	374	60	.06	.04	.9	34
—	—	—	6	193	45	2.5	308	8,120	.11	.20	.8	67
—	—	—	Trace	4	4	.1	7	—	—	—	—	—
—	—	—	26	—	—	—	—	—	—	—	—	—
—	—	—	37	16	94	1.4	70	110	.22	.13	1.9	0
.4	.8	.9	23	22	137	1.4	146	0	.19	.05	.2	0
—	—	—	19	44	102	2.9	—	1,180	.29	.35	2.9	9

(Table A.3, continued)

Item No.	Food	Approximate measure	Weight, g	Water, percent	Food energy, kcal	Protein, g	Fat, g
151	Ocean perch, breaded, fried	1 fillet	85	59	195	16	11
	Oils, salad or cooking:						
120	Corn	1 cup	218	0	1,925	0	218
121		1 tbsp	14	0	120	0	14
122	Olive	1 cup	216	0	1,910	0	216
123		1 tbsp	14	0	120	0	14
124	Peanut	1 cup	216	0	1,910	0	216
125		1 tbsp	14	0	120	0	14
126	Safflower	1 cup	218	0	1,925	0	218
127		1 tbsp	14	0	120	0	14
128	Soybean oil, hydrogenated (partially hardened)	1 cup	218	0	1,925	0	218
129		1 tbsp	14	0	120	0	14
130	Soybean-cottonseed oil blend, hydrogenated	1 cup	218	0	1,925	0	218
131		1 tbsp	14	0	120	0	14
632	Okra pods, 3 by ⅝ in., cooked	10 pods	106	91	30	2	Trace
	Olives, pickled, canned:						
701	Green	4 medium or 3 extra large or 2 giant[a]	16	78	15	Trace	2
702	Ripe, Mission	3 small or 2 large[a]	10	73	15	Trace	2
	Onions:						
	Mature:						
	Raw:						
633	Chopped	1 cup	170	89	65	3	Trace
634	Sliced	1 cup	115	89	45	2	Trace
635	Cooked (whole or sliced), drained	1 cup	210	92	60	3	Trace
636	Young green, bulb (⅜ in. diam.) and white portion of top	6 onions	30	88	15	Trace	Trace
	Oranges, all commercial varieties, raw:						
273	Whole, 2⅝-in. diam., without peel and seeds (about 2½ per lb with peel and seeds)	1 orange	131	86	65	1	Trace
274	Sections without membranes	1 cup	180	86	90	2	Trace

[a] Weight includes pits. Without pits, weight is 13 g for item 701, 9 g for item 702.
[b] Value based on white-fleshed varieties. For yellow-fleshed varieties, value in International Units (IU) is 70 for item 633, 50 for item 634, and 80 for item 635.

(Table A.3, continued)

Satu-rated (total), g	Fatty acids Unsaturated		Carbo-hydrate, g	Cal-cium, mg	Phos-phorus, mg	Iron, mg	Potas-sium, mg	Vitamin A value, IU	Thia-min, mg	Ribo-flavin, mg	Niacin, mg	Vitamin C, mg
	Oleic, g	Lino-leic, g										
2.7	4.4	2.3	6	28	192	1.1	242	—	.10	.10	1.6	—
27.7	53.6	125.1	0	0	0	0	0	—	0	0	0	0
1.7	3.3	7.8	0	0	0	0	0	—	0	0	0	0
30.7	154.4	17.7	0	0	0	0	0	—	0	0	0	0
1.9	9.7	1.1	0	0	0	0	0	—	0	0	0	0
37.4	98.5	67.0	0	0	0	0	0	—	0	0	0	0
2.3	6.2	4.2	0	0	0	0	0	—	0	0	0	0
20.5	25.9	159.8	0	0	0	0	0	—	0	0	0	0
1.3	1.6	10.0	0	0	0	0	0	—	0	0	0	0
31.8	93.1	75.6	0	0	0	0	0	—	0	0	0	0
2.0	5.8	4.7	0	0	0	0	0	—	0	0	0	0
38.2	63.0	99.6	0	0	0	0	0	—	0	0	0	0
2.4	3.9	6.2	0	0	0	0	0	—	0	0	0	0
—	—	—	6	98	43	.5	184	520	.14	.19	1.0	21
.2	1.2	.1	Trace	8	2	.2	7	40	—	—	—	—
.2	1.2	.1	Trace	9	1	.1	2	10	Trace	Trace	—	—
—	—	—	15	46	61	.9	267	Trace[b]	.05	.07	.3	17
—	—	—	10	31	41	.6	181	Trace[b]	.03	.05	.2	12
—	—	—	14	50	61	.8	231	Trace[b]	.06	.06	.4	15
—	—	—	3	12	12	.2	69	Trace	.02	.01	.1	8
—	—	—	16	54	26	.5	263	260	.13	.05	.5	66
—	—	—	22	74	36	.7	360	360	.18	.07	.7	90

(Table A.3, continued)

Item No.	Food	Approximate measure	Weight, g	Water, percent	Food energy, kcal	Protein, g	Fat, g
	Orange juice:						
275	Raw, all varieties	1 cup	248	88	110	2	Trace
276	Canned, unsweetened	1 cup	249	87	120	2	Trace
	Frozen concentrate:						
277	Undiluted, 6-fl oz can	1 can	213	55	360	5	Trace
278	Diluted with 3 parts water by volume	1 cup	249	87	120	2	Trace
279	Dehydrated crystals, prepared with water (1 lb yields about 1 gal)	1 cup	248	88	115	1	Trace
	Orange and grapefruit juice:						
	Frozen concentrate:						
280	Undiluted, 6-fl oz can	1 can	210	59	330	4	1
281	Diluted with 3 parts water by volume	1 cup	248	88	110	1	Trace
152	Oysters, raw, meat only (13-19 medium Selects)	1 cup	240	85	160	20	4
	Pancakes (4-in. diam.):						
450	Buckwheat, made from mix (with buckwheat and enriched flours), egg and milk added	1 cake	27	58	55	2	2
	Plain:						
451	Made from home recipe using enriched flour	1 cake	27	50	60	2	2
452	Made from mix with enriched flour, egg and milk added	1 cake	27	51	60	2	2
282	Papayas, raw, ½-in. cubes	1 cup	140	89	55	1	Trace
637	Parsley, raw, chopped	1 tbsp	4	85	Trace	Trace	Trace
638	Parsnips, cooked (diced or 2-in. lengths)	1 cup	155	82	100	2	1
	Peaches:						
	Raw:						
283	Whole, 2½-in. diam., peeled, pitted (about 4 per lb with peels and pits)	1 peach	100	89	40	1	Trace
284	Sliced	1 cup	170	89	65	1	Trace
	Canned, yellow-fleshed, solids and liquid (halves or slices):						
285	Sirup pack	1 cup	256	79	200	1	Trace
286	Water pack	1 cup	244	91	75	1	Trace
	Dried:						
287	Uncooked	1 cup	160	25	420	5	1
288	Cooked, unsweetened, halves and juice	1 cup	250	77	205	3	1

(Table A.3, continued)

Fatty acids												
Satu-rated	Unsaturated											
(total), g	Oleic, g	Lino-leic, g	Carbo-hydrate, g	Cal-cium, mg	Phos-phorus, mg	Iron, mg	Potas-sium, mg	Vitamin A value, IU	Thia-min, mg	Ribo-flavin, mg	Niacin, mg	Vitamin C, mg
—	—	—	26	27	42	.5	496	500	.22	.07	1.0	124
—	—	—	28	25	45	1.0	496	500	.17	.05	.7	100
—	—	—	87	75	126	.9	1,500	1,620	.68	.11	2.8	360
—	—	—	29	25	42	.2	503	540	.23	.03	.9	120
—	—	—	27	25	40	.5	518	500	.20	.07	1.0	109
—	—	—	78	61	99	.8	1,308	800	.48	.06	2.3	302
—	—	—	26	20	32	.2	439	270	.15	.02	.7	102
1.3	.2	.1	8	226	343	13.2	290	740	.34	.43	6.0	—
.8	.9	.4	6	59	91	.4	66	60	.04	.05	.2	Trace
.5	.8	.5	9	27	38	.4	33	30	.06	.07	.5	Trace
.7	.7	.3	9	58	70	.3	42	70	.04	.06	.2	Trace
—	—	—	14	28	22	.4	328	2,450	.06	.06	.4	78
—	—	—	Trace	7	2	.2	25	300	Trace	.01	Trace	6
—	—	—	23	70	96	.9	587	50	.11	.12	.2	16
—	—	—	10	9	19	.5	202	1,330	.02	.05	1.0	7
—	—	—	16	15	32	.9	343	2,260	.03	.09	1.7	12
—	—	—	51	10	31	.8	333	1,100	.03	.05	1.5	8
—	—	—	20	10	32	.7	334	1,100	.02	.07	1.5	7
—	—	—	109	77	187	9.6	1,520	6,240	.02	.30	8.5	29
—	—	—	54	38	93	4.8	743	3,050	.01	.15	3.8	5

(Table A.3, continued)

Item No.	Food	Approximate measure	Weight, g	Water, percent	Food energy, kcal	Protein, g	Fat, g
	Frozen, sliced, sweetened:						
289	10-oz container	1 container	284	77	250	1	Trace
290	Cup	1 cup	250	77	220	1	Trace
523	Peanuts, roasted in oil, salted (whole, halves, chopped)	1 cup	144	2	840	37	72
524	Peanut butter	1 tbsp	16	2	95	4	8
	Pears:						
	Raw, with skin, cored:						
291	Bartlett, 2½-in. diam. (about 2½ per lb with cores and stems	1 pear	164	83	100	1	1
292	Bosc, 2½-in. diam. (about 3 per lb with cores and stems)	1 pear	141	83	85	1	1
293	D'Anjou, 3-in. diam. (about 2 per lb with cores and stems)	1 pear	200	83	120	1	1
294	Canned, solids and liquid, sirup pack, heavy (halves or slices)	1 cup	255	80	195	1	1
	Peas, green						
	Canned:						
639	Whole, drained solids	1 cup	170	77	150	8	1
640	Strained (baby food)	1 oz (1¾ to 2 tbsp)	28	86	15	1	Trace
641	Frozen, cooked, drained	1 cup	160	82	110	8	Trace
525	Peas, split, dry, cooked	1 cup	200	70	230	16	1
526	Pecans, chopped or pieces (about 120 large halves)	1 cup	118	3	810	11	84
642	Peppers, hot, red, without seeds, dried (ground chili powder, added seasonings)	1 tsp	2	9	5	Trace	Trace
	Peppers, sweet (about 5 per lb, whole), stem and seeds removed:						
643	Raw	1 pod	74	93	15	1	Trace
644	Cooked, boiled, drained	1 pod	73	95	15	1	Trace
	Pickles, cucumber:						
703	Dill, medium, whole, 3¾ in. long, 1¼-in. diam.	1 pickle	65	93	5	Trace	Trace
704	Fresh-pack, slices 1½-in. diam., ¼ in. thick	2 slices	15	79	10	Trace	Trace
705	Sweet, gherkin, small, whole, about 2½ in. long, ¾-in. diam.	1 pickle	15	61	20	Trace	Trace
706	Relish, finely chopped, sweet	1 tbsp	15	63	20	Trace	Trace

548

(Table A.3, continued)

| | Fatty acids | | | | | | | | | | | | |
| Satu-rated *(total)*, g | Unsaturated | | Carbo-hydrate, g | Cal-cium, mg | Phos-phorus, mg | Iron, mg | Potas-sium, mg | Vitamin A value, IU | Thia-min, mg | Ribo-flavin, mg | Niacin, mg | Vitamin C, mg |
	Oleic, g	Lino-leic, g										
—	—	—	64	11	37	1.4	352	1,850	.03	.11	2.0	116
—	—	—	57	10	33	1.3	310	1,630	.03	.10	1.8	103
13.7	33.0	20.7	27	107	577	3.0	971	—	.46	.19	24.8	0
1.5	3.7	2.3	3	9	61	.3	100	—	.02	.02	2.4	0
—	—	—	25	13	18	.5	213	30	.03	.07	.2	7
—	—	—	22	11	16	.4	83	30	.03	.06	.1	6
—	—	—	31	16	22	.6	260	40	.04	.08	.2	8
—	—	—	50	13	18	.5	214	10	.03	.05	.3	3
—	—	—	29	44	129	3.2	163	1,170	.15	.10	1.4	14
—	—	—	3	3	18	.3	28	140	.02	.03	.3	3
—	—	—	19	30	138	3.0	216	960	.43	.14	2.7	21
—	—	—	42	22	178	3.4	592	80	.30	.18	1.8	—
7.2	50.5	20.0	17	86	341	2.8	712	150	1.01	.15	1.1	2
—	—	—	1	5	4	.3	20	1,300	Trace	.02	.2	Trace
—	—	—	4	7	16	.5	157	310	.06	.06	.4	94
—	—	—	3	7	12	.4	109	310	.05	.05	.4	70
—	—	—	1	17	14	.7	130	70	Trace	.01	Trace	4
—	—	—	3	5	4	.3	—	20	Trace	Trace	Trace	1
—	—	—	5	2	2	.2	—	10	Trace	Trace	Trace	1
—	—	—	5	3	2	.1	—	—	—	—	—	—

(Table A.3, continued)

Item No.	Food	Approximate measure	Weight, g	Water, percent	Food energy, kcal	Protein, g	Fat, g
	Pies, piecrust made with enriched flour, vegetable shortening (9-in. diam.):						
	Apple:						
453	Whole	1 pie	945	48	2,420	21	105
454	Sector, 1/7 of pie	1 sector	135	48	345	3	15
	Banana cream:						
455	Whole	1 pie	910	54	2,010	41	85
456	Sector, 1/7 of pie	1 sector	130	54	285	6	12
	Blueberry:						
457	Whole	1 pie	945	51	2,285	23	102
458	Sector, 1/7 of pie	1 sector	135	51	325	3	15
	Cherry:						
459	Whole	1 pie	945	47	2,465	25	107
460	Sector, 1/7 of pie	1 sector	135	47	350	4	15
	Custard:						
461	Whole	1 pie	910	58	1,985	56	101
462	Sector, 1/7 of pie	1 sector	130	58	285	8	14
	Lemon meringue:						
463	Whole	1 pie	840	47	2,140	31	86
464	Sector, 1/7 of pie	1 sector	120	47	305	4	12
	Mince:						
465	Whole	1 pie	945	43	2,560	24	109
466	Sector, 1/7 of pie	1 sector	135	43	365	3	16
	Peach:						
467	Whole	1 pie	945	48	2,410	24	101
468	Sector, 1/7 of pie	1 sector	135	48	345	3	14
	Pecan:						
469	Whole	1 pie	825	20	3,450	42	189
470	Sector, 1/7 of pie	1 sector	118	20	495	6	27
	Pumpkin:						
471	Whole	1 pie	910	59	1,920	36	102
472	Sector, 1/7 of pie	1 sector	130	59	275	5	15
473	Piecrust (home recipe) made with enriched flour and vegetable shortening, baked	1 pie shell, 9-in. diam.	180	15	900	11	60
474	Piecrust mix with enriched flour and vegetable shortening, 10-oz pkg. prepared and baked	Piecrust for 2-crust pie, 9-in. diam.	320	19	1,485	20	93

(Table A.3, continued)

Saturated (total), g	Fatty acids		Carbohydrate, g	Calcium, mg	Phosphorus, mg	Iron, mg	Potassium, mg	Vitamin A value, IU	Thiamin, mg	Riboflavin, mg	Niacin, mg	Vitamin C, mg
	Unsaturated											
	Oleic, g	Linoleic, g										
27.0	44.5	25.2	360	76	208	6.6	756	280	1.06	.79	9.3	9
3.9	6.4	3.6	51	11	30	.9	108	40	.15	.11	1.3	2
26.7	33.2	16.2	279	601	746	7.3	1,847	2,280	.77	1.51	7.0	9
3.8	4.7	2.3	40	86	107	1.0	264	330	.11	.22	1.0	1
24.8	43.7	25.1	330	104	217	9.5	614	280	1.03	.80	10.0	28
3.5	6.2	3.6	47	15	31	1.4	88	40	.15	.11	1.4	4
28.2	45.0	25.3	363	132	236	6.6	992	4,160	1.09	.84	9.8	Trace
4.0	6.4	3.6	52	19	34	.9	142	590	.16	.12	1.4	Trace
33.9	38.5	17.5	213	874	1,028	8.2	1,247	2,090	.79	1.92	5.6	0
4.8	5.5	2.5	30	125	147	1.2	178	300	.11	.27	.8	0
26.1	33.8	16.4	317	118	412	6.7	420	1,430	.61	.84	5.2	25
3.7	4.8	2.3	45	17	59	1.0	60	200	.09	.12	.7	4
28.0	45.9	25.2	389	265	359	13.3	1,682	20	.96	.86	9.8	9
4.0	6.6	3.6	56	38	51	1.9	240	Trace	.14	.12	1.4	1
24.8	43.7	25.1	361	95	274	8.5	1,408	6,900	1.04	.97	14.0	28
3.5	6.2	3.6	52	14	39	1.2	201	990	.15	.14	2.0	4
27.8	101.0	44.2	423	388	850	25.6	1,015	1,320	1.80	.95	6.9	Trace
4.0	14.4	6.3	61	55	122	3.7	145	190	.26	.14	1.0	Trace
37.4	37.5	16.6	223	464	628	7.3	1,456	22,480	.78	1.27	7.0	Trace
5.4	5.4	2.4	32	66	90	1.0	208	3,210	.11	.18	1.0	Trace
14.8	26.1	14.9	79	25	90	3.1	89	0	.47	.40	5.0	0
22.7	39.7	23.4	141	131	272	6.1	179	0	1.07	.79	9.9	0

Item No.	Food	Approximate measure	Weight, g	Water, percent	Food energy, kcal	Protein, g	Fat, g
	Pineapple:						
295	Raw, diced	1 cup	155	85	80	1	Trace
	Canned, heavy sirup pack, solids and liquid:						
296	Crushed, chunks, tidbits	1 cup	255	80	190	1	Trace
	Slices and liquid:						
297	Large	1 slice; 2¼ tbsp liquid	105	80	80	Trace	Trace
298	Medium	1 slice; 1¼ tbsp liquid	58	80	45	Trace	Trace
299	Pineapple juice, unsweetened, canned	1 cup	250	86	140	1	Trace
475	Pizza (cheese) baked, 4¾-in. sector; ⅛ of 12-in. diam. pie	1 sector	60	45	145	6	4
	Plums:						
	Raw, wthout pits:						
300	Japanese and hybrid (2⅛-in. diam., about 6½ per lb with pits)	1 plum	66	87	30	Trace	Trace
301	Prune-type (1½-in. diam., about 15 per lb with pits)	1 plum	28	79	20	Trace	Trace
	Canned, heavy sirup pack (Italian prunes), with pits and liquid:						
302	Cup	1 cup[a]	272	77	215	1	Trace
303	Portion	3 plums; 2¾ tbsp liquid[a]	140	77	110	1	Trace
	Popcorn, popped:						
476	Plain, large kernel	1 cup	6	4	25	1	Trace
477	With oil (coconut) and salt added, large kernel	1 cup	9	3	40	1	2
478	Sugar coated	1 cup	35	4	135	2	1
707	Popsicle, 3-fl oz size	1 popsicle	95	80	70	0	0
	Pork, cured, cooked:						
189	Ham, light cure, lean and fat, roasted (2 pieces, 4⅛ by 2¼ by ¼ in.)[b]	3 oz	85	54	245	18	19

[a] Weight includes pits. After removal of the pits, the weight of the edible portion is 258 g for item 302; 133 g for item 303.
[b] About one-fourth of the outer layer of fat on the cut was removed. Deposits of fat within the cut were not removed.

(Table A.3, continued)

Saturated (total), g	Unsaturated Oleic, g	Linoleic, g	Carbohydrate, g	Calcium, mg	Phosphorus, mg	Iron, mg	Potassium, mg	Vitamin A value, IU	Thiamin, mg	Riboflavin, mg	Niacin, mg	Vitamin C, mg
—	—	—	21	26	12	.8	226	110	.14	.05	.3	26
—	—	—	49	28	13	.8	245	130	.20	.05	.5	18
—	—	—	20	12	5	.3	101	50	.08	.02	.2	7
—	—	—	11	6	3	.2	56	30	.05	.01	.1	4
—	—	—	34	38	23	.8	373	130	.13	.05	.5	80
1.7	1.5	.6	22	86	89	1.1	67	230	.16	.18	1.6	4
—	—	—	8	8	12	.3	112	160	.02	.02	.3	4
—	—	—	6	3	5	.1	48	80	.01	.01	.1	1
—	—	—	56	23	26	2.3	367	3,130	.05	.05	1.0	5
—	—	—	29	12	13	1.2	189	1,610	.03	.03	.5	3
Trace	.1	.2	5	1	17	.2	—	—	—	.01	.1	0
1.5	.2	.2	5	1	19	.2	—	—	—	.01	.2	0
.5	.2	.4	30	2	47	.5	—	—	—	.02	.4	0
0	0	0	18	0	—	Trace	—	0	0	0	0	0
6.8	7.9	1.7	0	8	146	2.2	199	0	.40	.15	3.1	—

(Table A.3, continued)

Item No.	Food	Approximate measure	Weight, g	Water, percent	Food energy, kcal	Protein, g	Fat, g
	Luncheon meat:						
190	Boiled ham, slice (8 per 8-oz pkg.)	1 oz	28	59	65	5	5
	Canned, spiced or unspiced:						
191	Slice, approx. 3 by 2 by ½ in.	1 slice	60	55	175	9	15
	Pork, fresh,c cooked:						
	Chop, loin (cut 3 per lb with bone), broiled:						
192	Lean and fat	2.7 oz	78	42	305	19	25
193	Lean only from item 192	2 oz	56	53	150	17	9
	Roast, oven cooked, no liquid added:						
194	Lean and fat (piece, 2½ by 2½ by ¾ in.)	3 oz	85	46	310	21	24
195	Lean only from item 194	2.4 oz	68	55	175	20	10
	Shoulder cut, simmered:						
196	Lean and fat (3 pieces, 2½ by 2½ by ¼ in.)	3 oz	85	46	320	20	26
197	Lean only from item 196	2.2 oz.	63	60	135	18	6
	Potatoes, cooked:						
545	Baked, peeled after baking (about 2 per lb, raw)	1 potato	156	75	145	4	Trace
654	Potato chips, 1¾ by 2½ in. oval cross section	10 chips	20	2	115	1	8
655	Potato salad, made with cooked salad dressing	1 cup	250	76	250	7	7
	Pretzels, made with enriched flour:						
479	Dutch, twisted, 2¾ by 2⅝ in.	1 pretzel	16	5	60	2	1
	Boiled (about 3 per lb, raw):						
646	Peeled after boiling	1 potato	137	80	105	3	Trace
647	Peeled before boiling	1 potato	135	83	90	3	Trace
	Fresh-fried, strip, 2 to 3½ in. long:						
648	Prepared from raw	10 strips	50	45	135	2	7
649	Frozen, oven heated	10 strips	50	53	110	2	4
650	Hashed brown, prepared from frozen	1 cup	155	56	345	3	18
	Mashed, prepared from—						
	Raw:						
651	Milk added	1 cup	210	83	135	4	2
652	Milk and butter added	1 cup	210	80	195	4	9
653	Dehydrated flakes (without milk), water, milk, butter, and salt added	1 cup	210	79	195	4	7

c Outer layer of fat on the cut was removed to within approximately ½ in. of the lean. Deposits of fat within the cut were not removed.

(Table A.3, continued)

| Saturated (total), g | Fatty acids | | Carbo-hydrate, g | Cal-cium, mg | Phos-phorus, mg | Iron, mg | Potas-sium, mg | Vitamin A value, IU | Thia-min, mg | Ribo-flavin, mg | Niacin, mg | Vitamin C, mg |
| | Unsaturated | | | | | | | | | | | |
	Oleic, g	Lino-leic, g										
1.7	2.0	.4	0	3	47	.8	—	0	.12	.04	.7	—
5.4	6.7	1.0	1	5	65	1.3	133	0	.19	.13	1.8	—
8.9	10.4	2.2	0	9	209	2.7	216	0	.75	.22	4.5	—
3.1	3.6	.8	0	7	181	2.2	192	0	.63	.18	3.8	—
8.7	10.2	2.2	0	9	218	2.7	233	0	.78	.22	4.8	—
3.5	4.1	.8	0	9	211	2.6	224	0	.73	.21	4.4	—
9.3	10.9	2.3	0	9	118	2.6	158	0	.46	.21	4.1	—
2.2	2.6	.6	0	8	111	2.3	146	0	.42	.19	3.7	—
—	—	—	33	14	101	1.1	782	Trace	.15	.07	2.7	31
2.1	1.4	4.0	10	8	28	.4	226	Trace	.04	.01	1.0	3
2.0	2.7	1.3	41	80	160	1.5	798	350	.20	.18	2.8	28
—	—	—	12	4	21	.2	21	0	.05	.04	.7	0
—	—	—	23	10	72	.8	556	Trace	.12	.05	2.0	22
—	—	—	20	8	57	.7	385	Trace	.12	.05	1.6	22
1.7	1.2	3.3	18	8	56	.7	427	Trace	.07	.04	1.6	11
1.1	.8	2.1	17	5	43	.9	326	Trace	.07	.01	1.3	11
4.6	3.2	9.0	45	28	78	1.9	439	Trace	.11	.03	1.6	12
.7	.4	Trace	27	50	103	.8	548	40	.17	.11	2.1	21
5.6	2.3	.2	26	50	101	.8	525	360	.17	.11	2.1	19
3.6	2.1	.2	30	65	99	.6	601	270	.08	.08	1.9	11

(Table A.3, continued)

Item No.	Food	Approximate measure	Weight, g	Water, percent	Food energy, kcal	Protein, g	Fat, g
480	Thin, twisted, 3¼ by 2¼ by ¼ in.	10 pretzels	60	5	235	6	3
481	Stick, 2¼ in. long	10 pretzels	3	5	10	Trace	Trace
	Prunes, dried, "softenized," with pits:						
304	Uncooked	4 extra large or 5 large prunes*a*	49	28	110	1	Trace
305	Cooked, unsweetened, all sizes, fruit and liquid	1 cup*a*	250	66	255	2	1
306	Prune juice, canned or bottled	1 cup	256	80	195	1	Trace
656	Pumpkin, canned	1 cup	245	90	80	2	1
527	Pumpkin and squash kernels, dry, hulled	1 cup	140	4	775	41	65
657	Radishes, raw (prepackaged) stem ends, rootlets cut off	4 radishes	18	95	5	Trace	Trace
	Raisins, seedless:						
307	Cup, not pressed down	1 cup	145	18	420	4	Trace
308	Packet, ½ oz (1½ tbsp)	1 packet	14	18	40	Trace	Trace
	Raspberries, red:						
309	Raw, capped, whole	1 cup	123	84	70	1	1
310	Frozen, sweetened, 10-oz container	1 container	284	74	280	2	1
	Rhubarb, cooked, added sugar:						
311	From raw	1 cup	270	63	380	1	Trace
312	From frozen, sweetened	1 cup	270	63	385	1	1
	Rice, white, enriched:						
482	Instant, ready-to-serve, hot	1 cup	165	73	180	4	Trace
	Long grain:						
483	Raw	1 cup	185	12	670	12	1
484	Cooked, served hot	1 cup	205	73	225	4	Trace
	Parboiled:						
485	Raw	1 cup	185	10	685	14	1
486	Cooked, served hot	1 cup	175	73	185	4	Trace
	Puffed						
376	Plain, added iron, thiamin, niacin	1 cup	15	4	60	1	Trace
377	Presweetened, added salt, iron, vitamins	1 cup	28	3	115	1	0

a Weight includes pits. After removal of the pits, the weight of the edible portion is 43 g for item 304, and 213 g for item 305.

b Product may or may not be enriched with riboflavin. Consult the label.

c Value varies with the brand. Consult the label.

d Applies to product with added ascorbic acid. Without added ascorbic acid, value is trace.

(Table A.3, continued)

Saturated (total), g	Unsaturated Oleic, g	Linoleic, g	Carbohydrate, g	Calcium, mg	Phosphorus, mg	Iron, mg	Potassium, mg	Vitamin A value, IU	Thiamin, mg	Riboflavin, mg	Niacin, mg	Vitamin C, mg
—	—	—	46	13	79	.9	78	0	.20	.15	2.5	0
—	—	—	2	1	4	Trace	4	0	.01	.01	.1	0
—	—	—	29	22	34	1.7	298	690	.04	.07	.7	1
—	—	—	67	51	79	3.8	695	1,590	.07	.15	1.5	2
—	—	—	49	36	51	1.8	602	—	.03	.03	1.0	5
—	—	—	19	61	64	1.0	588	15,680	.07	.12	1.5	12
11.8	23.5	27.5	21	71	1,602	15.7	1,386	100	.34	.27	3.4	—
—	—	—	1	5	6	.2	58	Trace	.01	.01	.1	5
—	—	—	112	90	146	5.1	1,106	30	.16	.12	.7	1
—	—	—	11	9	14	.5	107	Trace	.02	.01	.1	Trace
—	—	—	17	27	27	1.1	207	160	.04	.11	1.1	31
—	—	—	70	37	48	1.7	284	200	.06	.17	1.7	60
—	—	—	97	211	41	1.6	548	220	.05	.14	.8	16
—	—	—	98	211	32	1.9	475	190	.05	.11	.5	16
Trace	Trace	Trace	40	5	31	1.3	—	0	.21	(b)	1.7	0
.2	.2	.2	149	44	174	5.4	170	0	.81	.06	6.5	0
.1	.1	.1	50	21	57	1.8	57	0	.23	.02	2.1	0
.2	.1	.2	150	111	370	5.4	278	0	.81	.07	6.5	0
.1	.1	.1	41	33	100	1.4	75	0	.19	.02	2.1	0
—	—	—	13	3	14	.3	15	0	.07	.01	.7	0
—	—	—	26	3	14	1.1[c]	43	1,250	.38	.43	5.0	15[d]

557

(Table A.3, continued)

Item No.	Food	Approximate measure	Weight, g	Water, percent	Food energy, kcal	Protein, g	Fat, g
	Rolls, enriched:						
	Commercial:						
487	Brown-and-serve (12 per 12-oz pkg.), browned	1 roll	26	27	85	2	2
488	Cloverleaf or pan, 2½-in. diam., 2 in. high	1 roll	28	31	85	2	2
489	Frankfurter and hamburger (8 per 11½-oz pkg.)	1 roll	40	31	120	3	2
490	Hard, 3¾-in. diam., 2 in. high	1 roll	50	25	155	5	2
491	Hoagie or submarine, 11½ by 3 by 2½ in.	1 roll	135	31	390	12	4
	From home recipe:						
492	Cloverleaf, 2½-in. diam., 2 in. high	1 roll	35	26	120	3	3
696	Root beer	12 fl oz	370	90	150	0	0
	Salad dressings:						
	Commercial:						
	Blue cheese:						
132	Regular	1 tbsp	15	32	75	1	8
133	Low calorie (5 Cal per tsp)	1 tbsp	16	84	10	Trace	1
	French:						
134	Regular	1 tbsp	16	39	65	Trace	6
135	Low calorie (5 Cal per tsp)	1 tbsp	16	77	15	Trace	1
	Italian:						
136	Regular	1 tbsp	15	28	85	Trace	9
137	Low calorie (2 Cal per tsp)	1 tbsp	15	90	10	Trace	1
138	Mayonnaise	1 tbsp	14	15	100	Trace	11
	Mayonnaise type:						
139	Regular	1 tbsp	15	41	65	Trace	6
140	Low calorie (8 Cal per tsp)	1 tbsp	16	81	20	Trace	2
141	Tartar sauce, regular	1 tbsp	14	34	75	Trace	8
	Thousand Island:						
142	Regular	1 tbsp	16	32	80	Trace	8
143	Low calorie (10 Cal per tsp)	1 tbsp	15	68	25	Trace	2
	From home recipe:						
144	Cooked type[a]	1 tbsp	16	68	25	1	2
153	Salmon, pink, canned, solids and liquid	3 oz	85	71	120	17	5
154	Sardines, Atlantic, canned in oil, drained solids:	3 oz	85	62	175	20	9
658	Sauerkraut, canned, solids and liquid	1 cup	235	93	40	2	Trace

[a] Fatty acid values apply to product made with regular-type margarine.

(Table A.3, continued)

Saturated (total), g	Fatty acids Unsaturated Oleic, g	Lino-leic, g	Carbo-hydrate, g	Cal-cium, mg	Phos-phorus, mg	Iron, mg	Potas-sium, mg	Vitamin A value, IU	Thia-min, mg	Ribo-flavin, mg	Niacin, mg	Vitamin C, mg
.4	.7	.5	14	20	23	.5	25	Trace	.10	.06	.9	Trace
.4	.6	.4	15	21	24	.5	27	Trace	.11	.07	.9	Trace
.5	.8	.6	21	30	34	.8	38	Trace	.16	.10	1.3	Trace
.4	.6	.5	30	24	46	1.2	49	Trace	.20	.12	1.7	Trace
.9	1.4	1.4	75	58	115	3.0	122	Trace	.54	.32	4.5	Trace
.8	1.1	.7	20	16	36	.7	41	30	.12	.12	1.2	Trace
0	0	0	39	—	—	—	0	0	0	0	0	0
1.6	1.7	3.8	1	12	11	Trace	6	30	Trace	.02	Trace	Trace
.5	.3	Trace	1	10	8	Trace	5	30	Trace	.01	Trace	Trace
1.1	1.3	3.2	3	2	2	.1	13	—	—	—	—	—
.1	.1	.4	2	2	2	.1	13	—	—	—	—	—
1.6	1.9	4.7	1	2	1	Trace	2	Trace	Trace	Trace	Trace	—
.1	.1	.4	Trace	Trace	1	Trace	2	Trace	Trace	Trace	Trace	—
2.0	2.4	5.6	Trace	3	4	.1	5	40	Trace	.01	Trace	—
1.1	1.4	3.2	2	2	4	Trace	1	30	Trace	Trace	Trace	—
.4	.4	1.0	2	3	4	Trace	1	40	Trace	Trace	Trace	—
1.5	1.8	4.1	1	3	4	.1	11	30	Trace	Trace	Trace	Trace
1.4	1.7	4.0	2	2	3	.1	18	50	Trace	Trace	Trace	Trace
.4	.4	1.0	2	2	3	.1	17	50	Trace	Trace	Trace	Trace
.5	.6	.3	2	14	15	.1	19	80	.01	.03	Trace	Trace
.9	.8	.1	0	167	243	.7	307	60	.03	.16	6.8	—
3.0	2.5	.5	0	372	424	2.5	502	190	.02	.17	4.6	—
—	—	—	9	85	42	1.2	329	120	.07	.09	.5	33

559

(Table A.3, continued)

Item No.	Food	Approximate measure	Weight, g	Water, percent	Food energy, kcal	Protein, g	Fat, g
	Sausages (see also Luncheon meat (items 190-191):						
198	Bologna, slice (8 per 8-oz pkg.)	1 slice	28	56	85	3	8
199	Braunschweiger, slice (6 per 6-oz pkg.)	1 slice	28	53	90	4	8
200	Brown and serve (10-11 per 8-oz pkg.), browned	1 link	17	40	70	3	6
201	Deviled ham, canned	1 tbsp	13	51	45	2	4
202	Frankfurter (8 per 1-lb pkg.), cooked (reheated)	1 frankfurter	56	57	170	7	15
203	Meat, potted (beef, chicken, turkey), canned	1 tbsp	13	61	30	2	2
204	Pork link (16 per 1-lb pkg.), cooked	1 link	13	35	60	2	6
	Salami:						
205	Dry type, slice (12 per 4-oz pkg.)	1 slice	10	30	45	2	4
206	Cooked type, slice (8 per 8-oz pkg.)	1 slice	28	51	90	5	7
207	Vienna sausage (7 per 4-oz can)	1 sausage	16	63	40	2	3
155	Scallops, frozen, breaded, fried, reheated	6 scallops	90	60	175	16	8
156	Shad, baked with butter or margarine, bacon	3 oz	85	64	170	20	10
84	Sherbet (about 2% fat)	½ gal	1,542	66	2,160	17	31
85		1 cup	193	66	270	2	4
	Shrimp:						
157	Canned meat	3 oz	85	70	100	21	1
158	French fried[b]	3 oz	85	57	190	17	9
	Sirups:						
	Chocolate-flavored sirup or topping:						
553	Thin type	1 fl oz or 2 tbsp	38	32	90	1	1
554	Fudge type	1 fl oz or 2 tbsp	38	25	125	2	5
	Molasses, cane:						
555	Light (first extraction)	1 tbsp	20	24	50	—	—
556	Blackstrap (third extraction)	1 tbsp	20	24	45	—	—
557	Sorghum	1 tbsp	21	23	55	—	—
558	Table blends, chiefly corn, light and dark	1 tbsp	21	24	60	0	0
	Soups:						
	Canned, condensed:						
	Prepared with equal volume of milk:						
708	Cream of chicken	1 cup	245	85	180	7	10
709	Cream of mushroom	1 cup	245	83	215	7	14
710	Tomato	1 cup	250	84	175	7	7

[b] Dipped in egg, breadcrumbs and flour or batter.

(Table A.3, continued)

Satu-rated (total), g	Oleic, g	Lino-leic, g	Carbo-hydrate, g	Cal-cium, mg	Phos-phorus, mg	Iron, mg	Potas-sium, mg	Vitamin A value, IU	Thia-min, mg	Ribo-flavin, mg	Niacin, mg	Vitamin C, mg
	Fatty acids Unsaturated											
3.0	3.4	.5	Trace	2	36	.5	65	—	.05	.06	.7	—
2.6	3.4	.8	1	3	69	1.7	—	1,850	.05	.41	2.3	—
2.3	2.8	.7	Trace	—	—	—	—	—	—	—	—	—
1.5	1.8	.4	0	1	12	.3	—	0	.02	.01	.2	—
5.6	6.5	1.2	1	3	57	.8	—	—	.08	.11	1.4	—
—	—	—	0	—	—	—	—	—	Trace	.03	.2	—
2.1	2.4	.5	Trace	1	21	.3	35	0	.10	.04	.5	—
1.6	1.6	.1	Trace	1	28	.4	—	—	.04	.03	.5	—
3.1	3.0	.2	Trace	3	57	.7	—	—	.07	.07	1.2	—
1.2	1.4	.2	Trace	1	24	.3	—	—	.01	.02	.4	—
—	—	—	9	—	—	—	—	—	—	—	—	—
—	—	—	0	20	266	.5	320	30	.11	.22	7.3	—
19.0	7.7	.7	469	827	594	2.5	1,585	1,480	.26	.71	1.0	31
2.4	1.0	.1	59	103	74	.3	198	190	.03	.09	.1	4
.1	.1	Trace	1	98	224	2.6	104	50	.01	.03	1.5	—
2.3	3.7	2.0	9	61	162	1.7	195	—	.03	.07	2.3	—
.5	.3	Trace	24	6	35	.6	106	Trace	.01	.03	.2	0
3.1	1.6	.1	20	48	60	.5	107	60	.02	.08	.2	Trace
—	—	—	13	33	9	.9	183	—	.01	.01	Trace	—
—	—	—	11	137	17	3.2	585	—	.02	.04	.4	—
—	—	—	14	35	5	2.6	—	—	—	.02	Trace	—
0	0	0	15	9	3	.8	1	0	0	0	0	0
4.2	3.6	1.3	15	172	152	.5	260	610	.05	.27	0.7	2
5.4	2.9	4.6	16	191	169	.5	279	250	.05	.34	.7	1
3.4	1.7	1.0	23	168	155	.8	418	1,200	.10	.25	1.3	15

(Table A.3, continued)

Item No.	Food	Approximate measure	Weight, g	Water, percent	Food energy, kcal	Protein, g	Fat, g
	Prepared with equal volume of water:						
711	Bean with pork	1 cup	250	84	170	8	6
712	Beef broth, bouillon, consomme	1 cup	240	96	30	5	0
713	Beef noodle	1 cup	240	93	65	4	3
714	Clam chowder, Manhattan type (with tomatoes, without milk)	1 cup	245	92	80	2	3
715	Cream of chicken	1 cup	240	92	95	3	6
716	Cream of mushroom	1 cup	240	90	135	2	10
717	Minestrone	1 cup	245	90	105	5	3
718	Split pea	1 cup	245	85	145	9	3
719	Tomato	1 cup	245	91	90	2	3
720	Vegetable beef	1 cup	245	92	80	5	2
721	Vegetarian	1 cup	245	92	80	2	2
	Dehydrated:						
722	Bouillon cube, ½ in.	1 cube	4	4	5	1	Trace
	Mixes:						
	Unprepared:						
723	Onion	1½-oz pkg	43	3	150	6	5
	Prepared with water:						
724	Chicken noodle	1 cup	240	95	55	2	1
725	Onion	1 cup	240	96	35	1	1
726	Tomato vegetable with noodles	1 cup	240	93	65	1	1
	Spaghetti, enriched, cooked:						
493	Firm stage, "al dente," served hot	1 cup	130	64	190	7	1
494	Tender stage, served hot	1 cup	140	73	155	5	1
	Spaghetti (enriched) in tomato sauce with cheese:						
495	From home recipe	1 cup	250	77	260	9	9
496	Canned	1 cup	250	80	190	6	2
	Spaghetti (enriched) with meat balls and tomato sauce:						
497	From home recipe	1 cup	248	70	330	19	12
498	Canned	1 cup	250	78	260	12	10
	Spinach:						
659	Raw, chopped	1 cup	55	91	15	2	Trace
	Cooked, drained:						
660	From raw	1 cup	180	92	40	5	1
	From frozen:						
661	Chopped	1 cup	205	92	45	6	1

(Table A.3, continued)

Saturated (total), g	Unsaturated Oleic, g	Linoleic, g	Carbohydrate, g	Calcium, mg	Phosphorus, mg	Iron, mg	Potassium, mg	Vitamin A value, IU	Thiamin, mg	Riboflavin, mg	Niacin, mg	Vitamin C, mg
1.2	1.8	2.4	22	63	128	2.3	395	650	.13	.08	1.0	3
0	0	0	3	Trace	31	.5	130	Trace	Trace	.02	1.2	—
.6	.7	.8	7	7	48	1.0	77	50	.05	.07	1.0	Trace
.5	.4	1.3	12	34	47	1.0	184	880	.02	.02	1.0	—
1.6	2.3	1.1	8	24	34	.5	79	410	.02	.05	.5	Trace
2.6	1.7	4.5	10	41	50	.5	98	70	.02	.12	.7	Trace
.7	.9	1.3	14	37	59	1.0	314	2,350	.07	.05	1.0	—
1.1	1.2	.4	21	29	149	1.5	270	440	.25	.15	1.5	1
.5	.5	1.0	16	15	34	.7	230	1,000	.05	.05	1.2	12
—	—	—	10	12	49	.7	162	2,700	.05	.05	1.0	—
—	—	—	13	20	39	1.0	172	2,940	.05	.05	1.0	—
—	—	—	Trace	—	—	—	4	—	—	—	—	—
1.1	2.3	1.0	23	42	49	.6	238	30	.05	.03	.3	6
—	—	—	8	7	19	.2	19	50	.07	.05	.5	Trace
—	—	—	6	10	12	.2	58	Trace	Trace	Trace	Trace	2
—	—	—	12	7	19	.2	29	480	.05	.02	.5	5
—	—	—	39	14	85	1.4	103	0	.23	.13	1.8	0
—	—	—	32	11	70	1.3	85	0	.20	.11	1.5	0
2.0	5.4	.7	37	80	135	2.3	408	1,080	.25	.18	2.3	13
.5	.3	.4	39	40	88	2.8	303	930	.35	.28	4.5	10
3.3	6.3	.9	39	124	236	3.7	665	1,590	.25	.30	4.0	22
2.2	3.3	3.9	29	53	113	3.3	245	1,000	.15	.18	2.3	5
—	—	—	2	51	28	1.7	259	4,460	.06	.11	.3	28
—	—	—	6	167	68	4.0	583	14,580	.13	.25	.9	50
—	—	—	8	232	90	4.3	683	16,200	.14	.31	.8	39

(Table A.3, continued)

Item No.	Food	Approximate measure	Weight, g	Water, percent	Food energy, kcal	Protein, g	Fat, g
662	Leaf	1 cup	190	92	45	6	1
663	Canned, drained solids	1 cup	205	91	50	6	1
	Squash, cooked:						
664	Summer (all varieties), diced, drained	1 cup	210	96	30	2	Trace
665	Winter (all varieties), baked, mashed	1 cup	205	81	130	4	1
	Strawberries:						
313	Raw, whole berries, capped	1 cup	149	90	55	1	1
	Frozen, sweetened:						
314	Sliced, 10-oz container	1 container	284	71	310	1	1
315	Whole, 1-lb container (about 1¾ cups)	1 container	454	76	415	2	1
	Sugars:						
559	Brown, pressed down	1 cup	220	2	820	0	0
	White:						
560	Granulated	1 cup	200	1	770	0	0
561		1 tbsp	12	1	45	0	0
562		1 packet	6	1	23	0	0
563	Powdered, sifted, spooned into cup	1 cup	100	1	385	0	0
528	Sunflower seeds, dry, hulled	1 cup	145	5	810	35	69
	Sweetpotatoes:						
	Cooked (raw, 5 by 2 in.; about 2½ per lb):						
666	Baked in skin, peeled	1 potato	114	64	160	2	1
667	Boiled in skin, peeled	1 potato	151	71	170	3	1
668	Candied, 2½ by 2-in. piece	1 piece	105	60	175	1	3
	Canned:						
669	Solid pack (mashed)	1 cup	255	72	275	5	1
670	Vacuum pack, piece 2¾ by 1 in.	1 piece	40	72	45	1	Trace
316	Tangerine, raw, 2⅜-in. diam., size 176, without peel (about 4 per lb with peels and seeds)	1 tangerine	86	87	40	1	Trace
317	Tangerine juice, canned, sweetened	1 cup	249	87	125	1	Trace
499	Toaster pastries	1 pastry	50	12	200	3	6
	Tomatoes:						
671	Raw, 2⅗-in. diam. (3 per 12 oz pkg.)	1 tomato[a]	135	94	25	1	Trace
672	Canned, solids and liquid	1 cup	241	94	50	2	Trace
673	Tomato catsup	1 cup	273	69	290	5	1
674		1 tbsp	15	69	15	Trace	Trace

[a] Weight includes cores and stem ends. Without these parts, weight is 123 g.
[b] Value varies with the brand. Consult the label.

(Table A.3, continued)

Saturated (total), g	Fatty acids — Unsaturated Oleic, g	Linoleic, g	Carbohydrate, g	Calcium, mg	Phosphorus, mg	Iron, mg	Potassium, mg	Vitamin A value, IU	Thiamin, mg	Riboflavin, mg	Niacin, mg	Vitamin C, mg
—	—	—	7	200	84	4.8	688	15,390	.15	.27	1.0	53
—	—	—	7	242	53	5.3	513	16,400	.04	.25	.6	29
—	—	—	7	53	53	.8	296	820	.11	.17	1.7	21
—	—	—	32	57	98	1.6	945	8,610	.10	.27	1.4	27
—	—	—	13	31	31	1.5	244	90	.04	.10	.9	88
—	—	—	79	40	48	2.0	318	90	.06	.17	1.4	151
—	—	—	107	59	73	2.7	472	140	.09	.27	2.3	249
0	0	0	212	187	42	7.5	757	0	.02	.07	.4	0
0	0	0	199	0	0	.2	6	0	0	0	0	0
0	0	0	12	0	0	Trace	Trace	0	0	0	0	0
0	0	0	6	0	0	Trace	Trace	0	0	0	0	0
0	0	0	100	0	0	.1	3	0	0	0	0	0
8.2	13.7	43.2	29	174	1,214	10.3	1,334	70	2.84	.33	7.8	—
—	—	—	37	46	66	1.0	342	9,230	.10	.08	.8	25
—	—	—	40	48	71	1.1	367	11,940	.14	.09	.9	26
2.0	.8	.1	36	39	45	.9	200	6,620	.06	.04	.4	11
—	—	—	63	64	105	2.0	510	19,890	.13	.10	1.5	36
—	—	—	10	10	16	.3	80	3,120	.02	.02	.2	6
—	—	—	10	34	15	.3	108	360	.05	.02	.1	27
—	—	—	30	44	35	.5	440	1,040	.15	.05	.2	54
—	—	—	36	54[b]	67[b]	1.9	74	500	.16	.17	2.1	(b)
—	—	—	6	16	33	.6	300	1,110	.07	.05	.9	28
—	—	—	10	14[c]	46	1.2	523	2,170	.12	.07	1.7	41
—	—	—	69	60	137	2.2	991	3,820	.25	.19	4.4	41
—	—	—	4	3	8	.1	54	210	.01	.01	.2	2

[c] Applies to product without calcium salts added. Value for products with calcium salts added may be as much as 63 mg for whole tomatoes, 241 mg for cut forms.

565

(Table A.3, continued)

Item No.	Food	Approximate measure	Weight, g	Water, percent	Food energy, kcal	Protein, g	Fat, g
	Tomato juice, canned:						
675	Cup	1 cup	243	94	45	2	Trace
676	Glass (6 fl oz)	1 glass	182	94	35	2	Trace
159	Tuna, canned in oil, drained solids	3 oz	85	61	170	24	7
	Turkey, roasted, flesh without skin:						
219	Dark meat, piece, 2½ by 1⅝ by ¼ in.	4 pieces	85	61	175	26	7
220	Light meat, piece, 4 by 2 by ¼ in.	2 pieces	85	62	150	28	3
	Light and dark meat:						
221	Chopped or diced	1 cup	140	61	265	44	9
222	Pieces (1 slice white meat, 4 by 2 by ¼ in. with 2 slices dark meat, 2½ by 1⅝ by ¼ in.)	3 pieces	85	61	160	27	5
677	Turnips, cooked, diced	1 cup	155	94	35	1	Trace
	Turnip greens, cooked, drained:						
678	From raw (leaves and stems)	1 cup	145	94	30	3	Trace
679	From frozen (chopped)	1 cup	165	93	40	4	Trace
	Veal, medium fat, cooked, bone removed:						
208	Cutlet (4⅛ by 2¼ by ½ in.), braised or broiled	3 oz	85	60	185	23	9
209	Rib (2 pieces, 4⅛ by 2¼ by ¼ in.), roasted	3 oz	85	55	230	23	14
680	Vegetables, mixed, frozen, cooked	1 cup	182	83	115	6	1
727	Vinegar, cider	1 tbsp	15	94	Trace	Trace	0
	Waffles, made with enriched flour, 7-in. diam.:						
500	From home recipe	1 waffle	75	41	210	7	7
501	From mix, egg and milk added	1 waffle	75	42	205	7	8
	Walnuts:						
	Black:						
529	Chopped or broken kernels	1 cup	125	3	785	26	74
530	Ground (finely)	1 cup	80	3	500	16	47
531	Persian or English, chopped (about 60 halves)	1 cup	120	4	780	18	77
318	Watermelon, raw, 4 by 8 in. wedge with rind and seeds (1/16 of 32⅔-lb melon, 10 by 16 in.)	1 wedge with rind and seeds	926	93	110	2	1
378	Wheat flakes, added sugar, salt, iron, vitamins	1 cup	30	4	105	3	Trace
	Wheat, puffed:						
379	Plain, added iron, thiamin, niacin	1 cup	15	3	55	2	Trace
380	Presweetened, added salt, iron, vitamins	1 cup	38	3	140	3	Trace

ᵃ Value varies with the brand. Consult the label.

(Table A.3, continued)

Saturated (total), g	Oleic, g	Linoleic, g	Carbohydrate, g	Calcium, mg	Phosphorus, mg	Iron, mg	Potassium, mg	Vitamin A value, IU	Thiamin, mg	Riboflavin, mg	Niacin, mg	Vitamin C, mg
—	—	—	10	17	44	2.2	552	1,940	.12	.07	1.9	39
—	—	—	8	13	33	1.6	413	1,460	.09	.05	1.5	29
1.7	1.7	.7	0	7	199	1.6	—	70	.04	.10	10.1	—
2.1	1.5	1.5	0	—	—	2.0	338	—	.03	.20	3.6	—
.9	.6	.7	0	—	—	1.0	349	—	.04	.12	9.4	—
2.5	1.7	1.8	0	11	351	2.5	514	—	.07	.25	10.8	—
1.5	1.0	1.1	0	7	213	1.5	312	—	.04	.15	6.5	—
—	—	—	8	54	37	.6	291	Trace	.06	.08	.5	34
—	—	—	5	252	49	1.5	—	8,270	.15	.33	.7	68
—	—	—	6	195	64	2.6	246	11,390	.08	.15	.7	31
4.0	3.4	.4	0	9	196	2.7	258	—	.06	.21	4.6	—
6.1	5.1	.6	0	10	211	2.9	259	—	.11	.26	6.6	—
—	—	—	24	46	115	2.4	348	9,010	.22	.13	2.0	15
0	0	0	1	1	1	.1	15	—	—	—	—	—
2.3	2.8	1.4	28	85	130	1.3	109	250	.17	.23	1.4	Trace
2.8	2.9	1.2	27	179	257	1.0	146	170	.14	.22	.9	Trace
6.3	13.3	45.7	19	Trace	713	7.5	575	380	.28	.14	.9	—
4.0	8.5	29.2	12	Trace	456	4.8	368	240	.18	.09	.6	—
8.4	11.8	42.2	19	119	456	3.7	540	40	.40	.16	1.1	2
—	—	—	27	30	43	2.1	426	2,510	.13	.13	.9	30
—	—	—	24	12	83	(a)	81	1,410	.35	.42	3.5	11
—	—	—	12	4	48	.6	51	0	.08	.03	1.2	0
—	—	—	33	7	52	1.6[a]	63	1,680	.50	.57	6.7	20

Item No.	Food	Approximate measure	Weight, g	Water, percent	Food energy, kcal	Protein, g	Fat, g
381	Wheat, shredded, plain	1 oblong biscuit or ½ cup spoon-size biscuits	25	7	90	2	1
382	Wheat germ, without salt and sugar, toasted	1 tbsp	6	4	25	2	1
	Wheat flours:						
	All-purpose or family flour, enriched:						
502	Sifted, spooned	1 cup	115	12	420	12	1
503	Unsifted, spooned	1 cup	125	12	455	13	1
504	Cake or pastry flour, enriched, sifted, spooned	1 cup	96	12	350	7	1
505	Self-rising, enriched, unsifted, spooned	1 cup	125	12	440	12	1
506	Whole-wheat, from hard wheats, stirred	1 cup	120	12	400	16	2
728	White sauce, medium, with enriched flour	1 cup	250	73	405	10	31
	Wines:						
690	Dessert	3½-fl oz glass	103	77	140	Trace	0
691	Table	3½-fl oz glass	102	86	85	Trace	0
	Yeast:						
729	Baker's, dry, active	1 pkg	7	5	20	3	Trace
730	Brewer's, dry	1 tbsp	8	5	25	3	Trace
	Yogurt:						
	With added milk solids:						
	Made with lowfat milk:						
92	Fruit-flavored^c	1 container, net wt., 8 oz	227	75	230	10	3
93	Plain	1 container, net wt., 8 oz	227	85	145	12	4
94	Made with nonfat milk	1 container, net wt., 8 oz	227	85	125	13	Trace
	Without added milk solids:						
95	Made with whole milk	1 container, net wt., 8 oz	227	88	140	8	7

[b] Value may vary from 6 to 60 mg.
[c] Content of fat, vitamin A, and carbohydrate varies. Consult the label when precise values are needed for special diets.
[d] Applies to product made with milk containing no added vitamin A.

(Table A.3, continued)

| Fatty acids | | | | | | | | | | | | |
| Satu-rated (total), g | Unsaturated | | Carbo-hydrate, g | Cal-cium, mg | Phos-phorus, mg | Iron, mg | Potas-sium, mg | Vitamin A value, IU | Thia-min, mg | Ribo-flavin, mg | Niacin, mg | Vitamin C, mg |
	Oleic, g	Lino-leic, g										
—	—	—	20	11	97	.9	87	0	.06	.03	1.1	0
—	—	—	3	3	70	.5	57	10	.11	.05	.3	1
.2	.1	.5	88	18	100	3.3	109	0	.74	.46	6.1	0
.2	.1	.5	95	20	109	3.6	119	0	.80	.50	6.6	0
.1	.1	.3	76	16	70	2.8	91	0	.61	.38	5.1	0
.2	.1	.5	93	331	583	3.6	—	0	.80	.50	6.6	0
.4	.2	1.0	85	49	446	4.0	444	0	.66	.14	5.2	0
19.3	7.8	.8	22	288	233	.5	348	1,150	.12	.43	.7	2
0	0	0	8	8	—	—	77	—	.01	.02	.2	—
0	0	0	4	9	10	.4	94	—	Trace	.01	.1	—
—	—	—	3	3	90	1.1	140	Trace	.16	.38	2.6	Trace
—	—	—	3	17[b]	140	1.4	152	Trace	1.25	.34	3.0	Trace
1.8	.6	.1	42	343	269	.2	439	120[d]	.08	.40	.2	1
2.3	.8	.1	16	415	326	.2	531	150[d]	.10	.49	.3	2
.3	.1	Trace	17	452	355	.2	579	20[d]	.11	.53	.3	2
4.8	1.7	.1	11	274	215	.1	351	280	.07	.32	.2	1

Table A.4 Thrifty Food Plan, Revised 1974–1975

Family member	Milk, cheese, ice cream,[b] qt	Meat, poultry, fish,[c] lb	Eggs, no	Dry beans and peas, nuts,[d] lb	Dark-green, deep-yellow vegetables, lb	Citrus fruit, tomatoes, lb	Potatoes, lb	Other vegetables, fruit, lb	Cereal, lb	Flour, lb	Bread, lb	Other bakery products, lb	Fats, oils, lb	Sugar, sweets, lb
Child:														
7 months to 1 year	5.0	0.39	1.2	0.15	0.41	0.55	0.09	2.49	1.02[e]	0.02	0.08	0.04	0.04	0.19
1–2 years	3.3	.83	3.3	.17	.22	.89	.65	2.26	1.02[e]	.31	.78	.24	.11	.30
3–5 years	3.5	.95	2.5	.28	.20	.92	.88	2.28	1.03	.37	.94	.53	.38	.74
6–8 years	4.2	1.27	2.4	.49	.22	1.10	1.23	2.50	1.12	.62	1.42	.79	.51	.94
9–11 years	4.9	1.61	3.4	.53	.28	1.52	1.48	3.38	1.34	.81	1.82	1.10	.60	1.20
Male:														
12–14 years	5.2	1.79	3.6	.67	.33	1.45	1.59	3.30	1.22	.81	2.07	1.13	.77	1.21
15–19 years	5.1	2.35	4.0	.43	.32	1.70	2.10	3.43	.98	.99	2.36	1.46	1.00	1.05
20–54 years	2.6	3.03	4.0	.44	.39	1.80	2.02	3.69	.89	.92	2.29	1.33	.95	.86
55 years and over	2.4	2.45	4.0	.25	.51	1.85	1.75	3.77	1.09	.80	1.90	1.12	.79	.94
Female:														
12–19 years	5.4	1.80	3.8	.28	.42	1.74	1.22	3.61	.72	.76	1.49	.84	.51	.74
20–54 years	2.8	2.41	4.0	.27	.52	1.86	1.51	3.39	.90	.67	1.41	.67	.57	.57
55 years and over	2.8	1.84	4.0	.19	.60	2.02	1.26	3.73	1.12	.68	1.30	.58	.37	.45
Pregnant	[f]5.2	2.69	4.0	.42	.56	2.17	1.89	4.03	1.13	.58	1.41	.66	.59	.58
Nursing	[f]5.2	3.00	4.0	.38	.57	2.36	1.92	4.27	.98	.63	1.56	.82	.80	.75

[a] Amounts are for food as purchased or brought into the kitchen from garden or farm. Amounts allow for a discard of about 5 percent of the edible food as plate waste, spoilage, etc. For general use, round the total amount of food groups for the family to the nearest tenth or quarter of a pound. In addition to groups shown, most families use some other foods: coffee, tea, cocoa, soft drinks, punches, ades, leavening agents, and seasonings.

[b] Fluid milk and beverage made from dry or evaporated milk. Cheese and ice cream may replace some milk. Count as equivalent to a quart of fluid milk: natural or processed Cheddar-type cheese, 6 ounces; cottage cheese, 2½ pounds; ice cream or ice milk, 1½ quarts; unflavored yogurt, 4 cups.

[c] Bacon and salt pork should not exceed ⅓ pound for each 5 pounds of this group.

[d] Weight in terms of dry beans and peas, shelled nuts, and peanut butter. Count 1 pound of canned dry beans, such as pork and beans or kidney beans, as .33 pound.

[e] Cereal fortified with iron is recommended.

[f] For pregnant and nursing teenagers, 7 quarts is recommended.

From B. Peterkin, *Family Food Budgeting, Home and Garden Bull. No. 94* (Washington, D.C.: Agr. Res. Service, U.S. Dept. Agr, 1976), p. 7.

Table A.5 Low-Cost Food Plan, Revised 1974–1975

Amounts of food for a week[a]

Family member	Milk, cheese, ice cream,[b] qt	Meat, poultry, fish,[c] lb	Eggs, no	Dry beans and peas, nuts,[d] lb	Dark-green, deep-yellow vegetables, lb	Citrus fruit, tomatoes, lb	Potatoes, lb	Other vegetables, fruit, lb	Cereal, Flour, lb	Bread, lb	Other bakery products, lb	Fats, oils, lb	Sugar, sweets, lb
Child:													
7 months to 1 year	5.7	0.56	2.1	0.15	0.35	0.42	0.06	3.43	[e]0.71	0.02	0.06	0.05	0.05	0.18
1–2 years	3.6	1.26	3.6	.16	.23	1.01	.60	2.88	[e].99	.27	.76	.33	.12	.36
3–5 years	3.9	1.52	2.7	.25	.25	1.20	.85	2.95	.90	.30	.91	.57	.38	.71
6–8 years	4.7	2.03	2.9	.39	.31	1.58	1.10	3.67	1.11	.45	1.27	.84	.52	.90
9–11 years	5.5	2.57	3.9	.44	.38	2.13	1.41	4.81	1.24	.62	1.65	1.20	.61	1.15
Male:													
12–14 years	5.7	2.98	4.0	.56	.40	1.99	1.50	3.90	1.15	.67	1.88	1.25	.77	1.15
15–19 years	5.5	3.74	4.0	.34	.39	2.20	1.87	4.50	.90	.75	2.10	1.55	1.05	1.04
20–54 years	2.7	4.56	4.0	.33	.48	2.32	1.87	4.81	.93	.71	2.10	1.47	.91	.81
55 years and over	2.6	3.63	4.0	.21	.61	2.38	1.72	4.92	1.02	.62	1.73	1.23	.77	.90
Female:													
12–19 years	5.6	2.55	4.0	.24	.46	2.17	1.17	4.57	.75	.63	1.44	1.05	.53	.88
20–54 years	3.0	3.21	4.0	.19	.55	2.34	1.40	4.17	.71	.55	1.31	.94	.59	.72
55 years and over	3.0	2.45	4.0	.15	.62	2.54	1.22	4.57	.97	.58	1.24	.86	.38	.64
Pregnant	[f]5.2	3.68	4.0	.29	.67	2.80	1.65	4.99	.95	.66	1.52	1.06	.55	.78
Nursing	[f]5.2	4.16	4.0	.26	.66	2.99	1.67	5.33	.78	.61	1.55	1.16	.76	.91

[a] Amounts are for food as purchased or brought into the kitchen from garden or farm. Amounts allow for a discard of about 5 percent of the edible food as plate waste, spoilage, etc. For general use, round the total amount of food groups for the family to the nearest tenth or quarter of a pound. In addition to groups shown, most families use some other foods: coffee, tea, cocoa, soft drinks, punches, ades, leavening agents, and seasonings.

[b] Fluid milk and beverage made from dry or evaporated milk. Cheese and ice cream may replace some milk. Count as equivalent to a quart of fluid milk: natural or processed Cheddar-type cheese, 6 ounces; cottage cheese, 2½ pounds; ice cream or ice milk, 1½ quarts; unflavored yogurt, 4 cups.

[c] Bacon and salt pork should not exceed ⅓ pound for each 5 pounds of this group.

[d] Weight in terms of dry beans and peas, shelled nuts, and peanut butter. Count 1 pound of canned dry beans, such as pork and beans or kidney beans, as .33 pound.

[e] Cereal fortified with iron is recommended.

[f] For pregnant and nursing teenagers, 7 quarts is recommended.

From B. Peterkin, Family Food Budgeting, Home and Garden Bull. No. 94 (Washington, D.C.: Agr. Res. Service, U.S. Dept. Agr, 1976), p. 7.

Table A.6 Moderate-Cost Food Plan, Revised 1974–1975

Family member	Milk, cheese, ice cream,[b] qt	Meat, poultry, fish,[c] lb	Eggs, no	Dry beans and peas, nuts,[d] lb	Dark-green, deep-yellow vege-tables, lb	Citrus fruit, to-matoes, lb	Po-tatoes, lb	Other vege-tables, fruit, lb	Cereal, lb	Flour, lb	Bread, lb	Other bakery prod-ucts, lb	Fats, oils, lb	Sugar, sweets, lb
Child:														
7 months to 1 year	6.5	0.80	2.2	0.13	0.41	0.49	0.06	3.98	[e]0.64	0.02	0.06	0.05	0.05	0.19
1–2 years	4.0	1.69	4.0	.15	.29	1.24	.59	3.44	[e]1.03	.26	.81	.33	.12	.28
3–5 years	4.7	1.88	3.0	.22	.30	1.46	.85	3.51	.74	.27	.82	.73	.41	.81
6–8 years	5.8	2.60	3.3	.34	.37	1.94	1.17	4.39	.84	.39	1.14	1.11	.56	1.03
9–11 years	6.7	3.31	4.0	.38	.45	2.61	1.40	5.76	1.03	.51	1.47	1.51	.66	1.31
Male:														
12–14 years	7.0	3.77	4.0	.48	.48	2.44	1.52	4.66	.94	.56	1.69	1.54	.85	1.34
15–19 years	6.6	4.65	4.0	.29	.47	2.73	2.00	5.45	.80	.67	1.98	1.82	1.05	1.15
20–54 years	3.4	5.73	4.0	.29	.59	2.92	1.94	5.93	.76	.65	1.97	1.65	.95	.96
55 years and over	3.0	4.64	4.0	.19	.70	2.91	1.69	5.88	.89	.53	1.58	1.45	.87	1.05
Female:														
12–19 years	6.2	3.32	4.0	.24	.53	2.62	1.21	5.38	.68	.56	1.34	1.22	.56	.97
20–54 years	3.4	4.12	4.0	.19	.62	2.84	1.35	4.94	.54	.49	1.28	1.08	.65	.81
55 years and over	3.4	3.21	4.0	.14	.72	3.09	1.17	5.50	.81	.52	1.20	.98	.45	.73
Pregnant	[f]5.4	4.57	4.0	.25	.91	3.52	1.60	6.13	.73	.83	1.77	1.28	.46	.85
Nursing	[f]5.3	5.01	4.0	.26	.91	3.76	1.73	6.52	.74	.81	1.84	1.42	.69	1.00

[a] Amounts are for food as purchased or brought into the kitchen from garden or farm. Amounts allow for a discard of about 5 percent of the edible food as plate waste, spoilage, etc. For general use, round the total amount of food groups for the family to the nearest tenth or quarter of a pound. In addition to groups shown, most families use some other foods: coffee, tea, cocoa, soft drinks, punches, ades, leavening agents, and seasonings.

[b] Fluid milk and beverage made from dry or evaporated milk. Cheese and ice cream may replace some milk. Count as equivalent to a quart of fluid milk: natural or processed Cheddar-type cheese, 6 ounces; cottage cheese, 2½ pounds; ice cream or ice milk, 1½ quarts; unflavored yogurt, 4 cups.

[c] Bacon and salt pork should not exceed ⅓ pound for each 5 pounds of this group.

[d] Weight in terms of dry beans and peas, shelled nuts, and peanut butter. Count 1 pound of canned dry beans, such as pork and beans or kidney beans, as .33 pound.

[e] Cereal fortified with iron is recommended.

[f] For pregnant and nursing teenagers, 7 quarts is recommended.

From B. Peterkin, *Family Food Budgeting*, Home and Garden Bull. No. 94 (Washington, D.C.: Agr. Res. Service, U.S. Dept. Agr, 1976), p. 7.

Table A.7 Liberal Food Plan, Revised 1974–1975

Amounts of food for a week[a]

Family member	Milk, cheese, ice cream,[b] qt	Meat, poultry, fish,[c] lb	Eggs, no	Dry beans and peas, nuts,[d] lb	Dark-green, deep-yellow vegetables, lb	Citrus fruit, tomatoes, lb	Potatoes, lb	Other vegetables, fruit, lb	Cereal, Flour, lb	Bread, lb	Other bakery products, lb	Fats, oils, lb	Sugar, sweets, lb
Child:													
7 months to 1 year	6.9	0.97	2.3	0.14	0.43	0.60	0.06	4.71	[e]0.64	0.05	0.06	0.05	0.20
1–2 years	4.3	2.07	4.0	.17	.31	1.50	.59	4.10	[e]1.07	.82	.35	.13	.27
3–5 years	5.1	2.35	3.1	.23	.32	1.77	.85	4.18	.76	.79	.78	.45	.85
6–8 years	6.2	3.18	3.4	.36	.40	2.35	1.18	5.21	.85	1.08	1.23	.60	1.08
9–11 years	7.2	4.04	4.0	.39	.48	3.15	1.41	6.83	1.04	1.39	1.67	.71	1.38
Male:													
12–14 years	7.6	4.57	4.0	.50	.51	2.94	1.52	5.52	.95	1.60	1.71	.92	1.40
15–19 years	7.2	5.59	4.0	.31	.50	3.29	2.01	6.45	.84	1.92	2.05	1.07	1.20
20–54 years	3.6	6.83	4.0	.32	.62	3.51	1.95	6.99	.79	1.91	1.86	.95	1.00
55 years and over	3.2	5.54	4.0	.19	.76	3.52	1.68	6.97	.89	1.49	1.57	.94	1.09
Female:													
12–19 years	6.7	3.97	4.0	.25	.56	3.15	1.21	6.34	.71	1.31	1.35	.54	.98
20–54 years	3.6	4.86	4.0	.20	.66	3.41	1.35	5.81	.56	1.24	1.22	.66	.84
55 years and over	3.6	3.79	4.0	.15	.76	3.71	1.14	6.42	.74	1.17	1.12	.48	.77
Pregnant	[f]5.9	5.43	4.0	.26	.96	4.22	1.57	7.17	.70	1.70	1.45	.46	.87
Nursing	[f]5.8	5.97	4.0	.28	.97	4.51	1.72	7.66	.75	1.76	1.58	.68	1.02

[a] Amounts are for food as purchased or brought into the kitchen from garden or farm. Amounts allow for a discard of about 5 percent of the edible food as plate waste, spoilage, etc. For general use, round the total amount of food groups for the family to the nearest tenth or quarter of a pound. In addition to groups shown, most families use some other foods: coffee, tea, cocoa, soft drinks, punches, ades, leavening agents, and seasonings.

[b] Fluid milk and beverage made from dry or evaporated milk. Cheese and ice cream may replace some milk. Count as equivalent to a quart of fluid milk: natural or processed Cheddar-type cheese, 6 ounces; cottage cheese, 2½ pounds; ice cream or ice milk, 1½ quarts; unflavored yogurt, 4 cups.

[c] Bacon and salt pork should not exceed ⅓ pound for each 5 pounds of this group.

[d] Weight in terms of dry beans and peas, shelled nuts, and peanut butter. Count 1 pound of canned dry beans, such as pork and beans or kidney beans, as .33 pound.

[e] Cereal fortified with iron is recommended.

[f] For pregnant and nursing teenagers, 7 quarts is recommended.

From B. Peterkin, *Family Food Budgeting, Home and Garden Bull. No. 94* (Washington, D.C.: Agr. Res. Service, U.S. Dept. Agr. 1976), p. 7.

Table A.8 Composition of Mature Human Milk and Cows' Milk (average values per 100 ml of whole milk)

Constituents	Human milk (after 30 days)	Cows' milk
Energy, kcal	71	69
Total solids, g	12.4	12.7
Fat, g	4.5	3.7
Lactose, g	6.8	4.8
Protein, g	1.1	3.3
casein, g	0.4	2.8
lactalbumin, g	0.3	0.4
ash, g	0.21	0.72
Minerals		
Calcium, mg	33	125
Magnesium, mg	4	12
Potassium, mg	55	138
Sodium, mg	15	58
Total electropositive, mEq	4.04	13.28
Chlorine, mg	43	103
Phosphorus, mg	15	96
Sulphur, mg	14	30
Total electronegative, mEq	2.95	10.55
Other minerals		
Iron, mg	0.15	0.10
Copper, mg	0.04	0.03
Zinc, mg	0.53	0.38
Iodine, mg	0.007	0.021
Amino acids		
Essential		
Arginine,[a] mg	51	124
Histidine,[b] mg	23	80
Isoleucine, mg	86	212
Leucine, mg	161	356
Lysine, mg	79	257
Methionine, mg	23	87
Phenylalanine, mg	64	173
Threonine, mg	62	152
Tryptophan, mg	22	50
Valine, mg	90	228
Nonessential		
Alanine, mg	35	75
Aspartic acid, mg	116	166
Cystine, mg	29	29
Glutamic acid, mg	230	680
Glycine, mg	0	11
Proline, mg	80	250
Serine, mg	69	160
Tyrosine, mg	62	190

(Table A.8, continued)

Constituents	Human milk (after 30 days)	Cows' milk
Fat distribution		
Lipid phosphorus, mg	4	4
Total cholesterol, mg	20	14
Lecithin, mg	78	57
Fatty acids distribution, g/100 g fat		
Essential		
Linoleic (octadecadienoic)	8.3	1.6
Nonessential		
Saturated		
Butyric	0.4	3.1
Caproic	0.1	1.0
Caprylic	0.3	1.2
Capric	1.7	2.6
Lauric	5.8	2.2
Myristic	8.6	10.5
Palmitic	22.6	26.3
Stearic	7.7	13.2
Unsaturated		
Oleic	36.4	32.2
Linolenic	0.4	
Arachidonic	0.8	1.0
Vitamins,[c] per liter		
Vitamin A, IU	1898	1025
Thiamin, μg	160	440
Riboflavin, μg	360	1750
Niacin, μg	1470	940
Pyridoxine, μg	100	640
Pantothenate, μg	1840	3460
Folic acid,[d] μg	54	54
Vitamin B 12, μg	0.3	4
Vitamin C, mg	43	11
Vitamin D, IU	21	13
Vitamin E, mg	6.6	1.0
Vitamin K, μg	15	60

[a] Essential for growth in young rats.
[b] Essential for growth in young children and young rats.
[c] The data on vitamins (except folic acid) from Fomon, S. J. (1967). *Infant Nutrition*. Philadelphia: W. B. Saunders Co., p. 199.
[d] The data on folic acid from Ford, J. E., and K. J. Scott (1961). The folic acid activity of some milk foods for babies. *J. Dairy Res.*, **35**, 85.
From Macy, I. G., and H. J. Kelly (1961). Human milk and cow's milk in infant nutrition. In *Milk: The Mammary Gland and Its Secretion*, Vol. 2, edited by S. K. Kon and A. T. Cowie. New York: Academic Press, pp. 268, 269, and 275–277.

Table A.9 Methods of Evaluating Protein Quality

a. Net Protein Utilization

$$NPU = \text{Food N} - \frac{\left(\begin{array}{c} \text{total urinary N} - \text{urinary N when N-free diet is fed} \\ + \\ \text{total fecal N} - \text{fecal N when N-free diet is fed} \end{array}\right)}{\text{Food N}}$$

b. Amino Acid Score (Chemical Score)

$$\text{Amino Acid Score} = \frac{\text{mg amino acid per g test protein (or N)} \times 100}{\text{mg amino acid per g reference protein (or N)}}$$

Table A.10 Provisional Amino Acid Scoring Pattern

Amino acid	Suggested level	
	mg per g of protein	mg per g of nitrogen
Isoleucine	40	250
Leucine	70	440
Lysine	55	340
Methionine and cystine	35	220
Phenylalanine and tyrosine	60	380
Threonine	40	250
Tryptophan	10	60
Valine	50	310
Total	360	2250

From *Energy and Protein Requirements*, FAO Nutrition Meetings Rept. Series 52, and WHO Tech. Rept. Series 522. Rome: Food and Agr. Organ., 1973, p. 63.

Table A.11 Amino Acid Abbreviations

Alanine	Ala	Lysine	Lys
Arginine	Arg	Methionine	Met
Asparagine	Asn	Phenylalanine	Phe
Aspartic acid	Asp	Proline	Pro
Cysteine	Cys	Serine	Ser
Glycine	Gly	Threonine	Thr
Histidine	His	Trypophan	Trp
Hydroxyproline	Hyp	Tyrosine	Tyr
Isoleucine	Ile	Valine	Val
Leucine	Leu		

Table A.12 Exchange Lists for Meal Planning

Exchange lists are groups of measured foods that have about the same nutritive value and can be substituted one for the other in meals. There are six major exchange lists: 1. milk exchanges, 2. vegetable exchanges, 3. fruit exchanges, 4. bread exchanges, 5. meat exchanges, and 6. fat exchanges.

1. *The Milk Exchanges*

One Exchange of Milk: carbohydrate, 12 g; protein, 8 g; fat, trace; kcalories, 80.

	One Milk Exchange
Nonfat fortified milk	
Skim or nonfat milk	1 cup
Powdered (nonfat dry, before adding liquid	⅓ cup
Canned, evaporated-skim milk	½ cup
Buttermilk made from skim milk	1 cup
Yogurt made from skim milk (plain, unflavored)	1 cup
Low-fat fortified milk	
1% fat fortified milk (omit ½ Fat Exchange)	1 cup
2% fat fortified milk (omit 1 Fat Exchange)	1 cup
Yogurt made from 2% fortified milk (plain, unflavored) (omit 1 Fat Exchange)	1 cup
Whole milk (omit 2 Fat Exchanges)	
Whole milk	1 cup
Canned, evaporated whole milk	½ cup
Buttermilk made from whole milk	1 cup
Yogurt made from whole milk (plain, unflavored)	1 cup

2. The Vegetable Exchanges

One Exchange of Vegetables: carbohydrate, 5 g; protein, 2 g; kcalories, 25.

Vegetables to use for one Vegetable Exchange: One Exchange: ½ cup.

Asparagus	Greens:
Bean sprouts	Mustard
Beets	Spinach
Broccoli	Turnip
Brussels sprouts	Mushrooms
Cabbage	Okra
Carrots	Onions
Cauliflower	Rhubarb
Celery	Rutabaga
Cucumbers	Sauerkraut
Eggplant	String beans, green or yellow
Green pepper	Summer squash
Greens:	Tomatoes
Beet	Tomato juice
Chard	Turnips
Collards	Vegetable juice cocktail
Dandelion	Zucchini
Kale	

The following raw vegetables may be used as desired:

Chicory	Lettuce
Chinese cabbage	Parsley
Endive	Radishes
Escarole	Watercress

Starchy vegetables are in the Bread Exchange list.

3. The Fruit Exchanges

One Exchange of Fruit: carbohydrate, 10 g; and 40 kcalories.

Kinds and amounts of fruits to use for one Fruit Exchange.

	One Fruit Exchange
Apple	1 small
Apple juice	⅓ cup
Applesauce (unsweetened)	½ cup
Apricots, fresh	2 medium
Apricots, dried	4 halves
Banana	½ small
Berries	
Blackberries	½ cup
Blueberries	½ cup
Raspberries	½ cup
Strawberries	¾ cup
Cherries	10 large
Cider	⅓ cup
Dates	2
Figs, fresh	1
Figs, dried	1
Grapefruit	1
Grapefruit juice	½ cup
Grapes	12
Grape juice	¼ cup
Mango	½ small
Melon	
Cantaloupe	¼ small
Honeydew	⅛ medium
Watermelon	1 cup
Nectarine	1 small
Orange	1 small
Orange juice	½ cup
Papaya	¾ cup
Peach	1 medium
Pear	1 small
Persimmon, native	1 medium
Pineapple	½ cup
Pineapple juice	⅓ cup
Plums	2 medium
Prunes	2 medium
Prune juice	¼ cup
Raisins	2 tablespoons
Tangerine	1 medium

Cranberries are negligible in carbohydrate content and calorie value if no sugar is added.

4. Bread Enchanges

(Includes bread, cereal, and starchy vegetables)
One Exchange of Bread: carbohydrate, 15 g; protein, 2 g; kcalories, 70.

	One Bread Exchange
Bread	
White (including French and Italian)	1 slice

Bread

	One Bread Exchange
Bread	
Whole wheat	1 slice
Rye or pumpernickel	1 slice
Raisin	1 slice
Bagel, small	½
English muffin, small	½
Plain roll, bread	1
Frankfurter, roll	½
Hamburger bun	½
Dried bread crumbs	3 tablespoons
Tortilla, 6″	1
Crackers	
Arrowroot	3
Graham, 2½″ square	2
Matzoth, 4″ x 6″	½
Oyster	20
Pretzels, 3⅛″ long x ⅛″ diameter	25
Rye wafers, 2″ x 3½″	3
Saltines	6
Soda, 2½″ square	4
Cereal	
Bran flakes	½ cup
Other ready-to-eat un-sweetened cereal	¾ cup
Puffed cereal (unfrosted)	1 cup
Cereal (cooked)	½ cup
Grits (cooked)	½ cup
Rice or barley (cooked)	½ cup
Pasta (cooked), spaghetti, noodles, macaroni	½ cup
Popcorn (popped no fat added)	3 cups
Cornmeal (dry)	2 tablespoons
Flour	2½ tablespoons
Wheat germ	¼ cup
Dried Beans, Peas, and Lentils	½ cup
Beans, peas, lentils (dried and cooked)	
Baked beans, no pork (canned)	¼ cup
Starchy vegetables	
Corn	⅓ cup

Corn on cob	1 small
Lima beans	½ cup
Parsnips	⅔ cup
Peas, green (canned or frozen)	½ cup
Potato, white	1 small
Potato, mashed	½ cup
Pumpkin	¾ cup
Winter squash (acorn or butternut)	½ cup
Yam or sweet potato	¼ cup
Prepared foods	
Biscuit 2″ diameter (omit 1 Fat Exchange)	1
Cornbread 2″ x 2″ x 1″ (omit 1 Fat Exchange)	1
Corn muffin, 2″ diameter (omit 1 Fat Exchange)	1
Crackers, round butter type (omit 1 Fat Exchange)	5
Muffin, plain small (omit 1 Fat Exchange)	1
Potatoes, French fried, length 2″ to 3½″ (omit 1 Fat Exchange)	8
Potato or corn chips (omit 2 Fat Exchanges)	15
Pancake, 5″ x ½″ (omit 1 Fat Exchange)	1
Waffle, 5″ x ½″ (omit 1 Fat Exchange)	1

5. *Meat Exchanges*
 (Lean Meat)
 One Exchange of Lean Meat (1 ounce or 30 gram): protein, 7 g; fat, 3 g; kcalories, 55.

	One Lean Meat Exchange
Beef: baby beef (very lean) chipped beef, chuck, flank steak, tenderloin, plate ribs, plate skirt steak, round (bottom, top), all cuts rump, spare ribs, tripe	1 ounce

(Table A.12, continued)

	One Lean Meat Exchange
Lamb: leg, rib, sirloin, loin (roast and chops), shank, shoulder	1 ounce
Pork: leg (whole rump, center shank), ham, smoked (center slices)	1 ounce
Veal: leg, loin, rib, shank, shoulder, cutlets	1 ounce
Poultry: meat without skin of chicken, turkey, cornish hen, guinea hen, pheasant	1 ounce
Fish:	
Any fresh or frozen	1 ounce
Canned salmon, tuna, mackerel, crab and lobster	¼ cup
Clams, oysters, scallops, shrimp	5 or 1 ounce
Sardines, drained	3
Cheeses containing less than 5 percent butterfat	1 ounce
Cottage cheese, dry and 2 percent butterfat	¼ cup
Dried beans and peas (omit 1 Bread Exchange)	½ cup

(Medium-Fat Meat) For each Exchange of Medium-Fat Meat omit ½ Fat Exchange.

	One Medium-Fat Meat Exchange
Beef: ground (15 percent fat), corned beef (canned), rib eye, round (ground commercial)	1 ounce
Pork: loin (all cuts tenderloin), shoulder arm (picnic), shoulder blade, Boston butt Canadian bacon, boiled ham	1 ounce
Liver, heart, kidney, and sweet-breads	1 ounce
Cottage cheese, creamed	¼ cup
Cheese: mozzarella, ricotta, farmer's cheese, neufchatel	1 ounce
parmesan	3 tablespoons
Egg	1
Peanut butter (omit 2 additional Fat Exchanges)	2 tablespoons

(Table A.12, continued)

Meat Exchanges

(Hight-Fat Meat) For each Exchange of high-fat meat omit 1 Fat Exchange.

	One High-Fat Meat Exchange
Beef: brisket, corned beef (brisket), ground beef (more than 20 percent fat), hamburger (commercial), chuck (ground commercial), roast (rib), steaks (club and rib)	1 ounce
Lamb: breast	1 ounce
Pork: spare ribs, loin (back ribs), pork (ground), country style ham, deviled ham	1 ounce
Veal: breast	1 ounce
Poultry: capon, duck (domestic), goose	1 ounce
Cheese: cheddar types	1 ounce
Cold cuts	4½″ x ⅛″ slice
Frankfurter	1 small

6. *Fat Exchanges*

One Exchange of Fat: 5 g; kcalories, 45.

	One Fat Exchange
Margarine, soft, tub, stick[1]	1 teaspoon
Avocado (4″ in diameter)[2]	⅛
Oil: corn, cottonseed, safflower, soy, sunflower	1 teaspoon
Oil, olive[2]	1 teaspoon
Oil, peanut[2]	1 teaspoon
Olives[2]	5 small
Almonds[2]	10 whole
Peacans[2]	2 large whole
Peanuts[2]	
Spanish	20 whole
Virginia	10 whole
Walnuts	6 small
Nuts, other[2]	6 small
Margarine, regular stick	1 teaspoon
Butter	1 teaspoon
Bacon fat	1 teaspoon
Bacon, crisp	1 strip

578

(Table A.12, continued)

	One Fat Exchange
Cream, light	2 tablespoons
Cream, sour	2 tablespoons
Cream, heavy	1 tablespoon
Cream cheese	1 tablespoon
French dressing[3]	1 tablespoon
Italian dressing[3]	1 tablespoon
Lard	1 teaspoon
Mayonnaise[3]	1 teaspoon
Salad dressing (mayonnaise type)[3]	2 teaspoons
Salt pork	¾″ cube

1. Made with corn, cottonseed, safflower, soy or sunflower oil only.
2. Fat content is primarily monounsaturated.
3. If made with corn, cottonseed, safflower, soy or sunflower oil can be used on fat modified diet.

Foods negligible in protein, carbohydrate, and fat content and consequently calorie value

Diet calorie free beverage	Salt and pepper	Mustard
	Red pepper	Chili powder
Coffee	Paprika	Onion salt or
Tea	Garlic	powder
Bouillon without fat	Celery salt	Horseradish
Unsweetened gelatin	Parsley	Vinegar
Unsweetened pickles	Nutmeg	Mint
	Lemon	Cinnamon
		Lime

Exchange Lists for Meal Planning prepared by Committees of the American Diabetes Association, Inc., and The American Dietetic Association in cooperation with The National Institute of Arthritis, Metabolism and Digestive Diseases and the National Heart and Lung Institute, National Institutes of Health, Public Health Service, U.S. Department of Health, Education, and Welfare, 1976.

Table A.13 Yield of Cooked Dried Foods

Food	Yield	Weight of 237-millimeter cup
		y
Cereals		
Cornmeal, yellow	1 cup uncooked	152
	= 5½ cups cooked	238
Cream of wheat	1 cup uncookd	—
	= 4 cups cooked	—
Farina	1 cup uncooked	151
	= 5 cups cooked	242
Hominy grits	1 cup uncooked	156
	= 3⅓ cups cooked	236
Oats, quick	1 cup uncooked	80
	= 1¾ cups cooked	—
Rice	1 cup uncooked	200
	= 3½ cups cooked	169
Fruits, dried		
Apricot, halves	1 cup uncooked	150
	= 2 cups cooked	—
Prunes, whole	1 cup uncooked	176
	= 1¾ cups cooked	229
Legumes, dried		
Chick peas (garbanzos)	1 cup uncooked	200
	= 2¾ cups cooked	—
Cowpeas (black-eyed)	1 cup uncooked	168
	= 2½ cups cooked	—
Kidney beans	1 cup uncooked	186
	= 2¾ cups cooked	185
Lentils	1 cup uncooked	191
	= 2¼ cups cooked	202
Lima beans, baby	1 cup uncooked	173
	= 2 cups cooked	178
Navy beans	1 cup uncooked	181
	= 2¼ cups cooked	180
Soybeans	1 cup uncooked	210
	= 2⅞ cups cooked	—
Split peas	1 cup uncooked	203
	= 2⅓ cups cooked	194

From: J. C. Gates (1976). *Basic Foods.* New York: Holt, Rinehart and Winston, p. 611.

Table A.14 Desirable Weights for Men of Age 25 and Over

Height (with shoes, 1-in. heels)		Weight in pounds according to frame (as ordinarily dressed)		
Feet	Inches	Small frame	Medium frame	Large frame
5	2	112–120	118–129	126–141
5	3	115–123	121–133	129–144
5	4	118–126	124–136	132–148
5	5	121–129	127–139	135–152
5	6	124–133	130–143	138–156
5	7	128–137	134–147	142–161
5	8	132–141	138–152	147–166
5	9	136–145	142–156	151–170
5	10	140–150	146–160	155–174
5	11	144–154	150–165	159–179
6	0	148–158	154–170	164–184
6	1	152–162	158–175	168–189
6	2	156–167	162–180	173–194
6	3	160–171	167–185	178–199
6	4	164–175	172–190	182–204

From the Metropolitan Life Insurance Company. Derived from data of the Body Build and Blood Pressure Study, 1959, Society of Actuaries.

Table A.15 Desirable Weights for Women of Age 25 and Over

Height (with shoes, 2-in. heels)		Weight in pounds according to frame (as ordinarily dressed)		
Feet	Inches	Small frame	Medium frame	Large frame
4	10	92–98	96–107	104–119
4	11	94–101	98–110	106–122
5	0	96–104	101–113	109–125
5	1	99–107	104–116	112–128
5	2	102–110	107–119	115–131
5	3	105–113	110–122	118–134
5	4	108–116	113–126	121–138
5	5	111–119	116–130	125–142
5	6	114–123	120–135	129–146
5	7	118–127	124–139	133–150
5	8	122–131	128–143	137–154
5	9	126–135	132–147	141–158
5	10	130–140	136–151	145–163
5	11	134–144	140–155	149–168
6	0	138–148	144–159	153–173

From the Metropolitan Life Insurance Company. Derived from data of the Body Build and Blood Pressure Study, 1959, Society of Actuaries.

Table A.16 Average Weights[1] for Men and Women Aged 18–74 Years, by Age Group and Height: United States, 1971–1974[2]

Sex and height	Age group in years					
	18–24	25–34	35–44	45–54	56–64	65–74
Men	Weight in pounds					
62 inches	130	141	143	147	143	143
63 inches	135	145	148	152	147	147
64 inches	140	150	153	156	153	151
65 inches	145	156	158	160	158	156
66 inches	150	160	163	164	163	160
67 inches	154	165	169	169	168	164
68 inches	159	170	174	173	173	169
69 inches	164	174	179	177	178	173
70 inches	168	179	184	182	183	177
71 inches	173	184	190	187	189	182
72 inches	178	189	194	191	193	186
73 inches	183	194	200	196	197	190
74 inches	188	199	205	200	203	194

Sex and height	Age group in years					
	18–24	25–34	35–44	45–54	56–64	65–74
Women	Weight in pounds					
57 inches	114	118	125	129	132	130
58 inches	117	121	129	133	136	134
59 inches	120	125	133	136	140	137
60 inches	123	128	137	140	143	140
61 inches	126	132	141	143	147	144
62 inches	129	136	144	147	150	147
63 inches	132	139	148	150	153	151
64 inches	135	142	152	154	157	154
65 inches	138	146	156	158	160	158
66 inches	141	150	159	161	164	161
67 inches	144	153	163	165	167	165
68 inches	147	157	167	168	171	169

[1] Estimated values from regression equations of weight on height for specified age groups.
[2] Height was measured without shoes. Total weights of all clothing for HANES ranged from 0.20 to 0.62 pound, which was not deducted from weights shown.

From S. Abraham, C. L. Johnson, and M. F. Najjar (1977). *Weight by Height and Age of Adults 18–74 years; United States, 1971–1974*. Advanced Data. Hyattsville, Md.; Natl. Center for Health Stat., U.S. Dept. Health, Educ., and Welfare, p. 9.

Table A.17 Observed Percentiles of Stature (in centimeters): National Center for Health Statistics, 2–24 years, Male

Sex and age	N[2]	Observed percentile[1]						
		5th	10th	25th	50th	75th	90th	95th
Male		Stature in centimeters						
2.00– 2.25 years	419	82.6	83.5	86.1	87.8	90.3	91.9	97.3
2.25– 2.75 years	945	86.1	87.0	89.0	91.2	93.8	97.3	98.3
2.75– 3.25 years	785	88.9	90.5	92.4	95.1	97.2	100.1	101.2
3.25– 3.75 years	857	92.1	93.3	95.7	98.2	101.1	102.8	104.4
3.75– 4.25 years	856	96.2	97.3	100.0	102.6	105.3	107.5	110.8
4.25– 4.75 years	937	98.0	100.2	103.4	105.8	108.6	111.8	113.2
4.75– 5.25 years	874	100.7	103.2	105.5	108.8	112.4	115.4	116.5
5.25– 5.75 years	878	106.2	107.7	110.1	113.5	116.1	118.2	119.5
5.75– 6.25 years	908	108.5	110.1	112.8	117.0	119.4	122.2	123.1
6.25– 6.75 years	1,033	108.9	110.0	114.8	118.2	121.9	125.0	127.1
6.75– 7.25 years	988	114.1	115.6	118.5	122.3	125.9	128.3	129.8
7.25– 7.75 years	1,120	115.6	118.3	120.8	124.5	127.9	131.4	133.4
7.75– 8.25 years	1,014	119.3	121.0	123.8	127.9	131.7	134.9	138.0
8.25– 8.75 years	902	121.2	123.4	126.2	129.6	133.2	136.4	138.8
8.75– 9.25 years	943	121.1	124.5	127.5	132.8	136.3	139.4	141.9
9.25– 9.75 years	958	125.2	127.7	131.2	135.0	138.7	142.7	144.7
9.75–10.25 years	1,030	127.3	130.0	133.7	138.6	142.1	145.9	149.0
10.25–10.75 years	1,070	130.5	132.5	135.8	139.4	144.1	148.4	151.4
10.75–11.25 years	1,052	132.5	135.3	138.7	143.5	147.9	151.4	154.0
11.25–11.75 years	952	135.1	138.0	141.4	145.8	150.8	154.5	156.1
11.75–12.25 years	1,010	138.5	140.1	144.1	148.6	153.7	159.4	162.6
12.25–12.75 years	1,092	139.3	141.8	146.4	152.1	157.2	162.6	165.5
12.75–13.25 years	1,155	142.2	144.8	149.7	154.8	159.6	165.3	167.8
13.25–13.75 years	1,056	145.6	148.6	153.6	160.0	166.5	172.2	175.5
13.75–14.25 years	954	149.2	153.0	157.7	164.4	169.9	175.1	177.6
14.25–14.75 years	1,019	152.9	156.4	161.1	167.6	173.1	177.8	179.4
14.75–15.25 years	1,112	155.0	157.6	163.0	169.4	173.8	178.2	181.8
15.25–15.75 years	914	158.8	161.4	166.6	171.6	175.4	180.4	183.4
15.75–16.25 years	1,051	160.5	164.3	169.0	173.5	177.8	181.5	185.8
16.25–16.75 years	876	163.8	165.5	170.6	174.9	179.5	183.3	186.4
16.75–17.25 years	1,054	164.4	166.2	170.7	176.8	181.8	184.6	187.3
17.25–17.75 years	935	163.3	167.7	172.1	176.4	181.0	185.0	187.8
17.75–18.25 years	866	166.5	170.1	173.1	176.0	180.2	186.1	187.3
18.25–19.00 years	1,067	166.8	169.3	172.0	175.8	180.1	185.9	186.8
19.00–20.00 years	1,770	162.8	166.9	171.6	177.2	180.8	185.0	186.2
20.00–21.00 years	1,668	159.4	168.4	172.2	177.4	181.2	183.6	185.8
21.00–22.00 years	1,703	166.2	168.3	172.5	177.3	181.1	184.8	190.0
22.00–23.00 years	1,662	167.2	167.7	171.3	177.1	180.6	187.1	192.0
23.00–24.00 years	1,589	161.3	165.3	172.3	176.8	183.0	188.5	189.2
24.00–25.00 years	1,595	165.4	168.5	172.9	178.1	183.0	186.7	189.5

[1] For explanation of percentile, see page 492.
[2] Sample size expressed in thousands.
From P. V. V. Hamill, T. A. Drizd, C. L. Johnson, R. B. Reed, and A. F. Roche (1977). *NCHS Growth Curves for Children Birth—18 years.* DHEW Publ. No. (PHS) 78-1650. Hyattsville, Md.: Natl. Center for Health Stat., U.S. Dept. Health, Educ., and Welfare, p. 28.

Table A.18 Observed Percentiles of Stature (in centimeters): National Center for Health Statistics, 2–24 years, Female

Sex and age	N[2]	Observed percentile[1]						
		5th	10th	25th	50th	75th	90th	95th
Female		Stature in centimeters						
2.00– 2.25 years	440	81.3	82.5	84.6	86.8	89.9	93.6	94.6
2.25– 2.75 years	972	84.2	85.3	87.1	90.3	93.4	94.8	96.4
2.75– 3.25 years	622	90.2	90.7	92.7	95.3	96.7	99.1	100.6
3.25– 3.75 years	887	91.8	92.8	95.0	97.4	99.8	102.1	103.6
3.75– 4.25 years	775	94.8	96.2	97.9	100.5	103.8	106.0	108.2
4.25– 4.75 years	848	96.8	97.6	100.5	103.8	106.2	109.4	112.0
4.75– 5.25 years	876	99.1	101.1	105.2	108.1	111.6	113.7	114.7
5.25– 5.75 years	890	103.8	106.1	108.4	111.8	115.5	118.7	121.3
5.75– 6.25 years	866	107.1	109.0	111.9	115.4	118.8	122.1	124.6
6.25– 6.75 years	1,025	109.3	111.6	114.3	117.7	121.7	125.2	126.9
6.75– 7.25 years	945	111.7	113.2	117.4	120.8	124.3	126.8	128.6
7.25– 7.75 years	952	115.8	117.2	120.0	123.7	127.9	131.7	134.2
7.75– 8.25 years	1,004	117.8	119.5	122.8	127.5	130.6	132.9	134.6
8.25– 8.75 years	968	118.9	121.4	124.4	129.2	133.4	135.8	138.0
8.75– 9.25 years	988	122.2	124.8	128.4	132.7	137.7	141.0	142.3
9.25– 9.75 years	885	126.6	127.6	131.1	135.1	139.8	144.4	147.6
9.75–10.25 years	1,092	129.0	130.3	134.4	138.5	143.0	147.0	149.8
10.25–10.75 years	1,086	129.4	131.1	135.2	140.6	144.7	149.8	152.4
10.75–11.25 years	870	132.1	134.8	139.5	143.9	148.8	153.7	157.0
11.25–11.75 years	862	134.5	135.8	141.7	147.3	152.6	157.1	158.8
11.75–12.25 years	1,082	139.4	142.2	146.7	151.8	156.4	161.4	165.9
12.25–12.75 years	1,019	141.7	145.9	150.8	154.8	159.7	164.0	165.7
12.75–13.25 years	1,058	143.7	147.7	153.0	157.5	161.4	165.5	167.4
13.25–13.75 years	1,120	149.4	151.6	155.4	159.6	163.8	165.9	169.2
13.75–14.25 years	1,080	149.8	151.6	155.7	160.0	163.4	167.1	168.7
14.25–14.75 years	951	150.3	153.2	157.4	161.6	165.4	169.5	171.1
14.75–15.25 years	1,012	151.5	153.3	157.2	161.2	166.3	171.2	174.9
15.25–15.75 years	980	152.6	154.8	157.9	162.9	167.6	172.1	176.2
15.75–16.25 years	959	152.5	154.8	158.2	163.6	167.7	170.7	172.3
16.25–16.75 years	836	150.7	153.3	157.6	162.1	166.5	171.5	172.6
16.75–17.25 years	1,108	151.8	154.6	158.0	161.8	166.5	171.6	173.8
17.25–17.75 years	810	150.7	154.3	158.0	162.6	166.6	170.0	172.5
17.75–18.25 years	826	152.2	155.5	159.8	163.9	168.0	171.0	171.8
18.25–19.00 years	1,420	154.9	157.8	161.2	165.3	167.2	172.4	174.2
19.00–20.00 years	1,384	155.0	155.9	159.9	163.0	166.8	170.6	173.1
20.00–21.00 years	1,771	152.3	155.1	159.0	163.2	168.8	172.4	175.3
21.00–22.00 years	1,818	152.0	154.6	158.5	162.5	167.0	170.8	173.0
22.00–23.00 years	1,734	150.4	153.0	156.9	162.8	167.2	171.2	174.5
23.00–24.00 years	1,800	154.2	156.0	158.6	163.1	166.8	170.5	172.6
24.00–25.00 years	1,776	152.3	155.4	158.3	162.3	167.4	170.4	171.6

[1] For explanation of percentile, see **page 492.**
[2] Sample size expressed in thousands.

From P. V. V. Hamill, T. A. Drizd, C. L. Johnson, R. B. Reed, and A. F. Roche (1977). *NCHS Growth Curves for Children Birth—18 years.* DHEW Publ. No. (PHS) 78-1650. Hyattsville, Md.: Natl. Center for Health Stat., U.S. Dept. Health, Educ., and Welfare, p. 29.

Table A.19 Observed Percentiles of Weight (in kilograms): National Center for Health Statistics, 2–24 years, Male

Sex and age	N[2]	Observed percentile[1]						
		5th	10th	25th	50th	75th	90th	95th
Male		Weight in kilograms						
2.00– 2.25 years	419	9.97	11.10	11.63	12.67	14.05	14.85	15.47
2.25– 2.75 years	945	11.31	11.89	12.63	13.53	14.57	15.69	16.80
2.75– 3.25 years	785	12.28	12.84	13.55	14.43	15.34	16.39	17.37
3.25– 3.75 years	857	12.70	13.34	14.33	15.39	16.46	17.77	18.63
3.75– 4.25 years	856	13.83	14.70	15.46	16.64	17.85	18.87	20.62
4.25– 4.75 years	937	14.42	15.09	16.02	17.71	19.17	20.45	21.51
4.75– 5.25 years	874	14.99	15.52	16.91	18.47	20.22	21.02	22.59
5.25– 5.75 years	878	17.01	17.31	18.33	19.88	21.39	23.21	25.32
5.75– 6.25 years	908	16.87	17.80	19.53	21.21	22.85	24.98	26.40
6.25– 6.75 years	1,033	17.21	17.82	19.70	21.59	23.41	26.21	28.18
6.75– 7.25 years	992	18.59	19.39	21.37	22.93	25.22	28.74	30.72
7.25– 7.75 years	1,120	18.76	20.07	22.04	24.33	26.48	29.08	32.31
7.75– 8.25 years	1,014	20.20	21.47	23.47	25.65	28.70	31.36	35.15
8.25– 8.75 years	902	21.71	22.63	24.35	26.31	29.27	33.08	34.96
8.75– 9.25 years	943	22.01	22.98	25.13	27.89	31.75	36.62	40.23
9.25– 9.75 years	958	23.11	24.30	26.40	29.65	33.63	38.58	45.67
9.75–10.25 years	1,030	24.40	25.63	27.98	31.83	36.09	41.08	43.69
10.25–10.75 years	1,070	26.09	27.73	29.49	32.57	36.39	40.75	45.66
10.75–11.25 years	1,052	27.98	28.79	31.23	35.86	39.68	44.71	51.83
11.25–11.75 years	952	28.17	30.14	34.07	37.48	41.94	47.16	52.45
11.75–12.25 years	1,010	30.10	31.18	34.21	38.75	46.43	55.24	62.43
12.25–12.75 years	1,092	31.72	32.98	36.18	41.98	47.30	54.05	58.45
12.75–13.25 years	1,155	32.17	34.61	38.43	43.62	50.17	59.22	64.29
13.25–13.75 years	1,056	36.24	37.80	42.92	49.23	58.38	63.44	68.39
13.75–14.25 years	954	38.25	41.47	46.98	51.65	60.77	67.04	76.61
14.25–14.75 years	1,019	40.52	43.64	49.70	55.32	62.62	72.69	77.03
14.75–15.25 years	1,112	42.14	44.93	50.35	56.35	63.63	71.27	76.91
15.25–15.75 years	914	46.26	49.12	54.29	58.92	66.68	75.40	81.81
15.75–16.25 years	1,051	46.83	51.29	55.79	61.74	69.33	76.78	86.07
16.25–16.75 years	876	50.46	53.22	56.77	64.71	72.28	81.62	87.57
16.75–17.25 years	1,054	52.15	55.42	60.65	65.90	73.76	81.72	91.23
17.25–17.75 years	935	51.80	55.53	60.81	66.64	75.36	83.35	92.16
17.75–18.25 years	866	54.76	58.18	62.04	68.96	75.49	88.36	94.71
18.25–19.00 years	1,067	54.96	60.35	63.62	69.88	78.67	92.66	99.60
19.00–20.00 years	1,770	55.40	57.38	65.91	70.66	76.43	87.01	96.48
20.00–21.00 years	1,668	55.86	57.71	65.04	71.89	78.44	88.86	94.84
21.00–22.00 years	1,703	52.66	58.17	65.29	72.12	80.96	89.04	96.13
22.00–23.00 years	1,662	55.02	59.14	65.09	71.77	79.66	90.57	96.93
23.00–24.00 years	1,589	59.16	60.69	65.54	74.71	82.44	94.05	105.35
24.00–25.00 years	1,595	60.87	63.96	67.96	79.37	85.69	97.60	103.19

[1] For explanation of percentile, see page 492.

[2] Sample size expressed in thousands.

From P. V. V. Hamill, T. A. Drizd, C. L. Johnson, R. B. Reed, and A. F. Roche (1977). *NCHS Growth Curves for Children Birth—18 years.* DHEW Publ. No. (PHS) 78-1650. Hyattsville, Md.: Natl. Center for Health Stat., U.S. Dept. Health, Educ., and Welfare, p. 30.

Table A.20 Observed Percentiles of Weight (in kilograms): National Center for Health Statistics, 2–24 years, Female

Sex and age	N[2]	Observed percentile[1]						
		5th	10th	25th	50th	75th	90th	95th
Female				Weight in kilograms				
2.00– 2.25 years	440	10.06	10.66	11.41	12.21	12.86	13.84	14.57
2.25– 2.75 years	972	10.77	11.20	11.98	12.76	13.94	14.74	15.09
2.75– 3.25 years	622	12.14	12.40	13.12	13.93	15.61	16.84	17.74
3.25– 3.75 years	887	12.29	13.03	13.58	14.60	15.93	17.54	18.28
3.75– 4.25 years	775	13.13	13.63	14.51	15.68	17.15	18.22	18.94
4.25– 4.75 years	848	13.45	14.05	15.04	16.57	17.78	19.35	20.26
4.75– 5.25 years	876	14.33	15.21	16.48	17.73	19.66	21.23	22.10
5.25– 5.75 years	890	15.18	16.20	17.47	18.92	20.96	23.44	25.01
5.75– 6.25 years	866	15.99	17.09	18.21	20.19	22.39	24.88	28.71
6.25– 6.75 years	1,025	17.02	17.71	19.24	21.06	23.55	26.17	27.89
6.75– 7.25 years	945	17.86	18.74	20.20	22.13	23.98	26.91	29.58
7.25– 7.75 years	952	18.84	19.60	21.33	23.72	26.54	29.61	31.55
7.75– 8.25 years	1,004	20.11	20.79	22.49	24.89	27.73	32.63	35.20
8.25– 8.75 years	968	20.47	21.50	23.30	26.39	29.69	33.65	36.45
8.75– 9.25 years	988	22.20	23.17	25.27	28.79	33.40	39.66	42.69
9.25– 9.75 years	885	23.29	24.72	26.92	30.26	34.54	39.87	43.62
9.75–10.25 years	1,092	24.34	25.25	28.03	31.68	36.38	43.16	45.92
10.25–10.75 years	1,086	25.28	26.69	29.42	33.00	37.63	45.90	48.37
10.75–11.25 years	870	26.73	28.32	32.09	36.13	42.27	47.72	54.49
11.25–11.75 years	862	27.44	29.45	32.88	37.97	44.38	50.77	58.09
11.75–12.25 years	1,082	29.72	32.74	36.42	41.70	48.78	57.77	64.79
12.25–12.75 years	1,019	32.59	34.97	39.46	45.37	51.40	58.10	63.21
12.75–13.25 years	1,058	34.21	37.17	41.44	47.06	54.79	62.20	66.61
13.25–13.75 years	1,120	37.72	39.45	45.00	50.30	56.81	67.05	75.78
13.75–14.25 years	1,080	37.74	39.86	44.86	50.22	56.44	66.44	74.70
14.25–14.75 years	951	40.77	42.96	47.21	53.03	60.95	68.88	78.43
14.75–15.25 years	1,012	41.14	43.65	47.48	53.29	59.72	71.57	75.36
15.25–15.75 years	980	42.99	46.11	48.98	55.25	60.80	71.45	77.78
15.75–16.25 years	959	43.64	45.74	49.22	54.92	61.58	67.70	78.03
16.25–16.75 years	836	43.86	45.69	49.46	54.97	62.64	72.37	83.10
16.75–17.25 years	1,108	43.87	45.57	50.76	56.49	62.22	72.45	84.19
17.25–17.75 years	810	42.90	45.36	50.56	55.23	61.59	70.62	84.82
17.75–18.25 years	826	45.05	47.89	52.68	57.68	62.32	69.62	75.86
18.25–19.00 years	1,420	44.83	45.89	51.03	56.97	63.16	72.62	78.70
19.00–20.00 years	1,384	48.65	48.83	51.62	57.24	63.48	76.33	83.48
20.00–21.00 years	1,771	44.40	47.23	51.70	57.22	63.94	72.15	75.89
21.00–22.00 years	1,818	46.08	48.54	52.15	58.36	64.64	72.88	81.76
22.00–23.00 years	1,734	42.86	46.18	51.35	58.82	67.38	75.54	85.35
23.00–24.00 years	1,800	45.59	47.77	52.16	59.87	64.64	72.80	84.62
24.00–25.00 years	1,796	46.65	48.13	52.06	58.88	66.33	77.17	86.04

[1] For explanation of percentile, see page 492.
[2] Sample size expressed in thousands.
From P. V. V. Hamill, T. A. Drizd, C. L. Johnson, R. B. Reed, and A. F. Roche (1977). *NCHS Growth Curves for Children Birth—18 years*. DHEW Publ. No. (PHS) 78-1650. Hyattsville, Md.: Natl. Center for Health Stat., U.S. Dept. Health, Educ., and Welfare, p. 31.

Table A.21 Triceps Skinfold of Children Aged 1–17 Years, United States, 1971–1972 (HANES Preliminary)

Sex and age	All income				
	Mean age	N	Mean	Median	Standard error of mean
Boys			In millimeters		
1 year	1.55	1,772	10.7	10.7	0.43
2 years	2.45	1,530	10.1	10.2	0.32
3 years	3.46	1,573	9.9	10.4	0.33
4 years	4.49	2,046	9.5	9.8	0.33
5 years	5.53	1,681	9.3	9.2	0.36
6 years	6.46	1,796	8.8	8.6	0.49
7 years	7.47	2,754	8.7	8.3	0.34
8 years	8.46	1,745	8.9	8.6	0.45
9 years	9.46	2,234	11.0	10.2	0.55
10 years	10.52	2,154	10.4	10.0	0.49
11 years	11.48	1,908	10.8	9.6	0.61
12 years	12.56	2,251	11.2	10.5	0.51
13 years	13.48	1,894	11.3	10.2	0.96
14 years	14.46	2,015	10.2	8.9	0.92
15 years	15.50	2,294	10.9	9.3	0.89
16 years	16.52	1,795	9.8	8.4	0.83
17 years	17.51	2,259	9.0	7.6	0.75
Girls					
1 year	1.49	1,509	10.3	10.6	0.43
2 years	2.45	1,647	10.4	10.5	0.28
3 years	3.50	1,534	11.3	11.8	0.36
4 years	4.54	1,785	10.5	10.7	0.29
5 years	5.55	1,801	10.7	10.3	0.29
6 years	6.47	1,885	10.2	10.7	0.42
7 years	7.51	2,135	10.7	10.9	0.59
8 years	8.47	1,716	12.8	11.6	0.70
9 years	9.52	2,070	13.5	13.4	0.61
10 years	10.47	2,403	13.4	12.6	0.52
11 years	11.55	2,033	13.9	13.1	0.83
12 years	12.49	1,742	14.8	15.1	0.56
13 years	13.52	2,389	16.6	15.7	0.87
14 years	14.50	2,189	17.6	17.1	0.83
15 years	15.48	1,997	17.6	17.2	1.05
16 years	16.55	2,062	17.8	17.1	1.25
17 years	17.46	1,860	19.7	18.9	1.42

N = estimated population in thousands.
Adapted from S. Abraham, F. W. Lowenstein, and D. E. O'Connell (1975). *Preliminary Findings of the First Health and Nutrition Examination Survey, United States, 1971–1972, Anthropometric and Clinical Findings.* DHEW Publ. No. (HRA) 75-1229. Rockville, Md.: Natl. Center for Health Stat., U.S. Dept. Health, Educ., and Welfare, p. 54.

Table A.22 Subscapular Skinfold of Children 1–17 Years, United States, 1971–1972 (HANES Preliminary)

Sex and age	All income				
	Mean age	N	Mean	Median	Standard error of mean
Boys			In millimeters		
1 year	1.55	1,772	6.4	6.4	0.25
2 years	2.45	1,530	5.5	5.5	0.28
3 years	3.46	1,573	5.5	5.5	0.29
4 years	4.49	2,046	5.2	5.3	0.22
5 years	5.53	1,681	5.0	5.0	0.18
6 years	6.46	1,796	5.1	4.8	0.27
7 years	7.47	2,754	5.4	4.8	0.38
8 years	8.46	1,745	5.0	4.9	0.26
9 years	9.46	2,234	7.7	5.8	0.72
10 years	10.52	2,154	7.2	5.9	0.62
11 years	11.48	1,908	7.1	6.1	0.51
12 years	12.56	2,251	7.7	6.0	0.53
13 years	13.48	1,894	8.9	6.8	1.05
14 years	14.46	2,015	8.8	7.0	1.16
15 years	15.50	2,294	10.4	7.7	0.79
16 years	16.52	1,795	10.4	8.4	0.94
17 years	17.51	2,259	10.0	8.3	0.66
Girls					
1 year	1.49	1,509	6.2	6.3	0.35
2 years	2.45	1,647	6.1	6.1	0.21
3 years	3.50	1,534	5.9	5.9	0.25
4 years	4.54	1,785	5.6	5.6	0.16
5 years	5.55	1,801	6.3	5.5	0.31
6 years	6.47	1,885	6.2	6.2	0.53
7 years	7.51	2,135	6.0	5.5	0.45
8 years	8.47	1,716	8.2	5.9	0.63
9 years	9.52	2,070	8.3	7.4	0.66
10 years	10.47	2,403	9.2	6.8	0.68
11 years	11.55	2,033	10.0	8.1	0.94
12 years	12.49	1,742	11.0	8.9	0.98
13 years	13.52	2,389	12.7	10.5	0.91
14 years	14.50	2,189	13.8	10.8	0.98
15 years	15.48	1,997	12.6	10.5	1.12
16 years	16.55	2,062	13.4	10.6	1.46
17 years	17.46	1,860	15.9	12.7	1.48

N = estimated population in thousands.
Adapted from S. Abraham, F. W. Lowenstein, and D. E. O'Connell (1975). *Preliminary Findings of the First Health and Nutrition Examination Survey, United States, 1971–1972, Anthropometric and Clinical Findings.* DHEW Publ. No. (HRA) 75-122g. Rockville, Md.; Natl. Center for Health State, U.S. Dept. Health, Educ., and Welfare, p. 56.

Table A.23 Right Arm Skinfold, Average, and Selected Percentiles for Adults, by Age and Sex: United States, 1960–1962

Sex, average, and percentile	Total 18–79 years	18–24 years	25–34 years	35–44 years	45–54 years	55–64 years	65–74 years	75–79 years
Men	Measurement (in centimeters)							
Average right arm skinfold	1.3	1.1	1.4	1.4	1.3	1.2	1.2	1.1
Percentile[1]								
99	4.1	3.7	4.5	4.0	3.8	3.3	3.2	3.0
95	2.8	2.6	3.3	2.9	2.8	2.4	2.7	2.0
90	2.3	2.4	2.6	2.4	2.2	2.0	2.2	1.7
80	1.8	1.7	2.0	1.9	1.8	1.6	1.7	1.5
70	1.5	1.3	1.6	1.6	1.5	1.4	1.4	1.3
60	1.3	1.1	1.4	1.4	1.3	1.3	1.3	1.1
50	1.1	0.9	1.2	1.2	1.1	1.2	1.1	1.0
40	1.0	0.8	1.0	1.1	1.0	1.0	1.0	0.9
30	0.8	0.7	0.8	1.0	0.9	0.9	0.8	0.8
20	0.7	0.6	0.7	0.8	0.7	0.8	0.7	0.7
10	0.5	0.5	0.5	0.6	0.6	0.6	0.6	0.6
5	0.5	0.5	0.5	0.5	0.5	0.5	0.5	0.5
1	0.4	0.4	0.4	0.4	0.4	0.4	0.3	0.4
Women								
Average right arm skinfold	2.2	1.8	2.1	2.3	2.4	2.5	2.4	2.0
Percentile[1]								
99	4.6	4.3	4.7	4.6	4.8	4.7	4.7	3.9
95	3.8	3.2	3.7	3.9	4.0	4.0	3.6	3.3
90	3.4	2.8	3.2	3.5	3.6	3.7	3.4	3.1
80	3.0	2.4	2.8	3.0	3.2	3.2	3.0	2.7
70	2.6	2.1	2.4	2.7	2.8	2.9	2.7	2.5
60	2.4	2.0	2.2	2.5	2.6	2.7	2.5	2.3
50	2.2	1.7	2.0	2.3	2.4	2.5	2.4	2.2
40	2.0	1.6	1.9	2.1	2.2	2.3	2.2	2.0
30	1.8	1.5	1.7	1.8	2.0	2.1	2.0	1.7
20	1.6	1.3	1.5	1.6	1.8	1.9	1.7	1.4
10	1.3	1.1	1.2	1.4	1.5	1.6	1.5	1.0
5	1.1	0.9	1.0	1.2	1.2	1.4	1.2	0.7
1	0.8	0.6	0.7	1.0	0.8	1.0	0.8	0.3

[1] Measurement below which the indicated percent of persons in the given age group fall.

From H. W. Stoudt, A. Damon, and R. A. McFarland, *Skinfolds, Body Girths, Biacromial Diameter, and Selected Anthropometric Indices of Adults* (1970). Vital and Health Statistics, Series 11, No. 35. Washington, D.C.: U.S. Dept. Health, Education, and Welfare, National Center for Health Statistics, p. 39.

Table A.24 Infrascapular Skinfold, Average, and Selected Percentiles for Adults, by Age and Sex: United States, 1960–1962

Sex, average, and percentile	Total 18–79 years	18–24 years	25–34 years	35–44 years	45–54 years	55–64 years	65–74 years	75–79 years
Men			Measurement (in centimeters)					
Average infrascapular skinfold	1.5	1.3	1.5	1.6	1.6	1.5	1.5	1.3
Percentile[1]								
99	4.1	4.3	4.1	4.2	3.9	4.0	3.5	3.3
95	3.0	2.4	3.1	3.1	3.0	2.9	2.9	2.7
90	2.6	2.2	2.7	2.8	2.6	2.5	2.6	2.2
80	2.1	1.6	2.2	2.2	2.3	2.1	2.1	1.8
70	1.8	1.3	1.9	1.9	1.9	1.8	1.8	1.6
60	1.6	1.2	1.6	1.7	1.7	1.6	1.6	1.3
50	1.4	1.1	1.3	1.5	1.5	1.4	1.4	1.2
40	1.2	1.0	1.2	1.3	1.3	1.3	1.2	1.1
30	1.0	0.9	1.0	1.1	1.1	1.1	1.0	0.9
20	0.9	0.8	0.9	1.0	1.0	1.0	0.9	0.8
10	0.8	0.7	0.8	0.8	0.8	0.8	0.7	0.7
5	0.7	0.7	0.7	0.7	0.7	0.7	0.6	0.6
1	0.6	0.6	0.5	0.6	0.6	0.6	0.5	0.5
Women								
Average infrascapular skinfold	1.8	1.3	1.5	1.8	2.0	2.2	2.0	1.7
Percentile[1]								
99	4.5	4.0	4.6	4.3	4.6	4.9	4.1	4.3
95	3.6	2.6	3.2	3.6	3.6	3.9	3.6	3.6
90	3.1	2.2	2.7	3.2	3.3	3.6	3.4	3.0
80	2.6	1.8	2.1	2.7	2.8	2.9	2.8	2.5
70	2.2	1.6	1.7	2.2	2.5	2.6	2.5	2.1
60	1.9	1.3	1.5	1.9	2.1	2.4	2.2	1.9
50	1.6	1.3	1.3	1.6	1.9	2.2	1.9	1.7
40	1.4	1.0	1.1	1.4	1.7	1.9	1.8	1.3
30	1.2	0.9	1.0	1.1	1.4	1.6	1.6	1.1
20	1.0	0.8	0.9	1.0	1.2	1.4	1.3	0.8
10	0.9	0.7	0.7	0.8	0.9	1.1	1.0	0.6
5	0.7	0.7	0.7	0.7	0.8	0.9	0.8	0.5
1	0.6	0.5	0.5	0.6	0.6	0.6	0.6	0.4

[1] Measurement below which the indicated percent of persons in the given age group fall.
From H. W. Stoudt, A. Damon, and R. A. McFarland, *Skinfolds, Body Girths, Biacromial Diameter, and Selected Anthropometric Indices of Adults* (1970). Vital and Health Statistics, Series 11, No. 35. Washington, D.C.: U.S. Dept. Health, Education, and Welfare, National Center for Health Statistics, p. 40.

Table A.25 Guidelines for Classification of Biochemical Determinations Used in the Health and Nutrition Examination Survey, United States, 1971–1972

Biochemical determination, age, and sex	Classification category		
	Low	Acceptable	High
Hemoglobin (gm/100 ml)			
1–5 years	<10.0	10.0–11.0	>11.0
12–17 years, female	<11.5	11.5–12.5	>12.5
18 years and over, male	<14.0	14.0–16.5	>16.5
18 years and over, female	<12.0	12.0–14.5	>14.5
6–11 years	<11.5	11.5–12.5	>12.5
12–17 years, male	<13.0	13.0–14.0	>14.0
Hematocrit (percent)			
1–5 years	<31	31–34	>34
6–11 years	<35	35–39	>39
12–17 years, male	<40	40–44	>44
12–17 years, female	<36	36–38	>38
18 years and over, male	<44	44–52	>52
18 years and over, female	<38	38–48	>48
Serum iron (μg/100 ml)			
1–5 years	<40	40–49	>49
6–11 years	<50	50–59	>59
12 years and over, male	<60	60–149	>149
12 years and over, female	>40	40–119	>119
Transferrin saturation (percent)			
1–5 years	<15	15–29	>30

Biochemical determination, age, and sex	Classification category		
	Low	Acceptable	High
6–11 years	<20	20–29	>30
12 years and over, male	<20	20–29	>30
12 years and over, female	<15	15–29	>30
Serum protein (gm/100 ml)			
1–5 years	< 5.0	5.0–6.0	>6.0
6–17 years	<6.0	6.0–8.0	>8.0
Adult	<6.5	6.5–8.5	>8.5
Serum albumin (gm/100 ml)			
1–5 years	< 2.5	2.5–3.5	>3.5
6–17 years	< 3.0	3.0–4.0	>4.0
Adult	< 3.5	3.5–5.5	>5.5
Serum vitamin A (μg/100 ml)			
All ages	<20	20–80	>80

1. less than
2. more than

From S. Abraham, F. W. Lowenstein, and C. L. Johnson (1974). *Preliminary Findings of the First Health and Nutrition Examination Survey, United States, 1971-1972; Dietary Intake and Biochemical Findings.* Rockville, Md.; Natonal Center for Health Stat., U.S. Dept. of Health, Educ., and Welfare, p. 182.

Table A.26 Clinical Signs of Nutrient Deficiency, United States, 1971–1972 (HANES Preliminary)

Nutrient	Clinical Sign	Nutrient	Clinical Sign
Protein	Dyspigmented hair		Bowed legs
	Abnormal texture or loss of curl of hair		Knock knees
	Visible or enlarged parotids		Epiphyseal enlargement, wrists
	Liver enlargement	Vitamin A	Bitot's spots
	Potbelly		Keratomalacia
	Apathy		Xerophthalmia
	Marked hyperirritability		Xerosis of the conjunctiva
Vitamin B Complex: Riboflavin	Angular inflammation of eyelids	Vitamin A and/or essential fatty acids	Follicular hyperkeratosis of upper back
	Angular lesions of lips ⎫ bilateral		Follicular hyperkeratosis, arms
	Angular scars of lips ⎭		Dry or scaling skin (xerosis)
	Cheilosis		Mosaic skin
	Magenta tongue	Vitamin C	Follicular keratosis
	Nasolabial seborrhea		Small subcutaneous hemorrhage
Vitamin B Complex other than Riboflavin: Niacin	Changes in tongue surface		Bleeding and swollen gums
	Fissures of tongue	Iodine	Enlarged thyroid gland, Group I
	Serrations or swelling of tongue		Enlarged thyroid gland, Group II
	Hyperpigmentation, hands and face	Calcium	Positive Chvostek's sign
	Pellagrous dermatitis		
	Scarlet beefy tongue		
Thiamin	Absent knee jerks		
	Absent ankle jerks		
Vitamin D	Bossing of skull		
	Beading of ribs		

Adapted from S. Abraham, F. W. Lowenstein, and D. E. O'Connell (1975). *Preliminary Findings of the First Health and Nutrition Examination Survey, United States, 1971–1972, Anthropometric and Clinical Findings.* DHEW Publ. No. (HRA) 75-1229. Rockville, Md.: Center for Health Stat., U.S. Dept. of Health, Educ., and Welfare, p. 81.

589

Table A.27 Standards for HANES Dietary Intake Data (Table II. Standards for evaluation of daily dietary intake used in the Health and Nutrition Examination Survey, by age, by sex, and physiological state: United States, 1971–1974.)

Age, sex, and physiological state		Calories (per kg)	Protein (g per kg)	Calcium (mg)	Iron (mg)	Vitamin A[1] (IU)	Vitamin C (mg)	B vitamins (all ages)
Age and sex								
1–5 years:								
12–23 months, male and female		90	1.9	450	15	2,000	40	Thiamin 0.4 mg
24–47 months, male and female		86	1.7	450	15	2,000	40	per 1,000
48–71 months, male and female		82	1.5	450	10	2,000	40	calories
6–7 years, male and female		82	1.3	450	10	2,500	40	
8–9 years, male and female		82	1.3	450	10	2,500	40	Riboflavin
10–12 years	Male	68	1.2	650	10	2,500	40	0.55 mg
	Female	64	1.2	650	18	2,500	40	per 1,000
13–16 years	Male	60	1.2	650	18	3,500	50	calories
	Female	48	1.2	650	18	3,500	50	
17–19 years	Male	44	1.1	550	18	3,500	55	Niacin
	Female	35	1.1	550	18	3,500	50	6.6 mg
20–29 years	Male	40	1.0	400	10	3,500	60	per 1,000
	Female	35	1.0	600	18	3,500	55	calories
30–39 years	Male	38	1.0	400	10	3,500	60	
	Female	33	1.0	600	18	3,500	55	
40–49 years	Male	37	1.0	400	10	3,500	60	
	Female	31	1.0	600	18	3,500	55	
50–54 years	Male	36	1.0	400	10	3,500	60	
	Female	30	1.0	600	18	3,500	55	
55–59 years	Male	36	1.0	400	10	3,500	60	
	Female	30	1.0	600	10	3,500	55	
60–69 years	Male	34	1.0	400	10	3,500	60	
	Female	29	1.0	600	10	3,500	55	
70 years and over	Male	34	1.0	400	10	3,500	60	
	Female	29	1.0	600	10	3,500	55	
Physiological state								
Pregnancy (5th month and beyond), add to basic standard		200	20	200		1,000	5[2]	
Lactating, add to basic standard		1,000	25	500		1,000	5	

[1] Assumed 70 percent carotene, 30 percent retinol.
[2] For all pregnancies.

From S. Abraham, M. D. Carroll, C. M. Dresser, and C. L. Johnson (1977). *Dietary Intake Findings*, United States, 1971–1974. DHEW Publ. No. (HRA) 77-1647. Hyattsville, Md.: Natl. Center for Health Stat., U.S. Dept. Health, Educ., and Welfare, p. 74.

Chapter Opening Photo Credits

Chapter 1   Tom McHugh/Photo Researchers.
Chapter 2   Jeanne M. Riddle, Ph.D.
Chapter 3   Ken Heyman.
Chapter 4   Kathy Bendo.
Chapter 5   American Heart Association.
Chapter 6   Kathy Bendo.
Chapter 7   Grant Heilman.
Chapter 8   James B. Johnson/D.P.I.
Chapter 9   Kathy Bendo.
Chapter 10   Grant Heilman.
Chapter 11   Hubertus Kanus/Rapho-Photo
                  Researchers.
Chapter 12   Grant Heilman.
Chapter 13   Macmillan Science Company.
Chapter 14   Kathy Bendo.
Chapter 15   Grant Heilman.
Chapter 16   Peter Southwick/Stock, Boston.
Chapter 17   Kathy Bendo.
Chapter 18   Jean Hollyman/Photo Researchers.
Chapter 19   Richard Frieman/Photo Researchers.
Chapter 20   Hugh Rogers/Monkmeyer.
Chapter 21   Christa Armstrong/Rapho-Photo
                  Researchers.

Index